HEALTH ECONOMICS AND FINANCING

HEALTH ECONOMICS AND FINANCING

Fifth Edition

Thomas E. Getzen
Temple University and iHEA

WILEY

VP & Executive Publisher	George Hoffman
Executive Editor	Joel Hollenbeck
Content Editor	Jennifer Manias
Assistant Editor	Courtney Luzzi
Senior Editorial Assistant	Erica Horowitz
Associate Director of Marketing	Amy Scholz
Senior Marketing Manager	Jesse Cruz
Marketing Assistant	Justine Kay
Product Designer	Greg Chaput
Media Specialist	Daniela DiMaggio
Senior Production Manager	Janis Soo
Associate Production Manager	Joel Balbin
Production Editor	Yee Lyn Song
Designer	Kenji Ngieng
Cover Photo	© Pawel Gaul/istockphoto

This book was set in Minion by Aptara, Inc. and printed and bound by Quad/Graphics. The cover was printed by Quad/Graphics.

This book is printed on acid-free paper. ∞

Founded in 1807, John Wiley & Sons, Inc. has been a valued source of knowledge and understanding for more than 200 years, helping people around the world meet their needs and fulfill their aspirations. Our company is built on a foundation of principles that include responsibility to the communities we serve and where we live and work. In 2008, we launched a Corporate Citizenship Initiative, a global effort to address the environmental, social, economic, and ethical challenges we face in our business. Among the issues we are addressing are carbon impact, paper specifications and procurement, ethical conduct within our business and among our vendors, and community and charitable support. For more information, please visit our website: www.wiley.com/go/citizenship.

Evaluation copies are provided to qualified academics and professionals for review purposes only, for use in their courses during the next academic year. These copies are licensed and may not be sold or transferred to a third party. Upon completion of the review period, please return the evaluation copy to Wiley. Return instructions and a free of charge return mailing label are available at www.wiley.com/go/returnlabel. If you have chosen to adopt this textbook for use in your course, please accept this book as your complimentary desk copy. Outside of the United States, please contact your local sales representative.

Library of Congress Cataloging-in-Publication Data

Getzen, Thomas E.
    Health economics and financing / Thomas E. Getzen.—5th ed.
        p. ; cm.
    Includes bibliographical references and index.
    ISBN 978-1-118-18490-5 (cloth : alk. paper)
    I. Title.
    [DNLM: 1. Economics, Medical—United States. 2. Delivery of Health Care—economics—United States. 3. Health Care Reform—economics—United States. W 74 AA1] 2013
        338.4′33621–dc23

                                                2012028595

Printed in the United States of America
SKY10026349_041621

—to Karen, Matt, Zoa, and Kayla

BRIEF CONTENTS

CONTENTS

15   History, Demography, and the Growth of Modern Medicine   347

PREFACE

Health Economics and Financing is a primer for the economic analysis of medical markets. Its intended audiences are students of medicine, public health, policy, and administration who wish to engage the central economic issues of their field without prolonged preparatory work; beginning students in economics who wish to study an applied area in detail without recourse to extensive mathematical manipulation; and more advanced students in economics who may be familiar with analytical techniques but lack knowledge of the many institutional features that make the study of health and health care so unique and rewarding.[1] This book draws upon the work of many scholars, but in keeping with its design as a primer for introducing students to the principles and concepts of health economics rather than its literature and research methods, the use of attribution, footnotes, and references is purposely limited. Suggestions for additional reading and more advanced source materials and databases are listed at the end of each chapter and are available on the text website at www.wiley.com/college/getzen or from the author at **getzen@temple.edu.**

The first eleven chapters use a flow-of-funds approach to investigate the sources and uses of financing and to explore the incentives and organizational structure of the health care system. Transactions between patients and physicians (and others) are examined to see how profits are made, costs covered, contracts written (or implied), and regulations formed. The long-term consequences of exchanging services for money in a particular way are revealed by exploring the historical development of those distinctive features that characterize the industrial organization of health care: licensure, third-party insurance, nonprofit hospitals, and government regulation. The last seven chapters take a wider macroeconomic perspective in order to explore the dynamics of change within the health care system and to explicitly consider determinants of national health spending and the role of governments in public and private health.

The introductory chapter lays out the overall flow of funds, schematically presents the complexity of medical care transactions, and introduces the basic principles that form the toolkit for economic analysis. Chapter 2 examines the economic concept of demand and compares it to the medical concept of need. Chapter 3 applies the basic principles of supply and demand, marginalism and equilibrium, using a cost–benefit approach in a clinical context. The more detailed investigation of medical care organization begins in Chapters 4 and 5 on insurance and third-party reimbursement, which has become the dominant source of funds in medical care. The physician whose role as the patient's agent and a central player in all medical care transactions is the subject of the next two chapters. Chapters 8 and 9 cover the reimbursement, regulation, and cost structure of hospitals. Nursing homes, long-term care, and the effects of aging on medical costs are covered in Chapter 10. In Chapter 11, pharmaceuticals provide an exemplar of the modern "information economy," where the fixed costs of research and marketing outweigh the cost of production and where competition relies on continuous

---

[1] The special features, which make medical care so interesting as a subject for economic analysis, also tend to make the application of simple models difficult or implausible. Students who have the desire and opportunity to do so are well advised to get a firm grasp of basic principles using a text such as Heyne's *The Economic Way of Thinking* or Samuelson's *Economics* before attempting to grapple with the complexities and ambiguities of medical care.

innovation. In Chapter 12, the means and consequences of access to capital for health care providers are briefly reviewed, with particular attention to the implication of nonprofit status and ownership structure.

To understand the interactions between component parts of the system, it is necessary to place health care in a macroeconomic context that includes redistribution, taxation, inflation, and growth. The dynamics of national health expenditure are presented in Chapter 13 as an application of the permanent income hypothesis. Chapter 14 explores the role of government, public goods, and public health. The economic history of health is traced in Chapter 15, drawing on the contributions of demography and the cliometric work of Fogel and North. Chapter 16 provides international comparisons of health and medical care expenditures, taking Ghana, Sudan, China, Mexico, Poland, Germany, and Japan as illustrative examples. Health policy, reform, and the Patient Protection and Affordable Care Act of 2010 are described and discussed at length in Chapter 17. A final chapter addresses the probable trends in health care spending, suggesting that the primary barrier to increased effectiveness and efficiency is poor allocation and problems of effective political alignment.

Health economics is fascinating to study, but it is not easily summarized or readily captured in neat equations. In part, this is because the study of health economics is relatively new and still in the process of refinement, but primarily it is because the transactions made by doctors and hospitals are not simple, and they cut to the heart of what it means to be human. What is the value of life? Who pays the price of pain, and what does it mean to trust a surgeon who profits because of a crisis? Because most medical care is funded through taxes and insurance, there is no direct linkage between the amount paid and the resources used in treatment. As a consequence, "prices" become more ambiguous and are often of less immediate relevance to the trading parties than ongoing relationships of trust and professional behavior. It is important to understand how economic forces continue to operate when markets are indirect and inefficient, and how other organizing principles (professionalism, licensure, agency, regulation) act as substitutes for prices. Although most of the special features of medical markets are there to make people better off, they have also been shaped by groups who had the power to modify the rules in their own interest, subject to the controls of economic and political competition. Tracing the economic rationale and development of medical care licensure and organization and making those forces more clearly visible and amenable to analysis is the purpose of this book.

CHANGES FOR THE FIFTH EDITION

As this preface is written (April 2012) the United States once again *appears* to be standing on the cusp of a major change in health care and medical financing—but such moments have come and gone before. The potential for change, and the well-grounded expectation that any changes will grow out of what has come before (a process known as "path dependence") is addressed in Chapter 18. Forecasts of the future are necessarily somewhat speculative, but this chapter does offer students and instructors some chance to step back and think about some general policy principles and the practical aspects of forecasting in an economy for which change is constant. It can also provide a brief introduction to behavioral economics, the dynamics of technological change, the expansion of welfare to include "happiness" and alternative valuations of "GDP," disequilibrium, and some other issues that are now at the forefront of contemporary economics research. Most students need to obtain a set of skills, an economics toolkit, in order to work. This fifth edition continues to emphasize basic "principles" (opportunity cost, scarcity, demand, marginal revenue, value, fundamental theory of exchange) in Chapters 1 and 2. For classes emphasizing economic evaluation, a more detailed quantitative and diagrammatic presentation can be quite useful. For general classes directed toward clinicians, administrators, or policy makers, it can be a bit too long and dry, severely taxing their enthusiasm for health economics before they have fully worked through the mechanics of determining the marginal rate of technical substitution. I usually find time to review this material in most classes by adjusting the length of the presentation and the number of illustrative examples to the extent of familiarity within that particular class setting. Teaching notes, presentation slides, and problem sets for all chapters can be found online at http://www.wiley.com/college/getzen. World Wide Web references are used throughout the text to provide access to constantly updated material. There are links to a variety of major sources of health economics data and commentary such as the National Center for Health Statistics, World Health Organization, Organisation for Economic Cooperation and Development, Centers for Disease Control and Prevention, Centers for Medicare and Medicaid Services, Government Accountability Office, and others. Your comments and queries are welcome. For adopting professors, online help, answers to all problems, and chapter teaching guidelines are available through the text website and also through email at **getzen@temple.edu.**

ACKNOWLEDGMENTS

The writing of this book incurred intellectual and personal debts sufficient to preclude any complete listing of those who have contributed. My family and extended family (Rufus and Beverley Getzen, Sydney White, Bill W.) come first. My initial research on these topics began at the University of Washington, with the assistance of Yoram Barzel, Gardner Brown, Steve Shortell, Bill Richardson, and Mike Morrisey and while working under Gordon Bergey, who was an exemplar of the concerned physician and administrator. I am indebted to the efforts of Joe Newhouse, Mark Pauly, Tony Culyer, Morris Barer, Mike Drummond, Bill Swan, and others who have done so much to build the field and create a rigorous body of literature in health economics, and I thank them for their service to *i*HEA. Patrick Bernet of Florida Atlantic University created and revised the Instructor's Manual, and Laura Shinn (CHERP) and Maia Platt of University of Detroit-Mercy created and updated the new Test Bank and PowerPoint slides. David Barton Smith, Bill Aaronson, Chuck Hall, Jackie Zinn, and other colleagues at Temple have shaped the health economics course as it was taught. Alan Maynard sheltered and inspired me during my sabbatical at York, during which the first edition was begun, Richard "Buz" Cooper schooled me on workforce projections, and Uwe Reinhardt has always kept me informed, amused, and concerned. The numerous reviewers over five editions have provided invaluable feedback and suggestions. The usual and heartfelt disclaimer applies: All remaining errors are mine.

ABOUT THE AUTHOR

Thomas E. Getzen is Emeritus Professor of Risk, Insurance, and Health Management at Temple University and the founder and Executive Director of *i*HEA, the International Health Economics Association. After receiving an undergraduate degree in literature from Yale University, he worked for the U.S. Public Health Service Centers for Disease Control venereal disease program in New York and Los Angeles, and then obtained a Master of Health Administration degree in Medical Care Organization and a Ph.D. in Economics from the University of Washington. Dr. Getzen's main research contributions have been in the areas of contracting, price indexes, and forecasting of health care spending. His consulting work has included employee benefit negotiations, projections of health care cost trends and premiums, laboratory diagnostics, risk assessment, and capital financing for managed care. Dr. Getzen has been a visiting professor at the University of Toronto, the Center for Health and Wellbeing of the Woodrow Wilson School at Princeton University, the Wharton School at the University of Pennsylvania, and the University of York (UK). He has served on the boards of Covenant House, a local community health center in northwest Philadelphia; MSI, a venture capital–financed managed behavioral health care corporation; and CHE, a multi-institutional health provider system with more than 30 hospitals and nursing homes. He is the editor-in-chief for the "*HEN*-Health Economics Network" in collaboration with SSRN, associate editor for *Health Economics,* and a reviewer for a number of medical, health services, and economics journals. Professor Getzen periodically updates the forecasting model of "Long Run Medical Cost Trends" for the Society of Actuaries, and he currently serves on the National Academy of Sciences IOM Committee on the Future of Public Health.

FOREWORD

Public policy in almost any field depends on specific knowledge of the field, but it usually also depends (or should depend) on general principles of economics. For example, the building of a bridge requires knowledge of engineering to know what is feasible; it requires knowledge of traffic patterns; and it requires knowledge of economic principles, to see whether the traffic that will use the bridge and the value of the time saving to that traffic will justify the costs imposed by the engineering requirements. So, too, there is a need of economic analysis to help in the construction of a system of health care. First of all, indeed, we must know what medical care can do, and how much in the way of skilled professionals, other workers, machinery, and buildings it takes to achieve any given level of medical care. But second, we must analyze how the payment mechanisms to compensate for these supplies affect the delivery of medical care.

Medical care is indeed a more complex economic problem than bridge-building. Like some other professions but unlike many other goods and even services, it is difficult for the consumer (here the patient) to evaluate the quality of the services received. Much depends on the self-control and reliability of the individual practitioner, the supplying group, and the medical profession as a whole in ways that the patient cannot readily check. Then, too, the service provided is needed only at unpredictable intervals, but it frequently is very important when it is needed. Further, the costs, a reflection of the resources used, are uncertain be very high. All these reasons lead to the use of some form of insurance, a natural economic institution for improving everyone's welfare. But insurance reduces the incentive of an individual patient or physician to seek the most economical means of treatment. As a result, new institutions and regulations develop to overcome this "moral hazard," as it has been termed—institutions such as health maintenance organizations, managed care by insurance companies, and regulations such as those that govern Medicare expenditures. The standard paradigms of economics have been enriched to discuss problems such as this.

The difficulties of quality evaluation and moral hazard are special cases of a more general phenomenon, differences in information between the two sides of a transaction. These differences, though not confined to medical practice, are especially important there, and have further consequences beyond those already noted, as in the need for licensing physicians or the specially important role of nonprofit institutions.

The economic problems of allocating resources to medical care have long been a major part of government economic policy, more in other countries than in the United States. The steady rise in the expenditures on medical care, outstripping the rise in national income by a considerable margin, has brought these issues to the fore of public attention. Equally important has been the increase of explicit consideration of costs within the medical profession; the historically unwelcome trade-off between costs and treatment has come forcibly to the fore. The need for good education and good texts has become acute, and Professor Getzen's book is a welcome attempt to meet this strongly felt need.

Kenneth J. Arrow

CHAPTER 1

CHOICES: MONEY, MEDICINE, AND HEALTH

QUESTIONS

1. Who pays when you skip a workout to watch television?
2. Is health scarce?
3. Do some people pay more (or less) than their fair share?
4. Does everyone get the same kind of care?
5. Who decides: the patient, the doctor, the hospital, or the government?
6. Who is made better off: the surgeon or the patient?
7. Why does health care cost so much?
8. Are there futures contracts in health care?
9. Why is health care bought and sold differently from other goods and services?

What to do, *how* to do it, and *for whom* are core issues of economics. Should Melanie go to the emergency department to have her twisted knee examined now, or should she wait until Tuesday when she already has an appointment with the doctor? Is it better to get medication or surgery for that injury? Which seriously ill patient should get the kidney transplant? Is it worth extending the Supplemental Children's Health Insurance Program (SCHIP) legislation to cover legal immigrants? Questions like these are dealt with every day in peoples' homes, in hospitals, and in the halls of Congress. They are the subject of health economics, along with more mundane decisions that cumulatively have an even greater impact on your health: partying until 3 A.M. or getting a good night's sleep, how much exercise to get, whom to vote for in the next election, whether to major in accounting or enlist in the army reserves, eating more vegetables or less cake, and so on.

Economics is often described as the "theory of choice," and health economics is about the choices people make with regard to health, choices medical providers make in order to care for people and earn money, and choices made collectively (by Congress, community groups, or professional associations). Making a choice means deciding that what is given up—the **opportunity cost**—is not worth as much as what is obtained. Choosing to go to the doctor for treatment means the time and money it will take is worth less to me than the benefit I expect to receive. A hospital choosing Mark rather than Mary to receive a heart transplant must expect that the therapeutic benefits to (and insurance payments from) Mark are greater than what is lost by leaving Mary on the waiting list. When a patient and a medical provider agree to a transaction, making a trade that exchanges money for services, both have decided that it will make them better off. When Congress votes to expand SCHIP, they have decided that running a temporary deficit, raising taxes, or cutting some other program is less important to the American public than the additional health coverage.

1.1   WHAT IS ECONOMICS?

Trade, "making a buck," is a quintessential economic activity. Its focal point is the market, the place where buyers and sellers exchange dollars for goods and services. Without buyers and sellers there would be no economy: no rich surgeons, no insurance companies, no hospital billing departments (or textbook royalties for economists). To say that there would be no rich surgeons is not a statement of envy but one of fact. Without an advanced economy, a person could not spend 15 years studying and practicing eye surgery, and hence could not provide a highly specialized form of labor that is so much more valuable than digging ditches; therefore, patients could not reap the benefits of so much knowledge and training.

For a surgeon to be a seller, the patient must be a buyer. They both must agree on a price so that an exchange can occur. The surgeon would probably prefer that the price be higher and the patient would probably prefer that it be lower, but both must be satisfied in order for a trade to take place. As economists, we can observe that because a transaction took place, there must have been mutual agreement that made both the buyer and the seller better off. If the surgeon would rather have watched television than perform another operation, she would have turned down the case. If the patient would rather have saved the money, or gone to a different surgeon, he could have done so. The insight that both parties must be benefiting if they freely agreed to make a trade is central to an economic vision of the world and is known as the *fundamental theorem of exchange*.

FUNDAMENTAL THEOREM OF EXCHANGE

The foundation of market economics is that trade makes both parties better off. People make a deal because they expect it will provide more satisfaction than not making the deal. The surgeon and the patient expect to gain from trade: the surgeon by receiving money and gratitude, the patient by being healed. It might turn out that the patient dies and the surgeon gets sued for malpractice, but both made the transaction with the expectation that they would become better off. Trade does not take advantage of people so that one party is made better off at the expense of the other (that is stealing). Trade takes advantage of differences in skills, endowments, and tastes so that people can make exchanges that are mutually advantageous.

Terms of Trade

The "terms of trade" specify what the buyer is to give to the seller and what the seller is to give to the buyer in return. When you buy a common item in a store, such as aspirin, a simple price of $1.29 per bottle of 50 might tell you everything you need to know about the transaction. For services, and for medical care in particular, the transaction is apt to be much more complex. For example, consider the transaction for an operation to implant an artificial intraocular lens (IOL) in a patient's eye to replace the natural lens that has become clouded by cataracts. The patient is to pay a $200 deposit up front and $800 more within 30 days after the surgery is completed and all sutures are removed. Reduced to its most simple element, the terms of trade in this exchange can be expressed as a monetary price of $1,000 for the IOL implant. Yet much more than the $1,000 is being agreed to in this transaction. The physician agrees to provide not just any artificial lens but to choose the correct one, continuously monitor the quality of the operation, and control adverse reactions to postoperative medications. The patient agrees to make payment in two parts, with a time limit, and may assume that the operation will be redone without further charges if the first attempt is not satisfactory. Many of the agreed-upon conditions (that the physician is licensed, will use only qualified assistants, will not try to boost the bill needlessly to increase her fees, and will keep the patient informed of any possible adverse consequences, and that the patient will wear bandages as long as necessary and not go skydiving) will never be specified explicitly unless some disagreement and subsequent legal action force the doctor and patient into court.

In the simplified neoclassical model of perfectly competitive behavior with which most textbooks begin, price is the only term that matters in a transaction and both the buyer and seller are "price takers." That is, there are so many buyers that whether one person buys or not has little influence on the price in the market; therefore, buyers must "take" the price as given. Similarly, there are so many firms selling the same product that no single firm can affect prices; hence, all firms must take the price as given. This uncomplicated model of perfectly competitive behavior is not too distant from reality when you buy a bottle of aspirin. The model works reasonably well for most of the purchases made by consumers, and thus it can be used to frame the analysis of the economy as a whole. However, buying a bottle of aspirin is not representative of most medical decisions, and an elementary model does not capture many of the essentials when life-and-death decisions are being made by doctors in the operating room (see the more detailed discussion in Section 6.4, "The Medical Transaction"). No one needs a prescription to buy a car or rent a movie. You don't have to have insurance or sign a consent form to have your car's fuel pump worked on, and almost anyone can cut your hair without a license. Treating disease requires knowledge and entails risks that are quite special, forcing a patient to trust the judgment of the surgeon and leading to special forms of economic organization and contracts in medicine: professional licensure, hospital staff bylaws, regulatory review. Studying such adaptations reveals the potential of economics as a discipline in a way that the analysis of more standard markets cannot.

Value

Why does health care cost so much? Because health is so precious that its value exceeds that of all the things we possess. What benefit do I get from spending my money on food or music or cars or clothes if I am dead? Sick and in pain, confronted with the possibility of death, people are willing to spend almost any amount of money to get their health back. Health care costs so much because people are willing to pay so much for it. The many years a surgeon spends in training, the billions of dollars government spends on public health, and the comprehensive health insurance plans provided by employers are consequences of the value we as a society place on health care. They are effects, rather than causes. We are willing to spend so much on physician training, public health, and health insurance because what they produce is valuable to us. If we stopped caring about (or paying for) health, no new magnetic resonance imaging (MRI) scanners are built, surgeons would stop spending years in training, and our taxes would go toward highways or national parks instead of AIDS and cancer research. Cows can get just as many diseases as humans do and we could put all those resources to work saving cows, but we don't. Cows, I am sure, would set priorities rather differently, but they are not paying the bills.

Can We Pay Somebody to Care?

Doctors and nurses want to care for patients. Given a chance, they will make extraordinary efforts on your behalf. Medicine is as much about caring as it is about curing. Does paying somebody make them care for you? Probably not. However, not paying people can make it impossible for them to care for you. If doctors and nurses had to find another way to make a living and pay the bills, then they could not spend their time looking after your health.

Do your friends expect to be paid because they care for you? Not precisely, but they do expect to be paid back in kind, by your caring for them. If you treat your friends as if you did not care, eventually you will not have any friends. Parents are a bit more understanding, but in part that is because they know that however ungrateful you may be for their help, you will probably be willing to help your own ungrateful kids (their grandchildren) someday. Medical professionals are even more compassionate. They work for many hours even when a case is nearly hopeless, knowing they will not get additional pay for all the extra effort. However, as professionals, they can expect respect and a reasonable income. The development of medicine as a **profession** (see Chapters 6 and 7), dedicated to science and caring, is a great social innovation, one of the adaptations of economic organization mentioned earlier. Sometimes it is only the professionalism of the helpers that keeps someone who is poor and sick from being left all alone to deal with an illness.

Doctors work on your behalf. Most importantly to an economist, it is doctors who decide what medicine is right or wrong, not you. Although patients do ultimately have the right to make their own decisions, in practice those decisions are made largely by the professionals who take care of the patient. In the operating room, it is not the patient who decides, but the surgeon (in some ways, it is a bit like a family, where the parents make decisions on behalf of their children). In basic trades, all that is required is that a buyer and a seller agree on a price. In medicine, the buyer–seller distinction is not clear. Is the doctor the one who is "buying" the surgery, or the one selling it? A medical "trade" is made on the patient's behalf by someone who cares about them, not by the patient acting on their own. The situation is complex and involves a set of professional expectations and external forces (quality regulations, consent forms, insurance) as well as the patient's illness or their personal tastes and preferences. Caring, from an economic point of view, means making decisions for someone else—to help them, rather than just to help yourself.

Financing Health Care

What does it mean "to finance" something: a house, a car, your education? When you finance a car, you have to make payments over many months. To buy a house, you go to a bank for a loan, which is then usually bundled with other mortgages by Fannie Mae or some other financial entity and sold to many investors. Financing your education often means making tuition payments over time, taking out student loans, getting money from parents, and maybe getting a scholarship from the university. If it is a public university, taxpayers are usually covering a large part of the costs. At a private college, donations and income from the endowment are used to supplement student fees (and are indirectly subsidized by tax breaks). Financing means that many parties are involved, not just the buyer and the seller. Often there are *financial intermediaries,* like banks, that help to make the transaction possible by providing guarantees over time and spreading the risks across many investors. For student loans, Sallie Mae (formerly the Student Loan Marketing Association) is the financial intermediary making loans possible with the backing of the federal government, which is the largest intermediary of all and makes possible the whole banking system as well as all the subsidies from taxpayers for national defense, schools, and health care.

The development of medicine as a caring profession is a kind of primitive financial intermediation. Those who can afford to pay extra do so, and therefore those who cannot pay are able to get professional care. With transplants and therapies costing hundreds of thousands of dollars, professional goodwill and charity alone are hardly sufficient, so there are public and private insurance plans pooling funds and sharing risks across millions of people, and these plans provide most of the financing for health care (see Chapters 4 and 5). Looking into the funding of research provides additional insight. The people who benefit from medical research are not usually the people who pay for it. A study of brain function or cell structure will do nothing for a patient in the hospital today and not much for the foundation that donated money or the taxpayers funding a research grant. Tomorrow's miracle drugs are paid for by adding overhead into the price of today's pharmaceuticals (see Chapter 11), and advances in surgical technique are paid for by adding overhead into the price of an operation. The basic discoveries that make all of this new technology possible are funded by federal grants and other forms of taxpayer support, with benefits coming far into the future, if at all. Only sometimes do the efforts succeed, and those few successes must provide sufficient rewards to make the overall returns on a risky investment worthwhile.

The two core concepts of financial analysis are **timing** and **risk**. Something that cannot be used until far into the future is not worth as much as something you can start using today (time discounting, or present value; see Chapter 3 and Chapter 12). Uncertainty also makes a thing less valuable (risk adjustment or discounting). Usually the longer you wait for something the more risky it is, so value is discounted both for time and risk. Discounting for uncertainty and the lapse of time are factors that make it hard for college sophomores to spend less so they will have more savings for retirement, or to stop eating french fries so that they can be healthier when they are in their 50s, or for a soldier being sent to war to give up smoking. In health care the benefits are almost never immediate or certain and thus must be discounted, and they are almost always financed by others rather than paid for directly, so that the patient rarely stops to compare costs and benefits before going to the doctor. The fundamental theorem of exchange becomes complicated and diffuse when trades involve millions of people in complex transactions with uncertain effects lasting for decades or generations.

Full Cost: Paying for Medical Care

All goods and services must be paid for. Many regular goods are paid for by consumers at the point of purchase. Some large purchases, such as cars and houses, are financed by paying over time. Then there are those, like medicine and college, that are mostly paid for with "other people's money"—from philanthropists, grandparents, or taxpayers.

Many people believe that because they pay something for medical care or college, they are bearing the full costs. Usually they are not. The total cost of health care in the United States was about $2.8 trillion in 2012. Thus the various providers that make up the U.S. health care "system" must take in an average of $8,936 from every person in America (man, woman, child; old, young; rich, poor; sick, well; working, disabled—everybody). The average household has 1.9 people and paid less than $350 per month on medications, doctor visits, copayments, and insurance premiums directly (termed "out-of-pocket" or OOP), meaning that most (>75%) of the financing came from "other people's money." College students and recent grads are less expensive than the average, but they also pay in much less (Table 1.1). The elderly tend to spend significantly more from their equally limited incomes, but they also cost the system much, much more (more than $3,000 per person; see Chapter 10). The only way we can begin to get a full financial picture of the whole health system is to carefully trace all the payments in and out.

TABLE 1.1	Monthly Household "Out-Of-Pocket" Spending		
	young <25	*25 to 64*	*old >65*
Total (All Goods & Services)	$3,039	$4,995	$3,015
Prescription Drugs	$ 13	$ 33	$ 72
Medical	$ 37	$ 89	$ 70
Health Insurance	$ 71	$ 153	$ 246
Health as % of Monthly Spending	*4.0%*	*5.5%*	*12.9%*

Source: U.S. Bureau of Labor Statistics, "Focus on Prices and Spending: Consumer Expenditure Survey," 1(8), August 2010.

1.2 THE FLOW OF FUNDS

Goods and services are provided in a market economy only if the people who want them are willing to pay for them and if suppliers are willing to accept those payments in return. Exchange is based on voluntary agreement, so that trade between a buyer and seller occurs only when both parties believe that they will be made better off by trading (the fundamental theorem of exchange). In the simplest form of trade, consumers buy from businesses, exchanging money for goods and services in a two-party transaction.

Consumers make up the demand side of this simple service market, and firms make up the supply side (see Chapter 2). In legal terms, firms are contractual entities that can own, buy, and sell property and pay taxes just as people do. To get the labor, land, and other inputs needed for production, the firm (the seller) in Figure 1.1 must also be a buyer, as shown in Figure 1.2. These secondary two-party transactions are characteristic of derived demand, purchases made as an intermediate step in production rather than for final consumption. Firms are owned by individuals (or other firms) that provide the capital, labor, and organizational effort necessary to get them started and keep them running. Thus, every dollar that a consumer gives to a firm, whether used for wages, profits, or purchase of input from another firm, ultimately ends up

FIGURE 1.1　　　Two-Party Transaction

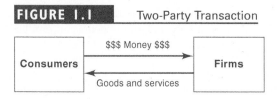

FIGURE 1.2　　　Derived Demand between Firms

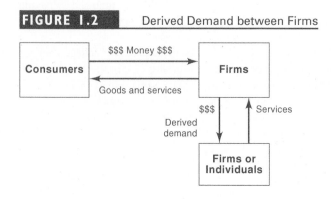

FIGURE 1.3　　　Circular Flow of Funds

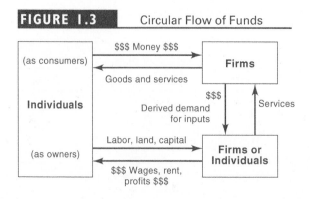

in the hands of someone who wants to spend it. When workers or owners spend money, they become consumers and therefore complete the circular flow of funds through the economy, as shown in Figure 1.3.

Health Care Spending in the United States

Medical care in the United States is a trillion-dollar business ($2,824,257,000,000), with an estimated average of $8,936 spent per person in 2012.[1] The 316 million citizens of the United States received services from more than 5,000 hospitals, 30,000 nursing homes, 800,000 physicians, 2.8 million registered nurses, and 10 million other health care workers. Financial flows, the major sources and uses of health care funding during 2012, are indicated in Table 1.2. Individuals paid $322 billion, or 11 percent of total funding; private (mostly employer-based) health insurance paid 31 percent; and government, the largest payer, paid 50 percent (20 percent Medicare, 16 percent Medicaid, 14 percent other government programs). The remaining 7 percent of total health care financing came from a variety of other private sources (philanthropy, industrial clinics, interest, and rental income of providers). The largest use of funds was the $873 billion spent on hospital care, 31 percent of the total.

Figure 1.4 presents this information graphically, highlighting a simple yet important fact about financial balances: the "sources (in)" and "uses (out)" bars are of equal height. Every dollar spent by a patient, insurance company, or government is recorded as a cost but is also recorded as income to a physician, hospital, agency, administrator, or other health employee. Therefore the totals must be equal: Financial flows in and out balance each other. The flow of money is circular. Money itself is only a way of keeping track of all the obligations within the economy. Every dollar spent by one person is, of necessity, a dollar of income for someone else. Tracing the flow of funds through this complex system provides some sense of the forces that shape the economy.

Sources of Financing

Health care spending has grown enormously. In 2012, it accounted for about 18 percent of the gross domestic product (GDP) and one of every nine employees in the labor force. That growth has been facilitated by the shift from individual payments to third-party financing.

TABLE 1.2   U.S. Health Care Spending, 2012

Uses of Funds	Percentage of Total	Amount per Person	Sources of Funds	Percentage of Total	Amount per Person
Hospital	31%	$ 2,763	Medicare	20%	$ 1,790
Physician	19%	1,718	*Paycheck deduction*		*590*
Dental	4%	347	Medicaid	16%	1,446
Other	8%	706	VA & DOD	3%	291
Nursing home	5%	477	Other government	11%	966
Home health	3%	254	*Total government*	*50%*	
Drugs	10%	918			
Products	3%	269	Employer insurance	31%	2,799
Administrative costs	7%	635	*Tax subsidy*		*455*
Public health	3%	289	Self-paid	11%	1,019
Research	2%	179	Charity, etc.	7%	626
Construction	4%	381			
Total	100%	$8,936	Total	100%	$8,936

Based on a projected U.S. population of 316 million.
Source: U.S. Office of the Actuary, National Health Projections, http://www.cms.gov/NationalHealthExpendData/.

FIGURE 1.4   Sources and Uses of Health Care Funds, United States, 2012

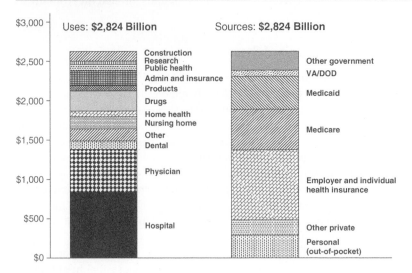

Source: CMS Office of the Actuary, www.cms.gov.

In 1929, 81 percent of medical expenditures were financed by individual out-of-pocket payments and only 19 percent from government and other third-party organizations (Table 1.3). By 2012, this ratio had been reversed, with individuals paying only 11 percent directly and the remaining 89 percent of financing coming from third-party transactions involving government, nonprofit organizations, and insurance.

All of the elements that characterized health care in 2012 were present in some form one hundred years ago, but their relative importance to the flow of funds has changed so much that the transactions look entirely different today.[2] Physicians, who in 1900 were tradespeople sometimes making do with partial payment in eggs or flour, have become highly paid and technologically sophisticated professionals who rarely talk to their patients about paying the bills (see Chapter 7). Hospitals, once minor supports for some disabled and disadvantaged people, are now technological palaces of intensive treatment and the largest users of U.S. health care funds (see Chapter 8). Whereas in 1900 hospitals were financed by a few donors and some patient fees, they are now financed almost entirely by third parties: either by government insurance

TABLE 1.3   Sources of Financing 1929, 1970, and 2012

Source	1929	1970	2012
Health Spending			
Total (millions of dollars)	$3,656	$74,894	$2,823,587
Adjusted for inflation (2012 dollars)	$40,070	$357,047	$2,823,587
Per capita (adjusted)	$330	$1,697	$8,936
As a percentage of GDP	3.5%	7.2%	17.9%
Percentage Paid by			
Self (out-of-pocket)	81%	33%	11%
Third parties	19%	67%	89%
Government	13%	38%	50%
Private insurance	<1%	21%	31%
Philanthropy, other	6%	8%	7%

Source: U.S. Office of the Actuary, National Health Projections, http://www.cms.gov/NationalHealthExpendData/.

FIGURE 1.5   Health Care Flow of Funds, circa 1900

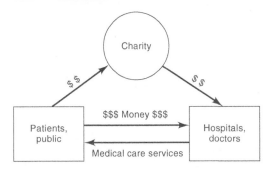

such as Medicare and Medicaid or by private insurance provided through employment or purchased directly by consumers (Figures 1.5 and 1.6). For every $100 spent in the hospital, less than 2 percent now comes from charitable donations. Even the 3 percent paid for by patients out-of-pocket does not really flow through a two-party transaction, because much of that 3 percent consists of copayments, deductibles, and other fees related to third-party insurance payments.

There are many reasons health care spending has grown rapidly. An increasingly wealthy population is willing to spend more on all goods and services. Extra spending on health care has a greater appeal after basic necessities such as food and housing are taken care of. Technological advances make modern medicine more desirable. An aging population favors health care over other goods. Insurance now finances more of the cost. Shifting the financial burden from individuals to third parties through insurance not only changed the way funds flowed but also made more funds available, so that the health care system could grow rapidly and absorb an ever-larger share of total economic output.

Such cost shifting has made the financing system complex and opaque: Almost no one knows who is paying for what.[3] Billed charges bear little resemblance to what is paid or what the provider receives, and provider revenues are usually identified not as "income" but as "reimbursement." Third-party payments are made with:

- Taxes paid to government agencies (Chapters 13 and 14)
- Employer and employee payments to commercial insurance companies (Chapters 4 and 5) and for-profit and nonprofit managed-care firms, including health maintenance organizations (HMOs), preferred provider organizations (PPOs), and other organizations
- Philanthropic contributions to charities (Chapters 9 and 12)

FIGURE 1.6   Health Care Flow of Funds, circa 2012

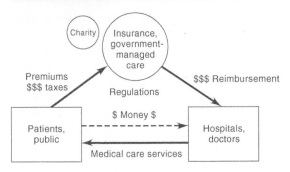

Each of these major categories of third-party payments exists in endless variations. The details differ widely, but from a financial perspective they all have a similar purpose: pooling funds from many people to pay the bills of the few patients who need major care.

Who gets care and what kind of care are decisions made according to embedded rules and the opinions of professionals who run the health care system. In each case, indirect third-party payment weakens the monetary linkage between buyer and seller that characterizes the direct two-party transactions typical in most other sectors of the economy. For most medical transactions, there is no exchange of money between the recipient of services and the provider. The patients (or their families) pay insurance premiums and taxes, and the doctors and hospitals are paid by the government and insurance companies. In the absence of a direct link between the amount paid and the resources used in treatment, "prices" become more ambiguous and less important to the transaction than ongoing relationships of trust and professional behavior. One of the purposes of this textbook is to explain how economic forces continue to operate when prices do not function in a normal way and how other organizing principles (professionalism, licensure, regulation) serve as replacements.

Health Care Providers: The Uses of Funds

Payments by patients, government, and insurance companies have increased 200-fold over the past seventy years; thus, payments received by doctors, hospitals, and other care providers have increased by the same amount. In general, both the public, as users of the system, and providers, as suppliers of care, have been happy with this large increase in spending. The public has gotten a health care system that is technologically advanced and responsive to their needs. Providers have gained glory in the fight against disease and substantial gains in income, making them eager to continue the struggle.

Part of the increase in health care spending from $4 billion in 1929 to $2,824 billion in 2012 is just an accounting fiction due to inflation, because $1 in 1929 is roughly the same as $13 in 2012. Also, some of the increase reflects a rise in the number of people who must be cared for. Yet even after adjusting for changes in population and inflation, real per capita spending is more than 25 times larger today than in 1929. Part is due to a real increase in wages. As per capita incomes rise, workers expect more goods and services per hour of work. Therefore, expenditures on labor-intensive services tend to rise more rapidly than expenditures on goods and capital-intensive commodities. Furthermore, the wages of health care workers have risen more rapidly than for other types of labor.[4] This probably reflects both the increased education of health professionals today and the increased demand for their services (Chapter 7). Increases in the quantity of services provided account for some of the growth in total expenditures, but the medical services most commonly counted, number of days spent in the hospital and number of visits to physicians, have actually declined since 1970 (see Table 1.4).[5] However, nursing home days and number of prescriptions per person have increased substantially.

After taking all these factors into account—inflation, higher health care wages, and use of services—there still has been a tremendous increase in expenditures over the last forty years, more than 500 percent. How can spending increase so much more rapidly than the number of services or the wages of those who provide them? By increasing the **intensity and quality of services**. More tests are done for a patient in a modern intensive care unit during a single day than were done for a patient over the course of a month in his or her wooden bed in 1929. Many of those tests (MRIs, blood glucose, heart monitoring) were not available back then. The physician who drove to the patient's house and worked alone out of a black bag has been replaced by a team of therapists, technicians, and support staff assisting a group of specialists using an array of medical equipment. Also, as some common, acute (short-term) diseases have

TABLE 1.4	Changes in the Use of Health Care Funds over 80 Years		
Category	**1929**	**1970**	**2012**
Spending per person (in 2012 dollars)	$329	$1,697	$8,936
Percent Use			
Hospital	23%	37%	31%
Physician	36	19	19
Dental	12	6	4
Drugs	18	7	10
Other	1	3	8
Nursing home	na	5	5
Home health	na	na	3
Products	3	6	3
Administration and insurance	3	4	7
Public health	3	2	3
Research	1	3	2
Construction	na	8	4
Total	*100%*	*100%*	*100%*
Per Person Use			
Hospital days per person	0.9	1.2	0.6
Hospital employees per patient	<0.5	2.0	7.8
Physician visits per person	2.6	5.0	4.0

become curable or preventable, medical care is increasingly applied to chronic diseases that once were considered hopeless. The shift from simple caring to technologically sophisticated curing is reflected by shifts in the categories of expenditure; more is going to institutional care in hospitals and nursing homes, while the share devoted to personal service by doctors has declined. The fraction of the health care dollar spent on manufactured goods such as drugs has also fallen as the cost of labor-intensive services has risen.

1.3   ECONOMIC PRINCIPLES AS CONCEPTUAL TOOLS

Tracing the flow of funds through the health care system makes it possible to apply principles of price theory to situations involving life and death, nonprofit organizations, professional licensure, addiction, and other issues. The powerful generalizations and concepts of microeconomics, macroeconomics, finance, and industrial organization allow us to see how medical transactions are like, and yet unlike, most of the rest of the economy. Chapters 1 through 3 use a simplified set of economic constructs common to most basic Econ 101 presentations. Chapters 4 and after move on to consider the complications (uncertainty, information asymmetry, life and death, etc.) necessary to understand medical transactions. As a practical matter, it will be helpful if you already have a basic grasp of economic theory and applications.

It is not easy to "think" like an economist. Doing so requires a certain amount of practice to develop the necessary twist of perspective and narrowness of focus that allows thinking in terms of incentives, fixed and variable costs, profit margins, and market power. Starting out with a complex subject such as art or marriage or medicine makes it more difficult to study basic economic forces. That is why most textbooks begin with a simplified and abstract process such as operating a lemonade stand or widget factory. Reviewing an introductory text like *Economics* by Samuelson and Nordhaus, *Principles of Economics* by Mankiw, *Microeconomics* by McConnell and Brue, or *The Economic Way of Thinking* by Heyne could prove useful. Students might wish to check the website at www.wiley.com/college/getzen for current links, updates, and other material, or contact the author directly at **getzen@temple.edu**. An instructor's manual is available to professors. Some of the most common principles used by economists as tools for understanding society and the decisions people make are listed below. Most of these will be evident to you based on your own experience or previous study.

Scarcity (Budget Constraints)

Why does a decision always involve giving something up? It is because reality imposes constraints or limits on what you can do. The most basic limit is time. You have only 24 hours in a day, and once your days are gone (owing to death) you have no more life to use in production or consumption. Your income and your bank balance, the place you live, the things and friends you have, and even your credit rating all put limits on what you can do to make yourself better off. Economists call these "budget constraints." This term applies not only to money but also to time, things, relationships, and any other limited resource.

Opportunity Cost

The best measure of what something costs is what you have to give up to get it. The trip to Cancun might cost you $750 in savings; an extra weekend date might cost you an A as your grade falls to a B+ because you gave up study time. Conversely, you might say that the decision to be a grind and get an A cost you a date. It is the decision you make, not the price tag or money, that really determines the cost of something. The primary cost of attending this class is the time and work it takes (the fun you could have had and/or the money you could have earned), not the amount spent on tuition and books.

Willingness to Pay

The best measure for the value of what you get is your "willingness to pay": the complement and mirror image of "opportunity cost." Value includes money, time, pleasure, relief from pain—all of those things that when given up are counted negatively as costs and that when received are considered positively as benefits. The only real difference between a "cost" and a "benefit" is the sign. Note however that value often differs depending on who gets and who gives, which is why trading can increase the total value to society even when all that happens is that some things (including dollars) are moved back and forth from one person to another.

Trade

People engage in trade, exchanging things, time, favors, money, and information, because it makes them better off. Both sides must benefit, or they would not agree to trade. This is the fundamental theorem of exchange and perhaps the most basic principle of economic reasoning.

Money Flows in a Circle

When someone buys something, the money spent must be received by someone else. The seller wants those dollars for what he or she, in turn, can buy. The dollar is almighty because it flows—because it can be changed into anything else—not because there is any inherent value in a wrinkled piece of paper. Circularity implies that every dollar of "cost" is also some provider's "income." Protecting income is one reason few cuts in spending are actually made in practice even though most doctors, hospitals, and insurance companies claim that they want to reduce costs.

The Margin: What Matters?

The "margin" is whatever is different between the options in the choice being made. If you are choosing how long to study before going out to eat, the margin is "hours." If you are choosing whether to eat another slice of pizza, then it is "the difference between four and five slices." If you are deciding between plain and pepperoni, then it is "pepperoni." If you are deciding whether or not to add mushrooms, then "mushrooms" become the margin. When deciding between a small and a large, then "size" is the margin. Deciding between two restaurants? Then perhaps "flavor" or "distance" is the relevant margin (and you might have to consider multiple margins when making a choice). Differences such as slices, minutes, miles, or dollars with uniformly measured units are often termed *quantity margins,* whereas flavor, brand name, hipness, and other incommensurables are called *quality margins.* The important point is that most **decisions are made at the margin.** The relevant question is not "Will I ever eat pizza?" but rather *"How many slices?"* or *"With mushrooms?"* or *"Which place?"*

Maximization: Marginal Costs and Marginal Benefits

Productive effort and exchange (trade) are ways people make themselves better off. What principle determines when to stop? When the incremental (marginal) benefits from the next step are outweighed by the incremental (marginal) costs. Each decision increment (read one more page, eat one more slice of pizza, play one more game) adds a little value (marginal benefit). Each step also takes a little more time or money (marginal cost). The real issue is not whether something (grades, food, playing time) is good, but whether you would be better off with more or less of it. As more and more is done a point is usually reached at which the benefits of each additional step become smaller and smaller (**diminishing marginal returns**) and the costs of each additional unit become greater. Maximum net benefits are obtained by pushing to the point at which rising marginal costs equal falling marginal benefits.

Choice: Are Benefits Greater than Costs?

Every decision involves a trade-off, giving something up to get something else, choosing the option that means more to you. This is obvious when you engage in trade with someone else. It is also true whenever you make a choice, even though you "trade" only with yourself (e.g., giving up a workout at the gym in order to study, passing up a new movie in order to buy dinner at a restaurant, giving up some of your savings in order to take a trip to Cancun). Economists assume that people tend to make choices that make them better off in a way they value (not necessarily financially). This is known as the "benefit–cost principle." In the abstract, economists assume that people behave perfectly rationally, precisely conforming to principles of maximization expressed mathematically in "rational choice theory." More realistically, we accept that people behave "sort of" rationally, not deviating too much from the model of perfect rationality but not exactly conforming to it or meeting that exact standard even in everyday affairs: smoking when they say they want to quit, failing to save enough for retirement, or morosely lamenting the sunk costs of the job they did not take (see "Social Science and Rational Choice Theory" in Section 1.6).

Investment

Investment increases future productivity by diverting current output to infrastructure improvement rather than to immediate consumption. The economic approach to *human capital* uses concepts such as depreciation and rate of return to analyze going to school, having children, getting married, brushing teeth, and other activities that depend upon a long-run perspective. Taking time to exercise and giving up sweets are forms of investment. It is difficult to improve your health once it has deteriorated. Spending money on medicine once you are seriously ill is a little like spending money on your car after the engine has begun to burn oil; regular maintenance is a lot cheaper. How healthy you are when you get old depends less on the medical care you get than on what you have done to and for your body over the years. Income at age 55 depends not on how hard you work then but on what you have done to advance in your career. Most readers of this textbook are studying now for a future reward: knowledge, grades, a degree, and enhanced earnings. Medical school is a form of investment, usually a very good one (see Chapters 7 and 12), as is the research done by pharmaceutical companies, using some current profits to discover new drug that will begin to sell in fifteen years (Chapter 11).

Contracts: Complex Exchanges to Deal with Timing and Risk

The seller must have faith that the money obtained in trade will have value. The buyer must have faith that the goods received are what they are supposed to be. Both buyer and seller must be able to trust each other. More complex transactions require more trust and external guarantees. Buying on credit or for future delivery (mail order, new custom home, knee surgery) creates potential problems and requires a financial intermediary, as does shared purchasing through insurance, cooperatives, or public funds. Acceptance of risk and uncertainties in value (a used car "as is," a share of stock in a start-up company, an experimental drug to treat your rash, trip insurance for your vacation) also force greater reliance on trust and contract specifications. Using a financial intermediary as a third party that handles the money (purchasing agent, broker, insurance company) can make a transaction easier and safer, but it also makes transactions complex and vulnerable. Two of the parties could collude to take advantage of the third party. Often, tracing the flow of funds helps reveal the underlying economic forces at work, even if the contracts are confusing or people lie.

Organizations Adapt and Evolve

Organizations evolve to build trust and increase the efficiency of exchange. Laws, rules, political parties, mandatory labels, certified measures, corporate financial statements, clubs, professions, and nonprofit organizations are all in a sense market responses to market failure, as difficulties in making simple price transactions are resolved by more comprehensive contracts. Government is the most comprehensive of such social structures. Exchange and economic potential remain limited until a solid base of personal trust, laws, contractual organization (markets, firms, credit, regulations), and social structure evolves. The growth and output of a modern economy have more to do with the efficiency of organization than the endowment of natural resources, numbers of people, financial aid, or any other factor.[6]

Distribution: Who Gets What

Laws, rules, and organized exchanges determine not only how much the economy produces but also *distribution:* who gets the benefits and who bears the cost. A society in which the top decile (10%) of the population took 10 percent of the money and goods, the next decile also had 10 percent, and the bottom half of the families had exactly 50 percent, would be described as having no inequality (and does not exist). Conversely, a society in which just 2 percent of the people took 20 percent of all the income and goods would be relatively unequal (and many nations are far less equal than that).[7] Make a change in the rules and you change the outcomes, the distribution. That is one reason laws and organizations are so resistant to change. Virtually any modification will make some people better off and some worse. Whether productivity goes up or down matters less than "what happens to me." Build a railroad bridge, ban cigarette ads, move the three-point line, redraw congressional boundaries: any change will create winners and losers. In theory, efficiency trumps inequality after all the gains and losses are redistributed to make everyone happy. In the real world, action is driven by perceived costs and benefits, profits and losses, by what each person thinks might happen to them—and a real-world economist excels at identifying those incentives and outcomes.

1.4 HEALTH DISPARITIES

Although most goods are distributed privately through markets to whoever can pay for them, anything considered vital to life and fundamental to human happiness (freedom, air and water, the right to vote, protection of the law) is usually made available to everyone by the government and paid for with taxes. One way of defining who belongs in a society and who is excluded is access to such services (see Chapters 13, 14, 15). Medical care can be viewed as a matter of life and death or, in other circumstances, as just one of many goods that it would be better to have more of. Few societies would stand aside and watch someone die when vital medical intervention was easily available, yet the extent to which medical care is made dependent upon ability to pay varies widely (see Chapter 16). In Australia, Canada, Japan, and many European countries every citizen (and often noncitizens as well) has access to high-quality medical care at minimal or no charge regardless of income. In most poor developing countries, only very wealthy families can obtain good care. In the United States the picture is somewhat mixed. Everyone has access to high-quality medical care, but responsibility for payment can vary widely depending upon insurance status, and medical bills are a not-infrequent cause of personal bankruptcy.

Spending money on medical care is only one of many ways that the economy affects people's health. Economic prosperity enables people to have a better diet, to avoid hazardous jobs, and to clean up the environment, as well as to purchase more medical care. A major benefit of higher incomes is education, which changes values and production possibilities in ways that are favorable to health. Chapter 15 provides a more detailed examination of the complex relationships among economic growth, income distribution, medical care, and health. An introductory example of some issues regarding distributional equity in health is provided in Table 1.5, which presents the results of research on 320,000 middle-aged men enrolled in a trial of cardiac risk reduction.[8] Income for this study is based not on individual wages but

TABLE 1.5   Annual Mortality Rate among Middle-Aged Men

Income Category	Mortality Rate	
	White	Black
<$9,999	0.918%	1.234%
$10,000–$14,999	0.840%	1.123%
$15,000–$19,999	0.706%	0.899%
$20,000–$24,999	0.660%	0.867%
$25,000–$29,999	0.591%	0.603%
$30,000+	0.542%	—

Source: G. D. Smith et al., *American Journal of Public Health* 86 (1996): 486–504.

on the community in which the person lived (average per capita income of the zip code of residence). Reading down the columns, it becomes evident that men in poorer communities face a much higher risk of death each year, a finding that holds even as the groups are adjusted for age, unemployment, use of medical care, and other factors. Indeed, those living in areas with average incomes below $10,000 per year were twice as likely to die as those in areas with average incomes above $30,000 per year. Blacks were more likely to die than whites, largely because of living in lower-income areas. Yet even after controlling for differences in income, black mortality is still significantly greater each year. Similar differences in morbidity and mortality rates by socioeconomic and ethnic grouping are observed among women, the elderly, and children.

Although insurance and government assistance have done much to equalize access to medical care, large disparities in actual health and life expectancy endure. Inequalities in health are found throughout the world. Countries such as Sweden and the United Kingdom, which have universal national health systems, also show substantial differences in mortality between groups, as do poorer countries such as Bangladesh and Ghana, where a national health infrastructure is almost nonexistent. Indigenous minority groups in Canada (Inuit), Australia (Aborigine), Brazil (Indian), and Finland (Sami) have much poorer health than recently arriving European populations. Health economists are still working to understand the persistence of excess mortality among disadvantaged groups despite tremendous increases and redistribution in health care spending.

1.5   WHOSE CHOICES: PERSONAL, GROUP, OR PUBLIC?

A common quip from geneticists is: "Want to live longer? Choose better parents!" Superficially silly, from another perspective this statement is quite sensible. Parents not only determine your genetic makeup, they also determine your nutrition and lifestyle during your formative years, provide for your education, and are the basis for many of the work and health habits you carry into later life. Your "personal" choices are as much a reflection of what they wanted for you, and the expectations of the social group where you were born, as of any purely individual preferences or effort. Do you smoke cigarettes? Is that a personal choice or a result of your background and social group? (See the box, "Do You Choose to Smoke?")

Choice occurs along a continuum from the purely private individual choices that do not involve anyone else to those that are purely public that must be made collectively and affect everyone (Chapters 13 and 14). Interstate highways, the law, water supply, air quality standards, 911 emergency help systems, and the TCP/IP protocol for the Internet are all examples of public goods. Every public choice represents a compromise because it includes many people who must all choose or agree to abide by the same decision. For many public goods, "quantity" is not very economically meaningful, but "quality" is. Air quality and pollution can be addressed through various improvements, each of which has a cost. Being universal does not exempt public goods from scarcity. Public funds, although much greater than those of any individual, are still subject to budget constraints. The price of better air must be paid by giving up some other public goods or by all of us giving up some of our private goods by paying higher taxes.

Smoking has been banned on airplanes, trains, and buses and in buildings of many firms, universities, and hospitals. Air quality has been improved without paying for pollution control equipment or raising taxes. Does this mean that these improvements in air quality came without a price tag or that no trade-offs had to be made? Of course not. Listen to the smokers gripe or to the complaints of nonsmoking libertarians who worry that the next distasteful behavior to be banned will be drinking, or sex, or gun ownership. While it does not appear that anything has been bought or sold, a transaction has in fact taken place. The opportunity cost of a smoke-free

---

DO YOU CHOOSE TO SMOKE? PERSONAL AND COLLECTIVE DECISIONS

Smoking is a personal choice. An individual's decision is influenced by inherent desires and genetic makeup, but it is often even more strongly shaped by the decisions of others. If many of your friends gather and smoke on Friday nights, it is more likely that you will do so. If you know few people who smoke, and most of your friends speak disparagingly of those who do, then you are less likely to do so. When smoking is considered cool, sophisticated, and a sign of maturity, it is more desired than when it is considered a pathetic habit born of ignorance. In the 19th century, smoking cigarettes was a form of conspicuous consumption by the wealthy, a way of showing that you had "money to burn." During the Depression it was the Hollywood stars (and doctors) who smoked, rather than the poor, and cigarettes were accordingly considered a sign of glamour and sophistication.

During the 1950s and 1960s scientific studies showed conclusively that cigarettes were harmful to health, and public opinion began to change. However, behavior and social norms changed only slowly. For many years after cigarettes were banned in hospitals, smoking was still allowed in airplanes, restaurants, and economics classes. Even in the 1970s it was inconceivable to professors that a university would try to regulate their behavior within their own personal offices, yet today most universities ban smoking from all buildings.

Peer pressure and the social norms created by group choices are powerful. Formal public choices such as a tax of $3 per pack or a ban on smoking in bars and restaurants can even have the force of law. Of course the choice of whether or not to smoke is a personal one, but group and public decisions set the context within which each individual choice is made, and they can overwhelm individual tastes and preferences.

---

workplace was a discernible, but small, loss of personal liberty. This is the "price" of the gain in air quality. People have made it clear that this is a price they are willing to pay, and they have made it just as clear that some measures advocated by health advisors are too costly to be implemented. Even though such collective relationships are inherently complex, involving millions of people, the fundamentals of opportunity cost, budget constraints, and trade-offs still apply.

"Private" and "public" are polar concepts. Few goods are so purely private that they are entirely unregulated regarding safety, ingredients, and disposal, and few goods are so public that there are no differences among individuals regarding use or quality.[9] The economic organization of medical care clusters more services toward the public end than is immediately apparent. Even though each of us goes individually to the hospital emergency department, in a small city we must all go to the same emergency department and get pretty much the same quality of care. The mayor might get better service than a homeless person who is brought in off the street, but the mayor will be operated on by the same surgeon, will be cared for by the same nursing staff, and might end up in the same room as the homeless person. In a large city with many hospitals, there is somewhat more variation, but patients are rarely able to choose their surgeon, nursing staff, or room. Contrast that with the purchase of a coat, a birthday cake, or even a wheelchair, in which there are many more choices and much more individual control over quality. Financing systems also tend to make medical care a public good. All employees in a firm often have the same insurance plan. Therefore, the mail clerk and the executive vice president are equally valued customers of the hospital. In Chapters 4 and 5 we will examine how the pooling of funds into insurance for payment of medical expenses can distort choices and obscure budget constraints.

Connecting the public and private spheres are choices made as a group. An informal group (seniors at Hilltop High, friends of the band, libertarians) can exert a powerful social influence, but only formally constituted groups (corporations) that have legal status as fictitious collective "persons" can enter into contracts and create the circular flow of funds (opening a bank account, buying or selling a truckload of cigarettes, hiring an employee, getting sued). Physician groups, insurance plans, hospitals, and nurses' unions are all corporate entities engaging in medical care. Of particular interest to health economists is why so many of the relevant organizations in medicine are different from those in other markets—licensed professions or nonprofit voluntary hospitals, for example.

1.6   SOCIAL SCIENCE AND RATIONAL CHOICE THEORY

Groups are a pervasive force because humans are social beings, working constantly to set up and maintain markets, clubs, governments, medical facilities, and other institutions. Economics, sociology, anthropology, and politics are often lumped together as "social sciences," but each emphasizes a different perspective for studying interpersonal exchange. Economists look first and foremost at markets and thus concentrate on the formal transactions between people and organizations using money. However, the economic principles developed in studying those transactions can also be used to study the family, group psychology, education, war, the behavior of birds, and health, even when no money is changing hands. The core conceptual tools of economic price theory—scarcity, investment, maximization, marginalism, equilibrium, cost versus benefit—are expressed mathematically as rational choice theory and have been popularly applied to other areas, invigorating new fields of study such as sociobiology and neuroeconomics.

"Rationality" in economics means that people make choices to make themselves better off (maximize utility, minimize risk) subject to constraints, and organizations make choices to meet their objectives (maximize profits, minimize cost, get elected). It does not mean that people are perfectly rational but that they tend to choose in ways that make them better off rather than worse. Rather like natural selection in biology, rationality is a concept that organizes and guides a field of study rather than a precisely specified term. Just as physics uses the equations of Newtonian mechanics to analyze motion, rational choice theory describes actions as if they occurred in a vacuum, without the complications and frictions of the real world. The equations tell us as much, and as little, as knowing that the force of gravity is 32 feet per second squared tells us about the trajectory of a home-run hit or a dancer leaping across the stage. Like gravity, economic rationality and self-interest is always there. It is not the whole story, though, and sometimes misses the human meaning even as it calculates the path traced by the baseball and the ballerina.

What makes health economics so special is the focus on humanity. Questions of life and death are as salient as buying and selling. It definitely matters that we are talking about people rather than things. Selling human tissue or attaching a patient to a ventilator is not the same as buying chicken fingers or attaching a car to a tow truck. Behavioral economics examines what it means that human beings rather than rational calculators are making these decisions, looking at consistently irrational behavior such as stock-market bubbles and why people's willingness to pay for X is often different from the amount they want to receive in compensation in order to give it up, or why a $1,500 bonus is spent differently than a $1,500 check from the insurance company. A widely noted application of behavioral economics has been that moving to automatic enrollment (*must check "no" to opt out* instead of *must check "yes" to opt in*) greatly increases the number of employees with 401k plans and total amount saved for retirement. A similar experiment with elderly Medicare part D (drug plan) recipients indicated that after directing seniors to the relevant price comparison website, those sent a printed letter listing their individual results were more likely (28 percent compared to 17 percent) to switch plans and save money. Just as the principles of economics have been used to study politics, mating behavior, and even baseball, the quirks of human psychology can be used to analyze the twists and turns in perception and monetary flows.[10]

The effects of medical care on the economy are as profound as the effects of economics on health. Not only has medicine led to better health, greater longevity, and increased productivity but it has also become one of the largest businesses in the world. Investments are made in hospital bonds and biotech stocks to make people better off monetarily, not just better off in terms of health. To those who directly or indirectly earn their living from medicine (physicians, nurses, hospital administrators, equipment vendors, and even health economists), the business aspects—the contracts that are used to allocate health services—are important. The invisible hand plays a role in creating a demand for health economics that is just as powerful, and more direct, than the desire to improve the standard of living and care for the sick.

SUGGESTIONS FOR FURTHER READING

U.S. Department of Health and Human Services, *Health United States, 2010* (annual), http://www.cdc.gov/nchs/hus.htm.

U.S. Department of Health and Human Services, Centers for Medicare and Medicaid, National Health Accounts, *National Health Expenditures 1960–2010 and National Health Expenditure Projections 2011–2021*, http://www.cms.gov/NationalHealthExpendData/.

Kaiser Family Foundation Health Policy Studies (www.kff.org).

Victor Fuchs, "Economics, Values and Health Care Reform," *American Economic Review* 86, no. 1 (1996): 1–24.

SUMMARY

1. **Trade** is not the goal of health care, it is the means. For people to get what they want from the system, exchanges between patients and providers must be made. **Health economics** is the study of how those transactions are made and of the bottom-line results.

2. The **terms of trade** are the specifics of a transaction. Only in a very simple exchange are all of the terms of trade captured in the money price. The **fundamental theorem of exchange** states that for a trade to take place, both the buyer and the seller must believe that it makes them better off.

3. **Value** is not inherent in a good but rather in the trading relationship. **Health care costs so much because people are willing to pay for it**. As a wealthy country, the United States was willing to spend more than $2.8 trillion in 2012, $8,936 per person, supporting a dynamic and technologically sophisticated health care system.

4. Health care costs have consistently **risen 2 to 5 percent more rapidly than incomes** and now account for **18 percent of GDP**. Costs are **unevenly distributed**. Seventy percent of total health care dollars are spent on the 10 percent of people who become most ill during a year. Owing to the uncertain and uneven distribution of medical costs, most health care is financed by **third-party insurance** intermediaries, which pool and transfer funds. This system replaces the direct exchange of money for services between two parties (consumers and providers), which is common to most markets.

5. Most choices in medicine are made by **professionals** such as doctors (rather than consumers), and these choices are mostly about quality rather than price or quantity, making the economics of this special market more interesting and complex. **Physicians** account for about 0.6 percent of the U.S. labor force, about the same percentage

as in 1880. However, the number of nurses and other health workers per physician has risen from 0.2 to 15. **Hospitals** (31 percent) are the largest users of health care funds.

6.   **Government** is the largest provider of health care funds (50 percent). Most **research** into new drugs and therapeutic techniques is financed directly by government or indirectly by cost-shifting overheads added to the prices of hospitals, drugs, and surgery. Although research is very expensive, the forgone **opportunity cost** of not innovating would be much greater. Research, health statistics, airline safety, environmental regulations, and malpractice laws are **public goods** and involve choices that must be made by society as a whole. Pooled financing through insurance can make medical care into a form of public good even though services are provided and consumed in private transactions between doctors and patients.

7.   Improvement in **health and longevity** has come mostly from **economic growth, more knowledge, social factors,** and inexpensive **public health** activities rather than the application of expensive medical technology. Insurance and government programs have greatly reduced disparities in the use of medical care between income groups, but **socioeconomic differentials in health status** have persisted. Residents of poor neighborhoods are twice as likely to die as are people of the same age and sex who live in wealthy neighborhoods.

PROBLEMS

1.   {*economic principles*} What is the opportunity cost of going to a doctor to be examined for skin cancer?

2.   {*economic principles*} What is the primary budget constraint facing an 84-year-old billionaire?

3.   {*planning resources per capita*} Using the data in Health United States 2011 (http://www.cdc.gov/nchs/hus.htm), calculate the number of physicians, nurses, hospitals, and nursing homes there would be in an average small town with 10,000 people (total U.S. population was approximately 311 million in 2011).

4.   {*local estimates*} Using the telephone listings for your city, try to determine whether the number of physicians, nurses, hospitals, and nursing homes is greater than or less than the number you calculated for Problem 3. Why is it more difficult to estimate the number of physicians than the number of hospitals? Why is it so difficult to estimate the number of nurses?

5.   {*distribution of health expenditures*} Ranking everyone by the amount spent on medical care, 30 percent of the total (all expenditures for all people) is accounted for by the top 1 percent of patients. Take the overall average per capita personal health expenditure and determine how much on average is spent on each of these high-cost patients. The top half of the population accounts for 90 percent of total spending. What is the average amount spent on the remaining people in the bottom half of the distribution? Is the median (i.e., amount spent on the person who is at the middle of distribution, with half of all people spending more, and half of all people spending less) higher or lower than the mean?

6.   {*philanthropy, dollars versus percentage*} Has the dollar amount of charitable giving for health increased or decreased since 1929? Has the percentage of health expenditures paid for by charity increased or decreased?

7.   {*workforce*} Which has increased more rapidly since 1929: the number of physicians or the number of ancillary health workers? As medicine becomes more technologically

advanced, which will grow faster: the number of more-skilled workers or the number of less-skilled workers?

8. {*utilization*} Did people go to the doctor more often or less often in 2012 than in 1970? In 1929? Did they spend more or fewer days in the hospital? Why?

9. {*causality*} Have health expenditures increased because the number of people employed in health care has increased, or has health employment increased because total health expenditures have increased?

10. {*causality*} Would eliminating research reduce or increase the cost of U.S. health care?

11. {*normative and positive judgments*} Are public choices better or worse than private choices?

12. {*fieldwork*} Contact three people and find out how much they spent on health care last year. Try to estimate how much they spent out of their own pockets and how much was spent by their employers, insurance companies, or the government. Did the people with more serious health problems always end up spending more of their own money on health care? Did they personally end up paying a larger or smaller percentage of their total health bills out of pocket?

ENDNOTES

1. U.S. Department of Health and Human Services, Centers for Medicare and Medicaid, National Health Accounts, *National Health Expenditures 1960–2010 and National Health Expenditure Projections 2011–2021*, http://www.cms.gov/NationalHealthExpendData/, accessed March 28, 2012. The CMS Office of the Actuary is the source for all expenditure estimates in this and subsequent chapters, unless noted otherwise. The figure of $8,936 is an estimate for 2012 that includes research, construction, and other overhead as well as personal health expenditures.

2. Committee on the Costs of Medical Care, *Medical Care for the American People* (Chicago: University of Chicago Press, 1932); Odin W. Anderson, *Health Services as a Growth Enterprise in the United States since 1875* (Ann Arbor: Health Administration Press, 1990).

3. The distribution of costs across individuals can be measured only for personal health care costs that are billed to individuals, not for overhead items such as public health, construction and insurance administration. Such overhead items make up about 15 percent of national health expenditures. Hence, the "personal health expenditures" account for only 85 percent of national health expenditures in Table 1.2 and elsewhere. In truth, even when charges are billed to an individual, many costs have overhead components and are difficult to assign unambiguously to a single person, although they are clearly concentrated on the most ill and are not evenly distributed. Many economists argue that costs are more concentrated than statistics indicate (see Figure 4.1 and Table 4.2) because hospitals and physicians typically overcharge the least complex patients to subsidize the most difficult and complex cases (see the discussion of cost shifting in Chapter 8).

4. Bureau of Labor Statistics, U.S. Department of Labor, Employment and Earnings (http://www.bls.gov). Bureau of Labor Statistics, U.S. Department of Labor, *Employment Cost Indexes and Levels, 1975–90*, Bulletin 2372, 1990.

5. U.S. Department of Health and Human Services, Health United States 1975, and Health United States 2010 (http://www.cdc.gov/nchs/hus.htm). See also L. A. Green et al., "The Ecology of Medical Care Revisited," *New England Journal of Medicine* 344, no. 26 (2021): 2021–2025, which provides statistics indicating that the number of people experiencing symptoms, consulting physicians, and being admitted to the hospital was roughly constant from 1961 to 1996.

6. Compare Japan and Nigeria. One is a resource-poor island that has become one of the wealthiest societies in the world, while the other is a resource-rich nation that flounders to escape poverty. See Dani Rodrk, Arvind Subramanian, and Francesco Trebbi, "Institutions Rule: The Primacy of Institutions over Geography . . . ," *Journal of Economic Growth* 9, no. 2 (2004): 131–165; Niall Ferguson, *Civilization: The West and the Rest* (London: Penguin, 2011); Philippe Aghion, Alberto Alesina, and Fraancesco Trebbi, "Democracy, Technology and Growth," NBER working paper # 13180, 2007.

7. Basic information about the distribution of wealth can be gleaned from standard sources such as the Census Bureau's Current Population Survey and the Federal Reserve Bank's Survey of Income and Assets. More refined measures of inequality commonly used by economists include the Gini coefficient and the Thiel index. Current information on income equality and inequality is provided in Thomas Piketty and Emmanuel Saez, "Income

Inequality in the U.S.," *Quarterly Journal of Economics* 118, no. 1 (2003): 1–39, with recent updates of income inequality data, wealth of top 1 percent, etc. from these two economists reported in the *Wall Street Journal, New York Times,* and other publications.

8. G. D. Smith, J. D. Neaton, D. Wentworth, R. Stamler, and J. Stamler, "Socioeconomic Differentials in Mortality Risk Among Men Screened for the Multiple Risk Factor Intervention Trial," *American Journal of Public Health* 86, no. 4 (1986): 486–504.

9. Joseph E. Stiglitz, *The Economics of the Public Sector* (New York: W.W. Norton, 1986). See Chapter 15.

10. Daniel Kahneman, *Thinking Fast and Slow* (New York: Farrar, Strauss, Giroux, 2011); Richard Thaler and Cass Sunstein, *Nudge: Improving Decisions About Health, Wealth and Happiness* (New Haven: Yale University Press, 2008); Michael M. Lewis, *Moneyball* (New York: W.W. Norton, 2003); Richard Frank, "Behavioral Economics and Health Economics," NBER working paper #10881, November 2004; Jeffrey R. Kling et al., "Comparison Friction: Experimental Evidence from Medicare Drug Plans," NBER working paper #17410, September 2011; Jeffrey Liebman, Richard Zeckhauser, "Simple Humans, Complex Insurance, Subtle Subsidies," NBER working paper #14330, September 2008.

CHAPTER **2**

DEMAND AND SUPPLY

QUESTIONS

1. What is the difference between Mr. Axel's **demand** for physical therapy and his **need** for physical therapy?

2. Is price the only thing that matters? What is the difference between *price* and *value*?

3. Why would a life-saving cardiac drug cost less than one providing temporary symptomatic relief?

4. Do buyers and sellers face the same demand curve?

5. Can better quality actually decrease demand?

6. Which is most sensitive to price changes: one person, one firm, or the whole market?

7. Is the price of a treatment determined by the cost or production? Or by the benefits it produces? Measured in total, on average, or *at the margin*?

8. Do politicians face demand curves?

The choices made by buyers constitute **demand**, whereas the choices made by sellers constitute **supply**. Most people are active on both sides, exchanging money for goods and services as demanders and exchanging labor and other assets for money as suppliers. It is important to understand how such trades create extra value as **consumers' surplus** on the demand side, and producers' surplus or **profit** on the supply side. Money is moved around continuously between people and organizations in the endless loop of linked transactions discussed as the *circular flow of funds* in Chapter 1. We are more apt to be most directly involved in health care on the demand side as patients, but to understand the system we must also analyze the supply side, made up of doctors and other health professions (Chapters 6 and 7), hospitals (Chapters 8 and 9), nursing homes and other long-term care providers (Chapter 10), and pharmaceuticals (Chapter 11), as well as the role of insurance companies as financial intermediaries (Chapters 4 and 5). In this chapter we simplify matters by staying within the microeconomic perspective of individual choice, waiting until later (Chapters 13 to 18) to consider public choice and collective action.

2.1 THE DEMAND CURVE

When a patient chooses to buy he or she becomes a part of demand. Wanting to buy (drugs, plastic surgery, artificial hip, etc.) but not doing so leaves that potential patient invisible, a part of *latent demand* that does not effectively participate in the market. That extra demand will be revealed if the price goes low enough. For example, consider the development of an

FIGURE 2.1   Demand Curve for Artificial Hearts

artificial heart. If each heart costs $1 million, artificial hearts would only be used in matters of life and death. If further development reduced the cost of artificial hearts to $100,000 each, more people would get them (Figure 2.1). The artificial hearts would still be used only for people with serious illnesses, but they might be implanted long before a person's natural heart gave out. If the cost of making an artificial heart dropped to $100, one would be readily available to anyone who needed it. Consider what would happen if the cost of an artificial heart dropped to $10 and could be easily implanted during a 15-minute visit to the doctor. Some people who had never been ill but were just worried, or people who thought that they were weak and wanted a supercharger to help them run faster, might have new hearts implanted.

The demand curve shows how many patients are willing to buy at the current price and also at other potential prices. Thus the demand curve can be used to calculate the total and incremental benefits of each additional artificial heart sold. At a price of $1 million, the artificial heart would be implanted in only two people who believed they would receive more than $1 million in benefits and were willing to pay that much. At a price of $100,000, the artificial heart would be implanted in 38 people, adding 36 people whose perceived benefit is less than $1 million but equal to or more than $100,000. At $60,000, the artificial heart would be implanted in one more person, whose marginal benefit falls between $100,000 and $60,000, and at a price of $20,000, it would be implanted in two more people whose incremental benefit falls between $60,000 and $20,000. If, owing to insurance, the effective price were reduced to $0, then a total of 42 people would receive artificial hearts.

There are two important observations to note here. First, the demand curve is downward sloping because as price continues to be reduced, more and more people will buy (assuming all other conditions remain constant), a generalization known as the **law of demand**. Second, there is no such thing as "the value" of an artificial heart. Its value depends on how many are used. If only a few hearts were available across the United States, their value would be fantastically high, many millions of dollars each. Once many artificial hearts were sold, their value would drop, and eventually, if a sufficiently large number (hundreds of thousands) were sold then the additional (marginal) value would be quite low.

The Diamonds–Water Paradox: An Example of Marginal Analysis

All ordinary economic goods show the same functional relationship between marginal benefit and quantity. The goods are extremely valuable when only a few units are available. They are of moderate value to a larger number of people, and each additional unit is of less and less value as more and more people receive them, with extra services being almost worthless or

FIGURE 2.2   The Diamonds–Water Paradox

even harmful. The founder of modern economics, Adam Smith, was intrigued by the following problem: If water, which is necessary for life itself, is so valuable, why does it cost so little, and why do diamonds, which are simply ornamental, cost so much? Although Smith was a brilliant economist, he was never able to explain this phenomenon. With the benefit of price theory using demand and supply curves, the situation is easily explained by making the distinction between marginal benefits and total benefits. The value of the first ounce of water is very high because it can save the life of a dehydrated person. The second ounce is worth less and the third still less. In many areas, water is so plentiful that there are literally millions of gallons available, and few people have to pay more than a few cents for a glass of water. The total benefit, the value indicated by the area under the entire demand curve, is very large. The marginal benefit, the value of one more glass of water at this point (price) on the demand curve, is very small.

For diamonds, the situation is quite different. The area under the demand curve (total benefit) is not large (I can live very well with no diamonds at all). However, diamonds are scarce enough that the incremental benefit from obtaining one more is still substantial. This is shown in Figure 2.2. Whether the purchase is a bottle of water or a diamond or surgery, the decision to purchase is a decision made at the margin. How much is it worth to pay for one more?

It is useful to keep the diamonds–water paradox in mind when analyzing health policy. Treatments that are highly beneficial to a few selected patients get supplied to so many people that the system is moved farther and farther down the marginal benefit curve. Eventually, most of the additional work is being done on patients for whom doctors can do little good. Efficiency in medical care is not just a matter of technical excellence and minimizing the cost of production. More often, efficiency depends on how much is produced and which patients get treated. Some of the nation's problems with the high cost of medical care come from using diamonds when a bandage around the finger would do just as well.

Consumer Surplus: Marginal versus Average Value of Medicine

The demand curve for artificial hearts can be used to illustrate the distinction between average and marginal value. With the price at $60,000 there are 39 hearts being bought (and sold). Anyone who values an artificial heart at $60,000 or more purchases one. What would be the incremental value of putting one additional heart on the market? Obviously something less than $60,000, because everyone who wants to pay that much already has done so. The demand curve in Figure 2.1 indicates that the price will have to drop down to $50,000 in order to sell one more heart—that is, to have 40 people voluntarily purchasing artificial hearts at the market price.

Thus the marginal value of that additional heart is about $50,000 in this particular market. Because the other 39 people were all willing to pay more than $50,000, they are receiving a consumer's surplus—extra value to them above and beyond what they had to pay. How much extra value? Well, two were willing to pay $1 million or more, the third was willing to pay almost that much ($975,000), and the next was willing to pay just a little bit less ($950,000), and so on, until we get to the 39th person who valued an artificial heart at $75,000, and finally to the last (marginal) buyer (the 40th), who was only willing to pay $50,000.

All except the last receives a consumer surplus. How much consumer surplus? Adding up the value to each of the 40 people who are buying ($1,025,000 + 1,000,000 + 975,000 + 950,000... + 50,000) indicates that the total value to all 40 people is $21,500,000. The person valuing the heart at $950,000 received $950,000 − $50,000 = $900,000 in consumer surplus. The person who thought the benefit to them was worth $125,000 gets a consumer surplus of $75,000. Because 40 hearts at a price of $50,000 cost a total of $2 million, these 40 people together gain consumers surplus of almost $20 million ($21,500,000 − 40 × $50,000). That indicates what a tremendous value the introduction of artificial hearts brings to this market. Note that some people (those who value the benefits near $1 million) receive much more of the consumer surplus than others, and the marginal buyer (the 40th) who values the benefits at just $50,000 and pays $50,000 for the heart gets little or no consumer surplus.

The distinction between average and marginal value is crucial to an understanding of how markets work. This case is not atypical. The top value, and even the average value, of benefits often greatly exceeds the costs and the marginal value of providing a few extra units of service. As we will see in "Chapter 3," where cost–benefit methods are discussed in more detail, the total value of modern medical care is gigantic, and average benefit (total ÷ number of people) is large. However, the additional benefit from providing treatment to a few more patients, or the incremental benefit of adding some more treatments when many are already available, is often quite small and less than the cost.

Angioplasty and Aspirin Diamonds–water pricing can be found in medical care as well. Angiography, the procedure in which a catheter (small tube) is inserted through an artery in the groin and threaded up into the heart, can be used to diagnose and treat heart disease. The procedure is difficult and expensive, costing $5,000 to $25,000. Yet angioplasty works well only some of the time, provides only a temporary cure, and must often be repeated or followed up with major surgery. Research has shown that a low-dose aspirin tablet, taken daily, prevents many heart attacks, yet the price is minimal. Because firms can produce tons of aspirin for less than 2¢ per tablet, it remains by far the cheapest way to reduce cardiac mortality.

Perceptions: A Water–Water Paradox Even water is not always priced the same. It may be available free from the tap or drinking fountains yet sell for $2 or more in a store or restaurant. It is what buyers believe they are getting—not what they actually get—that counts here. Even though some people claim that bottled water is healthier, most biological analyses show little difference between it and tap water (much bottled water comes from the same source as tap water). Yet the two kinds of water are not the same if we perceive them differently. If you think that Evian water is more pure and you value purity, you will pay extra for it.

The dominance of perception is evident when examining treatment for breast cancer. For many years, even small lesions were removed using a radical mastectomy, in which all breast tissue, underlying muscle, and surrounding lymph nodes were removed. Subsequent research showed that much less invasive surgery (a lumpectomy) was usually just as effective, and often a patient could wait to see whether any surgery at all was necessary. The fact that millions of women had painful, disfiguring, and expensive radical mastectomies does not mean that they or their doctors were irrational. At the moment they had to choose, they believed they were choosing the right treatment.[1]

Medicine always deals with uncertain outcomes. At the moment of decision, expectations are more important than results. People buy lottery tickets, go on dates, book vacations, buy stock, major in computer science, or make appointments for surgery based on what they expect to get, even though many times they will be disappointed. Similarly, the outcomes from chemotherapy, infertility treatment, and heart transplants are never certain. When the purchase decision is being made, it is the expected value, not realized value, that counts (see Chapters 3 and 4).

Ceteris Paribus

Expectation is just one of the factors that can affect demand. Income, population growth, taste (i.e., personal preferences), health status, the availability of other goods, thunderstorms, war, and a host of other factors can influence the quantity demanded even when price is held constant. Such factors, usually known as **demand shifters**, are, in turn, the subject of economic analysis. At this stage, it is necessary to limit our discussion so that the effects of price and price alone can be examined. We will make use of the notion of *ceteris paribus*, a Latin phrase that means "all other things held the same." This assumption—that all other factors besides the one under discussion are assumed to hold constant—is standard and usually unstated.

Individual, Firm, and Market Demand Curves

So far, we have been rather casual about exactly who is to be counted when constructing the demand curve. Economists define individual, firm, and market demand, with the distinction depending upon the decision being made. To determine how many times Alice Anderson will visit the doctor, we look only at Alice's behavior, her **individual demand**. To estimate the use of ambulance services in Lockport, Maine, we look only at people in the town and the surrounding area, not the entire state. To project how a change in the hospital deductible for Medicare will affect spending, it is necessary to look at the entire elderly population, some 35 million seniors. The **market demand** is the sum of all individuals in that market. The definition of "the market" depends entirely on the particular decision being made. It can correspond to a geographic area, a group of friends, or all the people who visit a particular website. If we count only how many units of service people will buy from a specific provider, then we analyze **firm demand**. At that point, however, we have moved beyond the discussion of consumer demand and on to the supply side.

2.2   THE SUPPLY CURVE

Just as market demand includes all individuals and organizations currently buying the specific good (artificial heart, aspirin, water), market supply includes all organizations that are currently selling that good or service to them. Because every unit that is bought must be sold, it is a tautological identity that quantity demanded equals quantity supplied. The market supply curve is usually upward sloping, with a higher price calling forth a higher quantity supplied. However, this might not be the case in some markets with substantial economies of scale (see Chapter 8). Whereas demand and willingness to pay depend upon the tastes and preferences of individuals and can be highly variable, the standard economic analysis of supply assumes that a firm is interested in just one thing, *profit*, and that external constraints such as the cost of inputs and the technology of production largely determine the shape and position of the supply curve.

If there were only one pharmacy in Lockport, it would be a **monopolist** (sole seller) and the demand of the market as a whole would be the same as the demand for the firm. Suppose instead that there are four pharmacies in Lockport. What demand curve is relevant to them? The pharmacies are concerned with more than individual demand, because each of them has many customers. Yet none of them fills all the prescriptions in Lockport; therefore, a pharmacy's own business is not the same as market demand. Rather, each pharmacy can sell a greater or lesser fraction of all the drugs sold in town by changing prices. Economists say that the pharmacy "faces a **firm demand** curve" of potential customers (which is some fraction of the entire market). If one pharmacy's prices are much cheaper than the others, it will get the bulk of business. Conversely, even a pharmacy charging high prices gets some business from customers who live nearby or if it is the only one open in the middle of the night.

Marginal Revenue

A firm's profits depend not on how many units are sold but on the amount of money they bring in (revenue). In deciding whether to sell more, not only does price matter, but also important is how much price must be lowered to increase sales. If a pharmacy sells two bandages at $10 each, its total revenue is $2 \times \$10 = \$20$. Suppose that to sell three bandages under the same circumstances, the pharmacy would have to lower the price to $8. At the lower price, the pharmacy's total revenue will rise to $3 \times \$8 = \$24$. The gain in total sales is just $\$24 - \$20$, or $4. This is the **marginal revenue** of the third unit of sale. One way of looking at marginal revenue is that to increase sales, the $8 received from the additional unit sold is partially offset by the $2 price reduction (from $10 to $8) of the other two units, so that the net gain is just $4.

Suppose your cousin Bob is a star plastic surgeon, doing rhinoplasties (nose reconstructions) for $10,000 each. He has bragged to you that each operation takes him only 2 hours, and that if he lost money in the stock market, he could make it up by doing more noses. Knowing how little he needs the money, you suggest he help out Aunt Martha, who has been struggling to save enough to pay for a nose job. "Give Aunt Martha a deal," you say, "Do her nose for $4,000." Bob explains the realities of business to you. "I really want to help Aunt Martha, I really do. But I can't do her nose for $4,000. That will make me look like I'm cheating all my other patients. And you know Aunt Martha—she'll have to tell everyone what a deal she got. Every other patient is going to come after me for a cut-rate price. Pretty soon, I'm just a run of the mill guy who gets $5,000 per nose job. Given my expenses, I'd be lucky to be able to keep the yacht, much less the beach house. If I have to do her a favor, I'll just do it for free." The threat to Bob's income is not the loss on one operation. It is the way that a change in price affects all units sold. Without ever having taken an economics course, Bob is focused on the information relevant to his decision: marginal revenue. It is not how much Aunt Martha pays that matters but rather how changing the price for her affects the revenues from all other patients.

It is total revenue and total cost, not the apparent "costs" and "charges" that appear on bills and accounting statements, that count. The way to maximize profits (Total Revenue minus Total Costs) is to sell additional units as long as the marginal revenue is greater than the marginal cost. Once marginal revenue is less than marginal cost, the sale is a loser, even if the price is still above cost. The concept of marginal revenue takes a while to grasp but is essential for understanding business decisions. The relevant decision is about a bit more or a bit less, and how total revenue will change as a result: a decision *at the margin*.

2.3   PRICE SENSITIVITY

The distinctive feature of the economic approach to demand is the emphasis on change itself rather than the amount. A measure is needed that focuses on movement and differences, on the sensitivity of the buying decision to an increase or decrease in price. Economists have borrowed a calculation from engineering, **elasticity**, to measure price sensitivity. A demand curve indicating that the quantity demanded will change a lot for any small change in price is said to be "price **elastic**." If the quantity demanded barely budges when the price rises, demand is said to be **inelastic**. More precisely, price elasticity is measured by the percentage change in quantity demanded for each 1 percent change in price.

$$Price\ Elasticity = \frac{\%\ Change\ in\ Quantity}{\%\ Change\ in\ Price}$$

The elasticity measure of price sensitivity can be used to investigate the similarities and differences in demand. If Alice's demand for Claritin is likely to decline by 25 percent if the price increases by 10 percent, then her elasticity is –2.5. If Alice's response is pretty much average, then even though we may be talking about thousands of prescriptions, the effect on the market as a whole will still be a 25 percent decline for a 10 percent price increase. That is, market price elasticity and average individual demand elasticity are the same, even though the total quantities are much different. This demonstrates one of the advantages of the elasticity measure: It is dimensionless. We could have measured quantity in terms of the number of pills or the number of bottles containing 50 doses for one person or for 10,000, and the percentage changes would still be the same.

What about the firm demand for Eastside Pharmacy in Lockport? Chances are, it will be more price sensitive than the individual or market demands. If Eastside Pharmacy raised prices, many customers would start buying from Central Pharmacy instead. Only if all four pharmacies in Lockport raised prices by 10 percent would it be likely that all four would experience a 25 percent decline in demand. Why is firm demand so much more price sensitive? Because the other firms in the market are good substitutes. The more substitutes available, the more price sensitive demand is.

SUBSTITUTES: ANOTHER WATER PARADOX

Why are there so few drinking fountains at sports arenas? By reducing the number of substitutes, soda vendors can increase demand and decrease the price sensitivity of consumers. Such attempts to shift demand are common in most commercial activity. At games, fans expect to pay more to eat and drink and park, and they understand that such overcharges are part of the price they pay to see their team in action. Are there analogues in the medical arena? What does this behavior suggest about the enthusiasm of pharmacists to provide information about massage, chiropractic treatment, or herbs as alternatives to a prescription for back pain?

To see how substitution affects price sensitivity, consider what would happen if there were 10 percent increases not just in the price of Claritin, but also in the prices of all allergy medications. Alice would not be so quick to cut her purchases of Claritin, because all of her alternatives had also increased in price. Considering the range of substitution provides more insight into why so much medical care is price inelastic. If I think that a particular medication is best for me, or that my doctor is the only one who can understand my headaches—that there are no good substitutes for the care she provides—I am not likely to be very sensitive to price. On the other hand, if I consider all doctors and allergy medications to be pretty much the same, I will be quite happy to switch to save a few dollars.

The change in demand due to a change in price also depends on the amount of time available to find a substitute. Acute need (heart attack, stroke) makes it impossible to shop around for the best price in medical care. However, you might have a long time to look for a surgeon to operate on your sore knee or to find a nursing home for your grandfather. With an extended time horizon, demand is more sensitive to price.

FIGURE 2.3   Effect of Reducing Price on Total Revenue: Elastic, Unitary, and Inelastic Demand

(a) Elastic Demand, Total Revenues Up, MR Positive

(b) Unit-Elastic Demand, Total Revenue Same, MR = 0

(c) Inelastic Demand, Total Revenue Down, MR Negative

The area within the dashed lines shows total revenue (Price × Quantity) at price of $10, the shaded area shows total revenues at price of $5.

Price Elasticity and Marginal Revenue

If the percentage change in price is equal to the percentage change in quantity, demand is said to be "unit elastic."[2] Such demand has a special property. If the price of drugs went up by 2 percent, causing the quantity of prescriptions filled to decline also by 2 percent, the total amount spent would remain unchanged (see Figure 2.3). Firms facing elastic demand find that revenues increase when prices are reduced to sell more units. Firms facing inelastic demand find that total revenue goes down when they reduce price to sell more units.

Most medical care is relatively insensitive to price. Pain, critical needs, fear of uncertainty, and the prevalence of insurance tend to attenuate the role of price in patients' decision making. Note what happens to a firm selling more of an inelastic good. Because increasing the quantity sold by 2 percent requires a large decline in price, perhaps 10 percent, the firm will actually lose money. For example, a firm that lowers price from $99 to $90 will see a 2 percent increase in units sold from 300 to 306, but it will find that total revenue declined from $29,700 to $27,540. If demand had been unit elastic so that quantity rose by 10 percent to 330, total revenue would have remained unchanged at $29,700. If demand were elastic, so that the 10 percent price reduction led to a 50 percent increase in quantity (from 300 to 450), then total revenue would rise from $29,700 to $40,500. Conversely, the firm that faces inelastic demand and sells fewer units will be able to raise the price by a larger percentage and will actually take in more, not less, total revenue for a smaller quantity sold. For example, if raising the price from $10 to $11 reduced sales only slightly, from 50 units to 48, the marginal revenue from raising the price and selling fewer units would be $(48 \times \$11) - (50 \times \$10) = +\$28$.

To summarize, raising prices (and reducing quantity) increases total revenue if demand is inelastic, and it decreases total revenue if demand is elastic. Because most hospitals face very inelastic demand, especially for emergency services, it follows that they are charging less than profit-maximizing prices. Why don't they charge more if it would increase profits? The reasons are many, ranging from a desire to help the poor to administrative controls over allowable changes. Also, the sensitivity to price change today is significantly less than the ultimate response to a price change in the long run (after people organize protests, build another hospital, or shift their business across town).

Some medical goods—especially those for which consumers have several choices and good information in advance of purchase, such as allergy medications—are price elastic. For these goods, firms would reduce total revenues if they raised prices. Thus, it is more likely that a medical provider facing elastic demand is behaving more like a standard profit-maximizing firm. However, price controls, informal norms about overcharging, and other deviations from perfect competition can still be significant even in the more price-sensitive medical markets.

Price Discrimination

A firm does not necessarily face the same price elasticity in each market in which it operates. Where should it try to raise prices? In the market that is least price sensitive. Consider a young radiologist, Dr. Almon, who is starting a practice in Los Angeles. He works at a posh Beverly Hills clinic on Tuesday and Thursday, seeing a few patients, and on Monday, Wednesday, and Friday he works in a crowded clinic in East L.A., seeing a multitude of patients. Initially, he charges $25 to read a routine x-ray in both places. He finds that raising prices to $35 makes little difference in Beverly Hills, but he loses half his clients in East L.A. He can increase the profits of his overall practice by raising prices in Beverly Hills to $45 and lowering prices to $20 in East L.A. He is just as busy as he was before, but he is making more money.

Charging different prices in different markets is a standard strategy used by both business and nonprofit organizations to increase revenues. The practice is known as "price discrimination." Hot dogs cost more in baseball parks, clothes cost less if you work in the store (being there gives you great information and increases price sensitivity, and you might get an employee discount), and scholarships reduce the price of a college education for students who have the most choices (athletes and scholars). Price discrimination is socially accepted and pervasive in medicine. The most common form, charging more to patients with higher incomes and/or better insurance has the advantage of appearing socially beneficial and fair. Even the federal government practices price discrimination, making higher-income states pay a higher proportion of Medicaid expenditures. It seems right to charge less to those who can afford less, but is it? Milk and bread are not sold at a discount to people with less money, so why should radiology or physical therapy be? One major reason is that any attempt to sell bread and milk cheaper would be undercut by **arbitrage** (the process of trading between high- and low-price locations eliminates difference); rich people would drive to East L.A. for low-priced groceries.

Why is there no arbitrage between Beverly Hills and East L.A. for Dr. Almon's services? Some patients will switch clinics to obtain a lower price, but only a few. Service markets are much easier to separate for purposes of price discrimination than goods markets because patients actually have to show up at the office to receive services. First, they must find out that the price differential exists, and then they must be willing to incur the extra travel costs.

The profit-maximizing price for a monopolist to charge in a market depends on the price elasticity. Dr. Almon can charge more in Beverly Hills because his patients are less price sensitive there, not because they have higher incomes, can afford more, or deserve to pay more (even though these reasons may count for something as well). He will choose to set prices in each market relative to the price-elasticity of demand among consumers there. Looking at Figure 2.3, we can see he would raise prices in (c) where demand is inelastic and reduce prices in (a) where demand is elastic. It would be a mistake to assume that rich people are always less price sensitive than poor people. For example, inner city patients often lack transportation, which makes it difficult to shop around for the best prices. Many pharmaceuticals are priced higher in low-mobility city neighborhoods than they are in suburbs, where patients can easily drive to several stores and price competition is intense.

Just as markets can be separated by distance, they can also be separated by time. All that is needed for price discrimination is that consumers not be able to arbitrage by easily transferring goods from a low-price period to a high-price period. Movies are cheaper in the afternoon because customers are more price sensitive then—and they cannot transfer the picture to view it later in the evening.[3] Dining out is often less expensive during the week than on Saturday night for the same reason. Computer makers routinely roll out the newest machines at a high price to pick up the dollars of customers who must have a new machine now, then gradually reduce prices. Many DVD and CD producers practice price discrimination over time in the same way. One interesting question is why some forms of temporal price discrimination are discouraged. For instance, it would be considered highly unethical for a doctor to charge a patient more during an emergency than for similar services on a routine visit, even though it is clear that patients are very price inelastic during a medical emergency.

The frequency with which price discrimination is practiced in medicine was one of the factors that first convinced economists that physicians had substantial monopoly power even though there are many physicians competing for patients in every city. The evidence that physicians use monopoly power to increase their incomes is well established, but it tells only a small part of the story because there is even more persuasive evidence that physicians do not behave as profit-maximizing monopolists. Charging lower prices in poor neighborhoods might help increase total revenues, but providing care for free (which many physicians routinely do) is altruistic behavior inconsistent with profit maximization. Physicians also tend not to exploit patients' willingness to pay more during medical emergencies. Even more interesting to many economists is the evidence that for much of the medical care provided in hospitals and doctors' offices every day, demand is inelastic, but prices do not rise. As demonstrated earlier, a profit-maximizing firm would keep raising prices in the face of inelastic demand until it reached an elastic portion higher up the demand curve. Demand and supply analysis can give us some insight into the economics of medicine, but it does not account for many of the features that make medicine a notable profession with a special place in human society rather than just another way to make money.

2.4   IS MONEY THE ONLY PRICE?

What does it mean to pay for something? To a politician, it might mean losing some votes or giving up a pet project. To a student going out partying on Sunday night, it might mean a headache and a lower grade on Monday's exam. To someone who wants a driver's license, it might mean hours of anxiety. In each case, something has to be given up to get something else. Economists often use the term "price" to refer to all of the things one has to give up to get some desirable good in trade. For medical care, it is common to talk about time, pain, and risk of death as part of the price of treatment. The concept of a **time price** was developed in recognition that the time spent traveling to and from the hospital, in treatment, and confined to bed in recovery has an opportunity cost. At the margin, the cost of time is roughly equivalent to the time price, and so a net price of time+money can be calculated. Pain is far more difficult to value, because there is no objective measure for it. A monk and a businessman can go through identical operations, and one has much more pain than the other. Furthermore, even if the pain were in some technical sense the same, the two patients might value it differently. Some people can function well with a level of pain that would make others miserable. For hazardous procedures such as thoracic surgery and chemotherapy, it may not be pain but the risk of death due to therapy that is the most important cost associated with treatment.

Services can be allocated to patients through time, pain, and risk just as they can through money. In Canada, where patients do not pay directly for most doctors' services, waiting times have increased. By discouraging those who are not willing to spend time waiting for care, the number of patients treated is limited just as effectively as it is when price is used to discourage those who are not willing to pay money for care. An example of allocation by pain is provided by pain clinics that insist on screening patients with an uncomfortable diagnostic procedure known as an electromyelogram (EMG). Patients who are not willing to undergo an EMG cannot obtain clinic services.

A fundamental difference between a money price and a "time price" or a "pain price" is that the money is transferred to the other party in the transaction. If an arm brace costs $10, the store receives $10. In contrast, if a patient has to wait six extra hours in the waiting room, no one receives those six hours. If an EMG is painful, a patient's willingness to undergo it might convince the therapist that the patient needs services, but the pain does not yield pleasure to the therapist. The patient's time and pain are personal costs that do not directly benefit the provider. Whereas every dollar spent on medicine by one person is income to someone else, contributing to GDP, there is no "circular flow of time" or "circular flow of pain." Economists tend to favor money prices as a rationing mechanism because they entail fewer such "dead weight" costs (waste) that provide no revenue or benefit to the supplier.

2.5 INPUTS AND PRODUCTION FUNCTIONS

The economic concept of supply is always that of a **supply curve**, emphasizing change, focusing on how firms vary the amount supplied as price increases or decreases. The supply curve also relies on the ceteris paribus assumption, implicitly holding constant many factors that are not being talked about. Just as the demand curve is a marginal benefit curve, showing how people in the market are willing to pay for one more unit of a good, under perfect competition *the supply curve is a marginal cost curve*, showing how much must be paid to induce firms in the market to supply one more unit.[4]

Production Functions

A table or formula showing exactly how much is produced with any possible combination of inputs is called a **production function**. Often the full set of relationships is so complex that only a few basic results—such as the formula below—are important in practice. Yet the concept of a production function provides a way of thinking about the economics of the situation even when quantification is imprecise and uncertain. The basic principles involved help us to analyze behavior, even if there is no money involved. Consider an athlete training for the Olympics. She must spend time both lifting weights and running in order to get in shape. If running an hour more is twice as helpful as lifting an hour more, then she will do more running and less lifting until the law of diminishing returns equalizes the rewards from each activity. If the "price" of running increases (perhaps because of an injury or because the weather gets cold) then she will optimize her workouts by shifting some time from running to lifting. Athletes, architects, financial firms and drug manufacturers all try to do their best—and doing so leads them to show the kind of behavior that economics analyzes.

Marginal Productivity

The cost of each additional unit, and thus the supply curve, is determined by the technology available to the firm, its managerial expertise, and the price of the inputs (labor, machinery, chemicals) that are used in production. A more complete discussion of supply and production is provided in any basic economics textbook, but one basic result from the theory of production should be made evident here. A firm will use more of input A and less of input B if that enables it to make the same amount of goods and services at lower cost (or to produce more for the same total cost). Thus an input that costs twice as much should be twice as productive. More precisely:

$$\frac{Price\ Input\ A}{Price\ Input\ B} = \frac{Marginal\ Productivity\ of\ A}{Marginal\ Productivity\ of\ B}$$

Why marginal productivity? Because we are analyzing the trade-off between using a bit more of A and a bit less of B, or using a bit more B and bit less A—that is, a decision at the margin. For example, producing tablets of a drug requires the use of both labor and machinery. It is not possible to run the factory without any labor, and it is barely possible to make drugs with no machinery. The company will choose the combination of labor and machinery that allows them to produce tablets at least cost. If each machine costs $150,000 and each technician costs $50,000, then the trade-off is 3:1, the incremental productivity of another machine is three times the incremental productivity of another person. One implication of the formula above is that if the price of labor increases, then the company will try to use more labor-saving machinery to cut costs. Conversely, in a low-wage country there will be lots of labor and fewer machines (or older, cheaper machinery that is less automated). Once again, we see the operation of the *law of diminishing marginal returns.*

2.6 MARKETS: THE INTERSECTION OF DEMAND AND SUPPLY

Competitive **markets** use prices to *allocate* goods and services to consumers who want them the most (in monetary terms) and to *pay* suppliers for producing those goods and services. Most real markets, and virtually all medical markets, depart to some degree from the model of perfect competition. Nevertheless, it is a useful starting point for analyzing the underlying economic forces that shape human transactions even when time, pain, uncertainty, and tradition cause substantial deviations from the simple model.

In most competitive markets with which you are familiar, supply and demand are quite distinct, and the process of organization and maximization is straightforward. The firms set whatever price they choose, and consumers decide how much to buy. Firms experiment with different prices to maximize profits, just as consumers experiment with different patterns of consumption to maximize the benefits they can obtain within their budgets. Market price is the point at which all the stresses are met and balanced. The decision rule for a profit-maximizing firm is simple. Sell more (lower your price) if the marginal revenue (MR) obtained is greater than the marginal cost (MC) of providing the goods. The firm will continue to lower price until the gains from additional sales are offset by the costs—that is, until MR = MC. In a perfectly competitive market with lots of buyers and sellers and perfect information and price transparency, the market demand curve is the same as the marginal revenue curve, and the marginal cost curve is the same as the supply curve. An increase in demand (owing to an increase in incomes, population, or the price of competing substitute services) shifts the demand curve outward, and then the market price and quantity both increase as in Figure 2.4a. A supply increase (owing to an improvement in productive technology or a reduction in input prices) shifts the supply curve outward, and then the market quantity increases while the price falls, as in Figure 2.4b.

FIGURE 2.4   Shifting Demand and Supply

Shifting Demand Curve up
(price increases, quantity increases)

Shifting Supply Curve out
(quantity increases, price falls)

(a)   (b)

| FIGURE 2.5 | Fixed Supply and Fixed Demand |

What would happen if the quantity supplied did not vary with price but were fixed? Then the supply "curve" would be a specific amount, as represented by the vertical line in Figure 2.5a. Because quantity is fixed by the vertical supply curve, only the demand curve can move, and all it can do is move price up and down. If, however, it was the quantity demanded that was fixed and not sensitive to price changes at all, then demand would be said to be "perfectly inelastic" and the demand curve would be the vertical line in Figure 2.5b. Only the supply curve could move, and all it would do is to move price up and down without changing quantity. A totally inelastic vertical demand curve seems to be an extreme case, but it corresponds rather closely to the concept of "medical need" (where treatment is determined totally by illness and prices are irrelevant). The other extreme case, a totally inelastic vertical supply curve, is fairly descriptive of the restricted entry into the profession controlled by licensure, as discussed in Chapter 7.

2.7 NEED VERSUS DEMAND

Decisions regarding who gets what medical services and when are made mostly by doctors.[5] Doctors tend to consider medical decisions in terms of **need**. This perspective frames each decision as a response to a technical question regarding the level of service required to adequately treat the illness of a particular patient. Such a need-based medical perspective focuses on differences in health status and ignores the role of prices and incomes in allocating scarce resources. To concentrate on patients' needs, physicians try not to think about who pays (employer, patient, taxpayer) and who gets paid (themselves, hospitals) so as not to be distracted by economic concerns. Their task is to operate within a given system to allocate resources and to advocate for patients. Because physicians are supposed to act in a patient's best interest, they try to behave as though prices are set anonymously by somebody else, as if the bills get paid to some agency unrelated to their personal incomes and as if insurance payments are really paid by some insurance company rather than taken out of wages.

For decisions regarding individual patients, a need-based medical perspective is suitable. Within the health care system, most physicians strive to do the best for their patients, not to change the system or help people they have never met. We do not ask doctors to determine what is best for taxpayers or employers or insurance companies, yet someone must address the question of financing. Economists are required to think about differences among systems: how choosing one set of insurance regulations means more children get immunized but fewer elderly receive home care, whereas another plan might protect accident victims, reduce taxes, or provide more incentives to work (see Chapter 17 "Economic Evaluation of Health Policy: The Patient Protection and Affordable Care Act of 2010"). The trade-offs between medical care and other goods, among different groups of patients and different types of care, are the issues that health economics is designed to address.

Although a *demand curve for medical care* is a concept that is awkward when applied to a specific individual who either is or is not sick, it is a tool that works well regarding groups of people or society as a whole. In large groups there is always a range of illnesses and a range of treatments available; therefore, the necessity for choices and balancing at the margin (i.e., an incremental adjustment of a little bit more or less) is obvious. Need and demand are different, yet complementary, perspectives on the complex set of human, financial, and scientific exchanges that constitute medicine. Done properly, the two perspectives can be combined to provide a fuller understanding of how the system works on different levels: the individual, the hospital, the company, the community, and society as a whole.

There is often an unnecessary and acrimonious division between economists and doctors in addressing medical care because the two are trying to answer different questions. For doctors, the question is: "If money is no problem, what should I do for *this patient*?" Economists, even health economists, have no particular skill at addressing such a question. They focus on a different issue: "Given that there is not enough for everyone to have all that they need, how can optimal decisions be made? Who should get treated? How should resources used for medical care vary across groups?" Doctors often think about the benefits of treatment in terms of the total or average, and economists focus on the margin: How much benefit would really come from treating a few more patients and what it would cost. It could be said that to some extent, doctors ignore economics, whereas economists ignore medicine. Bringing the science of medicine together with the structure of economics is the interdisciplinary task of health economics.

How Much is a Doctor Visit Worth?

From a microeconomic perspective, the problem with using the environment, genetics, and the state of medical technology to modify health is that there is not much that you personally can do about them: They are not objects of personal choice, and hence they are not analyzable as individual economic behavior. Even "lifestyle" is not much of a choice when the crucial medical decisions are being made. It does not really help to quit smoking, or eat more fruits and vegetables, the day after you have a heart attack or a stroke. Once an illness strikes, there is very little you can do except go to the doctor and seek treatment.

How much is that treatment worth to you? It depends, and it does not depend very much upon how healthy you are. It does depend on how rich you are, because the more money you have, the less it matters if you have to pay $5,000 for treatment. It also depends on what your options are. In 2012 your ranges of treatments, and prices, is much different than it was in 1985. If you can get free treatment through a Veterans Administration clinic, it might not be worth much to go to a private doctor. If just lying in bed and waiting will eventually allow you to get well, then it is only the time lost by being sick that makes it worthwhile to seek care. If the illness is life-threatening, treatment is worth a lot. Indeed, even if there is very little chance that some special new expensive drug will cure your cancer, you might quickly spend your life savings because it is the only chance you have. The "opportunity cost" principle is at work here. The value of medical care depends in part on what you get from treatment and on what you have to give up: what the best forgone alternative is.

The Demand for Medical Care is Derived Demand

You get medical care only if you need it, if you think that doing so will improve your health. No one buys heart surgery, chemotherapy, or x-rays just because these are fun things to have or because the hospital is having a sale. As economists, you would say that the demand for medical care is **derived demand** and depends on the usefulness of the treatment in providing health. This is the case with most goods. A cast-iron skillet is bought not for the metal, but as a utensil for cooking food. Skis are bought for skiing, not to take up space in the closet. The business of health, the actual transactions observed—doctor visits, surgery, prescriptions—are in the derived realm of medical care, they are not direct trades for health itself. If we could simply buy health—adding to life expectancy the way one picks up a three-year guarantee on a new computer—then much of what makes health economics special would simply fade away.

Intermediate microeconomic theory courses build from an abstract base that begins with the ultimate source of demand, the utility function. Indifference curves, budget lines, and production functions are used to explore the mechanics of optimization. Such an approach is necessary for extending theory. It is possible to approach health economics in this way, but to do so is to risk losing track of all the structural features and organizational details that make medicine worthy of special study.

The Demand for Health: What Makes Medical Care Different

Most markets are driven by differences in consumer tastes and preferences. People buy red or black or blue shoes in all different sizes; music by Beyonce, Bono, or Beethoven; and a great variety of books. If the price was right, you might even buy a shirt or a DVD that you were not all that sure you needed. Medical care is different. No one would get surgery unless they had suffered from progressive heart disease. Every patient may be different, but it is their illness rather than their preferences that distinguish them, and most patients with the same illness want the same medicine, not lots of variety to choose from. There is little individual variation in the "taste" for treatment (see Chapter 1, section 1.4).

When they are sick, patients expect to be cared for (which is hardly what they would expect from a visit to the mall), and they want someone to help them right now. At the moment of need, medical care is perhaps the only thing patients can buy to make themselves feel better. The other factors that determine health (genetics, lifestyle, accumulated exposure to pollutants, luck, nutritional history) cannot be purchased on demand. None of us can buy new parents. In the United States, however, most of us can buy the surgical care needed to mend and straighten a broken nose. In an emergency, we will spend a fortune on medical care that might or might not make a difference, but often we will not take the time to exercise, put down a pack of cigarettes, or buy low-dose aspirin for daily prevention. Life is the most important thing you have, and yet life-and-death decisions about yourself as a patient are largely made by a doctor, not by you. Furthermore someone else (insurance, government, charity) is usually paying the bill (see Chapters 4 and 5). These special features make medical care different enough that it is worthwhile to carefully study health economics. Although the demand for medical care is derived demand, like that for many other goods, the derivation is not so straightforward as it is for batteries or a new printer.

Hospitals and doctors are often not allowed to set their own prices but must accept prices that are set administratively by government or insurance companies. Patients buy what is needed (i.e., what providers think patients should buy), and they do not pay any price directly but rather pay some amount indirectly through taxes and premiums. The transactions are highly regulated, and some of the funding comes from grants and philanthropy rather than sales. This is so different from the model of perfect competition that legislators and actuaries want information that spells out what would happen if medical transactions were "normal." Chapter 3 provides cost–benefit and cost–effectiveness estimates that are used to derive the values that would be obtained ("shadow prices") and the decisions that would be made under regular economic principles (opportunity cost, marginalism, and so on). The practice of such methods of "economic evaluation" replicates on paper what a market would do if it existed, but with some of the rules changed: acting as if rich and poor had the same purchasing power, assuming that decisions are made in advance rather than at a time of crisis, and assuming that decisions are rationally based on medical evidence rather than on patients' expectations and fears.

2.8 DETERMINANTS OF HEALTH

The production of health is determined by many factors. A common estimate is that less than a quarter of the gain in life expectancy over the last 100 years is attributable to clinical treatment, with improvements in public health, scientific knowledge, education, income per capita, and nutrition of relatively greater importance (see Chapter 16).[6] This estimate understates the effect of medical science, because many improvements in nutrition, sanitation, and child rearing owe much to the discoveries made by doctors and physiologists. The list below is one way of categorizing the determinants of health.

- Biology, genetics
- Living conditions (economic, social)
- Health system
- Lifestyle, behavior
- Medical treatments

As living beings our biology, coded in our DNA, poses certain limits and potentials for a productive and healthy life. The environment we live in, including the ability to obtain food, shelter, clean water, work, and relationships with friends and family, is a major factor. One aspect of the broader social and physical environment is the current state of medical science and our ability to access it (Internet, hospitals, pharmacies). Given all of these conditions, there are the choices we make (diet, occupation, family, recreation) that have a cumulative impact over many years. Finally, there are specific treatments we receive that constitute medical care.

Because most people living in the United States always pay for the important types of care and because most medical care provided in the United States is pretty good, the remaining marginal choices—Branch Creek Hospital versus University Hospital, generic naproxen sodium versus brand name Aleve, doctor at the local health department clinic versus specialist in private practice—will not have a major impact on death rates, although they might have a lot to do with personal satisfaction and the quality of the experience.

2.9 EFFICIENCY

Every economy must address certain basic questions: What should it produce? How? For whom? These are never purely technical questions, but at this stage it is useful to concentrate on only partial answers, looking at the efficiency of production. Even if we assume away all conflict over values, distribution, and culture, the question of production efficiency can become very complicated. For the sake of clarity, the following discussion simplifies a complex interdependent process into a set of discrete steps (see Table 2.1).

TABLE 2.1	Efficiency: Steps in the Decision Process
Step	**Type of Efficiency**
How do we get the most out of these inputs?	*Supervisory efficiency*
What processes should be used?	*Technique efficiency*
What combination of inputs should be used?	*Cost minimization*
How much should be produced?	*Allocative efficiency (profit maximization)*
How should contracts be formed with customers and suppliers?	*Transaction efficiency*
How should production change over time?	*Dynamic efficiency*
What is best overall (externalities)?	*Social efficiency*

The first step, often forgotten, is *management*. Labor, capital, and other inputs do not produce anything unless effort is put into making them do so. If the machines or the workers are idle, if supplies are being pilfered, or if directions are not being followed, output falls. The second step concerns process: what *technology and techniques* to use. This decision depends not only on the state of knowledge at the time but also on the price of labor, capital, and other inputs, as well as on external conditions. A "just-in-time" inventory system is not very efficient for a field hospital operating in the Cambodian jungle. Given adequate management and a choice of technology, the third step is the choice of the optimal combination of inputs to produce a specified level of output at the lowest cost. In many textbooks, the first two steps are called the **production function**, and in combination with input choice, they are defined as **cost minimization**. Yet the production of output is not an end in itself.

What should that specified level of output be? The task of management is to provide benefits to customers and to satisfy salaried workers, unions, government, other interested parties, and vendors who supply inputs. Both demand- and supply-side considerations must enter into deciding how much to produce and how to distribute goods to consumers and income to producers. Jointly maximizing the total value of output is necessary to achieve *allocative efficiency*. In the abstract world of perfect competition, the optimum is identical to the profit-maximizing solution, in which marginal revenue equals marginal cost for all goods and services. In the real world, this is not always possible (see Chapter 14). We often care more about who gets care than about how much care is produced or about making it possible for the incomes of surgeons or pharmaceutical companies to rise.

Minimizing the cost of production and distributing output is not sufficient to guarantee efficiency. In health care, insurance, finance, and other complex systems, the costs of transacting and exchange are especially high and far exceed the direct costs of production. Salespeople, insurance agents, lawyers, clerks, computer programmers, and accountants are all components of *transaction costs*. Many of the chapters in this book address how an organization may be structured—through property rights, professional associations, and regulations—to economize on transaction costs and promote efficiency. Understanding *dynamic efficiency* (i.e., how to create technological and organizational change to improve economic efficiency in the future) is even more challenging. In his *History of Economic Analysis,* Joseph Schumpeter attributes growth in a mature market economy to a process of "creative destruction," yet little is known about how entrepreneurial renewal occurs, except that some current efficiency must be sacrificed.[7] A purely cost-minimizing organization is not likely to be the most creative. To make new discoveries, scientists need time to tinker undisturbed, whereas managers need free time to come up with ideas for new products and service-delivery systems. Finally, the effects of economic decisions on everything else that matters must be factored in. The externalities and social costs of cloning, antibiotic use (and overuse), the creation of bacteria that excrete gold (yes, it is possible), muscle and brain enhancements, and the extension of life beyond 200 years cannot be taken lightly.

How can an organization lower costs? Why would it want to? Do not assume that more competition and greater efficiency are always good and desired by everyone. Competition is beneficial for the system as a whole, but for any given individual, more competition means more anxiety, more work, and a higher chance of failure. Greater efficiency comes at a cost to the individuals involved. First of all, change itself is difficult and often painful. Some workers will not be able to make the transition. Those who do must be willing to try harder, spend time learning new techniques, and make mistake after mistake in order to improve the process. All of the effort required to increase efficiency is clearly beneficial to the firm and to the economy, but it is worthwhile to the worker only to the extent that he or she shares in the benefits (e.g., through higher wages, greater job security, or more time off). If workers are paid by the hour regardless of the organization's output, why should they innovate or exert themselves? Capturing the benefits of increased productivity requires managers who know what gains are possible, an awareness of the costs to all the people in the organization, and a willingness to share some of the gains with them.

SUGGESTIONS FOR FURTHER READING

Katherine Baker and Amitabh Chandra, "Aspirin, Angioplasty and Proton Beam Therapy: The Economics of Smarter Health Spending," Kansas City Federal Reserve Bank Publication (2011), download at http://www.kc.frb.org/publicat/sympos/2011/2011.BaickerandChandra.paper.pdf
Robert H. Frank, *The Economic Naturalist* (New York: Basic Books, 2008).
Paul Heyne, *The Economic Way of Thinking* (Upper Saddle River, N.J.: Prentice Hall, 2002).
Joseph Newhouse, *Pricing the Priceless* (Cambridge, Mass.: MIT Press, 2002).
Thomas Rice, *The Economics of Health Reconsidered* (Chicago: Health Administration Press, 2002).

SUMMARY

1. The **law of demand** states that a rise in prices will, ceteris paribus (all other things being constant), cause the quantity purchased to fall. It is a reflection of the most fundamental trade-off a buyer must make, recognizing that having more of one good means having less of something else.

2. The concept of **need**, a professional assessment of the quantity of services required regardless of price or other trade-offs, is appropriate for individual decision making when price, cost, budget constraint, and other monetary factors have already been decided—for example, within a fully insured system. The concept of **demand**, a functional relationship (curve) showing how quantity changes as price changes, is more useful for decisions balancing the need for medical care with other goods or allocating care among groups of people.

3. **Value** in trade is determined by supply and demand, not the inherent worth or usefulness of a medical treatment (the diamonds–water paradox).

4. The demand curve is a **marginal benefit** curve, tracing how much each additional unit of service is worth. Much of the total value of health care might lie in only a few units of service targeted to those most in need, with many subsequent services provided to a large number of people for little additional benefit. Some things that are essential to health (nutrition, exercise, preventive care) are plentiful and trade at a very low price in the market, whereas some services that make only a marginal contribution but are scarce (neurosurgery for someone who is already seriously ill) command a high price.

5. **Prices** arise from **transactions**, the actual exchange of money for service. Because most health care is funded by government or third-party insurance, there is no real price,

and therefore careful attention must be paid to the use of demand curve analysis, which assumes well-defined goods exchanged in markets that depend only on price.

6. The major **demand shifters** for most goods are income, prices of substitutes and complementary goods and services, population growth, and (the catch-all term for everything else) "taste." In medical care, **quality** and **illness status**, personal characteristics that would usually be lumped in with taste and not analyzed separately, are of greatest importance. In making a decision about value, **expectations** or perceptions, not actual results (which cannot be known in advance, or maybe ever) are what matter.

7. **Elasticities** measure the percentage change in one variable (quantity) with respect to the percentage change in another (price). Elasticities have the advantage of being dimensionless; they do not depend on units of measurement or the size of the market. Elasticity is larger the longer the **time allowed for adjustment**. The price elasticity facing a single firm that has competition from many other firms competing for the same customers is much greater than the price elasticity of the market as a whole or of any individual consumer. A monopolist may use **price discrimination**, charging higher prices for the same good to consumers in the market with less price sensitivity (New York City versus Mexico City, insured versus uninsured, midnight versus daytime) to increase total revenues.

8. Empirical estimates of the **demand for medical care** usually show that it is quite **inelastic**, in the range of 0 to 0.5. However, elasticity is greater for items that are viewed as discretionary (dentistry, counseling) and less fully covered by insurance, and it may well exceed 1.0 over the long period required to change health habits and beliefs.

9. **Marginal revenue**, the additional revenue that can be obtained by selling one more unit, is always less than average revenue (price), because a firm must reduce the price of goods to sell more. How much the price must be reduced depends on the elasticity of demand. A firm facing elastic demand that raises prices will see total revenues fall because the quantity demanded will fall by a larger percentage than the increase in price. A firm facing inelastic demand can raise prices and increase revenues because there will be only a small decrease in quantity sold.

10. The demand for medical care is **derived demand**. Even though other factors such as genetics, the environment, public health, lifestyle, and the state of technology are more important determinants of health, the only choice a patient can make at the time of need is whether or not to go to the hospital and which one. For ordinary manufactured goods, supply and demand are clearly separated, with interaction occurring only through market forces. For health care, several factors make such a separation untenable: a strong physician–patient relationship of trust, the difficulty of making choices and obtaining information about life and death matters, and pervasive uncertainty. The tools of supply and demand analysis must be used with care and sometimes must be modified to conform to the realities of the health care market.

11. **Management** is necessary to make labor and capital productive and requires **converting economic principles into rules of behavior** that can be clearly communicated to employees, bosses, clients, and other partners. Management is not simple, because people, not things, have to be managed and because **decisions** must be made under **uncertainty**, based on **expectations**, without ever really knowing all the facts one would like to have.

12. **Efficiency** of the health care system depends not only on how effectively it is producing medical services and reducing costs but also on its **dynamic** ability to generate new medical technology and on the performance of the system in meeting broader **social welfare** goals.

PROBLEMS

1. {*demand versus need*} What is the difference between Mr. Axel's demand for physical therapy and his need for physical therapy?

2. {*value, expected value*} What determines the value of a knee brace? How can an economist maintain that I am better off if I paid $7,000 for an operation that made my twisted knee worse rather than better?

3. {*elasticity*} Which are more elastic: dental visits or visits for the treatment of diabetes? Physician visits or hospital days? Psychiatry or orthopedics? Why?

4. {*elasticity*} If the price of office visits increases from $20 to $22 and the number of visits per family per year declines from 12 to 10, what is the price elasticity of demand?

5. {*measurement*} If most college students are poor, why do they spend so much on discretionary goods, such as video games? Are the ones who go on to medical school richer or poorer than the ones who take jobs right after graduation?

6. {*demand, marginal benefit*} In the year 2015, in Anytown, suppose that one person is willing to pay $1,000 for relief from hay fever; another two are willing to pay $350; about five more are willing to pay $50; one is willing to pay $40; one is willing to pay $35; one each is willing to pay $34, $32, $30, and $28; about a dozen are willing to pay $10; four are willing to pay $5; and half of the rest of the town (another 75 people) are willing to pay $1.

    a. Draw the demand curve for hay fever relief in Anytown.
    b. What is the potential total benefit from relief of hay fever if it is provided to everyone who asks? To everyone willing to pay $35 or more?
    c. If the price of hay fever medication is $20, what is the quantity demanded? What is the quantity demanded if the price is $50? $5?

7. {*demand, marginal benefit*} Suppose Betty's demand for physician visits is Quantity = $10 - (0.2 \times \text{Price})$.

    a. Draw Betty's demand curve.
    b. What is the quantity demanded at a price of $10 per visit? $25?
    c. At what price will she buy four visits? Eight visits?
    d. If the government agrees to pay half of her health care bills, what would her quantity demanded be at a price of $10 per visit? $25? Draw the new, subsidized demand curve.
    e. What is the elasticity between a price of $5 and $6 per visit? Around a price of $30? Around a quantity demanded of eight visits?
    f. Calculate the elasticity of the new, half-subsidized demand at a price of $30 per visit and compare it with the elasticity you obtained from the original demand curve. What is the new elasticity around eight visits?

8. {*substitutes and complements*} Is chemotherapy a substitute for or a complement to cancer surgery?

9. {*marginal benefit*} Provide your own example of a diamonds–water paradox in medicine, in which the clearly more valuable service is provided at a much lower price.

10. {*measurement, transactions*} In what units is Prozac purchased? What are the units in which psychotherapy is purchased?

11. {*elasticity*} If the price of a postoperative follow-up visit is reduced from $40 to $30, the number of patients returning for follow-up increases from 18 to 25.

    a. What is the marginal revenue (MR)?

    b. What is the price elasticity?

    c. What would your estimate of MR and price elasticity be if the quantity demanded moved from 18 to 20 (instead of 25)?

12. {*transactions, elasticity*} Dr. Old requires that all services be paid for at time of treatment, in cash. If he decides to allow patients to pay with credit cards, will this increase or decrease demand? Will it increase or decrease price elasticity?

13. {*elasticity, total versus marginal*} Which is more price elastic: the demand for cesarean sections or the demand for vaginal deliveries? Why?

14. {*transactions, prices*} Ask four people what they have paid for (a) a drug, (b) minor care (office visit, physical therapy session), and (c) major care (hospitalization, surgical procedure). Find out how price sensitive they think they were for each. Do they think that everyone else receiving similar care paid the same amount as they did?

15. {*elasticity, price discrimination*} Our Lady of Dollars Hospital needs to increase total revenue to build a new chapel. The hospital wants to keep the total number of patients in each service area (emergency department, obstetrics ward, operating room, laboratory, cardiac ward) the same. How can the hospital use price discrimination to achieve this objective?

16. {*efficiency*} Give an example that shows how the health care system is willing to give up some current efficiency in the production of medical services to (a) increase dynamic efficiency by providing money for research and (b) increase social welfare.

17. {*supply and demand*} Explain how current proposals to increase insurance for mental health services would affect the market for psychiatrists. Discuss short-term and long-term effects, equilibrium, and disequilibrium. Illustrate with supply and demand graphs.

18. {*demand*} If people are healthier, will their demand for medical care increase or decrease? (Be careful, this is a tricky question. Consider some analogies: If people become more coordinated, will their demand for athletic equipment rise or fall? If they become more knowledgeable, what happens to their demand for books?)

ENDNOTES

1. Barron H. Lerner, *Breast Cancer Wars* (New York: Oxford University Press, 2001); R. Rettig et al., *False Hope: Bone Marrow Transplantation for Breast Cancer* (Oxford, UK: Oxford University Press, 2007).

2. Although it is, of course, opposite in sign owing to the law of downward-sloping demand: As price goes up, quantity goes down.

3. Video rentals cost the same whether you get them in the morning (when demand is low) or in the evening, because the customer can hold on to the disc and play it when they want to. However, video stores can still practice a form of "time price discrimination." My local store allows you to return a video "late" (until noon the next day) without penalty, because almost no one wants to watch videos in the early hours.

4. This perfect correspondence holds only under many simplifying assumptions. Supply curves may deviate from marginal costs, may be flat or upward sloping as well as downward sloping, and so on. These are complexities that must be faced but that are beyond the scope of this textbook. Too much attention to technical details relying on unreal assumptions (constant technology, perfect information, no charity) tends to obfuscate rather than clarify the workings of medical markets for most readers. A useful overview of some of the issues is provided in *The Economics of Health Reconsidered* by Thomas Rice, which is listed among the suggestions for further reading.

5. John Eisenberg, *Doctor's Decisions and the Cost of Medical Care* (Ann Arbor, Mich.: Health Administration Press, 1986). Jerome Groopman, *How Doctors Think* (Boston: Houghton Mifflin, 2007). Atul Gawande, *Complications: A Surgeon's Notes on an Imperfect Science* (New York: Picador, 2002).

6. Robert Fogel, *The Escape from Hunger and Premature Death, 1700–2100: Europe, America and the Third World* (New York: Cambridge University Press, 2004). David Cutler, Angus Deaton, Adrianna Lleras-Muney, "The Determinants of Health," *Journal of Economics Perspectives* 20, no. 3 (2006): 97-120. See also the variety of sources cited in Chapter 16.

7. Joseph Schumpeter, *History of Economic Analysis* (New York: Oxford University Press, 1954).

CHAPTER **3**

COST–BENEFIT AND COST-EFFECTIVENESS ANALYSIS

QUESTIONS

1. How much is too much to spend to save someone's life? Is one life worth more than another?
2. Is the effort expended to save one more life a total, average, or marginal cost?
3. Is it more beneficial to screen high-risk or low-risk people for disease?
4. Can the statistical probability of death among teenagers be compared to ordinary mortality among the retired elderly?
5. Which are better measures of the value of care: patient choices or professional judgments?
6. Is there necessarily a trade-off between health and money?
7. Why do decisions based on the average benefit from treatment lead to too much medical care?

Every choice involves a trade-off, giving up something to get something else (see Section 1.3). **Cost–benefit analysis (CBA)** replicates on paper the balancing of pros and cons, of advantages and disadvantages, that occurs implicitly in the marketplace. In this chapter we will review basic economic principles such as total, average and marginal cost, expected value, diminishing marginal product, and maximization as applied in a health care context.

CBA is used where technical analysis is needed to supplement or replace the market for decision making. Many health care decisions are sufficiently complicated and threatening that the individual, even though otherwise competent, might have to depend on the judgment of physicians and other professionals to identify alternative treatments and determine the relative value of medical outcomes rather than depending on his or her own informed choices. Third-party financing by private insurance or government requires an explicit process such as CBA to decide what services are covered. **Cost-effectiveness analysis (CEA)** is a truncated form of CBA, fully analyzing the cost side but not translating the benefits (lives saved, illnesses prevented, a patient's additional days of activity, extent of a patient's sight restored) into dollars. CEA is used in decision making to determine which alternatives are cheaper. A study evaluating whether hypertension screening, nutrition counseling, medication, or cardiac bypass surgery would provide the most additional years of life expectancy for each dollar spent is a cost-effectiveness study. A study evaluating whether cardiac bypass surgery adds a sufficient number of years to life expectancy to justify the amount spent on care is a cost–benefit study.

3.1   COST–BENEFIT ANALYSIS IS ABOUT MAKING CHOICES

"It is best to think of the cost–benefit approach as a way of organizing thought rather than as a substitute for it."

— *Michael Drummond* [1]

Every decision—whether in the market, the public sector, or the family—involves a form of CBA. Usually the consideration of costs and benefits is informal and internal; therefore, we are not conscious of it. What economists can observe is the behavior that results from this internal weighing of costs and benefits. One study addressed the increase in traffic fatalities caused by the decision to raise speed limits on major interstate highways from 55 mph to 65 mph.[2] Raising speed limits allows cars to go faster and can reasonably be expected to cause more traffic fatalities. This study showed that higher speed limits led to slightly faster travel, about +2 mph (many people routinely exceed posted speed limits), saving approximately 45 million hours of travel time each year. However, faster travel led to more deaths—approximately 360 additional fatalities per year. Doing some simple calculations translates these findings into a cost of 125,000 hours per life. Valuing time at a wage rate of $12.80 per hour yields an estimate of the value of time gained per life lost of $1.6 million. Differences in assumptions or in the estimation procedure can lead to a higher or lower value (the range here was $940,000 to $10 million). The point of the study is that the lives lost were not the result of a mistake or bad luck—they were a choice. We, the public, decided that it is worthwhile to have more people die on the road to save travel time for the rest. While economic analysis reveals the implied dollar value of this legislative choice, it is people's behavior, not economic analysis, that puts a value on human life.

An Everyday Example: Knee Injury

Life, and the health care system in particular, confronts us with difficult choices every day. Is it worth taking three hours, and possibly paying $80, to go to the emergency department (ED) so that a doctor can examine the throbbing knee you injured playing soccer? Because pain makes it difficult to think, it can be helpful to make a list of the pros and cons, such as the one in Table 3.1.

If you believe that the benefits of going to the ED outweigh the costs, you will go to the ED. Even if you do not write down the pros and cons, a similar sort of balancing takes place inside your head. CBA is the explicit and formal presentation of that mental balance sheet. Economics does not provide answers or make it easier to take bitter medicine, but it does clarify *how to ask the questions* to make decisions more rational and more consistent. First you must *enumerate* the benefits and costs. Then you must *quantify* each benefit and cost as accurately as possible, given what is known about the situation. For example, it is impossible to tell exactly how much time you will spend in the ED, but you think a range of two to four hours is likely. You must then place a value on each benefit and cost. A balance sheet can be added up only if every line is

TABLE 3.1	Cost–Benefit Analysis of Knee Injury (First Step)
Pros (go to Emergency)	**Cons (don't go to Emergency)**
It might stop the pain.	It will cost $50, $100, or more.
It could prevent long-term injury.	It will take at least two hours, maybe four.
I will feel stupid if something was wrong and I did not go.	Even if the injury is serious, surgery could make it worse.
I can't get any work done anyway while I sit here worrying.	My friends on the team will think I am not tough.

expressed in the same terms, usually dollars. It does not make much sense to compare a benefit of $50 with a cost of ¥910 (yen), and there is no rule for determining how many hours of pain are worth avoiding a permanent limp; however, it is very clear that a cost of $500 is less than a benefit of $1,000.

This hypothetical knee injury can be used to illustrate CBA. The direct dollar cost of the ED visit is expected to be about $80, and you expect to wait for three hours. Because you could have been at a job where you were making $7 per hour, we can add $21 for the *opportunity cost* of the waiting time. (We will later consider the fact that surgery could make you worse instead of better.) Feeling that you are not as tough as other members of the team seems silly, but it is worth something. How much? Suppose that you were willing to pay $40 for crutches you really did not need, just to keep your friends from making fun of you. This $40 is your willingness to pay (WTP) to avoid a "wimp" label. Adding all the items, your estimated comprehensive total cost for going to the ED is $80 (charges) + $21 (time) + $40 (WTP fear) = $141 (see Table 3.2).

It is reasonable to assume that if your knee does not get better, you will eventually seek treatment, even if you don't go to the ED immediately. Let's suppose that before you injured your knee, you already had an appointment to go to the sports medicine clinic a week from Thursday. Therefore, the relevant costs and benefits are for treatment today versus treatment ten days from now, rather than for treatment versus no treatment. *Only count items that change as a result of your decision: the marginal benefits and costs.* The potential that an ED visit will stop the pain is counted on the list of pros and cons as a benefit. The labeling of pros and cons

| TABLE 3.2 | Knee Injury as an Example of Cost–Benefit Analysis |

Scenario: I injured my knee playing soccer this afternoon. I called and got an appointment to go to an orthopedics/sports medicine clinic in ten days, next Thursday. However, it has now begun to hurt a lot and wonder if I should go to the emergency department right away.

Pros (go to emergency now)		Cons (don't go)	
Consideration	Benefit	Consideration	Cost
Might stop the pain	$150 × 1/3 = $50 (pills stop pain with certainty, going to ED just a 1-in-3 chance)	Visit to ED will cost $50, $100, or more	Average = $80 (direct personal cost, ignores cost to insurance)
Could prevent long-term injury	$50,000 × 1/200 × .71 = $178 (WTP knee surgery $50,000, 1/200 chance, discount 7 years @ 5 percent)	I will have to wait for at least 2 hours, maybe 4	3 hours × $7 = $21 (opportunity cost)
Will feel stupid if something was wrong and I did not go	Willingness to pay = $20 ("worried well" WTP for regular office visit)	My buddies on the team will think I am a wimp	Willingness to pay = $40 (willing to pay $40 for crutches just to look good)
I can't get any work done anyway while I sit here worrying about it	6 hours × $7 = $42 (time has same $ value for benefits and costs)	Even if the injury is serious, surgery could make it worse	Sunk cost = $0 (the issue is treatment today vs. Thursday, rather than treatment vs. no treatment, so only incremental costs count)
	Total benefits: $290		**Total cost: $141**

Observed behavior just gives us a lower bound that benefits exceed costs (>$141). Another observation, that I did not go when the wait was five hours and ED charges were $250, could provide an upper bound as well (<$325).

is somewhat arbitrary, and it is equally correct to say that the potential for continued pain is a cost of not going to the ED. A reduction in cost is the same as a benefit when both are expressed in dollar terms. It is this equivalence that makes it possible to create a balance sheet for decision making. If benefits and costs are not expressed in the same terms (dollars) with opposite signs (+ or −), one cannot say which is greater.

What is it worth to stop the pain? Suppose that instead of going to the ED, you call the clinic and ask that someone phone in a prescription to the pharmacy. How much would you be **willing to pay (WTP)** to get the prescription rather than endure the pain? It is difficult to study, and may be impossible to work, when you are in pain. It is also difficult to sleep or even enjoy watching television. You might be willing to pay as much as $150 for relief from pain for the next ten days. This WTP is the correct measure of the value of benefits received. WTP is the mirror image of opportunity cost, the highest-valued opportunity forgone. Different people put different values on what it is worth to endure pain. Furthermore, your estimate of its worth to you will be imprecise, because you don't frequently make deals trading money for pain. However, let's assume that if the pills cost $200, you would not buy them. That refusal would demonstrate that the value of pain relief is less than $200 for you. The value is somewhere between the lower ($0) and upper ($200) bounds. Is pain relief worth $40, $50, or $150? There is no way to tell unless we observe your entire demand curve.

There is an overstatement of benefits here, because the pills are virtually certain to relieve pain, whereas the visit to the ED might not. Clearly a chance of reduced pain is worth less than the certainty of reduced pain, but how much less? An approximate **adjustment for risk** can be made by calculating the **expected value**. Assume that we have made enough observations to know that the average person would be willing to pay $150 for relief of knee pain. If we think there is a one-in-three chance that going to the ED now will stop the pain, the expected benefit of this one-third chance of pain reduction is one third of the $150 I would be willing to pay for certain pain reduction (i.e., $50).

The most important benefit of prompt treatment is probably a reduction in the risk of permanent injury. People are willing to pay thousands of dollars and undergo multiple operations to try to fix their knees. Although your personal valuation is the only one that is truly relevant, the values established by other people might provide a useful guide, because you have not had hundreds of opportunities to figure out how much an injury is worth. Let's say your estimate of the loss imposed by a bad knee is $50,000. This is a lot of money, but the possibility that going to the doctor this week rather than next week will make a difference is slight, maybe 0.5 percent (1 in 200). Thus, the expected value of prompt versus delayed treatment is 1/200 × $50,000, or $250. Furthermore, it is likely that if the knee does cause you a problem, it will be some years in the future. Although that is still bad, it is not as bad as being harmed today. To take into account the fact that the problem will not occur for a while, we should **time discount** the $250, using the methods provided in Section 3.6. This reduces the expected marginal benefit of prompt treatment to $178.

The fear of looking stupid for failing to seek treatment for a problem that could have been cured if treated promptly is common. Indeed, some studies have estimated that more than 70 percent of all initial visits to the doctor are made by the "worried well," people who have some vague symptom and just need evaluation and reassurance rather than treatment.[3] A modest lower bound for the value of worry reduction might be the price of a brief diagnostic office visit, or $20. What about the loss of work time owing to pain and worry? These hours should be valued the same as the waiting time in the ED, or $7 an hour (the assumed hourly wage). If you think that a prompt visit will help you avoid six hours of wasted time between now and the appointment next Thursday, the prompt visit is worth 6 × $7, or $42. The sum total of all the benefits is $50 (pain) + $178 (prevention) + $20 (worry) + $42 (time) = $290.

You go to the ED. You might not realize it, but you have done a CBA even if you never thought about the injury in these quantitative terms. Your action (going to the ED) reveals that your subjective estimate of total benefits ($290) outweighs your subjective estimate of total costs ($141). You don't find yourself being wheeled into the ED saying "I'm happy because I've got a projected consumer surplus of $149 ($290 − $141) from coming here." You just do it, or you don't. An economist considers your choice the true indicator of your personal and largely unconscious CBA. Your preferences would be revealed in more detail if we could observe you in another situation in which you chose not to go to the ED. Suppose you arrived at the ED and found that the wait would be five hours instead of three and that the clinic charge was $250 instead of $80, and you chose to leave without waiting to be seen. This would provide an analyst of your behavior with a second set of costs ($325), which in this case exceeded benefits and set an upper bound on estimated total benefits.

Stepwise Choices: Yes or No? How Much?

The initial decision, whether or not to do something, is decided by looking to see whether total benefits are likely to be greater than total costs. Given that you should seek medical care, the secondary decision then becomes "how much?" Suppose that going to a physical therapist two times per week helps to strengthen your knee, making it less painful to walk and run, and seems well worth the time and money involved. If two times a week helps enough that you feel that paying the $50 ($25 for each visit) and using three hours (45 minutes for each therapy, 45 minutes to get there and back each time) is worthwhile, the question then becomes: Would you be better off going three times a week? Perhaps going just once a week would be better? It is possible to make this secondary decision regarding "how much" by examining every possible course of action and evaluating which one gave the greatest net gains (Total benefits − Total costs). However, it is often easier to approach this decision incrementally by asking whether doing a bit more increases benefits more than it increases costs. Going three times per week might make your knee significantly better, more than enough to outweigh the incremental **marginal cost** of $25 and 1.5 hours. Marginal cost is defined as the cost (all costs, not just the money paid out) of one additional unit.

Suppose you try going four times per week, and you think maybe it feels better but not much different. In that case the marginal benefit (the incremental benefit of four visits compared to three visits) is small, less than the $25 and 1.5 hour marginal cost. Then consider going just once per week. You can save some time and money, but now you find that your knee does not seem to be healing properly, and it often hurts after walking. We can summarize the decision process as follows: Try increasing the visits a little, and if the additional (marginal) benefit is worth more than the additional (marginal) cost, keep going more and more as long as the marginal benefits exceed the marginal cost; stop at the point where marginal benefit = marginal cost. Conversely, when the increased visits result in the marginal cost being more than the marginal benefit, then you should reduce the quantity of medical care. Keep reducing as long as the marginal costs saved are greater than the marginal benefits given up; stop when marginal cost = marginal benefit.

Decision Rule:

Marginal Benefit > Marginal Cost   *Try doing more*

Marginal Benefit < Marginal Cost   *Try doing less*

Marginal Benefit = Marginal Cost   *Stop: this is the best one can do*

Notice how the additional benefits of therapy (usually) decline as more and more visits are used. This is an example of the principle of declining marginal productivity and of the first law of demand (see Chapter 2). The first visit each week is much more valuable than the second, and once a person is going twice per week, they get little benefit from a third. A fourth visit is worth almost nothing to the person—not even worth the time it takes to get to the clinic.

Therefore it is incorrect to ask what is "the" value of a physical therapy treatment, because it depends on how many the person is already receiving. Only rarely would we try to decide whether we should get "some" or "no" medical care, and that would be when the condition to be treated is considered not very serious. Most medical decisions are marginal: Should the patient get more medical care or less? The new pills or the old ones? It is important to recognize that *total*, *average*, and *marginal* costs convey different types of information for these decisions.

Calculating Marginal and Average Costs

Marginal and average cost per unit are accounting interpolations. The only definite "real" cost is "total cost." **The amount by which *total costs* increase as one additional unit of service is provided is defined as that unit's *marginal cost*.** Similarly, the amount of total costs divided by the total number of units is defined as the **average cost per unit.** (More thorough discussions of marginal, average, and total costs are found in most economics and accounting textbooks.) For any specific level of service, adding up all the bills (input costs plus fixed or sunk costs) provides an estimate of total cost for that level of production. If the quantity is increased (decreased), then total costs will increase (decrease). The *difference* in total costs (divided by the number of additional units) estimates *marginal cost* per unit at that level of production. The **amount** of total costs (divided by the total number of units) is an estimate of **average cost.** Because there are usually some costs just to have an organization (fixed or sunk cost) even when it is not producing any goods or services, and because the additional costs per unit tend to vary with the level of production, the marginal and average costs per unit only rarely are the same.

In Table 3.3, it can be seen that when the clinic has produced a quantity of 99 visits, the Total cost is $2,000. With 100 visits, the Total cost rises to $2,017, so the marginal cost of that visit is ($2,017 − $2,000)/(100 − 99) = $17. The average cost per visit of 100 visits is $2,017 ÷ 100 = $20.17 per visit. Similar calculations provide the marginal and average costs for the 101st and 102nd visits. Above that, the table provides larger leaps. To calculate the marginal cost per visit between 102 and 110 visits, the difference in cost must be divided by the 8-unit difference in units, and between 110 and 120 visits, the difference in total cost must be divided by the 10-unit difference in total units. Average cost is always calculated by the total cost divided by total quantity. Note, however, that this is only a calculation, an estimate based on total costs. There is no separate and definitive cost of the 105th visit because it depends on sunk costs, how many units were already produced, production of other services in the building, and other factors. "Costs per unit" are guidelines for making decisions based on accounting data, not elements of absolute truth.

Medical organizations tend to pose more difficulties when estimating marginal or average costs than do factories because many inputs are used in a wide variety of services and there is

TABLE 3.3	Calculating Marginal and Average Costs per Unit		
Number of Units	Total Cost (Sum of All Fixed and Variable Costs) ($)	Marginal Cost (Difference in Cost ÷ Difference in Units) ($)	Average Cost (Total Costs ÷ Total Units) ($)
99	$2,000		
100	2,017	$17.00	$20.17
101	2,034	17.00	20.14
102	2,052	18.00	20.12
110	2,200	18.50	20.00
120	2,390	19.00	19.92
130	2,600	21.00	20.00
140	2,900	30.00	20.71

no single satisfactory measure of "quantity" (Days of care? Admissions? Surgeries performed? Number of lab tests? Should the ICU be counted the same as the outpatient radiology? See Chapter 8 for more discussion).

Defining Marginal: What Is the Decision?

The term "marginal," much favored by economists, means "the change in X." The decision being made defines the margin. The change in *how much* treatment a patient receives is called the quantity margin. In the example above, quantity is measured by the number of physical therapy visits per week. It could be the number of lab tests, the number of pills taken in a week, or the number of milligrams of the drug in each pill, or whether the treatment was given by a family doctor, a specialist, a hospital, or the intensive care unit of a medical center. All represent increases where greater **quantity** of treatment costs more. The decision of *how many* patients to treat is often called the **severity** or risk margin, and is usually stated in terms of the qualifications for treatment: for example, those with blood pressure >200, between 160 and 199, between 140 and 159, between 120 and 139, or anything over 100. The looser the criteria, the more patients treated and the greater the costs. In an accident, the risk margin might be (a) all patients with open fractures and unconscious, (b) any patients with any fractures, (c) anyone bruised or hurt. For a screening program it could be (a) infants, (b) children, (c) mothers, (d) everyone else. The important point to recognize is that some patients will benefit more than others. Choices regarding *which* treatment to use (rather than "how much" or "whom") involve a change along the **quality** margin, and they are the most common and important for medical care.

Quality Margin Example: What Treatment?   Most diseases can be treated in different ways, but often the newest or most powerful treatment costs more than a commonly used treatment that is effective most of the time. Suppose that a patient is admitted with cancer, and without treatment there is only a 30 percent chance that the patient will be alive one year later (Table 3.4). With the standard drug A (generic) treatment, average one-year survival increases to 62 percent. Somewhat better results, 65 percent, are sometimes achieved with drug B, but it is still under patent and thus costs significantly more for a year's treatment: $5,500 instead of $400. There is a brand new drug C, just out, and a preliminary trial indicates that it might provide 67 percent one-year survival. The company claims, correctly, that survival is doubled and justifies a premium price of $80,000.

Using drug A provides a gain of 32 percent (from 30 percent to 62 percent), whereas for drugs B and C the gain (compared to no treatment) is 35 percent and 37 percent, respectively. The cost per year of life saved using drug A is $400 ÷ 32 percent = $1,250, an amount that no one would question is worthwhile.[4] For drug B and drug C the cost per year of life saved is

TABLE 3.4   Quality Margin Analysis: Which Treatment?

Treatment	Survival Rate	Cost ($)	Cost per Year of Life Saved ($)
None	30%	0	
Drug A	62%	400	1,250
Drug B	65%	5,500	15,714
Drug C	67%	80,000	216,216
Drug B vs. Drug A	3%	5,100	170,000
Drug C vs. Drug A	5%	79,600	1,592,000
Drug C vs. Drug B	2%	74,500	3,725,000

similarly calculated and is $15,714 and $216,216, respectively. The cost of drug C is high, but most people would agree that spending $200,000 or more to save a life is still worthwhile.

This initial analysis does not reflect the actual decision facing the doctor, which is whether to use drug C, drug B, or drug A; giving no treatment is not really an option, and thus it is not a valid basis for comparison. The doctor should compare drug C with the alternatives, as shown in the last two rows of Table 3.4. Compared to drug B, the expensive drug C provides only a 2 percent gain in survival (from 65 percent to 67 percent) at an additional cost of $74,500 (from $5,500 to $80,000), so each additional year of life saved has an estimated cost of $74,500 ÷ 0.02 = $3,725,000. To obtain such a small gain for so much expenditure might make many people hesitate and suggest that it might be worthwhile to use the extra $3 million for additional primary care or vaccinations, and stick with the less-expensive drug B or even drug A.

The benefits of drug C depend on what it is compared to. When compared to nothing at all, the cost ($80,000) seems high but not exorbitant relative to the gain (an increase in survival from 30 percent to 67 percent). By applying the concept of *opportunity cost*, the economic analyst makes a more valid comparison to the best-available alternative, drug B, and sees that the cost (an additional $74,500) is very large relative to the small potential gain (increasing survival from 65 percent to 67 percent). Comparing drug C to nothing gives the analyst average cost ($216,216 per year of life saved). The appropriate comparison is marginal (incremental), taking account of opportunity cost by comparing drug C to the best available alternative, and it shows an added cost of $3,725,000 per year of life added.

Severity Margin Example: Which Patients to Treat? How Many?   Is every patient the same? Obviously not. How should an economic evaluation account for the differences in patients? A therapy might benefit some patients a lot, whereas other patients obtain only moderate benefit and some very little. Usually it is the people who are most severely ill who stand to benefit most. Consider heart surgery and heart transplants. Treatment could be life saving for someone whose heart is very weak and about to give out. Severe angina can be a symptom of serious disease. Patients with mild angina are usually less ill. Sometimes three or four heart vessels are occluded, but those with only one-vessel occlusion do not stand to benefit as much. Malfunctions of the heart valves can cause death, but many minor valve malfunctions that do not seriously threaten one's health can be heard through a stethoscope.

Much of the work of medicine is diagnostic, trying to determine who will benefit, and how much, from a particular therapy. Imagine patients going into a hospital to receive surgery that restored their hearts to perfect health or to receive a transplanted heart that was totally healthy. The greatest benefit would accrue to those most seriously ill, the next largest benefit to those who are seriously ill but not quite as bad off, then those who are moderately ill, then to those with mild illness, and so forth. Hypothetically, let us classify patients by degree of illness and likelihood of benefit into groups called stage V, stage IV, stage III, stage II, and stage I disease. We can classify those who seem to have symptoms but on further examination are found not to have any heart disease as stage 0. Typically, there are a few patients who are very seriously ill and stand to benefit quite a lot, and there are a rather large number of patients with minor illness who stand to benefit only slightly. Table 3.5 presents the data for our hypothetical example illustrating changes in the criteria used to determine which patients receive treatment.

TABLE 3.5	Marginal Analysis: Severity (Which Patients to Treat? How Many?)						
	Stage V	Stage IV	Stage III	Stage II	Stage I	Stage 0	Cumulative Total
Gain (each person)	30	10	5	2	1	0	274
Number of Patients Coming to the Clinic	4	6	10	12	20	48	100

The "gain" is assumed to be additional years of life obtained from having a healthier heart. The most seriously ill patients (Stage V) gain a lot: 30 extra years of life. Seriously ill patients (Stage IV) gain 10 years, and ill patients (Stage III) gain half that much. Moderately ill patients (Stage II) gain just 2 years of life, and slightly ill patients (Stage I) gain 1 year. Diagnostic exams show that almost half, 48 percent, have no defects that would benefit from surgery (Stage 0). If the four patients with the most-severe illness were treated, the total gains would be 120 additional years of life (gain of 30 years each times 4). If all 100 patients were treated, the total gains would be 274 years of life, or an average of 2.74 each. Most clinics would be very happy if they could increase the lifespan of the average patient by more than 2 years, but note how much more effective the clinic would be if it did not treat the 48 people whose diagnostic workup showed no defects: The average gain for the remaining 52 patients would be 274 ÷ 52 = 5.3 years of life gained per person. The more the therapy is concentrated on those who benefit most, the greater the gains for each surgery performed. The marginal analysis shows that more than half of the total gains are obtained just by treating the two sickest groups of patients, Stage IV and Stage V.

Assuming that the clinic does what most doctors would want to do—treat first those patients who are sickest and stand to benefit most—then the total benefits obtained by treating more and more patients are displayed graphically in Figure 3.1. Because there are no additional benefits after 52 patients are treated, the total benefits line flattens out. This is what many analysts call "flat of the curve medicine": extending a useful therapy to so many patients (including those who do not need it very much or at all) that there are no additional benefits. Note that the average benefit is still large, because those few patients who really benefited a lot bring the average up even though the many patients with little or no benefit add little or nothing.

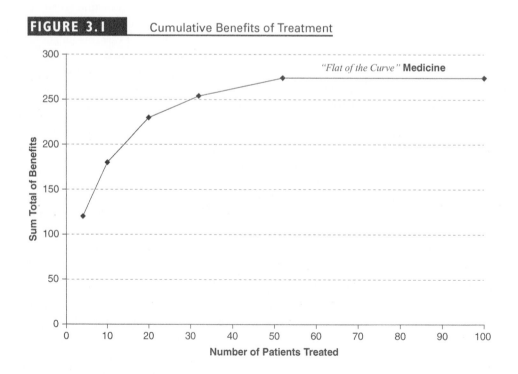

FIGURE 3.1   Cumulative Benefits of Treatment

IS IT BETTER TO LIVE NEAR A HIGH-TECH HOSPITAL?

A classic paper by Mark McClellan, Barbara McNeil, and Joseph Newhouse examined Medicare patients with acute myocardial infarction (MI).[5] This is a useful group to study because virtually all of them get admitted to the hospital and receive some treatment and thus have records that can be tabulated. The study separated the patients into two groups: those who lived close to hospitals with cardiac catheterization facilities and those who lived more than 2.5 miles from such hospitals. Many factors influence outcomes, but the major advantage to MI patients living closer to advanced hospitals is quicker treatment. Close patients were much more likely to be catheterized within 7 days and somewhat more likely within 90 days. They were also more likely to get a coronary artery bypass graft (CABG) or percutaneous transluminal coronary artery angioplasty (PCTA) within 90 days. Evaluation of outcomes showed slightly better (−1.4%) mortality at 24 hours but essentially no difference after 4 years. It is possible that rapid advanced treatment temporarily saved a few lives, but most of these patients were still seriously ill and did not fare much better over the long run.

Outcome of Treatment for MI by Distance from Hospital

	Close to Hospital	Far from Hospital
Treatment		
Catheterization within 1 day	20.7%	11.0%
Catheterization within 90 days	26.2	19.5
CABG within 90 days	8.6	6.9
PTCA within 90 days	6.4	4.3
Outcome		
Mortality within 1 day	7.5	8.9
Mortality within 30 days	24.9	26.4
Mortality within 1 year	39.8	40.5
Mortality within 2 years	47.2	47.9
Mortality within 3 years	53.1	53.6
Mortality within 4 years	58.1	58.5

Was it worthwhile to have more access to advanced catheterization treatment? One way to frame an answer is in terms of what had to be done (cost) and how much improvement (benefit) was gained. The 24-hour mortality was 1.4 percentage points less (7.5% − 8.9%), which implies that one out of every 72 (1 ÷ .014) MI patients living close to an advanced treatment hospital lived the first 24 hours who would not have done so if they had lived far away. Extrapolating from the annual mortality figures above (and assuming all of the extra days of life expectancy accrued to that one individual) that person would gain 2.55 days ([40.5% − 39.8%] × 365 days) the first year, another 2.55 days the 2nd year, 1.83 days the third year, and 1.46 days the fourth year for a total of +8.4 days. This gain of a bit more than a week comes at a cost of providing those 72 patients with an extra 4.8 catheterizations ([.262 − .195] × 72), 1.2 extra CABGs, and 1.5 extra PTCAs. Assuming that the cost of these procedures are approximately $2,500, $15,000, and $5,000, respectively, the implied extra cost is $29,250: (1.5 × $2,500) + (1.2 × $15,000) + (1.5 × $5,000). Is it worth almost $30,000 to get eight more days of life? That depends, and your answer might depend a lot on whether or not you just had an MI and how much $30,000 meant to you.

ARE SOME GOOD TREATMENTS REALLY OF NO BENEFIT?

Arthroscopic Surgery for Osteoarthritis of the Knee

Arthroscopic surgery carried out through a small incision using micro-tools is now preferred for many operations. Every Sunday in the fall we hear about a football player undergoing arthroscopic ACL surgery to fix an injured knee, or how that player is running so well just a few weeks after surgery. Osteoarthritis is perhaps the most common cause of knee pain, and it is a leading cause of disability often requiring total knee joint replacement. Because arthroscopic surgery has been so effective for injuries, and keeps many patients from requiring a joint replacement, it makes sense that similar surgery to debride and clean out the joint of osteoarthritic patients would be useful. In the year 2000, more than 650,000 such surgeries were performed at a cost of approximately $5,000 each.

Then a randomized, controlled trial at the Houston VA Hospital gave half the patients regular arthroscopic knee surgery and half placebo surgery (an incision but no actual cleaning or treatment of the knee joint) and evaluated pain and mobility over two years.[6] The patients receiving real surgery did no better than those receiving fake surgery (placebo) in terms of pain or mobility. Since then, the result has been confirmed in other studies.

Given the excellent record of arthroscopic surgery for knee injuries, it made sense to see how well it worked to help patients with osteoarthritis, but it might not have made sense to give surgery to 600,0000 people a year at a cost of $3 billion before knowing whether or not it worked. Arthroscopic surgery is not good or bad, or better or worse than medication or joint replacement, but it is much better for certain types of patients. Just as with cardiac angioplasty, treatment works well for some patients and not others, so that properly limiting treatment to those patients most likely to benefit is more important than simply treating more patients.

3.2 MAXIMIZATION: FINDING THE OPTIMUM

Economists use a powerful analytical rule to simplify decision making: **The decision between alternatives depends only on factors that change**. Therefore it is not necessary to examine the full range of possibilities but only to look at doing a little more or a little less (i.e., to consider changes at the margin) to determine whether a decision is optimal. If the marginal benefits of a therapy are greater than the marginal costs, more should be done. If marginal costs are greater than marginal benefits, less should be done.

If two alternatives share a common feature, that feature will not play a major role in determining which alternative to choose. For example, consider how many days a woman should remain in the hospital after delivering a baby. One proposal might be discharge from hospital after 24 hours ($10,000 for the delivery and $1,000 for one day in the hospital) and another proposal could be discharge after 48 hours ($10,000 for delivery and $2,000 for two days in the hospital). Both alternatives include the cost of delivery (and one day in the hospital), so their difference will cancel out the factor(s) that are the same. The extra cost of the 48-hour proposal is $1,000 ($12,000 − $11,000). The insight from economics is that it is the "extra" or "marginal" amounts that matter. Thus, the extra cost should be compared with the extra benefits.

More medical care usually makes people healthier. Physicians, rightly, concentrate on benefits as opposed to costs and often try to do as much as possible. However, people who use more resources to obtain medical care have fewer resources available for food, entertainment, housing, and other goods they want. Economics is concerned with trade-offs. What is the appropriate balance between medical care and other goods? How many doctors, nurses, and hospitals should there be? Economists insist that both costs and benefits be considered in making a decision. Economists also approach the decision differently from most physicians, asking not what is right or wrong, but whether a little more or a little less would make things better or worse. An economist uses marginal analysis to **optimize**, moving toward a maximum net benefit in small steps. To apply principles of maximization and use mathematics to estimate values, economists must abstract from other elements, ignoring some of the complexity of medical conditions and framing the issues in terms of dollars. Prices, costs, taxes, bids, contracts, and so on are the language used by economists to communicate human desires and limitations. The task of CBA is to make that language clear and applicable to the situation at hand and to present the essential facts and trade-offs in a way that is easily understood by physicians, the public, and politicians.

Declining Marginal Benefits

The **marginal benefit** is the value to consumers of one more unit of service. Willingness to pay for additional care declines as more and more is provided; therefore, the marginal benefit curve slopes downward. It looks like the demand curve; in fact, the marginal benefit curve and the demand curve are the same. To see why, remember that the demand curve is a schedule showing what quantity a consumer will buy at different prices. As long as marginal benefit exceeds the price, consumers will continue to buy. The quantity at which they have had enough and stop buying is the quantity at which the marginal benefit has fallen to the point where it is just equal to price. The quantity bought at price $P is the same as the quantity at which marginal benefit is $P; the marginal benefit (stated in dollars) of one more unit for a consumer who already has quantity Q is the same as the price they are willing to pay for one more unit.

Even though society benefits from having more medical care, the additional increment of benefit from each additional hospital day or doctor visit tends to become smaller and smaller as more services are provided. There are two reasons for declining marginal benefits. As more treatments are provided, they are given to less and less severely ill people, who are less likely to benefit. In EDs and Army field hospitals, the process of giving treatment first to those who are most likely to be helped is known as triage. Although it does not use mathematics or geometry, triage operates on the same principles as economic maximization, and both field triage and economic optimization suggest that efficiency is gained by treating first the patient most likely to benefit.

The other cause of declining marginal benefits is that for any single person, the benefit from having additional units of medical service tends to decline as more and more services are used, just as the benefit from consuming additional pizzas or sodas or pretzels per day tends to decline as the second, third, and fourth are consumed. In Figure 3.2 (top), the fact that more medical care will improve health is shown by the rise in the total benefit curve. The fact that marginal benefits become smaller as more and more services are used shows up as a lower rate of increase, reducing the slope to make it flatter.

Optimization: Maximum Net Benefits

Costs are the other side of the decision. Every additional unit of treatment adds to total costs. After start-up, the marginal cost of producing another unit of medical treatment is usually constant or rising as the total number of treatments increases. Each additional hospital bed tends to cost as much as or more than the last one, and each additional nurse who is hired expects to get paid as much as or more than the last one hired. At some point, the additional costs of extra treatments outweigh the additional benefits. An optimum is where the net gain (benefits minus costs) is largest. This can be found diagrammatically by plotting both benefits and costs on the horizontal axis and choosing the point where the distance between them is greatest (Figure 3.2, top), or equivalently by plotting net gains on the horizontal axis and choosing the quantity of care where it peaks (Figure 3.2, middle), or finally by plotting the marginal benefit and marginal cost curves and choosing the point where they cross (Figure 3.2, bottom).

FIGURE 3.2　　　Total, Net, and Marginal Benefits and Costs

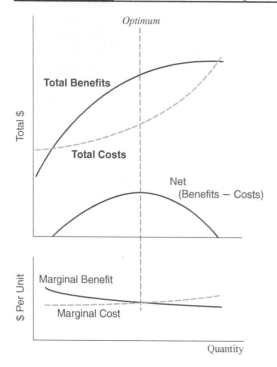

A geometric property in Figure 3.2 is used by economists to determine the point at which a maximum is reached: The "peak" of the net gains curve comes as it turns from going up to going down, where the slope is "0," i.e., horizontal (Figure 3.2, middle). The total benefit and total cost curves (Figure 3.2, top) have a corresponding property: at the point where net gains are maximized, their slopes are equal; therefore, the difference in the slopes is 0. More generally, because "net gains" are defined as (benefits − costs) and $slope_{net\ gains} = slope_{benefits} − slope_{costs}$, therefore at the maximum, $slope_{net\ gains} = 0$. These principles of maximization common to geometry and calculus can be stated in everyday terms. As any curve or function approaches a peak, the incremental increases become smaller and smaller. The maximum occurs at the turning point, where the curve goes from rising (positive) to falling (negative). Equivalently, one can state that to the left of the turning point, marginal gains are positive, and to the right of the turning point, marginal gains are negative. Here at the turning point, as the optimum is reached, the marginal gains from adding a bit more or a bit less are 0. Finally, considering the optimum as the maximum distance between two curves (Net Benefit), the focus is on the incremental or marginal change of one curve relative to another. If the additional (marginal) benefit from providing one more treatment is larger than the additional (marginal) cost of providing one more treatment, then providing more treatments will make society better off (Figure 3.2, bottom). If the additional benefit from providing one more treatment is smaller than the additional cost, providing more treatments will make society worse off. At the optimum, the additional benefit will just offset the marginal cost; therefore, there is no change in net gains (marginal gain = 0).

Maximum net gains at　Marginal Benefit = Marginal Cost　*so that*　MB − MC = 0

Expected Value

The general principle is to make a decision in which benefits (B) are greater than costs (C), or B > C. Suppose, however, that benefits or costs are uncertain. Five hundred grams of Xloxidine might cure you or leave you in the same condition. Surgery might cause you to miss one or five weeks of work. A choice must be made, based on the best possible information or the best guess, long before the outcome of treatment is revealed. The estimate of what is likely to happen is called the **expected value**, a core concept of risk analysis. If the analysis concerns many people, in which case the law of large numbers applies, the expected value is just the average.[7] For a single person facing an event that either will or will not happen, the expected value is the value of that event (benefit or cost) multiplied by the fraction of the time that the event will occur:

$$\text{Expected Value of } \mathbf{Z} = (\text{Probability that } \mathbf{Z} \text{ will occur}) \times (\text{Value of } \mathbf{Z})$$

A patient receiving chemotherapy with a 70 percent chance of death might live, while a patient receiving surgery with a 20 percent chance of death might not. Yet the decision must be made in advance and should maximize expected welfare in the face of this uncertainty. Of course, after the fact, the patient's family might wish that they had done something differently. To say that the optimal choice sometimes turns out worse is simply to recognize that life is full of risks. CBA is based on the best available estimate of probability. It may be a guess or, preferably, an extrapolation from well-designed studies reported in scientific journals to which the analyst refers. "I don't know," or "I need more information," are not valid responses, because a decision is going to be made regardless of how much is known. The job of the analyst is to get the best estimate and indicate the sources of information and the range of variability. A clear discussion of the alternatives in specific terms is required. Under this useful shorthand formula, an option is chosen if

$$(\textit{Probability of Gain}) \times (\text{Benefit}) > (\textit{Probability of Loss}) \times (\text{Cost})$$

In this formula, attention is focused separately on the uncertainty and the relative values that interact in the decision-making process. Judgmental advice, such as "it is better to get the operation and risk dying than not get the operation and remain impaired" jumbles probabilities and values together, hiding information and making communication more difficult. Such commingled statements do not make the patient think about how much it is worth to live impaired compared with dying or make the patient consider specifically the percentage probability of partial recovery or death. An explicit recognition of benefits, costs, and risks provides a better ground for shared decision making between physician and patient.

For situations involving many people and events with more than one outcome, the expected value is a weighted average of all possibilities. The calculation must be summed (Σ) across all categories of people and all possible outcomes to arrive at the expected value for the group as a whole:

$$\text{Expected Value} = \frac{\sum (\text{Number of people for whom } \mathbf{Z}_i \text{ occurs}) \times (\text{Value of } \mathbf{Z}_i)}{\text{Total number of people}}$$

The study of how heart attack outcomes varied in the box example (Is It Better to Live Near a High-Tech Hospital?) above illustrates an alternative form of this calculation: The expected value of the gain is +8.3 days, and the expected cost is $29,250. Of course, this still leaves the task of estimating the value of those extra days of life.

3.3   THE VALUE OF LIFE

"A man who knows the price of everything and the value of nothing."
                                    — *Oscar Wilde's definition of a cynic*

Isn't health priceless? Some patients and physicians protest that it is impossible to measure the value of an extra day of life or the priceless benefits of medical care with the crude yardstick of money. Regardless of whether people think it is right or proper, their actions place a dollar value on human life when they make a decision to provide or deny treatment. If an 87-year-old patient in heart failure is transferred from a nursing home to a cardiac care unit for 10 days, the physician affirms through this action that the potential gain in lifespan is worth more than the $25,000 cost of the hospital admission. Immediately discharging this patient with instructions to give him four aspirin every six hours affirms the physician's belief that it is not. Our actions place a dollar value on life even if we do not choose to recognize this fact. We live in a world of scarce resources and must make decisions within these limitations. We place a value on (and a limit on the value of) health whether we wish to or not, with money as a generalized expression of this value.[8] Perhaps the most important role of economists in the CBA of health care is pointing out this reality.

Valuing human life places special but unavoidable demands on economists. For activities that are traded in the market, such as medical care, work time, drugs, and transportation, valuation may be complicated by risk and discounting or blurred by overhead allocation and wage differentials. Nevertheless, the process of connecting resources and program effects to specific dollar amounts is understandable and familiar. Considerations of life and death or pain and suffering are not so clear. Because there is no explicit market for postoperative pain and mortality, a way must be found to reflect the value that people place on these events. By choosing to buy a car that is cheaper but less safe, a person is making an implicit trade between money and the risk of dying. That trade-off is also made when buying smoke detectors, choosing to accept a more dangerous job assignment for higher pay, refusing to fill a prescription because it costs too much, and flying to the Mayo Clinic to get the best possible treatment for a rare disease. People buy and sell health all the time, but they do not do so in an organized market like the New York Stock Exchange. **Economists do not put a value on life or illness; they measure the value that consumers put on life and illness as shown by their behavior.**

One attempt to provide an explicit dollar value for life is described by Michael Jones-Lee.[9] It was observed that people would run across a highway (at a small but noticeable risk of dying) rather than spend the time going around to a pedestrian overpass. Through observations and questionnaires, it was established that people were willing to accept a risk of 0.000002 of death to save seven minutes (0.117 hours) of walking. Valuing their time by an average wage rate of $20, the value of life as can be extrapolated as follows:

Value of Life: Jones-Lee Approach

$$\text{Value of Life} = \frac{(\text{Value of Time}) \times (\text{Hours used})}{(\text{Risk of death per hour saved})} = \frac{\$20 \times 0.117}{0.000002} = \$1,170,000$$

A more sophisticated approach is to consider the value of life as the additional wages required to get someone to take a more dangerous job. A statistical regression[10] of the association between wages and risk showed that for each 0.0001 increase in risk of death, there was an additional $240 in annual salary; therefore, the estimated value of life measured by the method used in this study was $240 ÷ 0.0001 = $2.4 million. Other studies using similar methods have estimated values of life from $800,000 to $6 million.[11] One problem with occupational risk estimates is selection bias: The people who are less risk-averse or who mistakenly underestimate the true risk are the ones most likely to apply for the more dangerous jobs. A study that captures the behavior of the more safety-conscious individuals was conducted by Rachel Dardis, a researcher who measured the number of people purchasing smoke detectors as a function of price.[12] From these data she constructed a demand curve (Figure 3.3). In 1974, the price of a smoke detector was $52, and only 1.8 million were sold (adjusted for inflation, $52 in 1974 is worth $198 in 2010, with an annualized operating cost per household of $27 in 2010 dollars). By 1979, the price had declined to $12, and 10 million were sold (which is $31, inflation adjusted,

FIGURE 3.3   Value of Life: Smoke Detector Study

Changes in the number of smoke detectors purchased as prices fell from $150 in 1974 to $24 in 1979 are interpreted as a derived demand for life saving, implying a "value of life" demand that exceeds $2,000,000 for early purchasers, and $305,000 for late purchasers.

Source: Rachel Dardis, *American Economic Review* 70 (1980): 1077–1082.

and yields an annualized cost of $4 a year). Each smoke detector was estimated to result in a 0.000036 reduction in the risk of death and a 0.000023 reduction in the risk of injury. Using these probabilities, Dardis estimated that those who purchased smoke detectors when they first came on the market at $198 made decisions consistent with a value of life of $2 million; those who waited until prices dropped to $30 implied a lower value of life—less than $400,000. This smoke detector study brings home the relevance of the first law of demand: even for life itself, people will buy more as the price decreases.

We must all die sometime; therefore no medical treatment can truly save a life forever. A problem with efforts to estimate the value of life is that the rhetoric itself reinforces denial, making it seem as if the purpose of medical care is to save lives. The real task of medicine is to reduce suffering and anxiety while extending the expected length of life by a few years. Glorified language can thwart clear thought and practical action. It can provide a convenient way to avoid admitting in public that the life of an eight-year-old child is valued more than the life of an 80-year-old grandparent. Such avoidance does not make the difference in valuation any less true. Economists use the decisions made by state legislatures, families, and patients to show that they value the length and quality of life, which can be changed by medical care, rather than the fact of mortality, which cannot.

3.4 QUALITY-ADJUSTED LIFE YEARS (QALYs)   *British   health care*
System

The extra dollar cost of providing one additional year of life expectancy has become a standard method for evaluating many health programs. Yet a year spent sick and in pain is worth less than a year lived in perfect health, free of symptoms. It is important to account for both quality and length of life when assessing the outcomes of new medical treatments. A significant risk of surgical mortality may be worth accepting to treat a disease and alleviate pain—but how much risk? Researchers use econometrics, surveys, and professional judgments to estimate the value of a year spent in different states of disability.[13] Such **quality-adjusted life years (QALYs)** rate quality of life between 0.0 (death) and 1.0 (good health). In the survey results presented in Table 3.6, respondents indicated that living for three months confined to a hospital for tuberculosis treatment was worth only 1.8 months (0.60 × 3 months) of regular time spent at home in

TABLE 3.6	Quality of Life Adjustment Factors	
Duration	**Health State**	**Adjustment**
	Perfect Health	1.00
3 months	Home confinement, tuberculosis	.68
3 months	Home confinement, contagious disease	.65
3 months	Hospital dialysis	.62
3 months	Hospital confinement, tuberculosis	.60
3 months	Hospital confinement, contagious disease	.56
3 months	Depression	.44
3 months	Home dialysis	.65
8 years	Mastectomy for injury	.63
8 years	Kidney transplant	.58
8 years	Hospital dialysis	.56
8 years	Mastectomy for breast cancer	.48
8 years	Hospital confinement, contagious disease	.33
Life	Home dialysis	.40
Life	Hospital dialysis	.32
Life	Hospital confinement, contagious disease	.16
	Reference State: Dead	.00

Source: D. L. Sackett and G. W. Torrance, "The Utility of Different Health States as Perceived by the General Public," *Journal of Chronic Diseases* 31, no. 11 (1978): 697–704.

good health.[14] The value of living in the hospital declines further when it is not temporary but permanent. Living 10 more years confined in a hospital being treated for a contagious disease was considered to be worth only 1.6 years of normal life. Although such conditions were not included in this survey, people consider some illnesses to be worse than death; therefore, each additional year lived in such misery could be counted as having negative value.

Discounting Over Time

The value of a dollar obtained 15 years from now is worth less than a dollar today. The value of potential increases in life expectancy 15 years from now is worth less than the same increase in the probability of living today. The *present value* of an additional year of life obtained 15 years from now is calculated by discounting over time, just like the present value of a dollar obtained 15 years from now is calculated. If the rate of discount (interest rate) is 5 percent, the present value of receiving a dollar next year is $1 \div (1.05) = \$0.952$, and the present value of receiving a dollar in 15 years is $1 \div (1.05)^{15} = \$0.481$. Analogously, the 5 percent discounted value of an additional year of life 15 years from now is about half the current value (see the further discussion of discounting and present value in Chapter 12).

QALY League Tables

The costs of medical care can be compared with benefits by calculating the cost per adjusted year of life gained. On the benefit side, each additional life year is discounted for risk (expected value), time, and quality of life. On the cost side, adjustments are made for any differences between charges and actual costs, expected reductions in days lost from work, and reductions in the cost of medical care for related conditions. Consider the hypothetical example in Table 3.7. The patient can expect to live three years with medications alone but will live five

TABLE 3.7			QALY Calculation: Hypothetical Example			
	Year 1	Year 2	Year 3	Year 4	Year 5	TOTAL Adjusted Life Expectancy
Time discounting factor	*1.00*	*.952*	*.907*	*.864*	*.823*	
Medication only *(baseline)*						
Quality of life	.60	.50	.40	(dead)	dead)	
Discounted value of QALY	.60	.48	.36	.00	.00	**1.44** years
100% of Medication Cases have quality-adjusted life expectancy of 1.44 years.						
Surgery						
3% **a) Surgical Mortality**						0.00 years
57% **b) Surgery not effective, but patient lives** *(QALYs same as baseline)*						1.44 years
40% **c) Surgery Successful**	.90	.80	.70	.60	.50	
discounted value of QALY	.90	.76	.63	.52	.41	3.23 years
Expected value with surgery	(probability weighted sum of a, b, c) =					**2.11** years
	$(.03 \times 0.00 + .57 \times 1.44 + .40 \times 3.23)$					
Gain in discounted QALYs with surgery			2.11 years − 1.44 years = **0.67 years**			
Cost per QALY gained			$30,000 / 0.67 = **$45,000**			

years, with a better quality of life, if the surgery is successful. However, the is effective only 40 percent of the time, it costs $30,000, and there is a 3 percent chance of immediate death from the surgery (surgical mortality). The estimated cost per QALY gained is $45,000. Similar estimates have been made for a number of medical interventions so that relative costs can be calculated and presented in QALY league tables, such as Table 3.8.[15] From these results, it can be seen that it costs more than seven times as much ($14,000 versus $1,900) to increase QALYs by one year with a heart transplant as it does with a pacemaker implant. Trying to extend and improve life by using coronary artery bypass grafting to treat minor two-vessel disease with mild angina is still more expensive, $35,000 per QALY gained.

QALY rankings can be used to assess which medical treatments should be expanded and which should be cut back to optimize system efficiency. When the state of Oregon decided in 1993 to enroll more poor residents in its Medicaid program, funding those extra people by eliminating coverage of medical services deemed to be of lowest benefit, legislators used a decision-making process analogous to the construction of a QALY league table.

TABLE 3.8	QALY League Table
Treatment	Present Value of Extra Cost per QALY ($)
Physician advice for smoking cessation	450
Pacemaker implantation for heart block	1,900
Hip replacement	2,000
CABG for severe angina LMD	2,800
Control of total serum cholesterol	4,600
CABG for severe angina 2VD	6,200
Kidney transplant	8,200
Breast cancer screening	9,500
Heart transplant	14,000
CABG for mild angina 2VD	35,000
Hospital hemodialysis	38,000

CABG, coronary artery bypass graft; LMD, left main disease; 2VD, two-vessel disease.
Source: A. Williams, "Economics of Coronary Artery Bypass Grafting," *British Medical Journal* 291, no. 6491 (1985): 326–329.

3.5   PERSPECTIVES: PATIENT, PROVIDER, PAYER, GOVERNMENT, SOCIETY

Costs (how much has to be paid for treatment) and benefits (how much the treatment is worth) depend on whose perspective the cost–benefit analyst is taking. From the individual's point of view, treatment that makes an infectious disease less communicable is of no direct benefit, and medical costs may be relatively unimportant because he or she has insurance. From a group perspective, reducing communicability to neighbors is a major benefit of treatment, and hospital charges are important because total insurance premiums for the group as a whole will rise. The broadest perspective is that of society as a whole, including future generations.

Many of the conflicts over health policy arise from the difference in perspectives of different groups. For gay men, research and prevention of AIDS may be the most important health issue of our time, whereas finding drugs to assist in stroke rehabilitation is not.[16] For women who are older than 65 and have hypertension, these priorities may be reversed. An economist hired by Medicare to do a CBA on whether a new type of surgery should be covered must ask, "Am I to consider primarily the effects on the Medicare budget, or should I also include benefits to hospitals, doctors, and state legislatures?" The treatment of taxes and transfers is crucial in this regard. If new Medicare regulations cost Medicare $100 but reduce state Medicaid expenditures by $40, is that reduction to be counted? From the state's perspective, it is a windfall gain of $40. From the perspective of the U.S. budget and the Medicare administrator, it is a cost of $100. From a social perspective, the shifting of costs from state to federal budgets is irrelevant, and the cost is the net amount, $60. Consider also the effect of taxes. If a 10 percent tax on health care raises the price of a visit to the doctor from $20 to $22, the extra $2 is a relevant cost to the patient or the insurance plan but not to society. If there were no "health taxes," that $2 would have to be obtained elsewhere by raising other taxes or by reducing government spending, perhaps on roads or defense.

Distribution: Whose Costs and Whose Benefits?

People tend to think first about the benefits and costs to themselves as individuals and then about the costs to the groups (teenagers, steelworkers, residents of Lancaster, Hispanics, senior citizens) to which they belong, rather than everyone else. A major barrier to actually implementing a project is raised by the following question: What about the losers? Laser surgery for cancer might help thousands of people who would not have survived with the chemotherapy previously used, but it will kill some people who would have lived. Development of a new home health system means that the hospital down the street will find even more of its beds empty and will have to lay off some employees. It is almost impossible to make a major change that hurts no one, and it is difficult for a politician to vote for a project that clearly hurts some identifiable person. Yet to objectively analyze "public" policy, an economist must take everyone into account, adopting the perspective of society as a whole.

Although apparently straightforward in principle, the admonition to treat everyone's costs and benefits alike can be problematic in practice. Should the heart attack of a investment banker count for much more than that of a farmworker because the banker has a greater willingness to pay for recovery and relief of pain? Should the lives of women lost in a flood count for less than men's because women's earnings are lower on average, or for more, because women's expected lifespan is longer? If a schoolbus for disabled children crashes, is that less costly than a regular bus crash because when disabled children die, the high cost of special medical care they would have needed in the future is avoided? If I am being paid by General Motors to study costs and benefits, why should they care about the health of the unemployed or the uninsured? Most analysts attempt to implement a social perspective by treating all persons "fairly," ignoring differences in sex, race, age, income, and occupation as they count costs and benefits. A good analysis points out how the distribution of costs and benefits is likely to affect the politics of a program and how the costs to be counted vary as different perspectives are considered.

CBA and Public Policy Decision Making

Cost–benefit analysis is a way of looking at past behavior, at decisions actually made, so that future decisions can become more clear, rational, and consistent. A decision being made by a single person was used in the knee injury example. In practice, CBAs are almost never done for a single case because it takes too long, costs too much, and depends on statistical assumptions that are more valid for large groups. Where a single person is concerned, that person knows his or her personal costs and willingness to pay better than any analyst. Formal analyses are apt to be most useful under the following circumstances:

- Large amounts of resources (millions or billions of dollars) are involved.
- Responsibility for decisions is fragmented (government agencies, large corporations).
- The goals and objectives of different groups are at odds or unclear.
- Alternative courses of action are radically different.
- The technology and risks underlying each alternative are well understood.
- A long time frame is involved (e.g., strategy versus management).

Econometrics, balance sheets, surveys, decision trees, and other tools of the economics trade are usually applied to large projects and long-standing problems. For example, is screening blood donors for HIV and hepatitis worthwhile? How often should they be screened, and with what tests? Is inpatient alcohol treatment better than outpatient treatment and, if so, is it enough to justify the increase in costs? The treatment of millions of people costing billions of dollars over many years is involved in these issues, each of which has been given full formal CBA. It might seem that so many questions and complications are brought out that the decision just becomes more confusing. That is because the real world is complex and full of unresolved questions. Even when analysis cannot deal with all of them perfectly, it can help to make decisions more informed and consistent. The test of what is important ultimately lies in the judgment of those who are most affected. Health CBA almost always counts two things, death and money, because they are routinely recorded. A good analysis is able to capture other factors that are significant and yet keep the presentation simple enough that the costs and benefits of alternative courses of action are clearly seen.

CBA Is a Limited Perspective

Although CBA is a powerful tool for policy analysis, it can be quite limited. It is difficult to do a useful economic analysis unless the medical facts are well known. How many people have the disease, what is the cure rate from therapy, and what levels of disability are likely to result? These clinical questions must be answered before any assessment of costs and benefits is attempted. The strength of CBA as a tool lies in its ability to interpret medical issues as choices in a market. Yet to do so, it must force health and human caring into such a rigid economic model that it tends to overemphasize efficiency and can entirely fail to recognize the most important ethical and social values that underlie medical practice. Medicine as a profession rests on the dignity and sanctity of life, a philosophy and practice that resists overt commercialization.

A social perspective must take all of these factors into account, including the way that the costs of an illness, which are often too great for any single individual to bear, are to be paid for and shared across a larger group. Risk pooling and insurance payment are the subject for the next two chapters.

SUGGESTIONS FOR FURTHER READING

Amitabh Chandra, Anupam Jena, Jonathan Skinner. "The Pragmatist's Guide to Comparative Effectiveness Research." NBER working Paper #16990, 2011.

David M. Cutler and Mark McClellan, "Is Technological Change in Medicine Worth It?" *Health Affairs* 20, no. 5 (2001): 11–29.

Michael F. Drummond, Mark J. Sculpher, George W. Torrance, Bernie J. O'Brien, and Greg L. Stoddart, *Methods for the Economic Evaluation of Health Programmes* (Oxford, U.K.: Oxford University Press, 2005).

Victor Fuchs, *Who Shall Live?* (New York: Basic Books, 1974).

Marthe Gold, JE Siegel, LB Russell, M Weinstein, *Cost Effectiveness in Health and Medicine* (Oxford, U.K.: Oxford University Press, 1995).

Mark McClellan, Barbara McNeil, and Joseph Newhouse, "Does More Intensive Treatment of Acute Myocardial Infarction in the Elderly Reduce Mortality?" *Journal of the American Medical Association* 272, no. 11 (1994): 859–866.

Martin I. Meltzer, "Introduction to Health Economics for Physicians," *Lancet* 358, no. 9286 (2001): 993–998.

M. A. Testa and D. C. Simonson, "Assessment of Quality of Life Outcomes," *New England Journal of Medicine* 334, no. 13 (1996): 835–840.

SUMMARY

1. **Every act is a judgment about value.** When people act, they show by that act that they think the gains are worth more than the costs. Economists look at decisions that patients and physicians have made in the past to estimate the value they place on health outcomes.

2. **Cost–benefit analysis (CBA)** does not make decisions. It is a **framework** that can be used to make the decision-making process more rational, more consistent, and more clearly communicated. The cost–benefit analyst organizes the facts provided by clinicians and the public's values to present data in a way that is useful for making policy decisions. Although some form of cost–benefit trade-off occurs in virtually all decisions made by consumers, a formal CBA is used only for large-scale government or corporate projects with a long time frame and many parties involved in the decision-making process.

3. **Cost-effectiveness analysis (CEA)** compares the cost of two different methods of reaching the same goal (immunizing 100 children, preventing 10 cases of flu, adding one extra year of life) but does not attempt to measure the benefits in dollars.

4. The appropriate measure of costs is the **opportunity cost** (i.e., what is given up). The appropriate measure of benefits is **willingness to pay (WTP)**, what the patient or society is willing to give up to attain an improvement in health.

5. In choosing between alternatives, it is the change in benefits **(marginal benefits)** and the change in costs **(marginal costs)** that matter, not the average value.

6. **Marginalism** is the process of trying out small adjustments and moving always in the direction of adjustments that make things better until no further improvements are possible. With marginalism, we do not need to know whether a decision is good or bad, only whether it makes things better or worse. If a manager keeps choosing in a way that makes things better, eventually the organization will reach the best possible decision (i.e., its **optimum**). Economists have found that to evaluate an organization they need not look at everything, but rather need only to examine the organization's **behavior at the margin** to determine whether it can do better.

7. The primary **benefits** to be accounted for in health care projects are as follows:

    a.   Health (extend life or reduce morbidity and pain)

b. Productivity (decrease time lost from work)

c. Reductions in future medical costs

8. Following are the major categories of **costs** to be accounted for:

a. Medical care and administration

b. Follow-up and treatment damages (side effects)

c. Time and pain of patient and family

d. Provider time and inconvenience

9. Because marginal benefits are usually declining and lower than the average benefits as health programs increase in size, it is important to **target treatment toward those most in need**. Many useful medical technologies become wasteful when they are expanded to include low-risk individuals.

10. Benefits are rarely certain. The **expected value** of a medical treatment is the product of the likelihood of success multiplied by the magnitude of the health gain that will occur if treatment is successful. A useful shorthand for dealing with risk is to examine whether:

Probability of Gain × Benefit > *Probability of Loss* × Cost

11. Years of life must be discounted if the quality of life is reduced. Questionnaires are used to estimate how many years of life a person with a disability would be willing to give up to gain one additional year of life without the disability or to reduce the risk of death. In this way, **comparisons can be made between treatment alternatives in terms of quality-adjusted life years (QALYs)**. Because an additional year of life expectancy in the distant future is worth less than an increase in health now, it is also necessary to use an interest rate to discount benefits over time.

12. Comparing medical therapies in standardized units, such as cost per QALY gained, can help decision makers determine which programs should be expanded and which should be cut back, and thus leads to better public policy.

PROBLEMS

1. {*expected value*}

a. Successful rehabilitation of a shoulder injury obviates the need for reconstructive surgery costing $6,000. However, rehabilitation is successful only 70 percent of the time. What is the expected value of rehabilitation?

b. Treatment for endocarditis is risky. The patient will either die in the hospital, partially recover, or fully recover. With full recovery, the patient can expect to live for another 20 years, but only 25 percent of patients fully recover. With partial recovery, the patient can expect to live 10 more years. However, 20 percent of patients die in the hospital. Assuming that patients usually live just one year without treatment, what is the expected value of the treatment expressed as additional years of life?

2. **a.** {*marginal cost*} A course of chemotherapy costs $8,000. If given to patient A, it will increase life expectancy by two months; for patient B, by six months; for patient C, by one month; for patient D, by five months; and for patient E, by four months. If all five patients are treated, what is the average cost per year of life gained? If only one patient can be treated, which one should it be? If only two patients are treated, which ones should they be? What is the marginal cost per additional year of life for the patient most likely to benefit? What is the marginal cost per additional year of

life for the patient least likely to benefit? Draw the total and marginal benefit curves (label the *y*-axis "Years of life gained" and the *x*-axis "Number of patients treated"). If all five patients are treated, what is the average cost per year of life gained? The marginal cost? If patients are treated in alphabetical order, which one determines the marginal cost per year of life gained: patient A, patient E, or some other patient?

b. {*demand curve*} Assuming that each additional year of life is worth $60,000, draw the demand curve for chemotherapy. Draw the supply curve. What is the relationship between the demand curve and the total and marginal benefit curves you drew in part A of this question?

3. {*marginal cost, quality dimension*} Those who suffer from allergies can take medicine to relieve their suffering. Without treatment, they will have 118 bad days per year. Generic drug G costs $76 for an annual prescription, whereas brand name drug B costs $680. With drug G, most people suffer only 42 days of allergy symptoms, whereas drug B seems a bit better, usually reducing symptomatic days to just 38. What is the average cost per day of symptom relief with drug G? With drug B? What is the marginal cost per additional day of relief if a patient is switched from drug G to drug B?

4. {*direct versus indirect costs*} A school district determines that less than 70 percent of first-grade students have completed all recommended immunizations. A task force suggests two ways to reach the goal of 95 percent immunization: (1) hire 20 visiting nurses to do outreach in the community or (2) pass a law mandating that children will not be allowed to attend school unless they bring documentation showing evidence of complete immunization. How is the distribution of costs and benefits different under the two plans? Which plan is more cost-effective?

5. {*need versus demand, opportunity cost*} Many experts recommend that people get at least 30 minutes of vigorous exercise three to five times a week; however, is actual participation in exercise less than the amount (a) needed or (b) demanded? Why do most college students get more exercise in summer than in winter? Does need, demand, or a difference in the opportunity cost of time account for the fact that most actors get more exercise than most accountants?

6. {*marginal, optimal*} The World Health Organization (WHO) is considering sending in a team of experts to deal with an outbreak of schistosomiasis in a distant country. Sending a larger team will allow WHO to prevent more fatalities, and they estimate the following effectiveness:

Number of Team Members	Number of Deaths
0 (i.e., no action)	1,200
5	500
10	200
15	100
20	60
25	40
30	30
35	25
40	22
45	20
50	20

a. It costs $5,000 for each team member sent. Calculate the *total*, *average*, and *marginal* cost of life saving through this effort and display it on a graph. If saving a life is valued at $100,000, what is the optimal number of people WHO should send to combat the epidemic? If saving a life is valued at $10,000, what is the optimal number? What team size gives the most "bang for the buck" (i.e., the largest number of lives saved per dollar spent)?

    b.   Each person sent must be taken away from a disease-fighting team at work elsewhere in the world. What is the appropriate opportunity cost measure of sending people to fight the new epidemic: the transportation cost of $5,000 or the reduction of life-saving efforts from the job they are pulled away from?

7.   {*willingness to pay*} What determines the value of a cure for acne? For ALS (amyotrophic lateral sclerosis, or Lou Gehrig's disease)? For Alzheimer's disease? Which discovery is worth more to a pharmaceutical firm that is able to patent a cure?

8.   {*QALYs*} Patient BN is a 36-year-old woman with a type of organ failure that reduces her quality of life to half of what it would be in good health. Without treatment she can expect to live only two years. With a successful transplant, BN can expect to live four years and have a quality of life that is near (80 percent) what she would enjoy in good health. However, the transplant costs $100,000, plus $10,000 each year for drugs and follow-up care, and it carries a 15 percent risk of rejection resulting in immediate death. What is the cost per additional year of life gained (without discounting for time or quality of life)? What is the cost per discounted QALY gained (assuming a 5 percent time discount rate)?

9.   {*interest rates and future value*} As a health economist for the CDC (U.S. Centers for Disease Control and Prevention), you have been asked to analyze a number of programs targeting different diseases and recommend which should receive priority, given that budgets are limited. As part of your analysis, you will have to determine what interest rate is appropriate for discounting future costs and benefits. You are going to be visited by an economist from AARP (formerly the American Association of Retired Persons) and another economist from the Children's Defense Fund. Which group will lobby harder for a lower discount rate? Why?

10.   {*incidence*} Should a new, expensive ($250,000+ per year) cancer drug be covered by insurance or not? Who might argue for covering the drug? Who might argue against coverage? What effect would the usefulness of this drug have? What effect would the quantity of patients who potentially would use this drug have? What role could the economic analysis play?

ENDNOTES

1. Michael Drummond, *Principles of Economic Appraisal in Health Care* (Cambridge: Oxford University Press, 1981), 17. Several sources and texts are listed at the end of this chapter as suggestions for further reading. Good current examples of cost–benefit analysis and reviews of the literature can be found in journals such as *Health Economics, American Journal of Public Health, Medical Decision Making, New England Journal of Medicine,* and *Journal of the American Medical Association.*
2. Orley Ashenfelter and Michael Greenstone, "Using Mandated Speed Limits to Measure the Value of a Statistical Life," *Journal of Political Economy* 112, no. 1 (2004): 226–267.
3. S. R. Garfield et al., "Evaluation of an Ambulatory Medical Care Delivery System," *New England Journal of Medicine* 294, no. 8 (1976): 426–431. P. J. Wagner and J. E. Hendrich, "Physician Views on Frequent Medical Use: Patient Beliefs and Demographic and Diagnostic Correlates," *Journal of Family Practice* 36, no. 4 (1993): 417–422.
4. The usual threshold for the value of adding one year of life is now usually considered to be somewhere in the range of $100,000 to $250,000, and certainly not less than $50,000.
5. Mark McClellan, Barbara McNeil, and Joseph Newhouse, "Does More Intensive Treatment of Acute Myocardial Infarction in the Elderly Reduce Mortality?" *Journal of the American Medical Association* 272, no. 11 (1994): 859–866.
6. JB Moseley et. al. "A Controlled Trial of Arthroscopic Surgery for Osteoarthritis of the Knee." *New England Journal of Medicine* 347, no. 2 (2002): 81–88.

7. The "law of large numbers" says that the observed average will be close to the "true" mean if the number of observations is large enough.

8. A decision maker's preferences are said to be "lexicographic" when everything depends on one factor, with other factors allowed to affect choice only when they are equal to the primary factor. For example, a parent might say to a physician, "Do whatever you can to minimize my child's chance of dying. Given that, if one treatment is less painful, or costs less, you can do that one." This decision is lexicographic because one factor, the probability of the child's survival, dominates all others. In such a case, there are no trade-offs and hence no necessity to make an economic analysis such as a CBA. Computers sort alphabetical lists lexicographically: by the first letter, then by the second, and so on. People often claim that one thing is important above all others (survival, honor, religious purity) even though most behavior indicates that trade-offs are made. Even saints respond to pain, and parents are not acting nobly if they do everything to try to save one child and in the process harm their other children and their own lives. Arguing that medical decisions should only be based on costs when there is no chance that doing so will affect quality or risk lives is the same as saying that money does not matter in the real world.

9. Michael W. Jones-Lee, *The Economics of Safety and Physical Risk* (Oxford: Blackwell, 1989), 67, based on data and extrapolations from S. J. Melinek, "A Method of Evaluating Human Life for Economic Purposes," *Accident Analysis and Prevention* 6, no. 2 (1974): 103–114.

10. Regression analysis is covered in virtually all standard statistics textbooks. There is also a short description provided in S. Folland, A. Goodman, and M. Stano, *The Economics of Health and Health Care* (Upper Saddle River, N.J.: Prentice Hall, 2001), 59–67.

11. M. Moore and W. Kip Viscusi, "Quality Adjusted Value of Life," *Economic Inquiry* 26, no. 3 (1998): 369–388.

12. Rachel Dardis, "The Value of a Life: New Evidence from the Marketplace," *American Economic Review* 70 (1980): 1077–1082.

13. M. E. Backhouse, R. J. Backhouse, and S. A. Edley, "Economic Evaluation Bibliography," *Health Economics* 1(Supplement): 1–236, 1992; John Hutton and Alan Maynard, "A NICE Challenge for Health Economics," *Health Economics* 9, no. 2 (2000): 89–94.

14. D. L. Sackett and D. W. Torrance, "The Utility of Different Health States as Perceived by the General Public," *Journal of Chronic Diseases* 31, no. 11 (1978): 697–704.

15. Alan Williams, "Economics of Coronary Artery Bypass Grafting," *British Medical Journal* 291, no. 6491 (1985): 326–329. Julia Fox-Rushby, Anne Mills, and Damian Walker, "Setting Health Priorities: The Development of Cost-Effectiveness League Tables," *Bulletin of the World Health Organization* 79, no. 7 (2001): 679–680, Tammy O. Tengs et al., "Five Hundred Life-Saving Interventions and Their Cost-Effectiveness," *Risk Analysis* 15, no. 3 (1995): 369–390.

16. T. R. Fanning et al., "The Epidemiology of AIDS in the New York and California Medicaid Programs," *Journal of Acquired Immune Deficiency Syndromes* 4, no. 10 (1991): 1025–1035.

CHAPTER 4

HEALTH INSURANCE: FINANCING MEDICAL CARE

QUESTIONS

1. Who pays for losses: insurance companies or the people who buy insurance?
2. What is an "actuarially fair" premium?
3. Does pooling of funds reduce losses or reduce variance?
4. Do insurance companies take risks, or do they just put a price on risks?
5. Who takes care of people when they need medical care they cannot afford?
6. Is a favor from a friend similar to a loan from a bank?
7. Are people who think they will become sick more likely to obtain insurance?
8. Are people with insurance more likely to sustain a financial loss?
9. Does company health insurance make people work more hours or fewer?
10. Does insurance increase or decrease the demand for medical care?

There are a dizzying array of risks that could disrupt your life: breaking an arm, catching pneumonia, having a heart attack. We hope none of these bad things will happen, but if they do, most of us can rely on insurance to cover some of our financial losses. From society's point of view, insurance is a method of pooling risk so that one person's loss is shared across many people rather than being borne by that person alone. If all people contribute, the pool of collected funds will be sufficient to compensate the unlucky few. All participants gain peace of mind, knowing that they can obtain necessary medical care with limited financial risk. From an individual perspective, insurance generates net benefits by allowing trade between two possible states of the world: in order to have plenty of money to pay medical bills in one state (when a person is sick), a little money in the usual state (when a person is healthy) is given up. Chapters 4 and 5 examine the operations, history, and theory of health insurance. To grasp how insurance works, it is necessary to understand that it is a means both for individual maximization of utility and for social promotion of group values such as respect for life, care of people with disabilities, equal opportunity, and political unity.

4.1 METHODS FOR COVERING RISKS

What would you do if you broke your arm? Who would take care of you? How would you eat and pay your rent while you were out of work? Who would pay for the doctor and hospital care? There are several ways this loss could be covered.

Savings

One consequence of a loss is that savings are used to pay for extra expenses. *Savings* can be thought of as a trade between time periods. People do not save to pile up money. They save so that they can consume more in the future, either because they plan to do so (e.g., for retirement or a vacation) or to protect themselves against the unexpected (e.g., accident, illness). Savings provide a buffer against random losses, smoothing out consumption over time so that you can still eat if you are not working, still pay the rent if you incur a $600 doctor bill immediately after your vacation, and still pay tuition bills if you need expensive prescription drugs to get you through your final exams. The ability to smooth out the amount of consumption over time improves utility. The difference between a planned variation (a vacation trip) and a risk (a broken leg) is the element of uncertainty. Saving is limited as a risk management tool because it allows individuals only to trade with themselves at different time periods; it does not spread a catastrophic loss over a large group of people so that it can be borne more easily. Although people can plan a vacation or retirement within their budgets, they might face an extraordinary loss (e.g., spinal injury, cranial fracture) that is far too expensive to be handled by their own resources.

Family and Friends

Young people who have not had a chance to accumulate their own savings must depend on their families' financial resources to carry them during an illness. Although family assistance may be freely and generously given, it creates an obligation to pay your family back when you are well, to be grateful, and to help other family members in the future when they need it. Thus, the family engages in a form of exchange among people as well as among time periods.[1] Your current loss is covered by someone else's current savings, which gives you an obligation to cover someone else's loss in the future. Whereas individual savings allow one person to trade among his or her own time periods to optimize consumption, families trade over time and over people; therefore, they can absorb the shock of a loss without a disastrous decline in living standards more effectively than an individual alone.

Favors that friends do for each other occur so often and unconsciously that it seems strange to look at them as trades. When I carry books for someone whose leg is in a cast or take notes for a classmate who has the flu, I am simply being nice and not looking to receive anything in return. Yet ultimately, families and friendship are based on a sense of mutual obligation and reciprocity. If someone consistently fails to help me, eventually I will stop being helpful to him or her. Furthermore, I might let others know how inconsiderate and selfish that person is so that they won't waste their time assisting him or her. It is by such means that the informal rules of exchange among friends and families are enforced. Helping out might not be legally binding, but it is socially binding.

Charity

The obligation to help extends beyond friends and family to people we have never met, whom we might never meet, and who can do nothing for us in return. We still care about people as human beings even if we don't know them. Mutual caring makes people a society rather than just a random collection of individuals.[2] The first hospitals were caring institutions, substitute homes for people who did not have a home and for people who were ill or had a disability but whose families were too poor to take care of them.[3] Charity as a means of social exchange predates formal insurance contracts by thousands of years and was far more important as a way to pay medical bills until the 20th century. Yet charity is limited in scope, and the extent to which most people feel responsible for someone else's misfortune has declined as formal market institutions have arisen to provide coverage for risks.

Private Market Insurance Contracts

Bad things happen. We cannot always do something about them. When we can do something, it often costs a great deal of money. Suppose that I am one of 100 middle-aged executives sent by XXumma Corp. to Eastern Europe for a year. We can assume that several of us will get sick during the year. Suppose we knew that one of us was going to have a heart attack. An operation could help, a coronary artery bypass graft (CABG, pronounced "cabbage"), but this operation, with all its attendant aftercare, costs about $50,000. The person who has the heart attack will suffer financially as well as physically. A way of making a bad situation a little better is for us to form a club. Each person puts in $500 and the unlucky one who has a heart attack gets the operation paid for. This is known as **risk pooling**, and it is the essential feature of all insurance.

Although no one can predict who will be the unlucky one, for large numbers of people, the **risk**—the variance and expected value of all losses averaged over all people—is quite predictable. From the individual perspective, insurance is a trade between two possible states of the universe: one in which the person has a heart attack and one in which he or she does not. Money is shifted from the state in which individuals have more (when they are healthy) to the state in which they have less (when they are sick), similar to the way saving shifts money from good periods to pay for the bad periods. From a societal point of view, insurance is a collection of trades between people. Money is shifted from people who have regular earnings (those who are healthy) to people who suffer losses (those who are sick).

Insurance pools losses; it does not get rid of the losses or even reduce them. The group members must pay for all losses (plus some administrative fees or "load") with the **premiums** they pay. Insurance companies do not like to take risks. They like to sell insurance to large groups of people with predictable (average) losses. This way the insurer's revenues and expenses, and therefore its profits, are very stable and predictable from year to year. Insurance companies specialize in pricing risks, not in taking risks. They try to predict exactly how large premiums need to be to cover all the predicted losses. This specialty, known as actuarial science, uses information on previous losses to make accurate predictions of the amount of money required to pay for future benefits. For this example, the probability (one in one hundred) and size ($50,000) of the loss is well known, so it is simple to determine the **actuarially fair premium**, $1/100 \times \$50,000 = \$500$. An actuarially fair premium is the same as the *expected value of a loss* discussed in Chapter 3 with regard to cost–benefit analysis.

Insurance must be priced above the actuarially fair premium to cover the expenses of administering the insurance plan, to provide a cushion for contingencies, and to provide profit to the owners who put up their expertise and capital. The difference between the actual premium and the actuarially fair premium is known as the **loading factor**. It may be as small as 5 percent or 10 percent for group policies covering large businesses and can exceed 60 percent for individual policies.

Traditional health insurance plans simply paid for all (or a defined part) of the medical bills a person incurred. Such **indemnity** plans have become rare. People want insurance companies to bargain for lower prices with hospitals and physicians, to evaluate whether new variations on an old drug are really worth twice as much, and to process all paperwork. **Managed-care** plans provide a package of services at a cost lower than people could obtain if they tried to do it all on their own (see Chapter 5).

Social Insurance

Market contracts are mutually beneficial to people who purchase insurance and to the companies that act as financial intermediaries. However, they do nothing for people who cannot afford to buy insurance or for people excluded from purchasing insurance (e.g., people with disabilities). Market contracts do not pay for medical research or education programs to promote healthy lifestyles, nor do they provide outreach to teenage mothers or people with mental illness. In short, they do nothing to strengthen the social contract that binds the people of a nation together in support of each other. The informal obligations of citizens to society expressed in charitable giving are extended and formalized in social insurance programs such as Medicare and Social Security in the United States, the National Health Service in the United Kingdom, universal Medicare in Canada, and the health care systems of most countries.[4] Contributions to social insurance are not voluntary but are mandatory through the tax system. Who will pay and who will receive are determined by concerns common to all and by the political process rather than through individual choices made in the marketplace.

WHY DO POLICE OFFICERS AND FIREFIGHTERS HAVE SUCH COMPREHENSIVE INSURANCE?

Medical coverage for those who put their lives on the line for the good of the community remains comprehensive even though many employers and government agencies are cutting back on benefits. There is a symbolic importance to this insurance that goes beyond financial considerations. If the community is not willing to do everything possible to protect the health of these public servants, why should these servants continue to risk it all to save lives? Similar considerations lie behind the willingness of an Army troop to go to great lengths to recover a wounded or dead comrade when such efforts don't seem to be worthwhile from a cost–benefit perspective and also have led to the creation of a $50 billion system to care for disabled veterans.

As explained in Chapter 1, the U.S. health care system is a blend of private and public financing. Medicare, a social insurance program that covers medical bills for most elderly people in the United States, is larger than the many private for-profit companies combined. Even when insurance is privately paid and managed by profit-making firms, government regulations mandate who is covered, what services are offered, and how prices are set. Therefore, even private insurance is forced into some conformity with social insurance principles.

Strengths and Weaknesses of Different Forms of Risk Spreading

Individual savings are quite limited as a form of risk management because the resources of only one person are used. There is no way that a person born with a genetic defect can save money to cover that risk. Most young people cannot save the $20,000 or so required to treat a broken leg, and a serious illness would exceed the financial capabilities of all but the wealthiest individuals. Trades involving more than one person are needed for coverage. Taking money from family and friends spreads the risk more widely, but this larger group might have difficulty telling whether you really need assistance. In addition, if family and friends do contribute toward your medical bills, they might also want to give you lots of unwelcome advice and intrude in your personal affairs. Charity brings in an even broader group, but the sick person has less incentive to minimize waste, because he or she is spending other people's money. Charity also tends to be unreliable and even more meddlesome. The extent of resources available is limited by how much people care, and charity alone could never fund a modern medical system.

Markets create impersonal contracts to pay for services. They can draw on financial resources from around the world. Your insurance may be handled by a company in the Netherlands that neither knows nor cares about you as a person but fully meets your needs as long as the doctor bills get paid on time. Yet markets are driven by profits, not love, and each participant must pay his or her own way. Nothing will be done for a child with a genetic defect unless a parent has a policy that includes dependents. A lawyer's interpretation of a contract replaces family concerns as the factor determining which kind of medical care will be provided. The

TABLE 4.1	Types of Risk Protection	
Method	**Reduces Effects of Loss By**	**Depends On**
Savings	Shifting consumption between periods	How much I personally have now
Family, friends, charity	Sharing between people	How much people care about me
Insurance contract	Trading between possible states of the world through financial markets	Ability to price risk
Social insurance	Pooling risks for all of the people	Political consensus

movement from individual to group to market financing reveals a trade-off: The individual is most sensitive to his or her own needs but has the smallest span for risk pooling (savings, trade over time periods). The market is global in reach but is impersonal and is willing to help only when there is a profit to be made (see Table 4.1).

Social insurance combines the humanitarian thrust of charity with the financial strengths of the market, but it provides only a compromise, not a reconciliation. Social insurance can be comprehensive only if contributions are made compulsory through taxes. As the financing base is broadened to include more people, social insurance grows ever more divorced from personal empathy and becomes a government service provided through the political process. As taxpayers, we are willing to provide some medical care for everyone, but not necessarily the best quality in the best rooms of the most modern hospitals. In addition, some taxpayers may be downright hostile about spending millions of dollars on patients who, for example, spent their money on entertainment rather than medical care or who have worsened their own illnesses through substance abuse or unhealthy lifestyles. Social insurance requires that society reach a consensus on who deserves what and how medical care should be delivered. Such a consensus currently exists in the United States only for the elderly under Medicare, and even that can fall apart, as it did in 1989 when revisions to cover pharmaceuticals and catastrophic expenses were passed, implemented, and then repealed by Congress after a revolt by older taxpayers.[5]

4.2   INSURANCE: THIRD-PARTY PAYMENT

As medical care became more expensive, the potential cost of illness went from burdensome to overwhelming. In 1929, $200 was an unusually large medical bill. In today's high-tech intensive care units (ICUs), hospital costs of $100,000 or more are common, with extra payments needed to cover surgery, anesthesia, laboratory tests, and drugs. Few individuals can afford to pay the high cost of advanced modern treatment for serious illness, but few are willing to forgo treatment if they become seriously ill. Insurance makes it possible for most people to obtain care when they need it without going bankrupt. Regular withholding of premiums and taxes spreads the financial risk across many people and makes catastrophic expenses bearable.

Why Third-Party Payment?

Insurance would not be necessary if everyone's medical expenses were near the average. Instead, there is a great deal of variation—much more than there is for food, housing, clothing, transportation, and other major expenses. Most people are healthy during any given year, so that more than half of them have minimal costs (less than $600) for medical care (see Table 4.2 and Figure 4.1).[6] However, each person in the top 1 percent had medical expenses around $200,000, and the average for the top 10 percent of the population, which includes most people that needed hospitalization during the year, was more than $50,000. Most people find that their actual costs for the year are much lower than the premiums for any reasonable health insurance policy, and 90 percent are well below average (i.e., less than $8,936). Yet who can

TABLE 4.2   The Concentration of Personal Health Expenditures

	All	Top 1%	Top Next 9%	Upper-Middle 40%	Bottom 50%
Persons (millions)	316	3	29	126	158
Health cost (millions)	$2,823,900	$595,843	$1,192,251	$945,442	$90,365
Per person	$ 8,936	$188,559	$ 41,922	$ 7,480	$ 572

afford the risk that they will be among the one in ten that requires significant medical care and end up paying $50,000 or more?

Although each of us would prefer to pay nothing, most of us can afford to pay for at least some of the cost of the care we expect to receive if we get sick. Even if we are healthy, it is reasonable to be asked to contribute something toward the expenses of those who are not—but how much? A $200,000 bill could be staggeringly difficult to pay. We might not even think that we can afford $8,936, which is the average annual cost of medical care per person. However, whether we wish to pay that much or not, an average of $8,936 per person must be extracted through taxes, bills paid by individuals, insurance premiums paid by employers (who must therefore reduce wages), or some other means, such as charitable giving, to keep the system running. These funds are needed to keep hospitals open; pay doctors, nurses, custodians, and clerks; keep research laboratories researching; and so forth.

Most of us are not aware of the financial burden we bear for health care provided to ourselves and others. For most workers, employers pay about $2.50 an hour (8 percent of total wage and benefit compensation) for health benefits, reducing the amount that can be paid out as wages.[7] Even if an employer does not provide health insurance, something is deducted each week as taxes, which is often labeled "H.I." or "FICA:M." This is hospital insurance, not for the employee but for the elderly and people with disabilities on Medicare. Every time we buy a candy bar or a gallon of gasoline, we pay state taxes that fund Medicaid for indigent people. On the other hand, senior citizens might complain bitterly about the cost of drugs and hospitals

FIGURE 4.1   Distribution of Individual Medical Care Expenditures

Note: The 1 percent of individuals with highest cost consume over 20 percent of total services, and the top 5 percent consume about 50 percent.

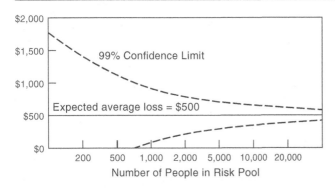

FIGURE 4.2   Variability Declines as the Size of the Risk-Sharing
Pool Increases

and nursing homes, with little awareness of how much subsidy they are receiving. Even if senior citizens pay thousands of dollars out of pocket, more than 90 percent of hospital bills, half of nursing home bills, and almost one third of the costs of their drugs are being borne by other people, mostly younger working people.

Variability

The chance that an insured group will have extraordinarily high or low losses declines sharply as the number of people in the group increases. Figure 4.2 shows how risk declines with the size of the risk-bearing pool. It assumes that each person in the group has a one in one hundred chance of sustaining a $50,000 loss. The expected loss ($500 per person) is the same regardless of the number of people insured. With just 10 people insured, it is virtually impossible for the loss to be equal to the expected loss of $500. With 100 people in the risk pool, it is possible (37 percent of the time, assuming a standard normal probability distribution) that one of them will get sick, thereby making the loss equal to the expected value of $500. Just as often (37 percent of the time), however, no one will get sick and losses will be 0. About 18 percent of the time two people in the group will get sick, making the average loss $1,000, and 8 percent of the time three or more people in the group will become ill. With 1,000 people in the group, it is unlikely (0.005 percent) that no one will have an illness. Most (99 percent) of the time the average loss will be between $100 and $900 per person. These are known as 99 percent confidence intervals, which are represented in Figure 4.2 by the dashed lines that start far from the mean and gradually move closer as the number of people in the group increases. With 10,000 people in the risk-pooling group, the chances of no one getting sick are vanishingly small, as are the chances that the average loss will exceed $1,000. The group will experience losses between $370 and $630 per person 99 percent of the time. An insurance company is quite confident doing business with a group this large. On the other hand, a company with fewer than 25 insureds has a sizable chance of losses that are more than double the expected value (about 22 percent of the time).

Third-Party Transactions

Insurance modifies the nature of economic exchange by redirecting the flow of money. It changes who negotiates prices, who bears responsibility for mistakes, and who has the right to profit from directing business to one hospital instead of another. The standard market model with one group (consumers) determining demand and a different group (firms) determining supply is left behind when we enter the medical world with patients (who receive care but do not

FIGURE 4.3   Third-Party Contracting

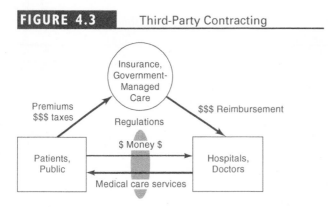

directly pay for it), insurance companies (who neither supply nor consume, but pool risk and profit from handling funds), and providers (who are reimbursed by a *third party*, insurance, on behalf of a group of patients rather than being paid directly (Figure 4.3 and Section 6.4 "The Medical Transaction").

What does each of the three parties in an insurance contracting network gain? *Patients* gain by pooling risks to eliminate financial uncertainty and to make expensive treatments affordable. Perhaps even more important, they gain peace of mind, not having to haggle over prices or worry about cost when a loved one is sick. *Insurance companies* benefit from profits. Even when the underwriting gains (the difference between premiums paid in and benefits paid out plus administrative costs) are negative, an apparent loss, companies might still make money because they hold the premiums for 6 to 24 months before paying out benefits. At 8 percent, the interest on $1 million dollars in premiums for two years is $(1.08) \times (1.08) \times (\$1,000,000) - (\$1,000,000) = \$166,400$, which is not a bad profit for a firm that some reports might claim made no money since benefit payouts exceeded premium revenues. In addition, insurance companies usually get higher returns on investments than individuals do because insurers are so large, with better opportunities and specialized investment staffs. Insurance companies are regulated and taxed as large financial investment institutions, with underwriting gains and losses treated as secondary. This does not mean that underwriting and risk selection are not important, only that expected investment returns are already built into the price of the premium.

Providers gain from an increase in demand and regularity of payment. When patients are covered by insurance, they are more apt to come in for care and less likely to argue about price. Traditionally, patients have expected doctors and hospitals to be more lenient than landlords and bankers about late payment, and many medical bills went unpaid or were paid only in part. Falling demand and irregular payment during the Great Depression in the 1930s forced many hospitals to close as a result of bankruptcy and led to the start-up of the nonprofit Blue Cross plans as a method of insuring patients so that provider revenues could continue.[8] Like all great ideas, insurance had to benefit all parties so that all parties would enthusiastically cooperate.

Benefits from Exchange

Patients	Insurers	Providers
Risk pooling	Cash flow	Increased demand
Purchasing	Profits	Ensured payment

Who Pays? How Much?

There is a popular misconception that when insurance pays for something, it is free. Unfortunately, although we might not realize who pays because third-party transactions are indirect, every dollar spent on medical care is paid by you, by me, or by someone just like us. Insurance companies and the government never really "pay" for anything. For the most part, individuals pay for medical care by paying higher taxes and/or taking home lower wages. Even the tax advantage for employee benefits does not mean that we are able to get something for nothing. (There are no free lunches!) The government still has to pay its bills. If fewer dollars are collected through wage taxes, more dollars must be collected through gasoline taxes, property taxes, income taxes, Social Security taxes, or other taxes to make up the difference. When a hospital provides "free" care to someone as charity, it must raise charges to those who are insured (and the few who cover their bills out of their own pockets) to pay for it. Insurance does not reduce the cost of medical care; rather, it redistributes costs so that different people end up paying.

Under third-party payment systems, the connection between what the first party (the patient) pays and what the second party (the provider) receives is indirect at best. The "charges billed" for a visit to the emergency department often bear little resemblance to what you have to pay or what the hospital receives. In health economics, one must give up the familiar realm of simple two-party transactions in which "bought" and "sold" happen at the same price. This chapter discusses how much the patient (or his or her family) pays, not how much the doctor or hospital actually receives, which is usually quite different (see Chapters 6 to 9). As pointed out in Chapter 1 (Figure 1.4), the total of all money paid by patients and families (as out-of-pocket charges, premiums, and taxes combined) automatically matches the total money received by all providers (e.g., hospitals, physicians, drug companies, nursing homes). However, for any particular subgroup or set of transactions, this equivalence is unlikely. Insurance breaks the linkage between what the patient pays and the amount the provider is paid.

People pay premiums to be insured, but they do not pay directly for the medical care they use. Health insurance is similar to having a credit card that allows you to buy whatever you need but for which payment is set at $100 per month regardless of the number of purchases you make. As you might expect, because one does not have to pay any extra for more purchases, the amount spent tends to rise uncontrollably (see Figure 9.6 for one illustration). That is why nearly all **indemnity insurance plans** providing unlimited reimbursements in return for a fixed premium have disappeared from the market. Most people are now covered by **managed-care** plans (see Section 5.4) in which they allow the insurer to exercise some control over the number and type of services covered in return for more affordable premiums. Managed-care plans use their control over purchasing to negotiate lower prices from hospitals, doctors, and drug companies. In a sense, managed care represents the evolution of the insurer from a passive financial intermediary to an active purchasing agent.

Over time, insurers modified contracts to create patient cost-sharing and reduce demand. A **deductible** is a provision that the patient pays the first $500 or $1000. **Copayments** require the patient to pay $10 or $20 for each visit to the doctor or day spent in the hospital. **Coinsurance** has the patient pay 10 percent or 20 percent of the bill. Moreover, the contract may specify that insurance will pay only up to a certain amount per visit or per day, with the doctor or hospital **balance-billing** the patient for anything above that amount. The policy could also have a **maximum** of $100,000 or $500,000 per year or per lifetime for the total of all reimbursements that the insurer will pay. However, some plans with significant copays and coinsurance move in the opposite direction by having a **stop-loss** provision, covering all bills in full after the patient has paid a certain amount, such as a total of $10,000 in a single year.

How Are Benefits Determined?

Insurance is a legal contract that is specific regarding how much will be paid, to which providers, under what conditions, the evidence of loss required, and who will arbitrate disputes. Health insurance isn't based on sickness at all but rather on incurring an expense for medical treatment. Most people never see the complete contract drawn up by their employer and the insurance company; they only see informational pamphlets, hear descriptions during new employee orientation, and so on. All such benefit descriptions, even in an advertisement or brochure written in Spanish or other language, are legally binding contracts. If a policy states that it covers eye examinations, it covers eye examinations. If a policy states that it will pay $36 for filling a tooth cavity, it will pay $36. In some sense, every set of documents constitutes a slightly different insurance plan. The insurance plan must pay any amount that a court decides a reasonable person reading such descriptions would expect the insurance plan to pay. Furthermore, any benefits routinely paid in previous years and not explicitly revoked become a precedent, even if those benefits are not mentioned in the contract. The use of fine print to leave the insured burdened with thousands of dollars of unexpected bills is simply not allowed. In fact, to do so would be self-defeating for an insurance company. Instead, if more money is needed to pay the bills, the insurer simply adjusts premiums upward over time as medical costs increase.

4.3 RISK AVERSION

Why would people be willing to pay even a 10 percent load (mark-up) just to get their premium money back as benefit payments? To the extent that people can easily fund routine losses through personal savings, they won't, which is why most routine losses are not insured. Only large and potentially catastrophic losses are worth paying extra to insure against.

Suppose the premiums required in the earlier heart attack example were not the actuarially fair $500, but $750, or $1,000, or even $1,500? This is still better than having to sell your house, being in debt for 20 years, or—perhaps worse—not being able to have an operation that could save your life if catastrophe strikes. To an economist, the fact that people are willing to pay more than the expected value of the loss for insurance is evidence that they think they are better off with insurance than without it. The desire to replace an uncertain loss with a steady and certain premium payment is known as **risk aversion**. Some people feel very strongly about risk and will go to great lengths to avoid it. Most people choose not to take financial chances unless they have to or are well paid for doing so (e.g., risky investments provide a higher rate of interest than safe government bonds). Others are willing to take some chances. To some extent this is a matter of taste, similar to how spicy you like your food. Your aversion to risk also depends to some extent on how much income you have: Going from $2 million a year to $50,000 is not nearly as scary as going from $200,000 to $5,000, which would provide you with less than $100 a week to spend on food, rent (forget it—you're living at your parent's place again or homeless), and travel (mostly by bus).

ARE YOU RISK AVERSE?

Here's an easy test. Imagine your boss offering to flip a coin to determine whether to double your monthly paycheck or take it away. If the prospect of losing your paycheck is much more unpleasant than the chance of doubling it, you, like most people, are risk averse and a good candidate for insurance.

With insurance, people can obtain medical care they otherwise could not afford. What if a $350,000 liver transplant could extend your life expectancy by 10 years? If you value your life at $100,000 per year (see Section 3.6), the benefit-to-cost ratio of treatment is 3:1 and clearly worthwhile. Yet you, like most people, do not have $350,000 in cash to spend and cannot get a bank loan for that amount, without collateral, just to possibly extend life. Insurance expands the choice set of patients facing serious illness and gives us all peace of mind. Economist John Nyman estimates that this **access to treatment** (affordability) gain is more valuable than pure risk sharing in ordinary financial insurance by an order of magnitude.[9] When it comes to life and death, being able to get help is extremely important.

Given that most people are risk averse, why aren't all risks insured? Life is full of risk. I buy an airplane ticket for a spring vacation even though I could die before I ever get to use it. My bicycle might be stolen. Some people study for a profession, such as accounting or computer science, only to find that job market conditions have changed by the time they graduate. As you take the exam for this course, at least some of the result (I hope not all) will be random (e.g., which questions were asked during class, when television commercial breaks occurred during your study time). Only a few risks in life are insured. Why? For one reason, it is costly to write up and specify insurance contracts, pay claims, and so on. Most small losses, on average, balance out over time and thus can be handled by savings. In addition, use of insurance to pay bills creates several structural incentive problems that reduce its value.[10]

4.4   ADVERSE SELECTION

Risk pooling works well because everyone in the group is at risk and therefore has an interest in making sure that solid insurance benefits are provided. Consider the heart attack example again, and suppose that instead of the risk being purely random, you knew that you were the one who would end up in the hospital. In this case, you would make sure that you got insurance and might even be willing to pay an astronomical premium to get it. However, if you were certain that you were not going to be the one ending up in the hospital, you would not try very hard to be part of the insurance group and might not be willing to pay $500 or even $50. Whenever the group of people actually insured is not average but disproportionately composed of those at higher risk, then adverse selection has occurred.

If higher risks result from something the insurance company can observe in advance and that both the insured and the company acknowledge, varying premiums by risk category causes no difficulties. For example, pricing by age is common, such as charging $300 per month for people 35 years old and younger, $500 for people 35 to 50, $650 for people 51 to 60, and $900 for people 61 and older. Adverse selection creates difficulties when some risk factors are known to the insured but not to the insurance company (e.g., my chest hurts every time I go walking, I enjoy fried foods and recreational drugs, my brother and sister recently died from heart attacks). Difficulties arise even when the risks are well known but it is considered "unfair" to charge for them (e.g., women employees paying less than men, doubling the premiums for people age 61 and older, charging unmarried men more because of the perceived higher risk of HIV/AIDS).

If an employer subsidizes an optional health plan for its workers, the ones most likely to buy insurance are those at high risk. This is called **adverse selection** and means that the average losses in the insured group will be larger than the expected value for the employees as a whole. If young, healthy workers do not participate, premiums have to increase. At the extreme, the plan may be left with only those who were ill to begin with and who knew that they would collect benefits, which is not considered insurance at all because there is no risk pooling. For this reason, insurance companies usually require that all or at least a majority of the employees in an organization be insured.

A subtler form of adverse selection occurs when a company offers two kinds of plans, a basic plan and a more comprehensive option for which employees pay extra. Who will choose the comprehensive plan? Some people will choose it because they are very risk averse and therefore willing to pay extra for the more comprehensive benefits. This causes no difficulty for the insurance plan because the actuarial risk (expected loss) of such people is about average. Financial difficulty arises because there will also be a disproportionate number of high-risk individuals (e.g., those who are older or overweight) who buy the comprehensive plan. As more and more high-risk people sign up for the comprehensive plan, their medical expenses will exceed the expected value, and even the "high" premium will not be sufficient to pay the bills. Thus, the extra premium for comprehensive insurance must be raised still higher. As the premium goes up, fewer and fewer average-risk people are willing to pay for the better coverage. Eventually, only the chronically ill who are certain to sustain a big loss will sign up for the comprehensive plan. As the difference in premiums between the basic and high-option plan becomes greater, fewer and fewer people at low risk are left in the high-option pool. The principle of risk sharing is defeated by the progressive separation of risks between the groups. This death spiral ends with the termination of the high-option plan (see the box "Adverse Selection at Harvard").

ADVERSE SELECTION AT HARVARD: GETTING PUSHED OUT OF THE PPO

In 1994, Harvard University faced a substantial deficit in the employee benefits budgets. For years, Harvard had offered both HMO and PPO health insurance plans, with the more expensive PPO plans being more generously subsidized by the university. To reduce cost, Harvard in 1995 implemented a new program in which it contributed the same dollar amount regardless of which plan an employee chose (with the fixed contribution amount set higher for low-income employees). Although the residual premium the employee had to pay went up for all plans, it went up more rapidly for the relatively generous PPO Flex plan (see Table 4.3). In response, enrollment in this high-option plan began to fall.

David Cutler and Sarah Reber examined the characteristics of those employees who switched out of the high-priced plan.[11] As theory predicts, those who switched were more likely to be healthy; they were younger on average and had spent less on medical care in prior years than those who elected to pay more and stay in the high-option plan. Hence it is not surprising that the high-option PPO Flex lost money in 1995. To compensate, PPO premiums were raised an additional 16 percent for 1996, which pushed even more young healthy employees into the HMO plans, and the PPO lost even more money. In 1997, the pattern was clear and the high-option plan was discontinued, completing an adverse-selection death spiral in only three years.

TABLE 4.3				Changes in Employee Premiums and Enrollment at Harvard			
	Employee Pays			**Enrollment**			
	Premium	**Old**	**New**	**1994**	**1995**	**1996**	**1997**
Individual							
PPO Flex	$2,773	$ 555	$1,152	16%	13%	8%	Discontinued
HMO	$1,980	$ 277	$ 421	84%	87%	92%	100%
Family							
PPO Flex	$6,238	$1,248	$2,208	22%	18%	11%	Discontinued
HMO	$5,395	$ 776	$1,191	78%	82%	89%	100%

Source: David M. Cutler and Sarah J. Rebler, "Paying for Health Insurance: The Trade-off Between Competition and Adverse Selection," *Quarterly Journal of Economics* 113, no. 2 (May 1988):433–466.

The more differences there are in expected medical costs and the more inside information people have about their own health, the greater the potential for adverse selection (see the box "Do People Choose to Die?"). The elderly are particularly problematic because many of their expenses are for chronic illnesses that are well known to them and not random. Insurers' major method for reducing adverse selection, insisting that all employees in a company be included in a group plan, is not available for the elderly because most of them are retired. The ultimate solution for adverse selection is to include everyone in a social insurance system, similar to what the United States did for the elderly by creating Medicare.

DO PEOPLE CHOOSE TO DIE?

Actuaries have found that people who buy life insurance are more likely than average to die prematurely.[12] The reasons have less to do with the drama depicted in Arthur Miller's *Death of a Salesman* (because suicide invalidates many policies) than with mundane adverse selection. For example, people who know that their parents died young or that their heart palpitates, or who worry about their lack of physical activity since they turned 50 are more apt to buy life insurance when it is offered. Conversely, those who buy annuities (policies that pay insureds a certain amount per year as long as they live) show positive selection and are less likely than average to die prematurely. Questionnaire respondents who reply "yes" when asked, "Do you expect to live a long time?" do, in fact, enjoy longer lives than those who respond "no," even after adjusting for the effects of age, blood pressure, cigarette smoking, and all other measurable health risks. This indicates that individuals do have private knowledge that they can use to select coverage that is most favorable to them but costly to the insurer.

Adverse selection is problematic for the insurance company, increasing losses without bringing in more premiums. Reverse or **positive selection** is the opposite: drawing in low-cost people who still pay regular premiums, which increases company profit margins. Providing a "gym benefit" creates positive selection, because the only people who care about getting a rebating for making 100 visits to the gym are active healthy people with below-average costs.[13] Similarly, extra benefits for wellness, nutrition classes, sports injuries, childcare, and so on can bring in better-than-average risks. Another way an insurance company can try to create positive selection is by discouraging bad risks. Reduced benefits for disabilities or expanded benefits for well-child visits, requiring a prequalifying examination, or even a lengthy application form all tend to differentially screen out the elderly and disabled. A study of 160,000 adults in Switzerland given the option of receiving a discount for a "restricted" plan in which they had to make a telephone call to the medical center prior to visiting the doctor found that those who chose the mandatory call option cost 50 percent less, primarily because they were younger and/or healthier.[14] Given the concentration and skewness of medical expenditures where just a few patients account for most of the spending, such positive selection can greatly increase insurance company profits and also greatly limit the use of insurance to provide universal coverage.

4.5 MORAL HAZARD

A person with medical insurance is more likely to go to the doctor because of a sore throat than someone who is not insured. If sent to the hospital, an insured person is more likely to pick a nicer and more expensive facility than an uninsured person. These changes in behavior cause the expenditures of people with insurance to be greater than what an actuary would have predicted from observing the records of people without insurance, and this increase in loss is known as **moral hazard**. One form of these behavioral changes can be illustrated using ordinary demand curve analysis (see Figure 4.4). The demand for physician visits by people without insurance is shown in line D. With insurance picking up 80 percent of the costs, the net "price"

FIGURE 4.4   Moral Hazard

"Moral hazard" increase in
consumption due to insurance

(P_i) that a patient has to pay personally is just 20 percent of the actual price; therefore, consumption will increase to Q_i. This increase in visits resulting from being insured is attributable to moral hazard.

Insurance obviously makes patients less aware of and sensitive to the price of care, but is it likely that people will use services having little or no health benefit just because they are free? For heart surgery, no. Pain and the loss of time are sufficient to keep people from undertaking surgery just for the fun of it. What about routine office visits? Many of them are for minor symptoms that will go away without treatment. Insurance makes people much more likely to seek treatment for minor symptoms and thus to increase the overall cost of insurance. Even some surgical procedures are of limited value and are likely to be undertaken only if insurance pays. Suppose 76-year-old Uncle Al has a liver infection. It is probable that he will die from the infection no matter what we do, but there is a chance that he could live several more months or even years with a liver transplant—at a cost of $100,000 for the surgery and $5,000 per month after that for drugs and after care. If Uncle Al or the family had to pay directly out of their own pockets, they would probably decide that it was not worth paying so much for such an expensive operation that is unlikely to be successful. However, if insurance is picking up the tab, or if Medicare is passing the cost on to all other taxpayers, Uncle Al and the family might go ahead and try for an improbable cure.

Figure 4.5 shows that the extent of expenditure due to moral hazard increases with the price elasticity of the demand curve. For services that are not very price sensitive (D_1), the fact that people are insured will not cause them to purchase many more services; therefore, there will not be much of a distortion in consumer behavior due to insurance. On the other hand, for services that are very price elastic (D_2), the fact that people are insured can cause a very large increase in the quantity they consume (which insurance will pay for), thereby making moral hazard a large problem. This theoretical result provides us with a hypothesis about which services will be covered by insurance. Because moral hazard reduces gains from risk pooling, types of medical care for which there is considerable moral hazard (services with high price elasticity) are less likely to be covered by insurance than services for which there is very little moral hazard (those with low price elasticity). A number of studies have shown that this is the case.[15] Services such as hospital care and surgery with lower price elasticity of demand are more likely to be insured than services such as nursing home care, physical therapy, behavioral counseling, dentistry, and drugs, which have a higher price elasticity of demand. Exchange

FIGURE 4.5   Amount of Moral Hazard Depends on Price

must make all parties better off, and when problems such as moral hazard reduce the value of transacting, there will be less pooling of risks through the insurance market.

Welfare Losses Due to Moral Hazard

The extra services people consume just because they are covered by insurance result in some economic waste. If it costs $20 to produce an x-ray, but the x-ray is only worth $5 to the patient, there is a net loss of value of $15. This loss of value is often called the **welfare triangle** because the area of the triangle between the price that the insurance company must pay and the demand curve yields a good measure of the size of the loss (see Figure 4.6). If insurance pays 80 percent of the bill, the number of x-rays consumed rises from five to nine. The cost of each x-ray stays the same, $20. The sixth x-ray is worth only $16, for a loss of $4; the seventh is worth $12, for a loss of $8; the eighth is worth $8, for a loss of $12; and the ninth is worth $4, for a loss of $16. The total amount paid for the four extra x-rays is $80, and the **welfare loss** is about half that, $40.[16]

Who loses? All members of the insured group lose because their premiums must be higher to cover this excess use of services. In fact, even the person getting the extra service probably

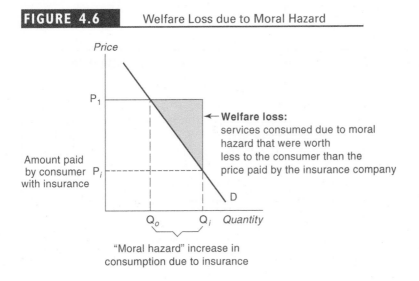

FIGURE 4.6   Welfare Loss due to Moral Hazard

would prefer a tighter contract that provided only worthwhile services at a lower premium. This is why so much work is done using contract exclusions, fee limits, second opinions, and so on to make sure that reimbursement is provided only for necessary services. There is a demand for the "hassle" of making patients and physicians justify their use of services—because it reduces premiums. Evidence of this demand is that consumers choose policies that include restrictive contractual language rather than policies that pay for everything without question but cost more. This does not mean that it is pleasant when you are sick to go through all sorts of bureaucratic hoops to get a claim paid; it does mean that the effort is justified in terms of reduced premiums—or else you would choose a different plan. Insurance companies give customers whatever they want, including aggravation, in order to make a profit.

Welfare losses due to moral hazard are to some extent unavoidable. They are part of the cost of insurance, the way that an unwanted orange peel is part of the cost of an orange. On net, people are better off with the insurance (including moral hazard) than without it. If people are buying insurance, the gains from trade due to risk pooling and access to high cost care must exceed the welfare losses from moral hazard. If the losses were larger than the gains, people would not buy. However, when the purchase of insurance is subsidized by the government, this might no longer be the case. The extra insurance bought because it is subsidized by taxes creates additional excess utilization of services that are not highly valued by consumers (see Section 4.6).[17]

There is a systemwide welfare loss caused by insurance that is more difficult to see. Insurance tends to increase demand and make patients less price sensitive, which increases prices overall. Whether or not one person becomes insured will have little effect on the price of x-rays. Yet if everyone who now has insurance had it taken away, demand would fall and the price of x-rays would surely decline. People who are uninsured are worse off because other people are insured, because those other people's insurance raises the price that uninsured people have to pay to obtain care.[18] It is even possible that we all would be better off if we were all uninsured, even though each one of us individually is better off with insurance. This paradoxical (and quite unlikely) result would only occur if the gains from risk pooling were smaller than the increase in prices resulting from universal insurance.[19] However, the systematic distortion of prices resulting from insurance raising overall demand can create a larger welfare loss than the moral hazard welfare triangle attributable to tax subsidy. Such systemwide effects are difficult to gauge, because looking at individual behavior might not tell us what is happening to the system as a whole. One way to measure systemwide effects is to compare different health care systems in different countries that use different types of insurance to see how well each one works and what they cost, but this ambitious effort is left for later (see Chapter 16).

WHAT HAPPENS WHEN YOUNG ADULTS LOSE HEALTH INSURANCE?

Before the passage of the Accountable Care Act of 2010 (see Chapter 17), young adults previously insured under a parent's health plan could lose coverage once they reached the age of 19 years unless they were deemed dependents or students. Anderson, Dobkin, and Gross used that reduction in coverage as a natural experiment to estimate the effects of a loss of insurance upon health care utilization.[20] They found that a 10 percent reduction in coverage led to a 4 percent decline in emergency department visits and a 6 percent decline in inpatient admissions. Further, their analysis indicated that most of the decline occurred in private voluntary and for-profit hospitals, with utilization of public "safety net" hospitals remaining the same as before.

Source: Michael Anderson, Carlos Dobkin, Tal Gross, "The Effect of Insurance Coverage on the Use of Medical Services," NBER Working paper #15823, March 2010.

Ex Ante Moral Hazard

Health economists make a distinction between *ex post* (after the fact) moral hazard resulting from extra dollars being spent on an existing illness because of insurance, and a change in *ex ante* (prior) behavior that increases the probability of getting sick. An example of ex ante moral hazard would be a person who, because they are insured, takes up the sport of parachuting, engages in risky sex, does not wear a seat belt, or does not bother to get a flu shot because "my insurance will pay for whatever happens." The term "moral hazard" originally came from such ex ante behavioral change among 19th century property owners with fire insurance that "lacked moral character" and did not provide adequate fire protection or even engaged in arson. Today "moral hazard" is most commonly applied to similar ex ante abuse when companies and banks that are "too big to fail" get bailed out by taxpayers and, since they do not bear the financial consequences of their actions, continue behave in ways that add to their profits by creating excessive risks that must eventually be paid for by the public.

   Although of considerable theoretical interest to economists, good evidence of such ex ante adoption of excessively risky behavior due to having insurance has not been reported very much in health studies. This is probably because the consequences to the individual outweigh any monetary advantage. Who wants to get sick just because an operation is paid for? There are hints that previously uninsured people who turn 65 and qualify for Medicare may be less likely to engage in exercise and control of bad habits, but it is difficult to separate the pure insurance incentives from other factors that might explain such differences in behavior.[21]

4.6   TAX BENEFITS

There is a less visible and more diffuse fourth party in most third-party insurance transactions: the government. Many governments take on the social obligation to provide medical care directly, as is done by the National Health Service in the United Kingdom and by the Swedish health system. Some countries have chosen to build on employee health insurance plans to create universal coverage for all citizens, such as the German Krankenkassen or the Japanese employment societies. The United States is somewhat unusual in that insurance is encouraged but not universally required. The U.S. government, through Medicare, directly provides insurance for all people 65 and older and, through Medicaid, it pays for many people who are classified as being indigent or disabled. The U.S. government also provides tax incentives for many others to be insured through the private sector. The primary tax incentive is that health benefits are nontaxable compensation for employees but still allowed as deductible expenses for the employer. Table 4.4 shows how this tax incentive works.

   The employer spends the same for labor either way and does not care whether insurance premiums are taken out of a paycheck or paid later from the employee's bank account. With

TABLE 4.4	Tax Incentives for Health Benefits	
Employee Pays for Medical Care		**Employer Pays for Insurance**
$1,000	Company labor cost	$1,000
none	Insurance premium	($200)
$1,000	Gross paycheck	$ 800
($350)	Taxes (at 35%)	($280)
$ 650	Net paycheck	$ 520
($200)	Medical bills	none
$ 450	**Available for spending**	$ 520

insurance taken out, the employees' gross income is less and therefore the amount of taxes paid is less. The employee with the larger paycheck, after paying for medical care with after-tax dollars, has less money left for spending than the employee whose health insurance premiums paid for the same amount of medical care on a pretax basis. As long as the administrative load is less than the tax rate, it is cheaper to buy medical care with pre-tax income using employer-paid insurance than for the employee to pay the bills directly. This tax break for employer-paid health insurance is a substantial ($250 billion per year) and important part of the voluntary system of health care that Americans have come to depend on.[22] Without the tax incentive, most working people would not have health insurance as an employee benefit.

4.7 EFFECTS OF HEALTH INSURANCE ON LABOR MARKETS

One of the reasons people take a job is to obtain health insurance. It is a benefit to them, but it is a cost to the employer. However, it is a fixed cost per person: the premiums do not go up if an employee works 48 hours rather than 40, or go down if only 30 hours are worked. Thus it is cheaper to hire 10 employees and have them work 20 percent harder than to hire 12 employees and pay for two additional insurance premiums (unless the wage rate has to go up for overtime). As the cost of health care rises, the employer has a greater and greater incentive to get each employee to work harder for more hours so as to avoid hiring more people.[23] Another way for a company to avoid the rising cost of health insurance is to replace full-time employees with part-timers who do not receive benefits. The costs of providing health insurance benefits is similarly reduced by using independent contractors, long-term temps, and adjunct instructors rather than regular faculty.

Looking at the supply and demand curves for labor, it is evident that increasing the benefits cost per person should reduce not only the quantity of regular labor but also its price. The total compensation (wage + benefits) rises, reducing quantity (number hired) and price (wage rates) (Figure 4.7). This result is confirmed by several studies showing that most, but not all, of an increase in health care premiums shows up as a decrease in take-home pay.[24]

Employers can also reduce their health insurance costs by having healthier employees. Whereas it is very difficult to get people to change their behavior by enough to significantly reduce the rate of costly illnesses, it is fairly easy to just not hire unhealthy employees (positive

---

FIGURE 4.7　　Effect of Increased Benefits Cost on Price (Wages) and Quantity of Labor

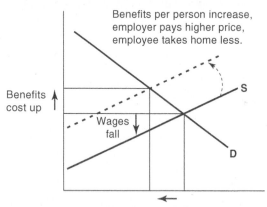

Quantity (number of employees) reduced

selection), which is why nondiscrimination laws and policies make it illegal to refuse to hire someone because they are old, overweight, have HIV, or could get pregnant. It is also why certain benefits are mandated and legally required. Rather than not hiring women, a restaurant could just refuse to pay for births or gynecology services. Although selecting only people who are healthy and inexpensive to cover might help the employer, it would make things worse not only for the people who are discriminated against but also for the government, hospitals, and all the rest of us who end up paying and caring for all the sick people who cannot get employer-provided health insurance.

Employees as well as employers respond to incentives. People who have health insurance through a spouse or family member are more likely to take time off, to switch jobs, or retire.[25] A poor single mother whose children are covered by Medicaid is not going to take a minimum-wage job that will cause her to lose her benefits. Studies have shown that potential loss of insurance benefits is a significant reason that people continue working when they would rather retire, and also stick with the same employer even when they would rather look for another job and switch.[26]

4.8 HISTORY OF HEALTH INSURANCE

In some sense, risk pooling has always existed: People have always taken care of each other during times of need. Financial contracts for pooling risk did not become important until the Industrial Revolution, when economies moved from the medieval manor system, where most people worked the land, to a wage-based economy centered in cities and towns. Freemen who left the medieval estates and gathered in town to practice skilled trades, such as printers and goldsmiths, often became quite wealthy, but they were potentially subject to catastrophic losses if they became ill. Although gaining freedom, they had given up the protection and security that went with being part of an estate. If they became sick, they might become destitute. The guilds were organized to further their interests collectively and became natural vehicles for sharing risks. Initially this took the form of soliciting donations from all other guild members: "passing the hat" when someone became ill or died. Then more formal institutions evolved that accumulated funds over time. A "subscription" would be regularly collected that could be used to pay benefits. In this early form of insurance, there was no distinction made between the loss of wages owing to illness and the costs of medical care (or burial). Insurance was simply a way to provide money in time of need. The guild members knew each other well, and therefore the definition of loss was made by a consensus of the leadership, not by the existence of a doctor's bill.[27]

Early industrialists also recognized the need to provide wages and medical care for workers when they were sick. It is unlikely that funds were set aside for this purpose. Rather, sickness funds were drawn out of daily business receipts. Most such benefits were informal, provided at the discretion of the business owner, and not part of the official employment contract. In this sense, early industrial benefits were quite similar to the paternalistic obligations owed to the serfs by the manorial lords who owned the land they worked on, except that as factories and wages replaced farms and tenant shares, the benefits were money payments rather than direct care.

By the 19th century, some industries that were especially dangerous and remote (mining, timber) had developed contracts with a "company doctor" so that regular medical care would always be available. In other industries, it was the workers who organized to provide sickness benefits. As unions became an important means for furthering the interests of workers, they found that they needed some way to keep the membership involved (and paying dues) throughout the year and not just when a strike was threatened. Medical coverage became the preferred union benefit. It was always needed, made the workers and their families grateful, and attracted newcomers. In those days care could be provided at relatively low cost through clinics or "dispensaries" staffed by young doctors hired by the union to practice several nights a week. Company and union clinics, mutual benefit societies, and other forms of prepayment had become common by 1850, but they still provided medical care financing to only a small fraction of the population, probably less than one-twentieth. As wages rose above the subsistence level and workers became more assertive, it became evident that insurance would have to be extended to cover more of the population.

The first national health insurance program was implemented in Germany in 1883. Bismarck, the chancellor who had unified the German Länder (provinces) into a nation, saw that his political successes were threatened by the popularity of socialist causes among workers. By putting together a social security system with medical insurance and retirement benefits for industrial workers, he preempted one of the main goals of the socialist movement and was able to maintain popular support.[28] National health plans were established in England in 1911, in Sweden in 1914, and in France in 1930. At first, only salaried workers in the major manufacturing plants were covered, usually with a lesser degree of coverage for dependents. Other workers, such as agricultural and retail workers, day laborers, shopkeepers, and the self-employed, had to take care of themselves.

Over the next 50 years, coverage was successively broadened. By 1980, almost every developed country had health insurance coverage for all citizens, either through a national health service (United Kingdom) or a universal insurance plan (Canada) or by coordinating all employer-based plans and providing government insurance for the rest of the population (Germany, Japan).[29] Evolution of health insurance in the United States was somewhat different, and a large segment of the population still lacks health insurance today.

The United States depended on voluntary private initiatives to develop health insurance, with much less reliance on government. There was a recognition that the population needed protection against losses due to illness, and in 1929 the independent Committee on the Costs of Medical Care began a fact-finding study, eventually producing a 28-volume report that was very influential in shaping the growth of voluntary insurance in the United States.[30] In the same year, Baylor Hospital proposed to the local teachers' association that it would provide all the care needed to anyone who would pay a premium of $0.50 a month. The plan proved to be very popular, and similar plans were started by other hospitals nearby. One problem with a "hospital prepayment" plan was that a patient whose doctor worked in a different hospital, or who needed a special type of care elsewhere, got no benefits. The solution was to combine all the separate plans under the sponsorship of the state hospital association so that one plan covered all hospitals; thus, Blue Cross was born. It grew rapidly, from 3,000 members in 1930, to 10,000 in 1932, and to 1,000,000 by 1936. In 2012 more than 100 million people were insured through 39 Blue Cross/Blue Shield plans, but many of these had changed during the last 10 years from local nonprofit community organizations to large multistate for-profit corporations.[31]

The imposition of wage and price controls during World War II provided an indirect, but powerful, boost to voluntary insurance. Employers were not allowed to raise wages, but they could provide additional benefits.[32] With wartime production booming and many laborers drafted into the military, most companies desperately needed to attract more workers. In less than 20 years, health insurance went from being an occasional perk that covered just 5 percent of the population to a routine benefit that was expected to be part of any good job and covered more than 50 percent of the population. Even with favorable tax treatments and active encouragement, however, voluntary insurance could not be extended to cover two of the groups who needed it most: the elderly and the poor. The poor were simply not able to afford health insurance. Furthermore, whereas policy makers and hospital administrators might think that paying premiums to prepare for future medical expenses was one of the most important things a family could do with its money, many of the poor did not. Because there was always some form of care available, usually in city clinics and hospitals, the poor often chose to spend what little discretionary money they had on better housing, better food, or some entertainment, rather than on insurance premiums.

The difficulties of the elderly in obtaining insurance were largely attributable to adverse selection and the discounting of consumption over time.[33] Younger people were formed into risk-pooling groups on the basis of employment, but many older people were not attached to an employer. There was no natural grouping by which risks could be shared, and there were no tax advantages to insurance premiums paid out of savings or retirement benefits rather than wages. Differences in the expected costs of medical care among individuals are much greater for older people, making it more difficult to constitute risk-sharing pools. Whereas many of the illnesses that strike younger people are essentially random events of low probability, many medical expenses of the elderly are for chronic conditions. There is no reason for a 72-year-old who is healthy to want to be in a group paying the same premium as someone with cancer or arthritis who is likely to have high medical expenses. Elderly people often know more about the potential cost of their own health conditions than any insurance company can, thus creating adverse selection problems when allowed to purchase insurance individually. These difficulties are exacerbated by the need to save early in one's career to pay for medical expenses that come after retirement. There must be a mechanism for transferring dollars from consumption at early ages toward old age. The Social Security Acts of 1965, which established the **Medicare** (Title XVI) program for the elderly and **Medicaid** (Title XVII) for the indigent, brought fundamental changes in the U.S. health care system and made government a major partner in financing medical care.[34] Adverse selection was no longer a problem for the elderly, because everyone age 65 or older was insured. Poverty no longer excluded the indigent from health insurance, because the government made these benefits available at no cost.[35]

After a century of development, health care financing in the United States is still in flux, with a mixed public and private system in which government accounts for 50 percent of total funds (56 percent once tax subsidies are included), private insurance accounts for 32 percent (including Blue Cross/Blue Shield, self-funded employer plans, commercial insurance companies, and HMOs), various programs and charitable contributions account for 7 percent, and the remaining 11 percent is paid directly by patients and family members out of pocket (of which more than half is for deductibles and coinsurance and could be considered part of the third-party insurance payments).

Among this variety of health insurance organizations, government (Medicare in particular) is now the dominant payer. During the 1950s, Blue Cross set the tone and structure for insurance coverage and Medicare copied the Blue Cross reimbursement system. Since then, the balance of power has changed dramatically. Blue Cross has fragmented, reducing what was once a pervasive community voluntary organization to a set of franchisees linked by a trademark, with the largest (California, New York) transformed into independent, and essentially faceless, for-profit insurance companies (Wellpoint, Anthem) with no specific ideology or geographic ties. Conversely, Medicare has become so large that no hospital and few doctors can afford to be without a Medicare contract. Every provider is thus compelled to use the complex and highly regulated Medicare cost and activity reporting scheme. Other insurers find it easier to adapt the Medicare payment system than to develop their own, making the influence of Medicare even greater than its percentage share of the market.

SUGGESTIONS FOR FURTHER READING

Michael Morrisey, *Health Insurance* (Chicago: AUPHA/Health Administration Press, 2007).

John Nyman, *Health Insurance* (Palo Alto: Stanford University Press, 2002).

Institute of Medicine, *Employment and Health Benefits: A Connection at Risk* (Washington, D.C.: National Academies Press, 1993).

AHIP (America's Health Insurance Plans), www.AHIP.org

Employee Benefit Research Institute, www.ebri.org

Paul Gertler and Jonathan Gruber, "Insuring Consumption Against Illness," *American Economic Review* 92, no. 1 (2002): 51–70, available at http://nber.org/papers/w6035.

Jonathan Gruber and Helen Levy, "The Evolution of Medical Spending Risk," *Journal of Economic Perspectives* 23, no. 4 (2009): 25–48.

Mark V. Pauly, "Risks and Benefits in Health Care: The View from Economics." *Health Affairs* 25, no. 3 (2007): 653–662.

SUMMARY

1. From an individual perspective, **insurance is a form of trade** between time periods or between different possible states (healthy or sick) in the future. From a societal perspective, insurance is a method of **pooling risks** so that the burden of financial loss is distributed over many people. An individual's **savings** can spread the cost of illness over time. **Family, friends, and charity** spread risk across people. **Private insurance contracts** spread risk through organized markets. **Social insurance** uses taxation to spread risk over all citizens.

2. Owing to the **uncertain and uneven distribution of medical care costs**, with 70 percent of total dollars being spent on behalf of the 10 percent of people who become most ill during a year, most health care payments flow through **third-party insurance** intermediaries that pool and transfer funds, which differs from the direct exchange of money for services between two parties (consumers and providers) common to most markets.

3. An **actuarially fair premium** is equal to the **expected value** of a loss, the dollar amount multiplied by the probability of occurrence. The "law of large numbers" means that higher losses for some will be offset by lower losses for others; therefore, for a large group the overall loss usually will be close to the expected value. If each person contributes an average amount, the pooled funds will be enough to pay for all the individual losses.

4. **Insurance companies do not pay for losses:** People do. The entire cost of medical care, including the costs of administration and use of financial capital, is paid through premiums, taxes, or patient coinsurance (e.g., deductibles, copayments) collected for each service rendered. Therefore, only large, random, infrequent losses are worth insuring. Insurance covering small, regular losses raises costs while providing few benefits from risk reduction.

5. People prefer having an income that is certain rather than the same average income subject to random fluctuations. Because of **risk aversion**, consumers are willing to pay more than the expected value of a loss to obtain insurance coverage. From the supply side, the excess of premiums received over benefits paid is called the load or **underwriting gains** of the insurance company.

6. People who know that they are likely to sustain a loss are more likely to purchase insurance, resulting in **adverse selection**, a change in the composition of the insured group. This difficulty in the grouping of people for insurance is to be distinguished from an increase in the average loss due to a change in the behavior of individuals.

7. **Moral hazard** occurs whenever having insurance leads individuals to increase the amount spent or to increase the risk of loss. In health economics, moral hazard most commonly refers to the increase in utilization of medical services that result from being insured. The **welfare loss due to insurance** occurs because people who do not have to pay the bills tend to consume some care that is worth less to them than what it costs to provide. The gains from risk reduction must be worth more than these welfare losses or people would choose to go without insurance. However, the subsidy provided by exempting employer-provided health insurance benefits from taxes encourages extra insurance coverage. There also may be a general rise in the price of medical care because insurance increases the demand for services. This clearly causes a loss of welfare to those who are

uninsured and, by increasing overall costs, creates a systemwide distortion that reduces economic efficiency.

8. The premiums for health insurance count as an expense to employers and are not counted as income to employees, thus generating **tax benefits** when medical expenses are paid through insurance rather than by patients directly out of pocket. Employer **tax subsidy**, wartime restriction on wage increases that favored benefits, and the ability of companies to avoid adverse selection through risk pools covering all employees are major reasons for the rise of employer-based health insurance.

9. Historically, the development of voluntary insurance plans in the United States was led by groups of hospitals and doctors who were interested in **assuring payment to providers** as well as in protecting patients from losses.

PROBLEMS

1. {*cost sharing*} Find four people who have been treated for illness in the past three years. Ask them the following questions.

    a. How much did you pay for insurance?
    b. How much did the insurance really cost (i.e., what you paid plus what the employer or government paid)?
    c. How much did you pay in medical bills?
    d. How much did the medical care really cost (i.e., what you paid plus what the insurance company or government paid)?

2. {*actuarially fair premium*} A company with 617 employees had the following experience this year:

Health Care	Cost Each
14 hospitalizations	$5,600
37 physical therapy sessions	$ 340
9 births	$1,800
4.1 physician visits per employee	$ 55
2.4 prescriptions filled per employee	$ 21

    Assuming that the cost of medical care rises 7 percent over the next year, what would the actuarially fair premium per employee be for the next year?

3. {*size of risk pool*} Use the information in Figure 4.2 pertaining to a loss of $50,000 that occurs randomly with a probability of 1/100. If the insurance company charges $750 per person per year, what is the load above the actuarially fair premium? If 100 people are in the group, will the insurance company show an underwriting profit? Will the insurance company ever break even? How likely is it that the plan will show a loss next year? With 50 people in the group, is it more or less likely that the plan will show a loss? What about with 500 people? How large does the group have to be before the insurance company can be 99 percent sure that it will show an underwriting gain for the year?

4. {*savings, social insurance*} Explain which mechanism (savings, charity and contributions from friends, private insurance, or social insurance) you believe would cover losses resulting from each of the following conditions:

    seasonal hay fever
    congenital birth defects
    schizophrenia

Alzheimer's disease

preventive dental cleaning

posttraumatic jaw reconstruction

cigarette-induced chronic pulmonary obstruction

5. {*load, gains from trade*} Give three good reasons why someone might choose to pay $1,150 for health insurance when the actuarially fair premium was only $900.

6. {*adverse selection*} In each of the following pairs, which situation (a) or (b) would pose the larger problems regarding adverse selection?

    i. (a)   A policy covering accidents for all children attending YMCA camps

    (b)   A policy covering accidents for college students traveling abroad

    ii. (a)   Inclusion of HIV/AIDS treatment in the standard benefit package offered to teachers

    (b)   An optional rider providing HIV/AIDS coverage for an additional premium

    iii. (a)   Basic medical services insurance package offered to students entering college

    (b)   Basic medical services package offered to professors seeking early retirement

    iv. (a)   Optional mental health coverage offered to employees of ABC Inc.

    iv. (b)   Optional mental health coverage offered to children of ABC Inc. employees

7. {*moral hazard*} Explain which types of insurance coverage (a) or (b) within each pair would be more likely to cause more problems resulting from moral hazard.

    i. (a)   Indemnity payments of $10,000 for each eye or limb lost

    (b)   Indemnity payments of $50 for each day spent in a nursing home

    ii. (a)   Treatment in an emergency department

    (b)   Treatment in an intensive care unit

    iii. (a)   Arthroscopic surgery for knee injuries

    (b)   Amputation for foot injuries

    iv. (a)   Family counseling

    (b)   Electroconvulsive therapy

    v. (a)   Decongestants

    (b)   Antibiotics

8. {*moral hazard*} The following table gives the demand curve for doctor visits for Ralph, who doesn't have health insurance. Assume that Ralph responds only to the amount he must pay out of pocket when deciding how much care to use. By filling in the blank lines, calculate Ralph's new demand curve if he obtained insurance coverage that paid 80 percent of the bill. If the charges are $100 (i.e., Ralph pays $20 out of pocket), how many of the additional services Ralph uses are worth less (to him) than what they cost? How many are worth less to him than what he pays?

Price per Visit	Number of Visits	Out-of-Pocket Cost with Insurance	Number of Visits with Insurance
$ 0	20	—	—
$ 20	18	—	—
$ 50	15	—	—
$100	10	—	—
$150	5	—	—

9. {*welfare loss*} Bill's new insurance policy contains a prescription plan that provides all drugs through a local pharmacy with a $2 copayment. Under the old insurance, Bill had to pay for his own medication and purchased nine inhalers at $16 apiece to help control his asthma. With the new plan, Bill purchased 15 inhalers, keeping some as spares in his glove compartment and desk, because he only had to pay a $2 copayment for each one. How much are the six additional inhalers worth to Bill? How much do they cost him? How much do they cost the insurance company? Is Bill better or worse off under the new plan? Who would be worse off?

10. {*incidence*} When medical care is reimbursed through employer-provided insurance, whose welfare is ultimately affected when the cost of medical care rises: the owners of the firm that pays the premiums (employer), the government whose revenues are reduced because insurance benefits are not taxable as wages, or the public in their roles as workers, consumers, and taxpayers? Is there any difference between short-term and long-term effects?

11. {*positive selection*} If an insurance company is able to discourage some of the sickest patients from enrolling, how much will that increase their profits? For this problem, assume average cost per person and concentration of costs are the same as in Table 4.2 but that the plan is able to discourage and "de-select" about one fifth of the top 1 percent and 9 percent, replacing them with enrollees having just average costs.

12. {*ownership*} Why was it more common for railroads and timber companies to provide health insurance in the early 1900s than for textile mills or accounting firms?

13. {*ownership*} Who controlled Blue Cross when it was formed? Did this form of insurance generate profits for its owners?

ENDNOTES

1. Gary Becker, *A Treatise on the Family* (Cambridge, Mass.: Harvard University Press, 1981); Robert H. Frank, *Passions within Reason: The Strategic Role of the Emotions* (New York: Norton, 1988).

2. Edward O. Wilson, *On Human Nature* (Cambridge, Mass.: Harvard University Press, 1976); Jerome H. Barkow, Leda Cosmides, John Tooby, eds., *The Adapted Mind: Evolutionary Psychology and the Generation of Culture* (New York: Oxford University Press, 1992).

3. Rosemary Stevens, *In Sickness and In Wealth: American Hospitals in the Twentieth Century* (New York: Basic Books, 1989); John D. Thompson, *The Hospital: A Social and Architectural History* (New Haven: Yale University Press, 1975).

4. William A. Glaser, *Health Insurance in Practice: International Variations in Financing, Benefits, and Problems* (San Francisco: Jossey-Bass, 1991).

5. William Aaronson, Jacqueline Zinn, and Michael Rosko, "The Success and Repeal of the Medicare Catastrophic Coverage Act," *Journal of Health Politics, Policy and Law* 19, no. 4 (1994): 753–771.

6. Agency for Healthcare Research Quality, *Distribution of Population by Percentile Ranking of Medical Expenditures and Insurance Coverage: United States and New York State, 2006* (Rockville, Md.: Agency for Healthcare Research Quality, 2006), http://www.ahrq.gov/data/meps/popdistabs.htm. Stephen Cohen and William Yu, "The Concentration and Persistence in the Level of Health Expenditures over Time: Estimates for the U.S. Population 2008–2009," Statistical Brief #354, January 2012, AHRQ, www.MEPS.ahrq.gov; *Health Care Financing Review,* Medicare and Medicaid Statistical Supplement, 1995, p. 35; Marc L. Berk and Alan Monheit, "The Concentration of Health Expenditures, Revisited," *Health Affairs* 20(2): 9–18, 2001. The distribution of costs across individuals can be measured only for personal health care costs that are billed to individuals, not overhead items such as public health, construction, insurance administration, etc. Such overhead items make up about 10 percent of national health expenditures, and hence the "all persons" average in Table 4.2 is only 90 percent as large as the per capita average for all national health expenditures reported elsewhere. In truth, many costs have overhead components and are difficult to unambiguously assign to a single person, although they are clearly concentrated on the most ill and not evenly distributed. Some economists would argue that costs are even more concentrated than Table 4.2 indicates, because hospitals and physicians typically overcharge the least-complex patients to subsidize the most difficult and complex cases (see the discussion of cost shifting in Chapter 8).

7. Bureau of Labor Statistics, U.S. Dept. of Labor, "Employer Costs for Employee Compensation," December 7, 2011, http://www.bls.gov/.

8. C. Rufus Rorem, "Sickness Insurance in the United States," *Bulletin of the American Hospital Association* (June 1932); Odin W. Anderson, *Health Services as a Growth Enterprise in the United States since 1875,* 2nd ed. (Ann Arbor: Health Administration Press, 1990).

9. John A. Nyman, *The Theory of Demand for Health Insurance* (Palo Alto: Stanford University Press, 2002) and "The Value of Health Insurance: The Access Motive," *Journal of Health Economics* 18, no. 2 (1999): 141–152.

10. The fact that we are not insured against all risks raises an interesting question: If people are so risk averse, why do they gamble (by playing the lottery or at casinos)? It is clear why people gamble on an investment in stock or land. They are compensated by getting (on average) higher returns than they can obtain with less-risky investments. However, in the casino form of gambling, you don't get paid for taking risks; you have to pay for the privilege of taking on risk. The truth is, people gamble this way mostly for fun. It is something exciting to do, like going to a sports event. Sometimes people gamble because they do not understand that the odds are against them—that if they keep playing long enough they are bound to lose. Then there are a few people who gamble because it is their job and, like casinos, they almost always win when we put our money on the table. Don't envy the professional gambler too much, though. For this person, gambling is work rather than a diversion, and the hardest thing is finding willing customers, which is also the case for insurance salespeople.

11. David M. Cutler and Sarah J. Reber, "Paying for Health Insurance: The Trade-Off Between Competition and Adverse Selection," *Quarterly Journal of Economics* 113, no. 2 (1998): 433–466.

12. Lewis C. Workman, "Life Annuities," in *Mathematical Foundations of Life Insurance* (Atlanta: Life Office Management Association, 1982), 155–195.

13. Alicia Cooper and Amal Trivedi, "Fitness Memberships and Favorable Selection in Medicare Advantage Plans," *New England Journal of Medicine* 366 (2012): 1448–1450.

14. Chantal Grandchamp and Lucien Gardiol, "Does A Mandatory Telemedicine Call Prior to Visiting a Physician Reduce Costs or Simply Attract Good Risks?" *Health Economics* 20, no. 10 (2011): 1257–1267.

15. Kevin F. O'Grady, Willard G. Manning, Joseph P. Newhouse, and Robert H. Brook, "The Impact of Cost Sharing on Emergency Department Use," *New England Journal of Medicine* 313, no. 8 (1985): 484–490; Mark V. Pauly, "Taxation, Health Insurance and Market Failure in the Medical Economy," *Journal of Economic Literature* 24, no. 2 (1968): 629–675.

16. The size of the welfare triangle is $(P_{original} - P_{insured}) \times (Q_{insured} - Q_{original}) \div 2$, which for this example would be $(\$20 - \$4) \times (9 - 5) \div 2 = \$32$. This is slightly less than in the numerical example because with discrete units (e.g., one, two, ... eight, nine x-rays, with no fractions) the demand curve is not a continuous straight line but a step function, and so the area between the original \$20 line and the demand curve is somewhat larger. In most cases, economists use the continuous formula, because with many consumers buying many units of service, the individual bumps are less important and the demand curve approximates a continuous line.

17. Martin S. Feldstein, "The Welfare Loss of Excess Health Insurance," *Journal of Political Economy* 81, no. 2 (1973): 251–280.

18. Gina Kolata, "Medical Fees Are Often Higher for Patients without Insurance," *New York Times,* April 1, 2001. However, it is sometimes the case that the profits that hospitals make from insured patients are used to provide charity services to the uninsured (see the discussion of cost shifting in Chapter 8). Whether or not an uninsured person is made better or worse off depends upon whether or not they receive services for free or with sufficient subsidy that the price to them is less than the market price would be without insurance.

19. Adam Wagstaff and Magnus Lindelow, "Can Insurance Increase Financial Risk? The Curious Case of Health Insurance in China," *Journal of Health Economics* 27, no. 4 (2008): 990–1005.

20. Michael Anderson, Carlos Dobkin, Tal Gross, "The Effect of Insurance Coverage on the Use of Medical Services," NBER working paper #15823, March 2010.

21. Laure De Preux, "Anticipatory Ex Ante Moral Hazard and the Effect of Medicare on Prevention," *Health Economics* 20, no. 9 (2011): 1056–1072; Teresa Longobardi, "Ex-Ante Moral Hazard in Health Care Insurance for Obese Populations," Presentation at iHEA World Congress July 2011; Dharval Dave and Robert Kaestner, "Health Insurance and Ex Ante Moral Hazard: Evidence from Medicare," *International Journal of Health Care Finance and Economics* 9, no. 4 (2009): 367–390; Peter Zweifel and Willard Manning, "Moral Hazard and Consumer Incentives in Health Care." in A. J. Culyer and J. P. Newhouse, eds., *Handbook of Health Economics* (Amsterdam: Elsevier, 2000).

22. J. Sheils and R. Haught, "The Cost of Tax Exempt Health Benefits in 2004," *Health Affairs* 23 2004: w106–w112; T. M. Selden and B. M. Gray, "Tax Subsidies for Employment-Related Health Insurance: Estimates for 2006," *Health Affairs* 25, no. 6 (2006): 1568–1579; Jonathan Gruber and Helen Levy, "The Evolution of Medical Spending Risk" *Journal of Economic Perspectives* 23, no. 4 (2009): 25–48.

23. David Cutler and Bridgette Madrian, "Labor Market Responses to Rising Health Insurance Costs: Evidence on Hours Worked." *RAND Journal of Economics* 29, no. 3 (1988): 509–530.

24. Kate Baicker and Amitabh Chandra, "The Labor Market Effects of Rising Health Insurance Premiums," NBER working paper #11160 (2005); Jonathan Gruber and Alan Krueger, "The Incidence of Mandated

Employer-Provided Insurance: Evidence from Worker's Compensation Insurance," in David Bradford, ed., *Tax Policy and the Economy,* Vol. 5, pp 111–143 (Cambridge Mass.: MIT Press, 1991).

25. Thomas Buchmueller and Robert Valetta, "The Effect of Health Insurance on Married Female Labor Supply," *Journal of Human Resources* 34, no. 1 (1999): 42–70.

26. David M. Blau and Donna Gilleskie, "Retiree Health Insurance and Labor Force Behavior of Older Men in the 1990s," *Review of Economics and Statistics* 83, no. 1 (2001): 64–80; Jeannette Rogowski and Lynn Karoly, "Health Insurance and Retirement Behavior: Evidence for the Health and Retirement Survey," *Journal of Health Economics* 19, no. 4 (2000): 529–539; Philip Cooper and Alan Monheit, "Does Employment-Related Health Insurance Inhibit Job Mobility?" *Inquiry* 30, no. 4 (1993): 400–416.

27. R. Munts, *Bargaining for Health: Labor Unions, Health Insurance and Medical Care* (Madison: University of Wisconsin Press, 1967); David T. Beito, *From Mutual Aid to the Welfare State: Fraternal Societies and Social Services 1890–1967* (Chapel Hill: UNC Press, 2000); Marco HD van Leeuwen, "Guilds and Middle-Class Welfare, 1550–1800," *Economic History Review* 65, no. 1 (2012): 61–90.

28. Peter A. Kohler and Hans F. Zacher, eds., *The Evolution of Social Insurance 1881–1991: Studies of Germany, France, Great Britain, Austria and Switzerland* (New York: St. Martin's Press, 1982).

29. William A. Glaser, *Health Insurance in Practice: International Variations in Financing, Benefits, and Problems* (San Francisco: Jossey-Bass, 1991).

30. Committee on the Costs of Medical Care, *Medical Care for the American People* (Chicago: University of Chicago Press, 1932).

31. Robert Cunningham III and Robert M. Cunningham, Jr., *The Blues: A History of the Blue Cross and Blue Shield System* (DeKalb: Northern Illinois University Press, 1997).

32. Institute of Medicine, *Employment and Health Benefits: A Connection at Risk* (Washington, D.C.: National Academies Press, 1993), 70; Melissa A. Thomasson, "The Importance of Group Coverage: How Tax Policy Shaped U.S. Health Insurance," *American Economic Review* 93, no. 4 (2003): 1373–84, and "From Sickness to Health: The Twentieth Century Development of U.S. Health Insurance" *Explorations in Economic History* 39, no. 3 (2002): 233–53.

33. Herman M. Somers and Anne R. Somers, *Medicare and the Hospitals: Issues and Prospects* (Washington, D.C.: Brookings Institution, 1967).

34. W. J. Cohen, "Reflections on the Enactment of Medicare and Medicaid," *Health Care Financing Review* (supplement): 3–16, 1985; Theodore Marmor, *The Politics of Medicare* (Chicago: Aldine, 1973).

35. Note, however, that many people you might consider "poor" are not eligible for Medicaid, a major reason that there are still 40 million uninsured. Typically the "working poor" have income above the poverty line but lack employer-provided insurance. Single persons without children usually do not qualify, even if their incomes are very low (hence the acronym TANF, Temporary Assistance to Needy Families).

CHAPTER 5

INSURANCE CONTRACTS AND MANAGED CARE

QUESTIONS

1. Who is the largest health insurer?
2. Which is better: individual insurance plans, employer-provided insurance, or government insurance?
3. How is a state mandate to cover alcoholism treatment similar to a tax?
4. Why are so many Americans uninsured?
5. Who pays when the cost of medical care rises: employers, employees, government, or insurance companies?
6. How much profit can an HMO make? At whose expense?
7. What is the underwriting cycle? A retention ratio? A self-insured ASO? ERISA?
8. Do managed care and health savings accounts (HSAs) reduce the cost of health insurance or just shift it around?
9. Who are the winners and losers in managed care? Do cost reductions mean that some doctors must earn lower incomes? Who are the winners and losers from HSAs?
10. Does a physician "gatekeeper" or "medical home" work for or against the patient?

5.1 SOURCES OF INSURANCE

Of the 316 million people in the United States, most have some form of health insurance, often as an employee or dependent benefit. Less than a tenth, 19 million people, purchase individual health insurance. Government covers one third of the people through Medicare, Medicaid, Department of Defense, Veterans' Affairs, or other plans, but it pays more than half of the total costs because it takes on many of the more expensive cases (disabled, elderly, nursing home residents) and provides extensive subsidies. However, there are still 50 million Americans without health insurance (Table 5.1).[1]

Health insurance is complicated. There are literally thousands of contracts. Even hospital administrators and insurance executives are often baffled and frustrated by the complexity. Most people are happy to just go along with whatever exists so long as they can get medical care when they need it and do not have to pay too much. Economists must dig deeper to understand the implications of third-party insurance financing for medical institutions, to see where the

TABLE 5.1	Health Insurance Coverage of the U.S. Population	
Population	**Non-Elderly**	**Elderly**
Total persons	274 million	42 million
With insurance	81.5%	98.1%
Employment	29.1	32.5
Employee (dependent)	29.6	—
Other private insurance	7.1	28.8
Military	3.3	8.1
Medicare	3.0	93.1
Medicaid	16.9	9.2
Uninsured	18.5	1.9

Note: Percentages add to more than 100% because some persons have multiple coverage.
Source: U.S. Census Bureau, Current Population Survey and EBRI.

incentives and unfunded liabilities are. To do so, this chapter looks at the sources of health insurance, contracting for consumer-directed and managed-care plans and provider networks. In conclusion, some conflicts and unresolved issues are briefly introduced before being subject to more extensive analysis and discussion in Chapters 17 and 18.

Employer-Based Group Health Insurance

Four factors explain why more than half of the U.S. population is covered by employer group health insurance:

- Covering a large group under a single contract reduces transaction costs.
- Group coverage mitigates adverse selection.
- Employer payment yields a tax benefit.
- Many of the most expensive patients are heavily subsidized or excluded.

An employer may offer one or many plans. The employee obtains insurance by choosing one, deciding whether to include children and other dependents, and contributing a fraction (usually around 20 percent) toward the total premium (see Table 5.2). Almost all large employers provide health insurance benefits, but only half of small companies with fewer than 10 employees do so (Figure 5.1). Employees who are part-time, temporary, or newly hired might not be eligible. Furthermore, some employees choose not to enroll because they already have health insurance through another health plan (covered spouse, Medicare, etc.) or just because they are healthy and do not want to have the monthly employee contribution taken from their paychecks.[2] In the end, about two-thirds of all workers obtain health insurance through their employer. The largest employee groups are self-insured (i.e., the employer bears the risk although it might use an insurance company to administer benefits). More than half of the population has coverage through an employer, but these plans pay less than one-third of the nation's health costs. This is because many of the expensive cases (elderly, disabled, nursing

TABLE 5.2	Annual Premiums for Employee Health Insurance Coverage, 2012			
	HMO, PPO, POS		**HD (HSA)**	
Premium	**Single**	**Family**	**Single**	**Family**
Total premium	$5,559	$15,353	$4,793	$13,704
Employee pays	$ 962	$ 4,230	$ 723	$ 3,634
Deductible	$ 800	$ 1,500	$2,000	$ 3,600
Max (Stop Loss)	$2,200	$ 4,500	$4,000	$ 7,000
Percentage of all insured employees	83%		17%	

Source: Kaiser/HRET Employer Health Benefits Survey, http://www.kff.org

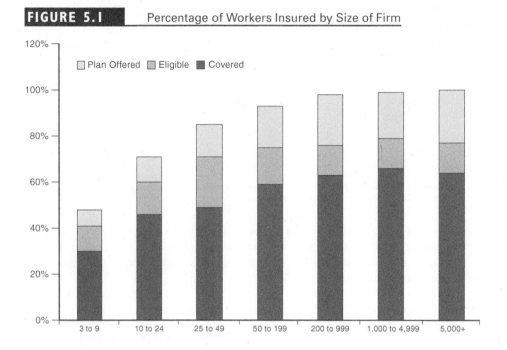

FIGURE 5.1   Percentage of Workers Insured by Size of Firm

home residents) are covered by Medicare, Medicaid, and other government programs and also because copays, coinsurance, and deductibles must be paid by patients out of pocket.

Medicare

Even though Medicare covers only 13 percent of the population, it is arguably the most important insurance plan in the United States because it pays the largest amount of money (more than $500 billion). Medicare sets a national standard, providing procedural definitions and payment levels used as references by hospitals, doctors, and private insurance companies in all 50 states to determine reimbursement. Created by Congress in 1965 to provide insurance for people older than 65 years and some people with disabilities, Medicare covered everyone in these categories and thereby overcame the adverse selection issues that made it so difficult for them as individuals to purchase private health insurance. A substantial portion of the money for Medicare comes from a tax of 2.9 percent on all wages, half paid by the employer and half paid by the employee, with the remainder coming from general tax revenues and premiums. Medicare financing thus redistributes resources from high-income wage earners to relatively needy elderly and disabled people with disproportionately large medical expenses (see Chapter 14).

Medicare is split into Part A (hospital), Part B (physician and outpatient services), and Part D (drugs). Although the specifics of coverage can be complex, clear and detailed descriptions of benefits are readily available at **www.medicare.gov**. Part A coverage is provided on application to people age 65 or older and to those entitled to Social Security Disability payments or patients with end-stage renal disease. To obtain Part B coverage, beneficiaries must pay a premium ($99.90 per month in 2012, or more if personal income is more than $85,000), which is supposed to cover a quarter of the actuarial cost but usually falls short because of the reluctance of politicians to offend groups that lobby for the elderly. Because Part B coverage is so heavily subsidized and Part A beneficiaries are usually enrolled unless they explicitly choose to opt out, almost all Medicare insureds (98 percent) have both Parts A and B. In addition, 88 percent of those with Medicare have supplemental "Medigap" insurance or "Medicare Advantage" plans that cover copayments, deductibles, drugs, and some other expenses (Table 5.3).[3]

TABLE 5.3   The Twelve Standard Medicare Supplement Plans

Basic Benefits must be included in all plans, and cover Part A coinsurance plus hospitalization for 365 days after Medicare benefits end; Part B coinsurance (generally 20% of Medicare-approved expenses) and copayments, and the first 3 pints of blood each year. Note that many people choose to purchase a comprehensive HMO benefit under the MEDICARE+CHOICE plan rather than Medigap insurance—you do not need both.

A	B	C	D	E	F*	G	H	I	J*
Basic benefits	Basic benefits	Basic benefits	Basic benefits	Basic benefits	Basic benefits	Basic benefits	Basic benefits	Basic benefits	Basic benefits
		Skilled nursing coinsurance	Skilled nursing coinsurance	Skilled nursing coinsurance	Skilled nursing coinsurance	Skilled nursing coinsurance	Skilled nursing coinsurance	Skilled nursing coinsurance	Skilled nursing coinsurance
	Medicare Part A deductible	Medicare Part A deductible	Medicare Part A deductible	Medicare Part A deductible	Medicare Part A deductible	Medicare Part A deductible	Medicare Part A deductible	Medicare Part A deductible	Medicare Part A deductible
		Medicare Part B deductible			Medicare Part B deductible				Medicare Part B deductible
					Medicare Part B excess charge (100%)	Medicare Part B excess charge (80%)		Medicare Part B excess charge (100%)	Medicare Part B excess charge (100%)
		Foreign travel emergency	Foreign travel emergency	Foreign travel emergency	Foreign travel emergency	Foreign travel emergency	Foreign travel emergency	Foreign travel emergency	Foreign travel emergency
			At-home recovery			At-home recovery		At-home recovery	At-home recovery
							Basic drug benefit ($1,250 Limit)	Basic drug benefit ($1,250 Limit)	Extended drug benefit ($3,000 Limit)
				Preventive care					Preventive care

*Plans F and J also have a high deductible option.

Note: Plans K and L offer lower premiums with higher out-of-pocket costs subject to an annual limit.

Source: 2002 Guide to Health Insurance for People with Medicare, CMS Publication No. 02110, www.medicare.gov.

Medicaid

Medicaid is actually fifty different state programs funded jointly by the states and the federal government to provide health insurance to those who are poor.[4] Although one could say that "Medicaid" is the largest category of health insurance because it covers more than 50 million people, the rules, benefits, and coverage vary so widely by state that it is hard to make generalizations. Depending on the state, Medicaid may be paying anywhere from 12 to 32 percent of total medical costs, with the federal government picking up half to 80 percent of the tab. Medicaid beneficiaries may have many options to choose from, or only one, and these health plans and programs may be statewide or limited to just a single area.

Initially designed to focus on the needs of small children and indigent mothers, much of Medicaid now pays for chronic illness and long-term care, and it has now become the major funding source for nursing homes. Many families who think they never need government benefits rely on Medicaid to keep Grandmother in a nursing home.

State Children's Health Insurance Program

The State Children's Health Insurance Program (SCHIP) was enacted by Congress in 1997 as Title XXI of the Social Security Act to provide $40 billion to increase coverage for the 10 million children younger than 18 years who were uninsured. However, the program works through state governments, and some have used available funding for other purposes, leading to great unevenness in implementation. Almost 5 million children eligible for SCHIP or Medicaid have not been enrolled. Less than 5 percent of children in Rhode Island, Connecticut, and Pennsylvania are uninsured, and almost 20 percent of children in Texas and New Mexico are left uninsured.[5] The fact that so many children are still uninsured reflects the choices made by the public and their elected representatives. In this regard, it is probably worth mentioning that children do not vote, and that the parents of poor children are much less likely to vote than the senior citizens who qualify for Medicare.

Other Government Programs and Charity

Charity paid for about $80 billion (3 percent) of health care in 2007. Workers' compensation, automobile accident insurance, and similar programs paid more than $25 billion. The Department of Veterans Affairs received $35 billion in funding, with a somewhat smaller amount being paid for dependents through the Department of Defense. Programs sponsored by the Maternal and Child Health Bureau, Substance Abuse and Mental Health Services Administration, Bureau of Indian Affairs, and a variety of other programs accounted for another $40 billion in health care. The government also provides a special tax break for families with very high medical costs (more than 7.5 percent of adjusted income).

The Uninsured

Despite the wide variety of health insurance plans, 50 million Americans (about 17 percent of the population) have no health insurance.[6] Uninsured persons needing care must try to pay with their own limited resources, find a special government program, depend on charity, or simply present themselves at a hospital or clinic and ask to be treated free of charge. The percentage of the population without coverage depends significantly on the efforts of local and state governments. States choosing expansive Medicaid programs and broad outreach to the working poor can reduce the number of uninsured individuals substantially. Wisconsin, Minnesota, Hawaii, and Massachusetts insure all but 8 percent of their citizens, whereas Texas leaves 24 percent of its population without insurance.

Although some uninsured persons pay large sums out of pocket when they get sick, a much greater number stay healthy and pocket the cash or, having no resources, depend on charity when they are ill. That is why the problem of the uninsured is so intractable. For many of the uninsured, not having insurance is a rational economic decision. Three fourths of the uninsured are younger than 35 years, and people this young tend to be healthy, to be enrolled in college, or to earn low wages. For them, paying $500 a month or even $50 a month for health insurance might not make sense.[7] People older than 35 who are working in low-paying jobs often need the money to eat and pay rent more than they need it to provide protection from uncertain medical bills that might never materialize. There are also a small number of people who are chronically ill and would not pass even a cursory medical exam and hence can be insured only if they take a job in a large firm that provides group coverage.

WHAT DO PEOPLE BUY WHEN THEY DON'T BUY HEALTH INSURANCE?

Most of the time, being uninsured is a matter of choice. It might not be a sensible choice or may be the result of a choice no one would want to face (buy the children food or buy health insurance), but it is a choice nonetheless. Knowing what people buy when they do not buy health insurance provides insight into their choice.

A study by Helen Levy and Thomas DeLeire from the University of Chicago indicates that what people buy with the money they save from not purchasing health insurance depends significantly on whether they are poor or relatively well off. According to the study, for people in the bottom quartile of the income distribution, the money they did not spend on health insurance went mostly toward food, rent, and other necessities. For people in the upper income quartile, the spending pattern was quite different: The largest type of spending increase was for transportation, specifically, for expensive used cars. The study indicates that programs trying to help people who are truly needy might inadvertently subsidize people who are uninsured simply because they want to spend on other things.

5.2 CONTRACTING AND PAYMENTS

Insurance Companies are Financial Intermediaries

A health insurance company is a financial intermediary. It makes money from transactions: collecting premiums, pricing risk, negotiating payments, pooling and investing funds. Health insurance does not "pay" for medical care any more than a bank "pays" a depositor's rent or utilities. Ultimately, it is people who pay, either through taxes, reduced wages, or cash out of pocket. The random loss due to severe illness that is financially ruinous to an individual patient is, in the big picture, of minor importance to an insurance company. So long as the insurer collects premiums from enough enrollees, correctly priced, it will consistently earn a share. "Risk" to an insurance company looks something like it does to a credit-card firm or a casino: Losses are a regular part of business, and what the house earns is a percentage.

Risk Bearing: From Fixed Premiums to Self-Insurance

Third-party health insurance has two functions: risk pooling and purchasing care. In the simple case where insurance is sold to individuals, the insurance company does both. However, a large employer already has a pooled group (employees) and can take premiums directly out of their paychecks, and hence it can take over these marketing functions to reduce costs. Indeed, if

FIGURE 5.2	Range of Insurance Contracts			

Insurer Bears Risk, ←——————————————————————————————→ Employer Bears Risk,
Processes Claims   Processes Own Claims

Fixed Premiums	Experience Related	Retention Ratio	ASO	Self-Insurance
Pay preset amount for coverage	Premiums changed each year to reflect last year's actual claims	If losses are less than expected, insurer gives back part of premium	Administrative services only, insurance company pays claims using the firms own funds	Firm pays claims, acts as their own insurance company

the employee group is large enough, the employer does not need any risk-pooling financial protection but only someone to work with the hospital and pay medical bills.

The range of risk bearing arrangements, from pure insurance at one end to an employer who does everything in-house (self-insured) at the other is depicted in Figure 5.2. An employer can purchase insurance at a fixed price and bear no risk, or it can pool its own funds, handle all claims, and self-insure while bearing all risks. In between these two options there are a range of contracts that split the risk and claims-processing burden: experience rated, retention ratio, minimum premium, and ASO plans. Negotiating a premium for the group can be a problem. **Experience rating** allows the group premium to rise or fall to match the amount during the previous year (total paid for all claims by employees, or "experience") and thus avoids costly and contentious haggling. A **retention ratio agreement** makes a similar adjustment, but in the current year. The employer and insurer estimate losses, and if claims turn out to be smaller than expected, the insurer returns most of the difference, retaining only a percentage (the retention ratio) for administrative expenses and profit.

Two things make it difficult for an employer to act as its own insurance company: catastrophic losses and claims processing. To some extent these difficulties can be ameliorated through contractual arrangements. Economies of scale in risk bearing can be obtained contractually through **reinsurance**, which is a type of major medical coverage for employers, a policy for the group as a whole that covers 90 percent of the cost of any individual above a specified amount (say $50,000) or an aggregate loss of the group as a whole that is above the expected value (say above $5 million). Of course, reinsurance is quite costly; therefore, coverage is usually purchased for extraordinary losses only. Claims processing is apt to create administrative difficulties, because a company is usually better at its own line of business than at the business of managing and paying insurance benefits. Economies of scale in claims processing can be obtained contractually through **administered services only** (ASO) contracts in which an insurance company processes the bills, pays the claims, and settles disputes for a set fee per year or per claim, but the funds for paying benefits come directly from the employer.[8]

Purchasing Medical Care For Groups

Financing health care with insurance fundamentally changes the flow of funds and business models of hospitals, physicians, pharmacies, nursing homes, and other health care providers. The contract is made by an insurance company, even though it is patients who are receiving the care and government or employers paying most of the costs. Later chapters take up each of the various provider types in detail, so only basic and common elements will be touched upon here. Payments by insurance companies to purchase care from providers can be categorized as follows:

Provider Payment Methods

- **Fee-for-service (FFS) charges:** Provider sets price for each item.
- **Bundled:** A single price for a package of services. For example, heart transplant and recovery; cancer treatment including surgery, drugs, and radiation; labor and delivery
- **Capitation:** Single price, usually *per member per month* (**PMPM**), for services. For example, gatekeeper physicians paid $20 to $50 PMPM for each patient choosing them for all primary care office visits; a laboratory contractor paid $3 PMPM for all lab testing
- **Carve out:** A subset of services (e.g., mental health, lab testing) is "carved out" and given to another provider or subcontractor, often on a capitation basis.
- **Administered:** Price per unit is set in advance by government. For example, cardiac catheterization is paid $23,391; follow-up office visit for flu, less than 15 minutes, is $61, and so on
- **Negotiated:** Contract between payer and provider, with simple or complex terms, where the financial arrangement is stated however the two parties agree.

Providers are economic organizations that must be able to meet a budget and maybe make a profit. Therefore they must adjust to the flow of revenues available. In 1960, Medicare and Medicaid did not exist, less than half of hospital funding came from insurance, and most of that was paid on the basis of fee-for-service charges through community Blue Cross plans or commercial indemnity insurance. Today, Medicare is the largest source of revenues, about 90 percent of hospital revenues come from insurance, and almost all private payments are made through negotiated payments that involve some form of managed care. The change in revenue sources for physicians is similar, but not quite as extreme (Medicare is 22 percent rather than 35 percent in hospitals, and insurance covers 80 percent rather than 90 percent). The system has changed, and it is still in the process of changing (see Chapter 18). Hospitals and physicians, which were mostly independent businesses setting their own prices back in the 1950s, are now part of a complex system that is not exactly led by the government but is dominated by administered and regulated insurance payments.

Medical Loss Ratios

Insurers usually take 15 to 20 percent of the premiums they receive for administration, marketing, and profit, with the bulk of the funds used to pay medical expenses. This fraction is known as the "**medical loss ratio**" (see Table 5.4). The largest expense category is physician services. Although hospitals are the largest expenditure item in the National Health Expenditure accounts (see Chapter 1), tight managed-care controls, favorable pricing, and coverage of a generally

TABLE 5.4	Medical Loss Ratio (% of Premium)	
Physician and outpatient	41%	
Inpatient	31%	"Medical loss ratio" = 82%
Outside referrals	7%	
Emergency	3%	
Administrative	13%	
Profit	5%	
Total Premium	100%	

younger and healthier population mean that less than a third of premiums are used to pay for inpatient hospital services. Some other expenses are reinsurance (to keep small plans solvent and ensure that patients' bills are paid even if the plans should have a catastrophic loss), taxes, emergency out-of-area services, and certain highly specialized treatments that must be paid for on a fee-for-service basis to noncontracted providers. Over time, health insurance has become fairly competitive. Administrative expenses and profit margins have been cut as plans become more efficient; therefore, the percentage of total dollars going to treatment (the medical loss ratio) has risen. In earlier years, wide variations of ±25 percent were not uncommon. With more experience and better information, competitive standards have been set so that most insurers offer a similar price (perhaps ±10 percent) for similar benefit packages. The Affordable Care Act of 2010 specifies that starting in 2014, all health insurance must pay out at least 80 percent of premiums for medical bills.

Claim Processing

Paying medical bills is a massive task. Even the government outsources claims processing. Although the fee schedule and format for "Medicare" billing is nationally regulated, the actual billing is handled regionally by large Blue Cross and commercial insurance plans rather than government employees. Standardized processing can be made very efficient. However, there are so many millions of bills paid that collecting even $1 or $0.50 for each claim is a lucrative business. Originally every provider created its own bills, causing much confusion and increasing administrative costs. The major processors now enforce electronic submission according to standardized formats for almost all medical insurance claims. Indeed, the rules and formulas (and exceptions and offsets) are now so complex that it would be virtually impossible to determine how much to pay for each bill without modern information technology.

The provider's fee-for-service charges are sent to the insurance company and reported to the patient in the **explanation of benefits (EOB)** letter but might have little or no effect on how much is actually paid. Uninsured persons or insurance companies with no provider contract (see below) would be liable for the full charges, which are usually 20 percent to 400 percent higher than Medicare and Medicaid are paying. That is one reason almost all insurance has contracts with providers to purchase care rather than simply reimbursing the bills, as was done under indemnity insurance (see "Provider Networks and Legal Structure" in Section 5.4).

The Underwriting Cycle

In the long run, the increases in premiums match the increases in underlying health care costs. However, in any given year the rate of increase could be higher or lower. Economists have observed that most insurance markets (e.g., property and casualty, malpractice, health) tend to have a cycle of overcharging and undercharging that lasts about 7 to 10 years.[9] At the peak of the cycle, premiums are high relative to costs, profits are fat, and competitors are attracted to start the cycle. As more insurance companies enter the market, premiums are driven downward. In the trough of the cycle, rates are low as insurance companies compete vigorously to gain market share. The lack of profitability eventually takes a toll, some insurance companies exit the market, and rates increase. Eventually, rising prices and good profits start the cycle over again.

Figure 5.3 shows how premiums and costs have risen and fallen since 1988. At the beginning of the 1990s, hefty double-digit premium increases built profitability. The rise of managed care and the overhanging threat of government intervention kept medical costs fairly low in the middle of the decade, but insurers trying to get a larger piece of the market drove premiums down below costs. The combination of low premiums and rising costs crushed profits, pushing several HMOs and insurance companies to the edge of insolvency. The years 2000 to 2004 were

FIGURE 5.3   The "Underwriting Cycle" of Health Insurance 1988–2011

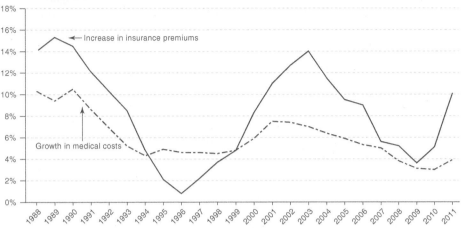

Source: Kaiser/HRET survey of employer health benefits and U.S. National Health Accounts.

catch-up time, with insurers once again trying to build reserves. After that, premiums started to fall, bottoming out in 2009. Since then, premiums and profits have once again been rising.

ERISA, Taxes, and Mandated Benefits

The benefits offered by a company are determined largely by competitive conditions in the labor market as the company tries to hire new workers or through negotiations with the unions that represent the workers. Companies view benefits as a way to retain workers, and workers view benefits as a way to protect themselves against losses. The interests of both companies and workers are represented in the final outcome.

Sometimes a broader public interest is imposed in the form of **mandated benefits**, regulations promulgated by the government stating that specific benefits (e.g., substance abuse treatment, AZT treatment for HIV infection) must be provided. If such benefits are a good thing, why don't they arise naturally in the course of competitive contracting? Consider the case of substance abuse benefits. Without such benefits, insurance will pay for treatment of liver damage, but not for treatment of the excessive drinking that caused it. From a social perspective, it is much more efficient to treat the underlying cause (alcoholism) than to treat just the symptom (liver damage). However, a company is not interested in the productivity of society as a whole but in the productivity of its workforce. A quite reasonable profit-maximizing response to alcoholism is to fire the employee and push him or her out onto the streets, where the burden is borne by the rest of society. Adverse selection can also play a role. A company with especially generous benefits for HIV/AIDS treatment will find its premiums going higher and higher as more chronically ill people try to get jobs there. Eventually, if adverse selection is severe enough, only people with a very high risk of HIV/AIDS would be willing to accept the low wages paid by this company in order to get the benefits.

Mental illness poses similar problems of adverse selection because the benefits are highly concentrated, with most of the dollars spent on just a few people, who, with their families, are much more aware of the risks than the insurance company. In a competitive market, insurance contracts reflect the interests of companies and most employees but not society as a whole. If such benefits are not mandatory, only a few companies will offer them.

Insurance is primarily regulated by the states. Some states, such as Arizona, impose very few mandates, while Massachusetts has more than thirty. Employers operating in multiple states need uniform national laws because it is difficult to maintain many different sets of benefit plans and give more or less to an employee depending on place of residence. Under the **Employee Retirement and Income Security Act of 1974 (ERISA)** and later amendments, self-insured firms are regulated under national ERISA rules and thus are exempt from state mandates. Because only large firms are able to self-insure, the attempt to increase coverage through mandates might have the paradoxical effect of reducing the number of people insured, as small firms opt to provide no health insurance at all.

State taxes provide another incentive to self-insure. Most states impose a premium tax of 1 to 2 percent that can be avoided through self-insurance or ASO contracts. Minimum premium plans in which the employer pays the first $X million (usually about 90 percent of estimated losses) and the insurer pays the rest exist primarily to avoid state taxes, because they are no different from fixed-premium full insurance with regard to risk or claims processing. Several innovative state health care financing plans have been challenged under ERISA. For example, New Jersey funded a special program for the uninsured through a 30 percent surcharge on all hospital bills. After large companies won ERISA exemption, only small employers and individuals were left paying the surcharge; therefore, the state was forced to dismantle its program.[10]

If mandated benefits are a good idea, why don't the states just pay for them? The answer is that they would have to raise taxes to do so. A mandated benefit, although it operates like a tax on firms, is counted as a regular cost of business to the firm. It does not appear on the government's budget and thus is not recognized by many voters. It seems as if the bills are being paid with *other people's money*. Although the public ultimately will lose more in forgone wages than in taxes avoided, this fact is not obvious to voters when they go to the polls. For this reason, any national insurance plan enacted in the United States is likely to be based on employer contributions. People who would never vote to increase taxes to fund national health insurance will calmly vote to have government insist that every employer provide benefits—and so our government will rationally follow the path of least resistance.

Other People's Money: Rising Costs and Mediocre Results

Insurance breaks the link between receiving care and paying for it. When a young driver is in a bad car accident, spends 22 days in intensive care, and requires three operations, these high costs are spread over a large group of people by his parents' insurance plan and also by charging most other patients in the hospital a bit extra. If he were uninsured, the care would be "free" only in the sense that he did not have an insurance card. Either way, most of the money comes from someone else. When Uncle Joe gets a heart transplant, Medicare funds are used by Blue Cross, Aetna, or some other third-party administrator to pay the bills; Medicare gets its funds from the 1.45 percent taken out of the paycheck at your summer job, as well as all sorts of other taxes, and then there is a small out-of-pocket contribution from Uncle Joe or his family.

Insurance does not pay for medical care; it prices risks and pools funds so that the bills can be paid more efficiently. "*Health*" insurance is somewhat of a misnomer. It is actually medical bills, rather than health, that are insured. This can be a problem. As with most purchases, you get what you pay for (more medical bills) but not much of what is not paid for (better health). If the procedure is billable, there is an incentive to provide it. There might even be too much of an incentive, because we are talking thousands and millions of dollars. Conversely, if giving better care does not produce a billable event, there is no financial reward for doing so. Hence the "aspirin and angioplasty" paradox discussed in Chapter 2: Each angioplasty provides payment of $5,000, whereas reminding a patient to take daily aspirin tablets, although valuable, takes time and provides no payments.

Traditional employer indemnity insurance, Medicare and Medicaid, were open-ended **entitlement** systems. Patients had no reason to worry about money.[11] As can be seen from

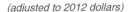

FIGURE 5.4   Real Per Capita Health Spending by Source 1960–2012

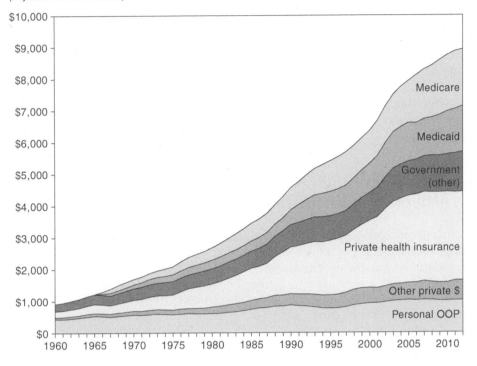

(adjusted to 2012 dollars)

Figure 5.4, almost all of the increase in costs came from more third-party spending, also called "other people's money." Fifty years ago, patients paid 2.5 percent of their average earnings out of pocket for medical care and insurance, whereas today the percentage is down to 2.0 percent ($147 out of $2,800 earned in 1960 compared to $1,019 out of $50,000 earnings in 2012). Because health care takes 18 percent of national income, most of the money must come from non-patient funds, through third-party payments.

Hospitals, doctors, and insurers, as recipients of funds, actually benefited from the increased spending, but businesses providing health insurance to employees were hurt. Health benefits took just 3.1 percent of compensation in 1970 but more than doubled to 8.4 percent in 2011.[12] The value of health benefits, equal to 36 percent of after-tax profits in 1970 and 43 percent in 1980, exceeded 108 percent of total corporate profits by 1990 and continued to soar over the next 20 years. Businesses became increasingly willing to turn to an outside contractor that could stabilize benefit costs, even if it meant having to accept some constraints and employee complaints. Premiums for regular Blue Cross and Blue Shield coverage rose as much as 30 percent a year in many markets during the early 1980s, and by 2010 indemnity insurance had become unaffordable and almost extinct (less than 1 percent of the market).

In a system characterized by a lack of financial restraints, it is not surprising that the United States was spending far more on health care than any other country in the world (Chapter 16); the surprise was how little health the nation was able to buy with all the extra money spent. Despite years of insistence by politicians and physicians that the United States had the best medical care in the world, there is scant evidence that the additional expenditures led to improvements in longevity, infant mortality, morbidity, or days lost from work relative to other countries spending less than half as much per person.[13] Instead, the United States ranks in the middle or lower end of the pack on most measures of health status and life expectancy.

The disparity between what Americans pay and their health status, relative to other advanced economies, is discussed at length in Chapter 16, "International Comparisons of Health and Health Expenditures," and suggests that health insurance reforms could lead to significant cost and value efficiencies.

What has become apparent is that the real inflation-adjusted hourly wages of workers have stagnated, or even declined, while the cost per hour of employer-provided health benefits has soared, that the federal government has been burdened by billions of dollars in deficits attributable to the soaring cost of Medicare, and that 50 million Americans are still uninsured. In attempting to reduce costs while improving quality of care, insurance contracts have been modified to increase demand-side patient cost sharing, to intensify supply-side provider management, or to find some combination that will be both effective and acceptable in the marketplace.

5.3 CONSUMER-DRIVEN HEALTH PLANS: HIGH DEDUCTIBLES AND HEALTH SAVINGS ACCOUNTS

The economic concept behind "consumer-directed" or consumer-driven health plans (**CDHP**) is that if patients have to pay enough of the bill, they will shop for lower prices and not use services wastefully, thus driving price competition and lowering the total costs of care. To create these incentives, patients must take "ownership" rather than escape the burdens of cost and decision making through insurance. Details of the various CDHP plans are somewhat fluid, but certain core elements are common[14]:

- Patients pay most small and medium medical expenses on their own.
- There is a high deductible (>$2,000) "catastrophic" coverage for major illness and costly care.
- HSA or similar tax-advantaged savings account is offered, which can only be used for medical expenses but can be invested and saved from year-to-year, hopefully growing large enough over time to cover major unanticipated losses.
- Employer contribution is limited to a specified dollar amount.

SAMPLE CONSUMER-DRIVEN PLAN (CDHP/HD-HSA)

Employer: Contributes $100 (before tax) per month and provides catastrophic major medical insurance that pays 90 percent of all expenses above $5,000 in a calendar year.
Employee: Pays all bills, first using money in his or her HSA, and when that is gone, uses own money for the rest up to $5,000 and 10 percent of all bills in excess of $5,000. Any savings left over earns interest and may be used for major illness or retirement.

Ninety percent of the under-65 population has medical expenses of less than $1,800 per year, and therefore a **high deductible (HD)** keeps most of them from submitting any claims. Their modest medical expenses can be paid from a **health savings account (HSA)** funded with pre-tax dollars so as to give them a subsidy equivalent to that provided by employer-paid benefits. If the person does have a major illness, the catastrophic plan protects them. If the person stays healthy, the investments in the HSA can grow tax-free and be used to supplement retirement benefits.[15]

HSAs, MSAs, and other consumer-directed plans based on high-deductible catastrophic insurance have become popular with employers as a way of cutting costs while continuing to offer coverage, yet they attract less than 15 percent of the market—mostly younger, healthier, and wealthier employees and dependents who are the least difficult to cover.[16] In part this is because the cost of insurance is reduced by having the patient pay more through deductibles, copays, and coinsurance. Demand-side cost sharing is painless until a person gets injured or sick, but then it hurts more and more as more care is needed.

Defined Contribution Health Plans

The cost of health care has created major problems for American industry. General Motors has been called "a health-insurance plan for retired auto-workers with a side business that tries to make and sell enough cars to pay the premiums." Rising health care costs have contributed to bankruptcies in all sorts of manufacturing, as well as airlines and some service industries. Employers have begun to get out of the business of providing pensions by replacing them with defined-contribution 401(k) retirement plans, and many would like to get out from under the responsibility of paying for ever-higher health care costs by making a fixed payment (defined contribution) of perhaps $400 or $800 per month. In this way, the responsibility for rising costs is shifted to the employees, who "own" their own health plan, just as they own a 401(k). This shifting of responsibility is clearly counted as a strength by employers, but it may be considered a weakness by employees, who could see even more of their future wage increases used to pay rising premiums or out-of-pocket medical expenses.

5.4 MANAGED CARE

Concern for rising cost has driven the evolution of health insurance plans over the last 50 years, slowly driving open-ended indemnity fee-for-service insurance to extinction. Unlike consumer-directed plans, where the task of cost control is placed on patients, managed care works with doctors, hospitals, and management to directly reduce the cost of care— to make both the production and allocation of medical services more efficient. Rather than making patients more sensitive to (and burdened by) price, these supply-side management controls reduce the cost directly.

Closed-Panel Group Practice HMOs

During the period 1930 to 1960 as health insurance spread across the United States, there were a few organizations (Kaiser, Group Health Cooperative, United Mine Workers) that integrated hospitals, physicians, and insurance within a single organization to provide comprehensive medical care, charging one monthly premium for all services (**capitation**) rather than separate prices for each visit or procedure. Although few, such **prepaid closed-panel group practice** plans were admired by many experts as offering coordinated care that was more efficient and less expensive than the fragmented system of private insurance with separate hospitals and independent physicians (see Chapter 10). To increase popular appeal, such plans were marketed as **health maintenance organizations (HMOs),** claiming that prepaid HMO plans benefitted financially by keeping patients healthy, while fee-for-service payments to hospitals and doctors under regular insurance created an incentive to give more treatment to sicker patients.

In this era, most Blue Cross/Blue Shield and commercial plans paid for all services at any hospital or physician (an "open" plan) with relatively minor coinsurance and copayments. In contrast, the closed-panel group practice HMO was "closed:" only members of the HMO who paid the monthly capitation were allowed to use the facility, the physicians treated only members of the HMO and worked on salary, the hospitals and clinics were owned by the HMO, and all of the drugs and supplies were purchased by the HMO. **A single entity** (a "closed HMO") **combined all the complex functions of providing and paying for medical care.**

Because a prepaid closed HMO offers a package rather than a set of parts, there are no meaningful prices and quantities and no distinction between insurance overhead and clinical management. It is like getting a package trip to Cancun rather than paying separately for airfare, hotels, meals, excursions, taxis, and a travel agent's fee. The challenge for a closed-HMO is to keep premiums low and satisfaction high; the itemized prices and quantities fade out of existence and relevance. Management and operations tend to be easier and cheaper because all the HMO doctors, nurses, technicians, and administrators work only for that HMO; they do not have to try to understand or accommodate the rules and procedures of other insurance plans, nor do the patients. In a regular community hospital, each doctor might have a different method for closing a wound during surgery, prefer a different type of bandage or topical ointment, use different terms when making notes in a patient chart, and have a different judgment as to whether a particular test result was "moderately high" or "serious." In a closed HMO, the head of surgery or medical director is the boss, able to hire and fire the medical staff—not a senior volunteering for the post who might or might not be highly regarded or listened to by the other doctors. Furthermore, many of the HMO doctors did their medical residency in the HMO, making them trained in the system and ready to comply with the approved clinical procedures.

The potential for organizational change to reconfigure consumption can perhaps best be grasped through a familiar example: music. For 200 years, people have listened to string quartets performing Brahms's compositions. To perform a 20-minute piece, it takes four musicians playing 20 minutes each (and practicing for years) to bring music to the audience. Whether it is 1710 or 2010, it still takes four musicians and 20 minutes. There is little room to cut price (musicians have never been all that well paid), and playing the entire prelude in 15 minutes is not a satisfactory way to achieve efficiency. However, focusing on the needs of the consumers rather than the producers reveals a new way, and a new organization: a recording company. The performance can be played around the world (OK, so it is not quite as good as being there) for a per-person cost that is a fraction of the four musicians' hourly wages. Indeed, once the music is digitized and placed on a compact disc, a person can listen to it at home, in the car, or at a picnic dinner on the beach rather inexpensively. If the revolution in musical consumption seems exceedingly far-fetched as an analogy, consider the health effects of smallpox vaccination, sanitation, heart pacemakers, and the Internet on the practice of medicine between 1910 and 2010.

Although structured organizations offer great potential for savings and quality improvement, they are hard to create or to replicate. There are parts of California where 10 percent to 20 percent of the insured population, and sometimes as much as 50 percent, are in closed HMOs. However, most states outside of the West still do not have any closed HMOs. In 1970 less than 5 percent of the privately insured population were in closed HMOs, and today the fraction is still under 5 percent, although the seeds of organizational change have spread widely through what has become known as "managed care."

IPA-HMOs and Open Contracts

In the areas where closed HMOs were popular, local doctors and hospitals had responded to the competitive threat by developing contractual entities known as "open HMOs" or independent practice associations (IPAs). In this way, employers and employees of a local firm could be offered a health plan that mimicked Kaiser: comprehensive care at a single fixed price per month (capitation). The associated hospitals and doctors used the contract to create a provider network, and so long as the patient used services within the network, there was no additional charge.

Hospital costs rose rapidly in the 1960s. The federal government thought it was facing a financial crisis when national health expenditures exceeded 7 percent of GDP. The bipartisan HMO Act of 1973, passed with the strong support of Senator Kennedy and President Nixon, set up grants and incentives to foster the growth of HMOs, required companies with more than 25 employees to offer an HMO plan as an option, and made the definition broad enough to

TABLE 5.5	Hypothetical PPO Payment	
Benefit	**Within Network**	**Outside Provider**
Hospital	100%	80%
Physician	90%	75%
Therapist	90%	50%
Pharmacies	No copay	$10 copay
Drugs		
In formulary	Covered	50%
Not in formulary	Not covered	Not covered

include IPA open HMOs. Growth was explosive. The number of people enrolled in HMOs rose from 3 million in 1970 to 9 million in 1980, 36 million in 1990, and 77 million in 2010.[17] However, almost all of this growth came in the form of open contractual HMOs created by Blue Cross/Blue Shield and commercial insurance companies, rather than Kaiser or other closed HMO organizations.

The first step in building an open HMO or other less restrictive **managed-care organization** is to make contracts with hospitals and physicians, forming a **provider network**, because an insurer can only exert control over an independent doctor or hospital if there is a contract between them. Patients desiring a little extra freedom of choice could enroll in a **preferred provider organization** (**PPO**) plan, which would allow them to occasionally use outside physicians or hospitals by paying extra (Table 5.5). Point-of-service (**POS**) plans are similar, but they have even fewer limits.

As the structure became less integrated and restrictive, it was less able to contain costs. The monitoring and control functions that had previously been carried out internally by management were replaced by a number of external procedures and contractual stipulations that are now known collectively as "managed care." Under a **gatekeeper** system, patients must receive all their primary care from a single physician, and any specialists, surgery, prescriptions, or hospitalization must be approved in advance. In this way, the plan is able to delegate responsibility for cost control and appropriateness to the gatekeeper **primary care physician** (PCP). A written **referral** signed by the PCP must be obtained before seeing a specialist, getting an x-ray, or being admitted to the hospital. **Preadmission testing** as an outpatient might be required in order to reduce the number of days in the hospital. Once the patient is admitted, the plan might call for **concurrent review** by a case management nurse every three days to make sure that the patient should not be sent home or transferred to a less-expensive bed in a nursing home. Before ordering surgery, the plan might require **precertification** that an operation was necessary, and perhaps it might also require a **second opinion** from another doctor before approving the procedure. After discharge, the patient might be limited to choice of drugs from a **formulary** or be required to pay extra to use a brand name rather than the equivalent generic (see box "Managing Pharmacy Costs").

Managed Care Contract Provisions

Some of the interventions used to control cost and utilization include the following:

- **Primary care provider (PCP):** A single doctor, clinic, or group practice has a contract with the plan and is chosen by the patient to provide all of their general medical care.
- **Referral:** A doctor is required to sign a form in advance before the patient can obtain certain kinds of care.
- **Gatekeeping:** Referrals are required for most nonprimary care, usually requiring authorization from the PCP.

- **Capitation:** A fixed amount is paid per member per month (PMPM) for a specified set of services. A PCP gatekeeper is often paid $25 to $45 for each person on their list, a large laboratory might receive $3 PMPM, and sometimes even specialty services (mental health, cardiac surgery) are capitated.

- **Carve-outs:** A subcontract is provided for a specified kind of services such a physical therapy, mental health, laboratory, diagnostic x-ray, or heart surgery.

- **Withholds:** Some of the budget for a carved-out service is held back to and paid only if the total bills stay under a specified amount. For example, the physical therapist might get 80 percent of agreed payment per visit, receiving the rest only if the total physical therapy bills were less than $2 million for the year.

- **Second opinion:** A second doctor must review the record and concur with the initial doctor's recommendation before surgery is performed.

- **Precertification:** Approval must be obtained in advance from the insurance company before elective surgery is performed.

- **Preadmission testing:** Many tests must be performed in advance on an outpatient basis so the patient spends fewer days in the hospital.

- **Concurrent review:** Regular evaluations are made by a case-control nurse to authorize a continued stay in the hospital or additional procedures.

- **Generic substitution:** A prescription for a brand-name drug is filled with a cheaper generic version if the two are deemed equivalent by the FDA.

- **Database profiling:** Graphs and charts indicating the number of services used per 1,000 patients by each doctor or hospital are maintained to identify abnormally high or low patterns of utilization.

- **Intensive case management:** A nurse in the insurance company follows and manages any case expected to cost more than $10,000.

- **Discharge planning:** A social worker meets with the patient and family early to facilitate rapid transfer back home or to a nursing home.

- **Retrospective review:** An evaluation is conducted after the patient is discharged from the hospital to deny payment for any medically unnecessary services.

- **Audits:** An insurance company representative ensures that all services billed for were actually performed.

MANAGING PHARMACY COSTS: CARVE-OUTS AND TRIPLE-TIER BENEFITS

In the past, Medicare and most employer indemnity insurance plans did not pay for the cost of pharmaceuticals taken by patients outside the hospital. Outpatient drugs were fairly inexpensive, billing information was hard to obtain, and therefore benefits were limited. As the cost of pharmaceuticals rose and information systems expanded, it became easier and more valuable to provide prescription coverage. It is now common for employer plans to have a pharmaceutical component, and Medicare has added drug coverage as "Part D." Yet dispensing prescriptions is sufficiently different from other types of medical services that most insurance companies subcontract with specialized firms called pharmacy benefit managers (PBMs). Thus, it is actually the PBM (not Blue Cross or Aetna) that processes the claims and pays the pharmacy. Drugs have become a carve-out benefit because the PBMs can do the job better and at lower cost.

How do PBMs manage care to save costs? First, they obtain **rebates** (payments for volume) and **price discounts**. PBMs are large, handling millions of prescriptions a year, and

(Continued)

MANAGING PHARMACY COSTS: CARVE-OUTS AND TRIPLE-TIER BENEFITS (CONTINUED)

can use their market power at both ends: manufacturing (pharmaceutical companies) and retail (pharmacy chains). Second, they can use **substitution.** A study showed that mandatory generic substitution (MGS) reduced average costs by 8 percent.[18] In such a contract, the insurance only pays for the generic version of a drug if the Food and Drug Administration (FDA) has deemed it equivalent to the more expensive brand-name version, regardless of how the prescription is written. Although 8 percent might not seem like a lot, it is larger than the profit margins in most retail businesses.

More sophisticated contracts divide drugs into tiers to provide incentives for patients to actively cooperate in **reducing the use** of expense drugs. In the three-tier plan shown here, the most favored tier 1 drugs have only a $2 copayment. These are generic versions of expensive brand-name drugs or brands for which the PBM has negotiated a large discount or rebate. Tier 2, with $10 copayments, is made up of drugs on an approved list (formulary): drugs with no generic equivalent, drugs with small discounts, and the like. Tier 3, in which patients face a hefty $30 copayment, is reserved for the expensive brand-name drugs that have a generic equivalent in tier 1, drugs of limited usefulness, drugs that are often prescribed for off-label (i.e., not approved by the FDA) purposes, or expensive drugs whose benefits seem relatively minor (Viagra, COX-2 inhibitor, and low-dose antihistamines might fall into this tier).

Triple-Tier Drug Benefit Plan

Category	Patient Copayment	Types of Drugs
Tier 1	$ 2	Generics, sole source
Tier 2	$10	Approved formulary
Tier 3	$30	Off-patent brands, lifestyle

Tiered pharmacy benefit plans were relatively rare a decade ago but are now found in 85 percent of large employee health insurance plans.[19] They have been shown to reduce total costs by increasing rates of generic substitution and by (slightly) reducing the number of prescriptions filled. What may be even more important to employers, though, is that they provide a relatively simple way of shifting more of the cost to the employee (all those copayments add up). Indeed, dissatisfaction with large and repeated copayments make the integrated CPGP HMO solution, in which the HMO has an in-house pharmacy and uses salaried pharmacists to distribute drugs, look more attractive, and it is one reason for the sudden influx of veterans who have other insurance plans moving into the Department of Veterans Affairs (VA) health system.

The Range of Managed Care Contracts: POS, PPO, HMO

Managed care contracts are too diverse for any single definition. It is better to think in terms of a range from unmanaged to tightly managed, as illustrated in Figure 5.5. At one extreme, under FFS medicine with indemnity insurance, the health plan takes all the financial risk but

FIGURE 5.5   Range of Managed Care Plans

Indemnity FFS	POS	PPO	Open HMO	Closed HMO

No management controls ←——————————————————→ *Tight management controls*

exercises no medical management. Whatever hospitalization, surgery, or drugs any physician decides to order are paid for by the insurance company without question. There is no haggling over prices. Any difference between premiums and expenses becomes a gain or loss to the insurance company but has no effect on the hospital or physician. The only "control" comes from making the patient pay for some deductibles, coinsurance, or excess over the plan maximums. At the other end is the closed HMO, in which a single organization combines the functions of medical provider and insurance company. It enrolls members; builds hospitals; employs physicians, nurses, and therapists on salary; purchases drugs, beds, cardiac pacemakers, and so on; and controls all finances. Any difference between premiums and expenses is a gain or loss to be shared with the physician group.[20] In between these two ends are a range of contracts that link medicine and insurance but do not combine them into a single organization. A preferred provider organization (**PPO**) limits the patient's choice of physicians and hospitals by paying in full (or a larger percentage) only for care received from approved providers within the network. Patients can choose to see a physician outside the network or to stay in a hospital that is not part of the preferred group if they are willing to pay a larger portion of the bill (see Table 5.5). A point-of-service (**POS**) plan is typically even looser, still having lower patient payments for in-network care but not requiring a gatekeeper, referrals, preadmission testing, or approvals for hospital admission. Many large insurers now offer **triple-option** plans, in which the enrollee can chose the HMO, the PPO, or "unlimited" insurance, with the premium increasing in steps as the controls over utilization become weaker.

The terms POS, PPO, and HMO are not standardized, and the differences can vary. For example, Independence Blue Cross in Philadelphia has a set of relatively unrestricted contracts ("personal choice") and a more restrictive set ("Keystone HMO"). Both are administered out of the same office and cover most of the same doctors and hospitals, but the Keystone HMO plans require referrals from the primary doctor, more often limit the choice of specialty care providers, and can require prior approval from Blue Cross for diagnostic procedures or hospital admission. Note also that the "Keystone HMO" for firefighters is not the same as it is for teachers or for employees of Tasty Baking: the coverage details depend upon the specific contract, which can differ widely from one employer to another.

Management: The Distinctive Feature of Managed Care

The fundamental difference between traditional fee-for-service (FFS) medical practice under indemnity insurance and managed care is that a **manager** with financial responsibility intervenes to monitor and control the transaction between doctor and patient (Figure 5.6).[21] An outside party, such as the plan medical director, a trained utilization review nurse, or a software program, identifies care that is potentially at variance with accepted clinical practice. This may be done through a statistical profile of each physician's practice, assessment of laboratory testing, a review of individual cases, or a combination of techniques. The manager examines the process of care and controls the flow of funds, facilitating payments in some circumstances and holding back in others. To remain viable, the managed care organization must compete on the basis of both cost and quality. A delicate balance must be maintained among expenditure control, administrative process, and medical uncertainty.

Figure 5.6 illustrates in simplified fashion the structural difference between (a) pure indemnity (insurer reimburses patient, not provider, and exercises no control over clinical matters), (b) contractual managed care, and (c) pure prepaid group practice closed HMOs (insurer and provider are integrated in same organization).

Provider Networks and Legal Structure

Under pure indemnity insurance, the contract is solely between the patient and the insurance company. Upon evidence of loss (a bill), the insurance company sends a check to the patient,

FIGURE 5.6   Flow of Funds with Managed Care

(a) Pure indemnity insurance
    (2 separate two-party transactions)

(b) Closed PPGP HMO
    (1 two-party transaction with integrated
    insurance/provider)

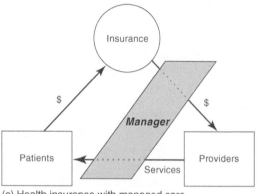

(c) Health insurance with managed care
    (3+ party transaction)

who is responsible for all relationships with the providers. A managed care organization arises when the insurance company begins to make contracts with physicians and hospitals, forming a network of providers. A participating provider network, also called a preferred provider organization or PPO, is a contractual intermediary: A corporate entity created by a group of doctors, an entrepreneur, a hospital chain, a union, an employer coalition, or the insurer links group of providers (the network) so that all can be negotiated with under a single contract.[22] It has procedures to certify providers (check license validity, meet standards, produce reports and statistics) and set specifications for reimbursement (per diems, discounted fees, other), some of which can depend on restrictions ("we get all of your heart surgery") or volume discounts. Contracts may be open or exclusive: A physician or hospital may belong to more than one network, and an insurance company may contract with several, one, or no networks in an area.

The legal differences and distinctions among PPOs, POS, HMOs, and other managed-care contracts usually do not matter much to the average consumer. Patients are concerned about getting the care they need and how much their family has to pay, not the background or commercial structure. Why, then, should health economists bother? Because such details are vital to business, to solvency, to profit margins, and to whether the insurer makes or loses tens of millions of dollars. Not thinking about contracts or incentives has led toward an untenable situation in which Medicare and Medicaid portend to vastly increase an already burdensome federal deficit and where many working families can no longer afford health insurance.

Contractual Reforms to Control Costs

Insurance is a contract to pay for care. The premium must be sufficient to pay for all medical care provided and administrative overhead:

$$\text{Total Premiums} = \Sigma(\text{Price} \times \text{Quantity}) + \text{Overhead (load)}$$

Of these three elements, *prices are the easiest to cut.* Most of the early successes of managed care plans came from the ability to cut the amounts paid to doctors and hospitals. Sometimes these prices were reduced because of excess supply; sometimes because the MCO became a big buyer and could exercise market power; sometimes because the mere threat of taking patients away, or sending more, was sufficient to obtain discounts; and sometimes just because no buyer had ever before haggled aggressively in a system that had grown fat and soft. It is worth remembering that during the reign of the indemnity insurance plans, no one, not even the insurance company, stood to gain very much from hard bargaining, so all parties avoided it. To the insurance company, higher medical costs meant larger premiums; to employers, cost of benefits were offset by declines in wages, not profits; to employees, the gains from reducing costs were seen as too distant, or barely perceived, even though ultimately it was the employees who paid the cost.

Cutting prices does not change the amount of actual resources used (physician hours, x-ray machines, hospital beds). It simply means that one group (buyers) is paying less, and thus another group (sellers) receives less money. In economic terms, it is a pure transfer. Presumably buyers are happy to pay less but sellers are not happy to receive less. In a regular two-party transaction, price cuts would put money directly into the pocket of patients. With third-party insurance, the savings go the government or the employer, who might eventually use those savings in ways that benefit taxpayers or employees, but the immediate effects on the patient are negative: more paperwork, restrictive rules, and unhappy doctors. Indeed, faced with an onslaught of discounts, hospitals and physicians finally revolted, creating a backlash that blamed managed care for all sorts of evil in the service of greed. Thus, while price cuts are the most readily used method to reduce costs, and the source of most savings that HMOs have achieved,[23] there are clear limitations to such a strategy.

More promising savings from lower prices can be obtained by **substituting cheaper forms of care**: prescribe generic rather than brand-name drugs, have patients see a nurse practitioner rather than a doctor, treat patients with medicine rather than surgery, perform hip replacement rather than long-term nursing home care, and so on. The idea that a manager could identify an alternative form of care that was just as (or almost as) effective but significantly less expensive sounds good, but it has proved difficult to execute in practice. Rarely will doctors or patients accept that a cheap therapy is really "just as good as the more expensive one" except in the case of pharmaceuticals where generics are chemically identical to the brand-name pills. Even for pharmaceuticals, the savings from use of cheaper generic substitutes has been more than offset by the rise in the total number of prescriptions and increased use of expensive new compounds, so total drug costs per patient have continued to rise.

The second method for reducing costs, cutting the quantity of medical services, has proved to be extremely difficult to perform. Despite the rhetoric of "restrictive" HMO rules, the reality is that the total volume of services is rarely reduced by enough to make a substantial difference in total spending. To reduce quantity of services, both the patient and the physician must agree to the reduction. The initial idea was that medical services that do not have much of an impact on health could be removed without conflict ("cutting out the fat"). Yet whether a service is medically useful or not has little to do with its effect on physician income: Both vital and merely marginal services bring in the same fee. Thus, physicians are harmed (by reduced incomes) even if patients are not. Furthermore, although it is relatively easy to discover services that are relatively unimportant ("the need for this service results from a rare side effect"), it is almost impossible to say that such services would never be helpful, that they would not be important in one in a hundred (or one in a million) cases.

What did happen was that the use of services was bent to follow the contract more closely. For example, because many contracts with hospitals specified a set payment per day, the number of days a patient could stay in the hospital was reduced. However, patients still needed the same amount of surgery, aftercare, drugs, and so on, so the intensity of services was increased: more hours of nursing care and more procedures performed each day. The net result of fewer days and more inputs per day was that the total cost of hospital care was not reduced. As long as more nurses are hired, more drugs are used, and more tests are performed, total expenses cannot fall even though the number of patient days is falling. Over time, the reduction in ALOS (average length of stay = number of days per patient admission) was more than offset by an increase in the cost per day (see Chapters 8 and 9).

The rigid equation of Cost = (Price × Quantity + Overhead) holds as long as one considers managed care only as a contractual modification that leaves the underlying organization of medical practice the same. More radical reform and greater cost savings are potentially available by changing the structure of production and eliminating the mass of almost incomprehensible medical bills that clog the system (see the box "How Managed Care Can Reduce Total Costs"). The challenge for such a plan is to keep premiums low and satisfaction high as itemized prices and quantities fade out of existence and relevance. Despite initial success, great promise, and high expectations, Kaiser and other closed HMO plans have rather timidly tried to stay close to "regular" medical practice and have been lacking in terms of both innovation and performance in recent years (see the discussion of Kaiser in Chapter 12). Some integrated health systems (Mayo, Henry Ford, Cleveland Clinic, Intermountain, Geisinger) seem to have potential, but all are currently engaged in a variety of contracts with only small comprehensive capitated HMOs as a limited part of the organization.

HOW MANAGED CARE CAN REDUCE TOTAL COSTS

Reduce Total P × Q by:

- Reducing prices
- Reducing quantities
- Substituting cheaper inputs
- Reorganization (e.g., integrated closed HMO collects capitation and provides comprehensive care with no prices or quantities)

5.5   UNRESOLVED ISSUES: SPLIT INCENTIVES, DIVIDED LOYALTIES

Incentives matter. Economics can say only a little about the practice of medicine, but it has a lot to say about how payments affect the price and quantity of the care provided. If insurance covers hospital care but not physician office visits, patients show up at the emergency department rather than the local doctor's office. If there is an extra $30 charge for a brand-name pill, patients usually opt for the chemically identical generic. A physician paid by the visit sees more patients (and sees them more often) than a physician on a fixed salary. A hospital that gets paid more for each test done (fee-for-service) orders more tests than a hospital paid on a fixed rate (capitated, bundled, or negotiated). Unregulated insurance entitlements lead to excessive costs and unwarranted profits.

Insurance, like many other business arrangements, tends to serve the interests of those who write the contracts. Thus, the original Blue Cross plans, developed by hospital associations, were beneficial to hospitals; the generous reimbursement with no patient charges and community rating kept hospital beds full and revenues flowing. The entry of commercial insurers depended on their ability to offer a lower-priced product using copayments and deductibles to reduce premiums and reduce services (not something in the interest of hospitals, which wanted more business, not less). If these contractual stipulations caused "positive selection"—discouraging sick people from purchasing commercial insurance and making them stick with Blue Cross— this was fine with the for-profit insurance companies, and also with businesses that purchased employee health benefits; neither had a desire to pay extra to cover the high-cost chronically ill people who could not work. In the long run, contracts must meet the needs of all parties, but it can take a long time to get there. Also, it is possible to structure contracts so that the interests of those lacking influence are ignored. For example, a corporation may be willing to eliminate coverage for alcoholism because it could just fire those employees rather than rehabilitating them, or it may be willing to put an annual maximum on the number of days of hospital treatment to discourage people with HIV/AIDS from taking a job there. This helps the corporate bottom line, but only by increasing the burden on the family and the rest of society.

Contractual pathologies and perverse incentives are almost inherent in the process: encouraging angioplasty rather than aspirin, denying coverage to those who need it most, paying extra for higher charges and wasteful testing rather than personalized care or better health. Third-party contracting is complex. It is difficult to align the interests of all the parties and create a smoothly functioning system that is both efficient and transparent. Even though put into place with good intentions, both "consumer-driven" and "managed-care" insurance contracts fell into a common trap. The direct benefits (cost savings) went to the employer, and the problems (restrictions, payments, documentation) went elsewhere: to the patient and the physician. Such split incentives frustrate providers and create angry backlash among consumers. Even if the changes create cost efficiencies, they are seen as unfair.

The lack of transparency in third-party transactions is one of the worst aspects of the complex system of health insurance that has arisen in the United States. Channeling funds through different organizations and contractual arrangements obscures the cost of medicine and keeps doctors, patients, and the government from accepting appropriate responsibility. It makes it possible to go on believing that other people's money can be used to solve the problems of rising costs, expensive new drugs, affordable premiums, the uninsured, and care for the disabled. Insurance breaks the link between payment and receiving care. Eventually, all parties must confront reality: *"How much medicine can we afford and who will pay?"* That question balancing costs and benefits, reconnecting what we as patients want to receive with what we as citizens are willing to contribute, will be deferred for more extensive discussion in Chapters 17 and 18.

SUGGESTIONS FOR FURTHER READING

Kaiser Family Foundation and HRET, *Employer Health Benefits, 2011* Annual Survey, (www.kff.org).

Employee Benefit Research Institute, *Employment Based Health Benefits, 2012* (serial publication available at www.ebri.org); and Paul Frontsin "Sources of Health Insurance and Characteristics of the Uninsured," EBRI Issue Brief #362, September 2011.

www.medicare.gov

John K. Iglehart, "Expanding Eligibility, Cutting Costs—A Medicaid Update." *New England Journal of Medicine* 366, no. 2 (2012): 105–107.

Diane Rowland, "Medicaid at Forty," *Health Care Financing Review* 27, no. 2 (2006): 63–78, http://www.cms.hhs.gov/HealthCareFinancingReview/.

David M. Cutler, Mark McClellan, and Joseph P. Newhouse, "How Does Managed Care Do It?" *RAND Journal of Economics* 31, no. 3 (2000): 526–548.

Peter R. Kongstvedt, *Managed Care: What It Is and How It Works* (Sudbury, Mass.: Jones & Bartlett, 2008).

SUMMARY

1. Paying medical bills with **insurance makes health care a third-party transaction**. All three parties—patients, providers, and insurers—must benefit from the transaction. However, **separating the flow of funds from the flow of services obscures the real cost** of medical care. Health care is paid for by people (as patients, taxpayers, or employees giving up some wages to get health benefits), not by corporations.

2. The **government is the single largest insurer**, paying for 48 percent of all medical care. **Medicare**, which pays for the medical care of the elderly, is the largest and most influential government program, although the state and federal **Medicaid** program dominates long-term care reimbursement. Tax advantages have fostered the growth of health insurance as an employee benefit. Private health insurance covers 60 percent of the population but pays only 34 percent of the total bills. About 12 percent is paid for out of pocket by patients or their families.

3. About 46 million Americans, **16 percent of the population, are uninsured**. For many of them it is a rational decision to go without insurance based on their youth, good health, and/or low current earning power. For some, going without insurance is the result of a chronic disease, bad luck, or the size of the company they work for.

4. Insurance comes in a range of contractual forms, from pure insurance with fixed premiums, to various forms of risk sharing, to administered services only, to self-insurance plans in which the employer bears all the risk. Obtaining **tax benefits and exemption from state-mandated coverage** under ERISA has been a major reason for companies to self-insure.

5. **Managed care** is a diverse set of contractual and management methods used to arrange the financing and delivery of medical services. Its distinctive feature is that a *manager* intervenes to monitor and control the transaction between doctor and patient. Traditional insurance provides value through risk pooling so that medical expenses can be covered by an actuarially fair premium equal to the expected average loss. Managed care adds value by systematically **reducing the average loss** through utilization review, negotiating discounts, preauthorization, formularies, case management, statistical profiling, and other process controls.

6. **Escalation in costs** under open-ended entitlement financing from Medicare, Medicaid, and employer-provided health insurance has been the primary force driving the development of managed care. HMOs **reduce costs** by saving money on both the demand and the supply side. They obtain **discounts** by contracting in volume with physicians and hospitals, **substitute** less-expensive services (e.g., home care instead of hospital stays), and **control utilization** through the approval process. HMO members can use one-third to two-thirds fewer inpatient hospital days per thousand people than traditional fee-for-service insurance, although they often use more ambulatory services.

7. A **pharmacy formulary** limiting payment to drugs listed, a **preferred provider network** that makes patients pay extra for using hospitals and physicians not on the list, **capitation**, primary care **gatekeepers**, and **utilization review** are some of the ways that managed-care firms control costs. However, simple **price cuts** obtained through hard bargaining appear to be the major source of savings. Managed care has made many doctors bitter, because these savings reduce the income and professional autonomy of physicians.

8. Managed care attempts to create a much greater degree of **vertical and horizontal integration** in a medical system that has resisted organizational change. Changes in telecommunications and **information technology** make it possible for management to practice utilization review and monitor quality of care. Managed care has been shown to **reduce**

costs, but it is probably not the answer to all of America's health care problems. Some HMOs have made money by **risk selection**, accepting mostly healthier patients. Other HMOs may find it hard to maintain **quality of care** once the easy savings from discounting and substitution have been taken, and thus they may be tempted to reduce services in precisely those areas where patients, hampered by information asymmetry, depend most on professionals for monitoring quality.

9. Insurance **contracts create incentives** for patients, providers, and insurance companies to behave in ways that affects the market. Almost any contract favors some interests and harms others.

PROBLEMS

1. {*gains from trade*} Who benefits from a three-party transaction?

2. {*accounting, incidence*} How can a patient benefit if the premiums paid are more than the cost of the medical care received? How can an insurance company benefit if the medical care it provides costs more than the premiums paid in?

3. {*marginal incentives*} Explain how one insurance contract can provide incentives to:
   a. Choose a more or less expensive hospital.
   b. Spend more or fewer days in the hospital.
   c. Choose a more or less expensive surgeon.
   d. Use more or fewer drugs.
   e. Use more- or less-expensive drugs.

4. {*uninsured*} The law now gives a worker who becomes unemployed the right to buy continuing health insurance coverage after leaving the company. Why might it be rational for a factory worker who loses his or her job to give up this legal right to purchase coverage and become uninsured, even knowing that he or she is at risk for high medical expenditures?

5. {*mandated benefits*} Prior to 1970, maternity was usually treated differently from other medical expenses, either excluded entirely from coverage or subject to a flat lump-sum cash (indemnity) benefit. Why? During the 1970s, 23 states mandated that treatment related to pregnancy be covered the same as any other type of treatment, and in 1978, such coverage became uniform throughout the United States. Would mandated maternity benefits make working in a salaried position more or less attractive to women? Would it make women of childbearing age more or less attractive as employees? Would it increase or decrease the number of births performed by cesarean section? Whom do you think bore the expense of implementing this mandate? (For a discussion of these issues see Jonathan Gruber, "The Incidence of Mandated Maternity Benefits," *American Economic Review* 84, no. 3 (1994): 622–641.

6. {*adverse selection*} Which government insurance program is more affected by adverse selection: Medicare or Medicaid?

7. {*incentives*} Which surgeons are more subject to financial incentives when deciding between alternative courses of therapy: FFS physicians who own their own practices or salaried physicians working for an HMO?

8. {*industrial organization*} If an HMO reduces the patient's marginal cost of surgery, hospitalization, chemotherapy, and other expensive items to zero, how can it provide incentives for reduced utilization?

9. {*industrial organization*} Is an HMO able to obtain the biggest discounts where it has a large market share or where it has a smaller market share?

10. {*transaction costs*} Because managed care firms must hire managers to review all hospitalizations and surgeries, isn't managed care necessarily more expensive than unmanaged FFS care owing to this extra administrative cost?

11. {*incidence*} If ABC Corporation shifts from an indemnity plan to an HMO plan that lowers its cost of employee benefits by 35 percent over three years, who benefits? Who loses?

12. {*selection bias*} If a company offers both an HMO and an indemnity plan, which employees will choose which? (Assume the company pays 80 percent of the premiums and the employee pays 20 percent).

13. {*selection*} Would an HMO entering the Medicare market expect to experience favorable or adverse selection? Would the magnitude of the selection bias be larger or smaller for an HMO entering the commercial employee benefit market? The Medicaid market?

14. {*costs*} What are the three main ways HMOs act to reduce the cost of care? What is the fourth way?

15. {*dynamics*} Will a contract that lowers the amount an HMO pays providers be more important with regard to the HMO's short-run or long-run profitability? The providers' short-run or long-run profitability? Why?

16. {*information*} In what ways can an HMO use information to increase profits? As information technology has become more efficient and cheaper to use, have health care firms invested more or less in computers?

17. {*distribution*} Why do "star" surgeons rarely work for HMOs, even the largest and wealthiest ones?

18. {*physician behavior*} Do HMOs have substitutes for financial incentives in controlling physician behavior? What factors make these substitutes more or less effective?

19. {*dynamics*} What technological change has been most important in fostering the growth of managed care?

20. {*selection*} Is a person who is chronically ill and has a long-term relationship with a physician more likely to choose an HMO, PPO, or indemnity plan? How will this affect HMO capitation rates?

21. {*incentives*} What incentives does a capitated physician have to keep his patients happy? What incentive does an FFS physician have? If Mr. Jones is a cranky old man who smokes and drinks so much that his liver and other organs are going downhill, which payment system provides more incentive to keep Mr. Jones satisfied? Which provides the most incentive to render extra care? Which provides the most incentive to make sure that the level of care is optimized?

22. {*marginal cost*} Ralph says he pays $960 per month for his employer's HMO plan. Because the employer also offers a PPO and POS plan from another insurance company, why doesn't Ralph switch plans?

23. {*marginal cost*} Suppose a family physician has HMO patients who are capitated for primary care, HMO patients who are capitated using a withhold for hospital care, and FFS patients. For which patients is the marginal cost to the physician of doing additional laboratory services highest? For which patients is the marginal cost to the physician of admitting them to the hospital the highest?

24. {*incidence*} Which groups tend to win by a general move toward capitated managed care? Which groups tend to lose?

ENDNOTES

1. Estimates of coverage from EBRI and the Kaiser Family Foundation 2011 annual publications, based primarily on the U.S. Census Bureau "Current Population Survey."

2. Kaiser and HRET, *Employer Health Benefits, 2011* Annual Survey.

3. Mary A. Laschober et al., "Trends in Medicare Supplemental Insurance and Prescription Drug Coverage, 1996–1999," *Health Affairs* 21, no. 2 (2002): 11; Gretchen Jacobson et al., "Medigap Reform," *KFF Issue Brief,* September 2011; Marsha Gold et al, "Medicare Advantage 2012 Spotlight: Plan Availability and Premiums." KFF.org (November 2011). See also www.Medicare.gov.

4. John K. Iglehart, "Expanding Eligibility, Cutting Costs—A Medicaid Update." *New England Journal of Medicine* 366, no. 2 (2012): 105–107; Diane Rowland, "Medicaid at Forty," *Health Care Financing Review* 27, no. 2 (2006): 63–78 http://www.cms.hhs.gov/HealthCareFinancingReview/; Mariacristina De Nardi et al, "Medicaid and the Elderly," NBER working paper #17689, December 2011.

5. Lisa Dubay, Ian Hill, and Genevieve Kenney, "Five Things Everyone Should Know About SCHIP," Series A, No.A-55, The Urban Institute, October 2002, www.urban.org/url.cfm?ID=3105707; Elizabeth Thompson Beckley, "Missing the SCHIP," *Modern Physician,* (September 2002): 10; also see www.insurekidsnow.gov.

6. John Holahan, "The 2007–2009 Recession and Health Insurance Coverage," *Health Affairs* 30, no. 1 (2011): 145–152; C. DeNavas-Walt, B. D. Proctor, C. H. Lee, "Income, Poverty and Health Insurance Coverage in the United States, 2004," http://www.census.gov/prod/2005pubs/p60-229.pdf, and Kaiser Family Foundation, "The Uninsured and Their Access to Health Care" Publication 1420-07, November 4, 2005, www.kff.org.

7. The 19 to 24 age group is more than twice as likely to be uninsured as other age groups (35 percent versus 15 percent). J. P. Vistnes and S. H. Zuvekas, *Health Insurance Status of the Civilian Noninstitutionalized Population, 1997* (Rockville, Md.: Agency for Health Care Policy and Research, 1999); MEPS Research Findings #8, AHCPR Pub. No.99-0030; Helen Levy and Thomas DeLeire, "What Do People Buy When They Don't Buy Health Insurance?" *Inquiry* 45, no. 4 (2008): 365–379.

8. Under "normal" circumstances the costs of experience-rated, retention ratio, ASO, and self-insurance contracts should converge toward the same amount; however, circumstances are rarely normal. When a firm accepts bids for an experience-rated plan, it is not uncommon for an insurance company to try to "buy the business" by setting the premiums very low in the first year. Then it uses the bad experience during that year to force a high premium in the following year. The employer who got such a good deal is now stuck and must accept a substantial premium increase or incur the costs of going out to bid again, often finding that with such a record of underwriting losses, few insurers want to bid. Also, a group with higher-than-expected losses might find that their insurer starts to give poor service and gets very nasty about paying claims (and thus is able to hold onto premium dollars longer). On the other hand, employee groups often try to take advantage of insurance companies by dropping them after a bad year (thus allowing no time to make up the extraordinary losses through experience rating) or repeatedly going into the market to search for low bids. The more flexible retention ratio agreement is like a partnership. The insurance company and the employee group get together in a long-term arrangement in which initial pricing is not so important. Year-to-year conflicts are avoided. However, the downside of this more integrated contract is that if things do go wrong, it is much worse for both parties.

9. J. Grossman and P. Ginsburg, "As The Health Insurance Underwriting Cycle Turns" *Health Affairs* 23, no. 6 (2004): 91–102; Alice Rosenblatt, "The Underwriting Cycle: the Rule of Six," *Health Affairs* 23, no. 6 (2004):103–106.

10. Howard S. Berliner and Sonia Delgada, "From DRGs to Deregulation: New Jersey Takes the Road Less Traveled," *Journal of American Health Policy* 3, no. 4 (1993): 44–48.

11. Jonathan Gruber and Helen Levy, "The Evolution of Medical Spending Risk," *Journal of Economic Perspectives* 23, no. 4 (2009): 25–48.

12. U.S. Bureau of Labor Statistics, "Employer Costs for Employee Compensation," news release March 14, 2012, www.bls.gov/ncs/ect/. The BLS employee compensation measures have varied over the years, and the various issues of the *BLS Handbook of Methods* should be examined to understand the vagaries of comparison (www.bls.gov). Bradley R. Braden and Stephanie L. Hyland, "Cost of Employee Compensation in Public and Private Sectors," *Monthly Labor Review* 116, no. 5 (1993): 14–21.

13. The United States ranked 26th in male life expectancy among 191 nations in 2000 (28th for females), a bit behind most other developed countries. The risk of dying between ages 15 and 59, a perhaps more significant measure, was even worse (36th for males, 38th for females). Overall, the World Health Organization ranked performance of the U.S. health system 37th, *World Health Report 2000* (www.who.int/whr). See also Victor Fuchs, "The Best Health Care System in the World?" *Journal of the American Medical Association* 268, no. 7 (1992): 916–917; Jack Hadley, *More Medical Care, Better Health?* (Washington, D.C.: Urban Institute Press, 1982); Organisation for Economic Cooperation and Development, *OECD Health Data: Comparative Analysis of Health Systems* (Paris: Organization for Economic Cooperation and Development, 2002). Eileen M. Crimmins, Samuel Preston, Barney Cohen, eds., *Explaining Divergent Levels of Longevity in High-Income Countries* (Washington, D.C.: National Academies Press, 2011).

14. James C. Robinson and Paul Ginsburg, "Consumer-Driven Health Care: Promise and Performance," *Health Affairs* 28, no. 2 (2009): w272–w281; Gary Claxton et al., "What High-Deductible Plans Look Like: Findings From a National Survey of Employers, 2005," *Health Affairs* Web exclusive W5, September 14 2005: 434–441; Debbie Welle-Powell, "HSAs—Friends or Foes?" *Healthcare Financial Management,* March 2006: 76–79. There are a number of regulatory changes in the Accountable Care Act of 2010 that will significantly affect consumer driven health plans starting in 2014.

15. Health savings accounts (HSAs), although authorized by the Medicare Modernization Act of 2003, which established Part D coverage for prescription drugs, have really been in operation only since 2005 because the rules and regulations for implementation are complex and took many months to work out. In essence, an HSA is a tax-favored savings account coupled with a high-deductible health plan. Patients must pay all of their expenses below the deductible (at least $1,000 for singles and $2,000 for families, rising with inflation after 2005) either out of pocket or from the HSA savings account. Any money left in the savings account can be carried forward to the next year, and any earnings on the savings are exempt from federal taxes. The savings account can be funded by either the person or the employer (in an amount less than or equal to the deductible), and such contributions are exempt from federal income taxes for both the employee and the company. Health reimbursement accounts (HRAs), established by a series of U.S. Internal Revenue Service rulings in 2002, are similar to HSAs but differ in that they are funded solely by the employer and can be offered with any type of health insurance plan (not only high-deductible plans), and any savings in the HRA account stays with the company if the employee changes jobs. Medical savings accounts (MSAs), an earlier type, linked a tax-advantaged savings account to a high-deductible health insurance plan and was limited primarily to self-employed persons. The argument for creating MSAs was that self-employed persons should be able to get the tax benefits available to people receiving insurance through their employer. Somewhat related are the pretax spending accounts where money is regularly deducted and deposited in accounts to be used for medical or dependent care and avoids income taxes. Pretax spending accounts have become very common, but they suffer from the disadvantage that any money not spent by the end of the year is taken away rather than rolling over from year to year or earning interest.

16. Colleen M. Barry et al. "Who Chooses a Consumer-Directed Health Plan?" *Health Affairs* 27, no. 6 (2008): 1671–1679.

17. Aventis Pharmaceuticals, 2005 HMO-PPO Medicare/Medicaid Digest, www.managedcaredigest.com.

18. Geoffrey F. Joyce, Jose J. Escarce, Matthew D. Solomon, and Dana Goldman, "Employer Drug Benefit Plans and Spending on Prescription Drugs," *Journal of the American Medical Association* 288, no. 14 (2002): 1733–1739. See also the comment on the article by Donald M. Steinwachs, "Pharmacy Benefit Plans and Prescription Drug Spending," on pages 1773–1774.

19. Kaiser Family Foundation and HRET, "Prescription Drugs Benefits," pages 156–166 in *Employee Health Benefits, 2011* Annual Survey, 2011.

20. In principle, an integrated closed HMO could be run as a for-profit corporation benefiting stockholders, a division of a voluntary hospital chain, or a consumer co-op with all profits used to increase community benefits. In practice, the residual ownership interest has de facto resided primarily with the senior physician group, even when they are technically employees of the HMO.

21. The term "PPO" is commonly used to refer to two things: an insurance plan and a corporate entity. The two are distinct. Your "PPO" insurance might actually have contracts with a dozen PPO organizations. Conversely, a single PPO organization with 50 physicians might have contracts with more than one insurance company (and at different prices).

22. Peter R. Kongstvedt, *Managed Care: What It Is and How It Works* (Sudbury, Mass.: Jones & Bartlett, 2008); Neelam K. Sekhri, "Managed Care: The U.S. Experience," *Bulletin of the World Health Organization* 78, no. 6 (2000): 830–844, www.who.org or www.who.int; C. Liu, R. Frank, and T. McGuire, "Demand Response of Mental Health Services to Cost Sharing under Managed Care," *Journal of Mental Health Policy and Economics* 11, no. 3 (2008): 113–125. Technically, any contract between insurer and provider might be called a "managed-care organization" (MCO), and many insurers have maintained such contracts even under indemnity plans so as to allow providers to accept payments and bill the insurer directly. Also, even closed plans that are completely integrated operationally are often legally structured as independent medical, financial, and hospital corporations, similar to the subsidiaries and holding entities found in many large firms.

23. David M. Cutler, Mark McClellan, and Joseph P. Newhouse, "How Does Managed Care Do It?" *RAND Journal of Economics* 31, no. 3 (2000): 526–548; Daniel Alman, Richard Zeckhauser, and David M. Cutler, "Enrollee Mix, Treatment Intensity and Cost in Competing Indemnity and HMO Plans," NBER working paper #7832, August 2000; Ann Barry Flood et al., "How Do HMOs Achieve Savings?" *Health Services Research* 33, no. 1 (1998): 79–99. Marsha Gold et al., "A National Survey of the Arrangements Managed-Care Plans Make With Physicians," *New England Journal of Medicine* 333 (1995): 1678–1683; Gerard Anderson et al., "Setting Payment Rates for Capitated Systems: A Comparison of Various Alternatives," *Inquiry* 27, no. 3 (1990): 225–233. For a hilarious and heartbreaking dramatization of HMO backlash, watch the Oscar award-winning *As Good As It Gets* with Jack Nicholson and Helen Hunt.

CHAPTER **6**

PHYSICIANS

QUESTIONS

1. How are physicians paid?
2. Which types of physicians earn the highest incomes?
3. How much does it cost to practice medicine?
4. Are malpractice insurance premiums a major cause of higher doctor bills?
5. Is medical care sold like other goods and services?
6. Who chooses which treatment to use, the patient or the doctor?
7. Why are licensure restrictions more strongly enforced for some types of medical care than for others?
8. Is the American Medical Association (AMA) a professional society serving science or a union serving the economic interests of its members? Is it both?
9. Which is more competitive: the market for health insurance or the market for medical care?

At the center of medical practice stands the physician. Physicians direct the flow of patients by controlling admissions, referrals, regulations, insurance reimbursements, and prescriptions. A very powerful and special bond exists between doctor and patient. This relationship is based on medical science—and ethics and emotions—as well as economics.[1] Even when a transaction does not directly involve a physician financially, the physician still plays a dominant role. In the preceding chapters we discussed health care from the perspective of the patient. Now we switch to the perspective of the provider: not the payer but the payee. For the physician, medical expenditures are not *costs*, they are *revenues*.

6.1 FINANCING PHYSICIAN SERVICES: REVENUES

Whereas most of the labor force is employed and paid a salary by a large organization, many physicians are independent entrepreneurs or partners running what are, in effect, small businesses.[2] The income of physicians in solo or group private practices mostly comes from **fee-for-service** payments, a specified amount paid for each visit or procedure, although an increasing amount is coming from complex, negotiated third-party contracts. In the 1930s, physicians were essentially free to charge whatever they decided was appropriate but they often collected much less than what they charged. Today, 89 percent of physician revenues come from third-party payments,[3] and most fees are subject to some form of external review or control (see box "Types of Physician Payment").

TYPES OF PHYSICIAN PAYMENT

Charges: The amount appearing on the bill, without insurance.

Fee-for-Service: A specified payment for each unit of service provided.

Fee Schedule: A set "menu" of prices for each service agreed upon in advance.

UCR: A method for denying bills that are out of line with the "usual, customary and reasonable charges made by this and other physicians for the same service last year."

RVS: A schedule based on objective standards showing relative value points for each service compared to a common unit (i.e., regular office visit). Deciding a dollar value per point converts it into a fee schedule.

RBRVS: The relative value schedule set by Medicare for physician fees.

Capitation: A set payment per person per month regardless of the number of services used.

Salary: A paycheck from an employer.

It is important to distinguish between what the physician **charges** (i.e., the amount that appears on the bill) and the actual payments made by the insurance company, which may be considerably less. One of the initial steps in the evolution of physician payment in the United States was the development of **usual, customary, and reasonable (UCR)** fee schedules. The Blue Shield plans, which then provided the largest portion of physician insurance and operated with the support of local medical societies, collected information on what each physician charged for each service in a local area during the previous year. When a physician submitted a bill, it was checked to determine whether it was above his or her median charge for the same service the previous year (usual), above the 75th percentile of charges by all doctors in the area (customary), or justifiably higher because of a patient's complicating secondary illness or another acceptable reason (reasonable). When Medicare was implemented in 1966, it adopted the Blue Shield UCR method of paying physicians.

An effort to reduce payments, particularly for certain services, led insurers to promulgate **fee schedules**. A fee schedule is like a menu that specifies how much the insurance company will pay physicians for particular services. Fee schedules can be proposed by the sellers (physicians) to try to keep prices up, or by the buyers (Medicare, insurance companies) to try to keep prices down. A major difficulty with fee schedules is the amazingly large number of services that must be priced. It is easy to come up with a reasonable price for a coronary artery bypass operation or services associated with a normal birth, but what about for oblique lateral pelvic x-rays, measurement of bilirubin or potassium levels, management of schizophrenia, and a host of other medical services?

To bring order to fee schedules, organizations have devised **relative value scales**, which give each service a point value. A common service (e.g., standard office visit, hernia repair surgery) is usually given a weight of 1 point, and all other services are given point values relative to that standard unit of service (e.g., 5 points, 0.2 point). After the physician and insurance company agree on the value per point, payment for each service is determined (e.g., if value per point is $20, a physician providing a 3.5-point service is paid 3.5 × $20 =$70). In 1992, the Medicare **resource-based relative value scale (RBRVS)** was implemented. A team of health economists led by William Hsiao of Harvard University studied the resources used in providing physician care to estimate a point value for each service based on (1) physician time, (2) intensity of effort, (3) practice costs, and (4) costs of advanced specialty training.[4] The Centers for Medicare and Medicaid Services (CMS) of the U.S. Department of Health and Human Services, which administers the Medicare program, set the dollars per point for

2003 at $34.59, with adjustments for geographic variation in practice costs and for malpractice insurance (see box "RBRVS Fee Schedule").

The Medicare physician reimbursement system provides a kind of "public good" (see Chapter 15) for other insurance programs; that is, a universally understood and practiced standard fee schedule they can adopt or easily modify by changing the dollar conversion factor or separating certain categories. Medicaid, Blue Cross, and commercial insurance contracts that cover the 87 percent of the population younger than 65 years often base their payments on a modified form of the Medicare RBRVS or use Medicare payment levels as a benchmark.

RBRVS FEE SCHEDULE

Medicare relies on a resource-based relative value scale (RBRVS) to determine the fees it will pay physicians to treat its beneficiaries. A fee is calculated by multiplying a service's relative value units (RVUs) by a conversion factor and adjusting for geographic cost variations. Medicare also uses the RBRVS to pay for certain services furnished by allied health professionals (e.g., physician assistants, nurse practitioners, certified registered nurse anesthetists, and physical therapists).

Relative Value Scale

An RBRVS is a list of physician services with RVUs assigned to each service. The units indicate a service's cost relative to that of the typical physician service, which has a relative value of 1.0 units. A service with 1.559 units is therefore 55.9 percent more costly to provide than the typical service, whereas a service with 0.693 units is 30.7 percent less costly to provide than the typical service.

A service's total RVUs are spread over the following three major components:

- *Physician work (pw)* is the time spent, effort exerted, and skills used by the physician to furnish the service. This component includes preservice, intraservice, and postservice work related to the physician's encounter with the patient.

- *Practice expenses (pe)* is the wages, salaries, and fringe benefits the physician provides office staff and money spent on other office expenses, such as rent and supplies. Many physician services have two practice expense RVUs: facility practice expense units and nonfacility practice expense units, the latter almost always higher than the former. This site-of-service differential recognizes that the physician does not absorb the full cost of services provided in a facility setting. Part of the cost is paid by the facility and therefore is included in the amount the facility is reimbursed.

- *Malpractice insurance (mi)* is separated from other practice expenses, largely because it varies significantly among specialties and across states and fluctuates markedly with oscillations in malpractice awards. Recently, malpractice expenses have significantly increased.

Physician work accounts for approximately 55 percent of total RVUs, followed by 42 percent for practice expenses and 3 percent for malpractice insurance.

Level 1 of the CMS Common Procedure Coding System is used to identify the physician services a patient receives. Level 1—*Current Procedural Terminology,* fourth edition (CPT-4)—is the most widely used coding system for office visits, consultations, surgery, imaging, and other physician services. Approximately 7,500 CPT codes are paid under the RBRVS

(Continued)

RBRVS FEE SCHEDULE (CONTINUED)

fee schedule. Certain physician services may be performed by nurse practitioners, nurse midwives, or other midlevel or nonphysician practitioners. These practitioners may practice independently or under a physician's supervision, depending on state law. The same CPT code is used to document a service, regardless of who performs it.

The Table 6.1 shows Medicare's RVUs for calendar year (CY) 2003 for selected physician services, which range from less than 1.0 to nearly 29. The table shows the following:

- The RVUs for a new patient's office visit exceed those for an established patient's office visit; the units for both types of visit vary directly with the level of care.

- The RVUs for major surgical procedures (e.g., CPT 69501) include the cost of services and items that are bundled with the procedure, such as the surgeon's initial consultation, preoperative visits, treatment for complications after surgery, and postoperative visits to the surgeon for 10 to 90 days after surgery.

- Diagnostic and therapeutic radiology services have a professional and technical component. The professional component represents the portion of the service associated with the interpretation of the test. The technical component is the portion associated with performing the test. Often, a physician is paid for the professional component and the hospital where the service is furnished is paid for the technical component.

The RVUs are adjusted for geographic variations in wage rates and other prices that physicians pay for the resources used to produce patient care. The adjustment is based on geographic practice cost indexes (GPCIs) for physician work, practice expenses, and malpractice insurance. As of January 1, 2003, there were about 90 Medicare payment areas nationally, including statewide areas and metropolitan statistical areas. GPCIs vary noticeably across payment areas.

TABLE 6.1　　　Proposed Relative Value Units for Ten Physician Services, CY 2003

HCPCS/CPT Code	Description	Physician Work	Practice Expense		Malpractice Insurance	Total Units	
			Facility	Nonfacility		Facility	Nonfacility
99202	Office or other outpatient visit, new patient, level 2	0.88	0.32	0.77	0.05	1.25	1.70
99204	Office or other outpatient visit, new patient, level 4	2.00	0.72	1.49	0.10	2.82	3.59
99212	Office or other outpatient visit, established patient, level 2	0.45	0.16	0.52	0.02	0.63	0.99
99214	Office or other outpatient visit, established patient, level 4	1.10	0.40	1.03	0.04	1.54	2.17
99283	Emergency department services, level 3	1.24	0.32	NA	0.08	1.64	NA
30400	Reconstruction of nose	9.83	8.81	NA	0.80	19.44	NA
35501	Artery bypass graft	19.19	7.43	NA	2.33	28.95	NA
42800	Biopsy of throat	1.39	2.62	3.09	0.10	4.11	4.58
69501	Mastoidectomy	9.07	8.07	NA	0.65	17.79	NA
70336	Magnetic image, jaw joint	1.48	NA	11.67	0.56	NA	13.71
	Professional component	1.48	0.51	0.51	0.07	2.06	2.06
	Technical component	0.00	NA	11.16	0.49	NA	11.65

NA = not applicable; nonfacility = outside of hospital.
Source: Federal Register, "Medicare Program," 67 (December 31, 2002), Appendix B.

(Continued)

RBRVS FEE SCHEDULE (CONTINUED)

Conversion Factor

The dollar value of an RVU is called the conversion factor (CF). This factor ($34.59 for CY 2003 for all physician services except anesthesia) is multiplied by the RVUs to calculate the fee for a given service. At times, Medicare's conversion factor serves as a floor for private health plans and a ceiling for state Medicaid programs. Given the following assumptions for CPT 99283, CF = $34.59, RVU_{pw} = 1.24 (RVUs for *physician work*), RVU_{pe} = 0.32 (RVUs for *practice expenses*), RVU_{mi} = 0.08 (RVUs for *malpractice insurance*), $GPCI_{pw}$ = 1.032 (GPCI for *physician work*), $GPCI_{pe}$ = 1.109 (GPCI for *practice expenses*), and $GPCI_{mi}$ = 1.215 (GPCI for *malpractice insurance*), the fee would be $59.90.

$$Fee = CF \times [(RVU_{pw} \times GPCI_{pw}) + (RVU_{pe} \times GPCI_{pe}) + (RVU_{mi} \times GPCI_{mi})]$$
$$\$59.90 = \$34.59 \times [(1.24 \times 1.032) + (0.32 \times 1.109) + (0.08 \times 1.215)]$$

If the annual Medicare Part B deductible has been met, Medicare would pay 80 percent of the lower of the calculated fee or the amount the physician actually charged for the service (see Section 5.1). The patient would be responsible for paying the balance plus any extra amount that Medicare allows a nonparticipating physician to charge.

Fee Updates

In general, the conversion factor is updated annually for changes in the costs physicians incur to provide patient care. Medicare's update factor equals the compound rate of change in the following items:

- *Medicare economic index* measures the weighted rate of change in the cost of physician and nonphysician labor, supplies, and other resources used to produce patient care. The calculation includes a downward adjustment for pro-ductivity growth.

- *Performance adjustment* is made when actual and allowed Medicare expenditures for physician services differ. The allowed amount is a target designed to slow spending growth. Spending above the target is deducted from future fee increases; spending below the target is added to future fee increases.

- *Other factors* can cause Medicare spending to increase or decrease. Examples include an expansion of the physician services that Medicare covers or new statutory or regulatory requirements that affect practice costs (e.g., the Health Insurance Portability and Accountability Act [HIPAA]).

Note: This box on RBRVS was prepared by health finance consultant and lecturer Paul L. Grimaldi, Ph.D., © 2003. For additional discussion on this topic, see Paul L. Grimaldi, "Medicare Fees for Physician Services are Resource-Based," *Journal of Health Care Finance* 28, no. 3 (2002): 88–104.

Copayments, Assignment, and Balance Billing

Medicare and other insurers' contracts not only state what they will pay the physician, but they also often specify what the patient must pay. A **copayment** of $5 or $10 per visit is often required, both to reduce premiums and, by forcing the patient to bear some costs, to reduce the number of services utilized. Some plans also have a **deductible**, which requires the patient to pay the first $100 to $500 out of pocket per year or per illness. **Coinsurance**, with patients paying 10 percent or 20 percent of the bill, is a common part of major medical benefits. The contracts are so complex that it is often difficult for either the patient or the physician to know exactly who is responsible for which part of the bill. Two forms of payment can be distinguished: individual reimbursement and assignment. Under **individual reimbursement**, the patient pays all the charges, sends copies of the bills to the insurer, and is reimbursed for the medical expenses that are covered. Under **assignment**, the physician sends the bill to the insurer. The patient is charged for the copayment and may be **balance billed** for the difference if the physician's charges exceed the maximum fee allowed by the insurance contract. Under the Medicare participation agreement, a physician who accepts the assignment agrees not to balance bill for any charges over the Medicare payment. Patients like assignment because they do not have to handle paperwork and are not stuck with additional fees. Physicians like the fact that they are paid directly and more rapidly, but they do not like being denied the right to charge as much as they believe their services are worth. Indeed, the prohibition of balance billing in Canada led to a national physician's strike when the rule was first imposed.

Under current U.S. Medicare rules, physicians are limited to an additional 15 percent above the Medicare fee for balance billing if they choose not to accept assignment and are penalized by receiving only 95 percent of the regular fee schedule for services. In effect, Medicare has ruled out balance billing by making it economically unattractive. Medicaid rules are often more stringent and have significantly lower payment rates, which is why many physicians choose not to participate in the Medicaid program. Some physicians choose not to participate in Medicare to avoid the payment limits imposed by the RBRVS system, but because 25 percent of all physician bills are paid for by Medicare, this is difficult to do unless their practice is mostly obstetrics, sports medicine, or another specialty in which they treat few elderly clients.

Physician Payment in Managed Care Plans

As insurance companies have tried to control their costs by exercising market power, the passive payment of bills has given way to a system of **negotiated fees**. For some common and easily specified services purchased in large volume (intraocular lens implants, psychiatric evaluations for drug abuse), the insurance company can often obtain a low fixed price set in advance in return for guaranteeing the physician a certain number of patients or procedures. When individual fees are not negotiated, it is common for managed care contracts to specify **discounted fees**, offering perhaps 75 percent of what the physician would ordinarily bill other patients.

The complexities of per-unit service pricing are bypassed completely under **capitation**, a fixed payment per person per month regardless of the number of services used (see Chapter 5). A health maintenance organization (HMO) using a capitation rate of $100 per month pays that amount to the physician for each of the HMO members enrolled with that physician whether the member visits the doctor's office once, twice, ten times, or not at all. Open independent practice HMOs that contract with many physicians use capitation rates to pay physicians, but a closed-panel staff HMO hires physicians to work exclusively in the HMO's facility and pays physicians a **salary**, with perhaps some bonus based on productivity or on the profitability of the HMO. With this arrangement, the physician, in effect, becomes an employee of a large medical care firm (even though legally the physician might still be considered an independent practitioner because of laws in many states prohibiting the corporate practice of medicine).

Salaried physicians are also found in hospitals providing emergency department and inpatient care, in administrative posts, and in research and teaching organizations. About 40 percent of physicians are now salaried employees, and the number continues to grow as health care organizations become larger and more complex. Chapter 5 presents a more extensive discussion of managed care contracting.

Incentives: Why Differences in the Type of Payment Matter

How physicians are paid determines the incentives they face to work harder, raise prices, or admit patients to the hospital. Under fee-for-service insurance, a physician gets paid more for doing more. Under HMO capitation, the payment is the same regardless of the number of services provided; therefore, a physician may do less. Under a relative value scale, payment is based on the number of points; therefore, physicians might push to classify the service in a higher point category (the ensuing gradual rise in total points while the number of services provided remains constant is known as "code creep").[5] In an intriguing experiment, half the doctors in a pediatric clinic were randomly selected to be paid on a fee-for-service basis and half were selected to be paid a salary.[6] The fees were set so that the average doctor seeing the average number of patients would earn the same on either a fee-for-service or salary basis. In practice, the fee-for-service doctors saw more patients, recalled them for more visits, and generally exceeded the normal guidelines for the amount of services, whereas the doctors who were on salary saw fewer patients, had them return less frequently, and were in less conformity with standard guidelines. This randomized, controlled trial demonstrates that economic predictions regarding the incentive effects of different types of payment are borne out in a practice setting. Similar increases in surgical utilization occur when physicians move from capitation to fee-for-service.

Payment type can affect patients' access to physician care as well. The Medicaid program has come under severe budgetary constraints and thus tends to pay physicians less well than Blue Shield, HMOs, and commercial insurance. Although physicians are constrained by ethics and law to provide high-quality care to all who need it, economic theory predicts that government imposition of mandatory price controls leads to shortages. A group of experimenters called 300 physician offices and requested an appointment, identifying their type of insurance as Medicaid.[7] Almost half the physician offices said that they were not accepting new patients, and when the experimenters did get an appointment, the average wait was two weeks. The experimenters then called back, identifying themselves as having commercial insurance, and 78 percent of the doctor's offices gave them an appointment within two days. Physicians try hard to provide adequate care to the poor, but if the payment levels are consistently lower, the level of service will be lower.

A Progression: From Prices to Reimbursement Mechanisms

As the medical care system moved away from individual fee-for-service toward third-party insurance, the financial linkage between patients and physicians was attenuated and finally severed. Although there may be some "price" attached to each service under Medicare RBRVS, the price bears almost no resemblance to what that would mean in a normal market: the patient does not pay the price, nor does the price allow the supplier to match output to demand, because it is imposed externally by the government. In such an environment, equilibrating varied interests through individual decisions based on price is replaced by a collective political market. Who is paid and how much is determined in part by concerns about how the elderly will vote in the next presidential election, the effectiveness of insurance lobbies, or a need to find the least difficult way of balancing the budget. Tracking the flow of funds to and from physicians is further obscured by referring to all payments as *reimbursement*, even though insurance companies do not "reimburse" physician costs (physician time is the bulk of the expense) and payments are more accurately termed *physician fees* or *revenues* or *salary*.

6.2 PHYSICIAN INCOMES

Physicians are among the most highly trained and well-compensated workers in the United States. The median physician income was about $225,000 in 2010, five times the average worker's salary. Physician earnings grew more rapidly than average workers' earnings for most of the 20th century. During the period 1982 to 2004, when average workers' earnings were almost flat (up only 3 percent in 22 years after adjustment for inflation), real physician earnings rose more than 25 percent. To a large extent, these high earnings were attributable to the quality of those who entered the profession (almost all were in the top quarter of their college graduating classes), the long years of post-college training required, the extra effort (most physicians worked about 50 percent more hours than the average salaried worker), and compensation for having to act as entrepreneurs and manage a medical business (self-employed physicians earned 50 percent more than those who chose to work on salary). However, even after adjusting for all these factors, there is still a premium obtained for becoming a physician. Perhaps even more important than higher incomes is the implied "floor"; physicians virtually never face unemployment, and many are able to accept "low-paid" positions (i.e., those that pay less than $100,000 per year) to follow their own interests in helping the poor, working with children, traveling to exotic locations, or studying interesting diseases.

Even during training in residency programs, physicians earn about $42,000 a year, which is about the same as the average worker, although it is certainly less than the opportunity cost of their time (see the discussion of the costs of time and returns in Chapter 12). As with most workers, physicians' earnings grow rapidly early in their careers, rise to a peak around age 50 years, and decline thereafter (see Table 6.2 and 6.3).

There is a marked difference in earnings by specialty. Pediatricians and family practitioners are at the low end, with psychiatrists only slightly above. The high end is made up of the surgeons, cardiologists, and radiologists. Although numerous factors are involved, much of the difference in incomes among specialties is attributable to the reimbursement system: physicians get paid more for doing something (e.g., reading an x-ray, performing an operation) than for caring or thinking (e.g., listening to a patient's history, deciding which path of treatment to follow, helping the family of a dying person). The reimbursement system is driven by the "billable event." Although a colleague or a manager might be able to assess all the work a physician does on behalf of patients, the financial system is not able to do so. A physician always finds it easier to get paid for a procedure, because it is observable and has a standard billing code, than for a personal interaction or conceptual effort.

A desire to rebalance incomes across specialties and provide more payment for thinking and caring was a goal of the Medicare RBRVS system, but it was not very successful at doing so. Health insurance is designed to protect individuals against potentially large but infrequent losses while minimizing moral hazard from excess purchase of discretionary services. Although correct from a risk-management perspective, in practice this means that fees for some specialties are almost fully covered (e.g., surgery, anesthesia), leading to increased demand and higher incomes, whereas other specialties are subject to copayments and deductibles that limit demand and incomes (e.g., pediatrics, psychiatry). The bottom line for the physician is that the income potential from choosing a particular specialty has more to do with how the services of that specialty are treated by insurance than with the work or training involved.

TABLE 6.2	Physician Supply
Category	**Number**
Total U.S. physicians	972,000
Active in patient care	838,000
Residents in training programs	102,000
International medical graduates	252,000

TABLE 6.3	Physician Incomes	
Type	**Median Income ($)**	*Percentage of All Physicians*
By Specialty		
All Physicians	$240,000	*100*
General/family practice	185,000	*10*
Pediatrics	191,000	*8*
Internal medicine	208,000	*17*
Psychiatry	210,000	*5*
Emergency medicine	272,000	*3*
Obstetrics/gynecology	291,000	*5*
General surgery	357,000	*4*
Dermatology	365,000	*1*
Anesthesiology	384,000	*4*
Plastic surgery	401,000	*1*
Cardiology	393,000	*2*
Radiology	445,000	*4*
Orthopedic surgery	495,000	*3*
By Type of Practice		
Self-employed solo	201,000	*22*
Employee or contractor	207,000	*45*
Self-employed group	319,000	*33*
2 physician partners	255,000	
3 physician group	288,000	
4 physician group	291,000	
5–25 physician group	331,000	
25+ physician group	322,000	
By Age		
35 years	186,000	*15*
35–44 years	227,000	*23*
45–54 years	265,000	*24*
55–64 years	240,000	*18*
65 and older	193,000	*20*

Sources: AMA Physician Characteristics and Distribution in the U.S., 2009, 2011. AMA Physician Socioeconomic Statistics, 2000–2002 and earlier years; Medical Economics and Modern Healthcare compensation surveys.

6.3   PHYSICIAN FINANCING: EXPENSES

Physician Practice Expenses

The expenses of maintaining a practice take up about half of all the funds flowing into physician offices. Physicians must pay for other medical professionals and assistants who help them take care of patients, as well as taxes, rent, utilities, supplies, malpractice insurance, and so on, as shown in Table 6.4. In addition to all these ongoing expenses, it usually takes at least $100,000 in start-up capital to equip even the most basic office, and an elaborate suite housing an active practice in specialties such as plastic surgery could cost several million dollars. One reason for physicians to work together in group practices is to obtain economies of scale from sharing office space, equipment, and information systems. Only a large group can afford to have assistants who specialize in support functions, such as laboratory technicians, billing and appointment clerks, physical therapists, and so on. Yet closer examination of the data reveals an apparently anomalous finding: Even though it seems that a large group practice would use ancillary help and equipment more efficiently, such expenses take a greater percentage of total revenues for

TABLE 6.4	Physicians' Office Practice Income and Expenses		
Category		Revenue ($)	Percentage
GROSS REVENUES		$470,000	100%
Private insurance			53%
Medicare			25%
Medicaid			11%
Patients paid			11%
Net income		$240,000	51%
EXPENSES			
Nonphysician employee wages (4 FTE per physician)		$ 79,900	17%
Employee physicians		$ 15,200	3%
Office rent and expenses		$ 56,400	12%
Medical supplies		$ 18,800	4%
Malpractice liability insurance		$ 23,500	5%
Equipment		$ 9,400	2%
Other expenses		$ 26,800	6%

Worked an average of 57 hours per week, seeing 105 patients, and giving 4 hours of charity or uncompensated care. The average charge for a patient visit was about $100 in 2006.
Source: AMA Physician Socioeconomic Statistics, 2000–2002, *Medical Economics* survey, 2006; *Modern Healthcare* Compensation Surveys, 2005–2011.

groups than for physicians who practice alone. To understand why a more efficient practice uses more rather than less nonphysician inputs, it is necessary to consider a basic result from the microeconomic analysis of firm production. To reduce per-unit costs, firms must use more of the inputs whose output per dollar is higher and/or use less of the input whose output per dollar is lower (see Section 2.5).[7] At the optimum, the ratio of marginal productivity to input price is the same for all inputs.

$$\frac{\text{Marginal Productivity}_{\text{input}A}}{\text{Price}_{\text{input}A}} = \frac{\text{Marginal Productivity}_{\text{input}B}}{\text{Price}_{\text{input}B}} = \ldots$$

$$= \frac{\text{Marginal Productivity}_{\text{input}Z}}{\text{Price}_{\text{input}Z}}$$

Larger and more organized physician groups are able to make better use of nonphysician inputs, raising their marginal productivity. Therefore, groups use more of these inputs relative to physician time. Efficiency is not defined as having the lowest amount of overhead, or even the highest number of patient visits per physician hour, but rather the lowest cost (physician and nonphysician) per visit. This raises the following question: What "price" should be applied to physician time?

The Labor versus Leisure Choice

A physician-entrepreneur has an income of revenues less expenses, which is called profit by the Internal Revenue Service (IRS). Most of the income is not economic profit but compensation for all the hours of work put in. How should this time be valued? What is its opportunity cost? For a young physician starting out with relatively few patients, it is common to take on a temporary part-time moonlighting job in a hospital emergency department or in a well established senior practice with many patients for wages of $75 to $150 per hour. Because doctors give up those jobs as their practices become established, their time must be worth more than that, but what forgone opportunity defines this higher hourly rate?

What a busy physician gives up is leisure: time to be with family, time to run and swim and watch television, and even time to sleep. The more lucrative each hour of practice and the more hours the physician puts in, the more each hour of forgone leisure is worth. Most doctors work very hard, averaging more than 50 hours per week. Furthermore, once they make $150,000 or $250,000 per year, a little time off may well be worth more to them than earning an extra $5,000 by working late. This is one reason the supply of physician time is not very elastic; even doubling or quadrupling physicians' income could not get them to double the number of hours worked. Indeed, it is even possible that for some physicians, supply is "backward bending": Higher income per hour might make them feel sufficiently rich that they work fewer rather than more hours.[8] If backward-bending supply seems difficult to understand, think about how much you would work if I paid you $100 per hour, $1,000 per hour, or $100,000 per hour. Eventually you would decide to work less and enjoy leisure more because additional money simply would not mean that much to you.

One difficulty physicians have in making the labor versus leisure choice is that their income often depends on putting in many hours per week early in their careers, when the rate of pay is low or even zero. This is similar to the problem facing most college students: Getting into the best business or law school and making partner depends on excess hours put in now to obtain future income. To fully analyze the trade-off between labor and leisure, it is necessary to recognize that some work is done more for its value as investment in future earnings than for current earnings.

The Doctor's Workshop and Unpaid Hospital Inputs

Almost every doctor needs to use a hospital to provide patient care. Some specialties (anesthesiology, thoracic surgery, pathology) are practiced almost entirely inside hospitals. Yet physicians do not pay the hospital for the privilege of working there and usually are not employees of the hospital. In terms of an influential model proposed by Mark Pauly and Michael Redisch, the hospital functions as the "doctor's workshop" and is a source of unpaid inputs in production.[9] Because the efforts of hospital nurses, laboratory technicians, and record keeping professionals do not "cost" the physician anything, physicians tend to overuse them to supplant the use of similar inputs in their offices. It is easy to see how they might favor a system of nonprofit hospitals supported by the community and government subsidy because the value added to their practices by these hospitals far exceeds the hours physicians are expected to "give" to hospital educational and administrative functions.

The hospital-based specialties of radiology and pathology are a special case, with high incomes that clearly depend on hospital practice. Because physicians in these specialties spend virtually all their professional time within the hospital, have a regular flow of work, and do not meet individually with patients, it appears that they might most readily be paid on salary. Yet historically, radiologists have strongly opposed salaried practice, favoring fee-for-service arrangements, contracts in which they operate the diagnostic facility for a percentage of gross revenues or pay rent to the hospital. Their opposition was sufficient to force Medicare to separate the professional fee for reviewing x-rays and specimens from the hospital charges for producing them. The primary issue is control—over professional activity and over money. If the pathologist runs the lab, he or she in effect "owns" the captive block of business constituted by the hospital's patients. However, if the hospital runs the lab, pathologists must compete on the basis of price (i.e., take a lower salary) and accept hospital direction over their working conditions. Consider the case of a 60-year-old pathologist who has been head of the lab for 20 years and is friendly with most of the surgeons on staff. If it is his lab, he can bring in a junior pathologist to do the day-to-day work and go into semi-retirement to play golf with the hospital administrator and his surgeon friends, living off the "rents" he collects as an owner of the practice. If it is the hospital's lab and he is on salary, the hospital can threaten to fire him and hire the junior pathologist to save money, unless the senior pathologist is willing to accept a pay cut and work harder. The issue of who "owns" the patient's business and can collect the additional income (rents) arising from control over volume and referrals arises repeatedly in our examination of the organization of medicine and is central to managed care (see Chapters 5 and 12).

Malpractice

One of the most contentious physician practice expenses is malpractice insurance. The rationale for allowing medical malpractice suits is that they improve incentives for safety by forcing doctors to behave more carefully when treating patients. Malpractice is not a good way of compensating patients for harm done to them, since it costs $1.20 in legal fees for every $1 a patient receives.[10] About one in twenty physicians will incur a malpractice claim in any given year, and two in five will be sued at least once during their careers. The premium for a physician's malpractice insurance averages about $23,500 (5 percent of gross revenues), but it ranges from just $7,000 or less for family practitioners to $100,000 and more for orthopedic and neurosurgeons. Although malpractice premiums have risen rapidly in some years, virtually all the additional costs are quickly passed on to patients and their insurance companies in the form of higher fees, and one recent study showed that after adjustment for inflation over the last 30 years, premiums were actually level or lower in a majority of specialties.

Malpractice is a real problem, but the current malpractice system might not be the best solution. Studies have shown that a negligent iatrogenic injury (i.e., caused by the physician) occurs approximately once in every 100 hospital admissions. Only a tenth of those injured will file a claim, and less than half will gain compensation through the courts. At the same time, a larger number of suits are filed when there was no negligence, and some of these patients win despite the lack of any physician error. The randomness of the legal process, as well as the fact that most physicians are almost fully insured for losses due to malpractice, limits the effectiveness of the system to change behavior. However, being sued is costly in terms of lost time and increased anxiety, and most physicians exercise extraordinary care in treating patients. After all, they became physicians because they wanted to care for patients, not because they wanted a job that was easy. Although some physicians have claimed that the fear of being sued has raised medical costs by forcing them to practice "defensive medicine," some studies have shown that higher levels of liability or a greater number of suits do not necessarily lead to much higher numbers of tests per patient, more admissions, or more prescriptions.[11] Because most suits are filed for a procedure that a doctor has done, rather than for something not done or for a diagnosis that was missed, the lack of excessive testing or other medical treatment attributable to malpractice is not surprising.

Does the malpractice system deter negligence by physicians? Only to a limited extent, and at considerable cost. Yet while the ability of malpractice suits to compensate patients for damages or to force doctors to practice better medicine has been roundly criticized with good reason, it has not been easy to find a solution that is clearly more efficient or acceptable to both doctors and patients.

6.4 THE MEDICAL TRANSACTION

People do not purchase medical care: they go to the doctor because they are sick. Patients enter the health system to get care, not to "buy" something, yet somebody must pay. When patients show up at a doctor's office, they are apt to ask two questions: "What is wrong with me?" and "What should I do about it?" If told that they have a disease, most patients trust the doctor to perform the right diagnostic tests and therapeutic procedures, with little idea of what those might be or what the charges will add up to.[12] If a surgeon is called in, he or she is likely to be a complete stranger who asks for thousands of dollars to make an evaluation and incision.

Patients who agree to surgery can only hope that in the long run it will do some good, because postoperative pain and mortality will make them worse off in the short run. Unlike a person shopping for a car, a suit, or a haircut, patients do not know what they need, what it should cost, and even, once paid for, how much good the treatment actually did. Instead of a clear specification of what is to be expected from both parties, the patient must trust the doctor to do what is right and to bill fairly for the necessary care (which will mostly be paid for by insurance).

Asymmetric Information

It is the superior ability of the physician to answer those two questions that tends to make the doctor–patient relationship so much different from an ordinary commercial transaction. Although the physician's information is not perfect, it is much better than that of the patient, and the physician is able to seek additional information required for treating an illness at much lower cost. This disparity is known as **information asymmetry**. When it is necessary to decide which test to perform, which drug to prescribe, and whether to perform surgery, all these choices can be made better and at lower cost by a physician. An exchange relationship in which one party makes choices on behalf of the other is known as **agency**.[13] Just as a purchasing agent buys supplies for a company and an actor's agent represents the actor in negotiations, a physician is the patient's agent in deciding which treatment is appropriate and which medical services to buy. The reason that agents act on behalf of another is that the agent's information and transaction costs are lower. It is cheaper for a physician to make medical choices on behalf of a patient than for the patient to go to medical school to make a decision.

Agency: Whose Choices?

When ordering food or renting a movie, personal tastes and preferences determine the best choice. Markets excel at matching myriads of consumers with thousands of products. Complex tradeoffs among price, quality, and individual desires are made with little difficulty or cost. Medicine is different. The best choice of treatment depends upon illness, not tastes and preferences. Value for money is achieved in the markets for food and movies by allowing consumers to choose among the many alternatives available in the marketplace. In medicine, most choices must be made by the doctor. Patients often would not even know what illness they have, much less the pros and cons of each treatment option, without expert advice. The patient cannot choose his or her own medicine but must have a prescription written by the doctor. The choice among specialists and diagnostic facilities is called a referral because it is made by the doctor, not the patient.

Although many goods and services are transacted under conditions of less-than-perfect information, it is the magnitude of the disparity that sets medical care apart. For example, although I might not know what my mechanic is doing, I can readily observe whether my automobile is working better when it comes back from the shop. Poor quality parts can be repaired or replaced. At most, I might ask for my money back. Bad surgery is not only difficult to detect, it also can be disabling or even fatal. Once you are dead, repairs, replacements, and even outrageously large malpractice settlements are irrelevant. To an extraordinary degree, the demand-side choices normally made by consumers are delegated to providers in medical markets.

6.5 UNCERTAINTY

In what is perhaps the most well-known and often-cited paper on health economics, Nobel laureate Kenneth Arrow stated: "The special economic problems of medical care can be explained as adaptations to the existence of uncertainty in the incidence of disease and in the efficacy of treatment."[14]

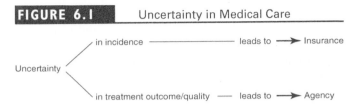

FIGURE 6.1   Uncertainty in Medical Care

Uncertainty in the incidence of illness can be ameliorated by the use of insurance. Uncertainty in the outcome and quality of treatment can be ameliorated by exchange using an agency relationship; licensure and trust in physicians, nonprofit ownership, and government regulation.

As discussed in Chapter 4, uncertainty "in the incidence of disease" refers to the random occurrence of illness: One never knows when one will get sick or how bad the illness will be. The problem of randomly occurring losses can be offset to some extent by pooling risks through insurance. The losses still occur and must be paid for, but the financial uncertainty is removed.

Uncertainty "in the efficacy of treatment" refers to the inability to know whether the chosen treatment will work. In theory, it might be possible to "insure" against such losses, but in the real world there are no meaningful guarantees for medical care. A cardiologist treating you for a heart attack does not guarantee that you will be able to run marathons again, nor does an oncologist guarantee that she can cure your cancer. The most either will promise is to provide you with everything modern medicine has to offer. Why can't they give a guarantee? First of all, because it is so difficult to tell how ill you were in the first place, it is often impossible to tell whether treatment has improved your health. Second, unlike a car or a house, there is no way to replace your body. Although almost any ordinary loss can be fixed with sufficient compensation, a monetary guarantee is an empty promise if you are dead.[15]

The distinction between the two types of uncertainty and the economic response to them is shown in Figure 6.1. Note that in each case, there is a transfer of responsibility away from the patient. Under insurance, the responsibility for payment is transferred to the insurance company, relieving all actual and potential patients of the uncertainty of financial losses due to illness. Under agency, the responsibility for making a decision on appropriate care is transferred from the patient to the physician. Agency creates gains because it substitutes professional control for costly patient monitoring of quality. It is much cheaper for an experienced and highly educated physician to determine which treatment is best than for a patient to try to do so.

6.6   LICENSURE: QUALITY OR PROFITS?

Licensure is a collective extension of the doctor–patient relationship of agency. Not only do individual patients trust their physicians to act as their personal agents, all of us together have collectively chosen to let the medical profession act as our public agent, deciding who is qualified to practice medicine. Through the institution of **licensure**, the medical profession serves as a sort of quasi-governmental body making decisions of behalf of all consumers.[16] Consumers do not examine each doctor's credentials and legal records, they turn that responsibility over to licensure boards. It is cheaper for knowledgeable professionals to do this once for all consumers rather than having each patient individually try to determine whether the person listed as a "doctor" in the directory is qualified to practice medicine. The government does not make laws regarding the practice of medicine, but it uses laws to enforce the decisions made by voluntary and independent professional boards.

It is often debated in the media and among economists whether licensure serves the interests of patients (by improving the quality of care) or of physicians (by raising prices and incomes).[17] Such a debate, framed in terms of one side or the other, misses the point: Any public policy in a democracy is in fact a form of trade that must serve the interests of both parties if the policy is to be upheld. By the fundamental theorem of exchange, both physicians and patients must be made better off by licensure.

How Does Licensure Increase Physician Profits?

Licensure radically changes the market structure. A flexible supply curve is replaced by a fixed supply—diagrammatically a vertical line, because the number of doctors does not change as prices rise or fall (see Figure 6.2). To the extent that the supply of doctor services is reduced under licensure, prices are pushed higher so that all doctors enjoy higher incomes (of course, this means that some people who wished to become doctors are not allowed to do so). These profits are maximized if the profession acts as a monopoly in determining how many doctors are allowed to practice. Supply can also be reduced by work rules that control total productivity. For example, it is common for dental practice regulations to determine how many assistants each dentist can supervise (and therefore the number of total patients who can be seen). Extending the physician's training period also serves to reduce the effective doctor supply, because each graduate has fewer remaining years of productivity.

Thinking of the demand for physician services as derived demand suggests two further possibilities for raising income: (1) increasing the price of substitutes such as chiropractors or nurses and (2) increasing demand for output. The effective price of many physician substitutes can be made prohibitively large by forbidding them to perform some acts (prescribing drugs, performing surgery, admitting a patient to the hospital). Less extreme, but also effective, are rules that limit health insurance to reimbursement for services performed by or under the supervision of a physician. Even if a substitute provider is willing to provide services at a much lower price, it will still cost patients more because they will have to pay the entire bill out of pocket. Insurance has been the most important factor in increasing the overall demand for medical care. Physicians have played a major role in the spread of insurance and the creation of payment system rules (e.g., UCR fees, separate professional fees for radiologists and pathologists) which increase physicians' economic power. Hospital-based specialists such as radiologists and pathologists have fought the implementation of RBRVS and bulk-purchase managed-care contracts that tend to give more control to payers and increase price competition among suppliers. Professional activities also directly increase demand both through new

FIGURE 6.2   Demand and Supply with Licensure

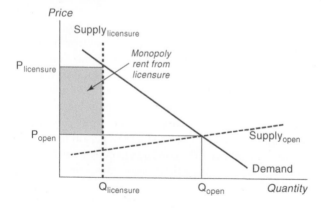

medical discoveries and by monitoring and controlling quality so that patients are more willing to visit any licensed practitioner.

Supply and Demand Response in Licensed versus Unlicensed Professions

To illustrate the differences in market dynamics between licensed and unlicensed labor supply, physicians are compared with health administrators in Figure 6.3. Health administrators often earn a master of health administration (M.H.A.) degree early in their careers, but many rise through the ranks without attending graduate school and others obtain master of business administration (M.B.A.) or master of science (M.S.) degrees in schools of business, medicine, public health, public policy, or human services.[18] The crucial point is that there is no central control over the number of people who can enter the profession, no licensure or specific educational requirement, and no legal restriction on practice by outsiders. Administrators usually start at modest salaries ranging from $40,000 to $80,000, like most people with an M.B.A. degree, and work their way up the organizational ranks. Although some administrators eventually earn large salaries, many tend to get stuck in the middle ranges and some are pushed out of the field entirely. Thus, administrator earnings are related to individual characteristics and experience and hence are rather variable. Physician earnings are in part monopoly "rents," increased profits shared by the profession as a whole, and thus are not only higher but are also more stable. Although both physicians and administrators see their earnings increase as they gain more experience, for physicians, the growth is more regular and virtually never interrupted by unemployment.

The comparative effects of an increase in demand are shown in Figure 6.3. For physicians, who are licensed, virtually all the increase in demand goes into higher incomes because there is no flexibility for supply to increase. For unlicensed administrators, higher wages attract more and better entrants so that part of the increase in demand goes into an increase in the quantity of labor supplied and only partly into an increase in incomes. Although increased demand leads to more applicants to medical schools, no new medical schools will be built because these numbers are controlled by the AMA, American Association of Medical Colleges (AAMC), and affiliated professional bodies. In contrast, increasing demand for health administrators has caused graduate programs to spring up around the country as universities compete to attract students.

FIGURE 6.3   Comparison of Demand Increase with and without Licensure

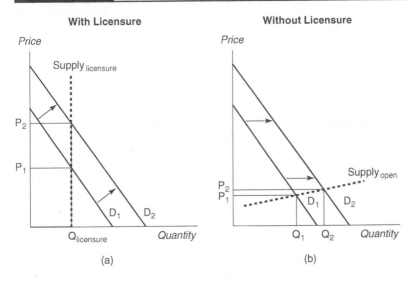

How Does Licensure Improve Quality?

It is possible to improve quality by revoking the licenses of physicians whose medical practices are shown to be inferior, but such removals are rare.[19] The quality of physicians in practice depends much more on the initial selection of who is allowed to enter the profession, the training they receive, and efforts by practicing physicians to monitor one another and impose informal sanctions (ostracism from professional groups, denial of hospital privileges, refusal to refer new patients or share business opportunities).[20] *The ability of sanctions and selection to improve quality would be greatly reduced if there were no monopoly profits.* Because licensure restrictions guarantee successful applicants a career with high income and prestige, many outstanding students seek admission to medical school. After becoming doctors, they work very hard not to lose that title. The money and power that come with being a physician, a form of monopoly profits, are too attractive to give up. If a doctor could earn more money and satisfaction working in a bank, an insurance company, or another career, why worry about losing a medical license? The opportunity cost of losing a license is so significant that the threat is sufficient deterrent, making rather rare for the profession to actually revoke a license and terminate a physician's right to practice.

The value of a license depends on the prestige of the medical profession as a whole; therefore, each doctor has an incentive to maintain the professional franchise by selecting only the best candidates to enter the profession and by continuing to make sure that all doctors are as good as they can be at caring for patients so that demand remains high.[21]

Choosing only the best candidates for admission to medical school means that the graduates will be superior regardless of how much they learn during medical school. Prestige and income play a large part in attracting outstanding students. The incentive for a student to train long and hard is also related to the expectation of high income in the future. After graduation, the threat of losing these extraordinary returns provides an incentive to maintain competency and support licensing boards. The existence of monopoly profits serves as a monetary performance bond that can be lost, a kind of collective collateral put up by the profession to ensure good service on the part of all its members.

Observing that some specific restrictions on medical practice have no direct bearing on quality has led some economists to question whether licensure boards are committed to protecting the public interest or the private economic interests of their members. Application of the fundamental theorem of exchange indicates that there is no conflict between the two objectives and that they can reinforce each other. A particular restriction on medical practice might not directly improve quality, but removing it could cause quality to deteriorate by reducing the monopoly profits that provide incentives for the profession to police itself. A better test of whether licensure improves quality is to look at how the strength of licensure restrictions varies by type of medical practice—where and when the "licensure contract" is most apt to be approved by both patients and physicians.

A Test of the Quality Hypothesis: Strong versus Weak Licensure

The timing of licensure legislation suggests that until the level of a doctor's training can significantly affect quality and the probable outcome of treatment, effective professional licensure is unlikely to occur or will be very weakly enforced. Before 1900, licensure was clearly desired by physicians to improve their economic status, as demonstrated by their vociferous support of such laws in state legislatures. Yet licensure laws could not get popular political support until medical science advanced to the point at which knowledge made a real difference.[22] The strength of licensure was related not only to the increased effectiveness of new treatments but also to the increased danger posed by the use of surgery and powerful drugs.

TABLE 6.5	Weak versus Strong Licensure
Weak ◄──────── Licensure ────────►	**Strong**
Consumers can choose	Only trained professionals choose well
Low risk	High risk
Uncertainty small	Information asymmetry high
Examples: podiatry, eyeglasses	*Examples: neurosurgery, organ transplants*

Some types of medical care, such as cardiac surgery, are inherently dangerous and demand great skill. Bad heart surgeons can have a mortality rate five times higher than good heart surgeons.[23] Given the great impact of measurable indicators of physician quality (training, medical practice records, opinions of peers), we would expect licensure restrictions to be very strong for heart surgery (see Table 6.5). That is indeed the case. Although legally one need only be licensed as a physician in order to perform heart surgery, in practice doctors are virtually prohibited from doing so unless they have completed a residency, completed a fellowship in the specialty, and been given special hospital privileges after a review by peers who have observed them acting as assistants on a number of operations. These additional mandatory checks make it evident that heart surgery has strong licensure restrictions.

Conversely, other types of medical care are much less dangerous and demanding, such as surgery to remove corns from the foot. Although such surgery can be practiced with greater or lesser skill, it is not likely to cost a life. One does not need a residency or hospital medical staff review to remove corns, and indeed corns are often removed by podiatrists, who are not licensed doctors of medicine (M.D.s), although they are usually licensed doctors of podiatric medicine (D.P.M.s). The lack of special medical staff restrictions and the existence of alternative professional certification show that care of the foot has weak licensure. Refractions to prescribe eyeglasses are similarly performed by competing professions (M.D. ophthalmologists and O.D. optometrists) under weak licensure. Mental health is a specialty with a wide array of professionals—psychiatrists (M.D.s), psychologists (Psy.D. doctors of psychology or Ph.D. doctors of philosophy), family therapists and counselors (C.A.C., M.S.W., A.A.M.F.T., and other designations), and even psychics (palm readers, speakers for past lives, aura visionaries)—and such weak licensure that virtually anyone can offer to help you with your problems. There are substantial risks to life in mental illness, and more people die from substance abuse and depression than from many other conditions, but the professional does not always have substantial advantage over the client in choosing therapies and therapists, because personality match is so important. It is hard to gain insight from a psychologist you despise, or who despises you, but a cardiac surgeon can be totally lacking in human interpersonal skills and still perform a good operation.

As the extent and value of the information asymmetry between patients and professionals increases, licensure becomes stronger. For heart surgery, technical quality is paramount and is well evaluated by professional standards. Medical licensure is supplemented by hospital privilege reviews, insurance restrictions, and other forceful measures. However, for types of care in which the information differential is small, licensure is weak. For a broken heart, an MD psychiatrist may be no more effective than a sympathetic psychic whom the patient trusts, and for counseling, there are multiple forms of licensure, all rather weakly enforced.

SUGGESTIONS FOR FURTHER READING

American Medical Association, *Socioeconomic Characteristics of Medical Practice and Physician Characteristics and Distribution in the United States,* published annually.

Kenneth Arrow, "Uncertainty and the Welfare Economics of Medical Care," *American Economic Review* 53, no. 3 (1963): 941–973

Atul Gawande, *Complications: A Surgeon's Notes on an Imperfect Science* (New York: Holt & Co., 2002) and "The Velluvial Matrix." *The New Yorker,* June 16, 2010.

Paul L. Grimaldi, "Medicare's Physician Fees Are Resource Based," *Journal of Health Care Finance,* (Spring 2002): 88–104.

Institute of Medicine, *To Err Is Human* (Washington, D.C.: National Academies Press, 2000); *Crossing the Quality Chasm* (Washington, D.C.: National Academies Press, 2001).

George D. Lundberg, *Severed Trust: Why American Medicine Hasn't Been Fixed* (New York: Basic Books, 2001).

Michael Millenson, *Demanding Medical Excellence: Doctors and Accountability in the Information Age* (Chicago: University of Chicago Press, 2000).

Roy Porter, *The Greatest Benefit of Mankind: A Medical History of Humanity* (New York: WW Norton, 1999).

SUMMARY

1. The **doctor–patient relationship** stands at the center of the medical care system. Although payments to physicians constitute only 20 percent of total health care expenditures, special characteristics of this exchange influence the organization and financing of all other parts of the system. The bond of **trust** between doctor and patient is one of the strongest professional relationships in society.

2. Over time, physician payment has changed from fee-for-service prices similar to prices of most other economic goods and services to complex reimbursement plans based on administrative formulas and negotiation. Increasingly, physicians are involved with managed care plans that pay a **capitation** rate (physicians receive a certain amount per member per month) or **discounted fee schedules** based on **relative value scales**.

3. Most physicians are owners or partners in small businesses rather than employees. They work long hours but do not face much business risk. On average, **self-employed physicians earn about $260,000**, and those who work as employees and are somewhat younger earn $210,000. Physicians who practiced in cognitive and caring specialties (family practice, psychiatry, pediatrics, internal medicine) earned less than those who practiced in procedure-oriented specialties (surgery, obstetrics/gynecology, radiology).

4. The average office medical practice hired **four allied health workers per physician** and had overall expenses equal to 51 percent of gross patient revenues. Although malpractice insurance is the expense category most commonly complained about, **malpractice takes only 3 to 7 percent of gross** revenues for most physician practices.

5. **Uncertainty** creates or exacerbates most of the information problems in medical care. Whereas financial uncertainty due to the random occurrence of illness can be reduced by insurance, uncertainty about the quality of care and outcome of treatment cannot. Therefore collective agency mechanisms such as licensure and strong ethical traditions for physicians have been established.

6. **Information asymmetry** arises from the difference between the physician's and the patient's knowledge of medical treatments. Because of this disparity in the cost of knowledge, patients must trust physicians to act as their agents and make decisions on their behalf. In most economic exchanges, the point at which goods and services are transacted is the point at which information cost differentials are lowest. Because a low-cost valuation of well-defined goods is not possible in medicine, a trust relationship of agency has been established to ameliorate this potential market failure.

7. **Licensure** is a collective extension of the doctor–patient relationship of agency. It helps solve the problems caused by uncertainty and information asymmetry. **Licensure increases profits** by restricting supply, thus changing the traditional supply and demand curve analysis. The supply curve is fixed, or vertical, and increases in demand do not result

in an increase in quantity but in increased profits for suppliers known by economists as "rents." **Licensure increases quality** by ensuring that only the best students are selected to enter medical school, mandating that students have four years of medical school, three years of residency, and periodical refresher courses thereafter, and having physicians monitor one another. All these depend on having some excess profits or monopoly rents to serve as an incentive. Licensure is intended both to increase profits and to increase quality. Like any law, it **must satisfy both parties** (physicians and the public/patients) to be a self-enforcing political exchange. The importance of quality concerns is evidenced by comparing the types of care for which licensure is strong (cardiac surgery, chemotherapy) with those for which it is weak (removing corns, prescribing eyeglasses, counseling).

PROBLEMS

1. {*incentives*} Which type of payment gives a physician the most incentive to do the following:
    a. Spend more time with each patient? Spend less?
    b. Provide more laboratory services to each patient? Provide less?
    c. Modify the listing of diagnoses to increase revenues? Be objective?
    d. Reduce hospital utilization? Increase hospital utilization?
    e. Ask patients to return frequently? Try to handle problems once and for all?

2. {*compensation*} Do you believe that radiologists prefer to be compensated in a fee-for-service manner, by relative value scale, on salary, or as part of a capitated rate? Why? Why might practitioners of different specialties prefer different forms of payment?

3. {*organization*} Which organization provides the largest amount of payment to physicians in the United States? How does this organization choose to make these payments? Has the form of payment changed over time? Why?

4. {*earnings differentials*} What are some of the reasons that most pediatricians earn less than most neurosurgeons?

5. {*age earnings profile*} Generally, most physicians' incomes increase as they get older. Is the rate of earnings increase greater for some specialties than others? Why? Do you expect that male and female physicians have the same age-earnings profile? Why or why not?

6. {*earnings differentials*} Would you expect that physicians who earn significantly more than their peers have office practice costs that are above or below average? Are they more or less likely to hire other physicians?

7. {*valuation*} How are the values determined in setting up a relative value scale?

8. {*malpractice*} What are the objectives of the current medical malpractice system in the United States? How well does it work in achieving these objectives?

9. {*uncertainty*} If uncertainty regarding the occurrence of losses can be dealt with through insurance markets, why can't uncertainty regarding the outcome or quality of medical care be similarly priced and transferred?

10. {*agency*} What is an agent? How does employing an agent reduce the costs of making a transaction? Does employing an agent create any problems that would not occur if the consumer acted alone?

11. {*licensure*} Does licensure raise the quality of medical care, or does it raise the profitability of medical practice?

12. {*information asymmetry*} How do agency and information asymmetry lead to licensure? Are there more or fewer gains from trade as the degree of information asymmetry increases?

13. {*information asymmetry*} What does it mean to say that licensure is weak or strong? Why does the strength of licensure vary?

ENDNOTES

1. Atul Gawande, "Piecework: Medicine's Money Problem," *The New Yorker,* April 4, 2005: 44–53; Eliot Freidson, *Profession of Medicine* (New York: Dodd, Mead, 1970); Victor R. Fuchs, *Who Shall Live? Health, Economics and Social Choice* (New York: Basic Books, 1983).

2. Most of the information here is from surveys done by the American Medical Association and reported in *Socioeconomic Characteristics of Medical Practice,* an annual/biennial monograph. A good sense of the entrepreneurial flavor of medical practice can be obtained by perusing several issues of *Medical Economics,* the "Business Week" of physicians.

3. U.S. National Health Accounts (www.cms.gov/statistics/nhe), see discussion and references in Chapter 1.

4. W. C. Hsiao, P. Braun, D. Dunn, and E. R. Becker, "Resource-Based Relative Values: An Overview," *Journal of the American Medical Association* 260, no. 16 (1988): 2347–2353; William C. Hsiao et al., "Results and Impacts of the Resource-Based Relative Value Scale," *Medical Care* 30(11 Supplement): NS61–NS79, 1992.

5. Christopher S. Brunt, "CPT Fee Differentials and Visit Upcoding under Medicare Part B." *Health Economics* 20, 2011: 831-841.

6. GB. Hickson, WA. Altmeier, and JM. Perris, "Physician Reimbursement by Salary or Fee-For-Service: Effect on Physician Practice Behavior in a Randomized Prospective Study," *Pediatrics* 80, no. 3 (1987): 344–350; LA Helmchen and AT Lo Sasso, "How Sensitive is Physician Performance to Alternative Compensation Schedules?" *Health Economics* 19, no. 11 (2010): 1300–1317; Jason Shafrin, "Operating on Commission: Analyzing How Physician Financial Incentives Affect Surgery Rates," *Health Economics* 19, no. 5 (2010): 562–589.

7. Medicaid Access Study Group, "Access of Medicaid Recipients to Outpatient Care," *New England Journal of Medicine* 330, no. 20 (1994): 1426–1430.

8. Frank A. Sloan, "Physician Supply Behavior in the Short Run," *Industrial and Labor Relations Review* 28, no. 4 (1975): 549–569.

9. Mark V. Pauly and Michael Redisch, "The Not-for-Profit Hospital as a Physician Cooperative," *American Economic Review* 63, no. 1 (1973): 87–99.

10. Patricia Danzon, "Liability for Medical Malpractice," *Journal of Economic Perspectives* 5, no. 3 (1995): 51–69; A. J. Culyer and J. P. Newhouse, eds., *Handbook of Health Economics* (Amsterdam: Elsevier, 2000), 1339–1404; MA Rodwin, HJ Chang, and J Clause, "Malpractice Premiums and Physicians' Income Perceptions of a Crisis Conflict with Empirical Evidence," *Health Affairs* 25, no. 3 (2005): 750–758; Marc A. Rodwin et al., "Malpractice Premiums in Massachusetts, a High-Risk State: 1975–2005," *Health Affairs* 27, no. 3 (2008): 835–844; M. M. Mello et al., "National Costs of the Medical Liability System," *Health Affairs* 29, no. 9 (2010): 1569–1582.

11. Peter A. Glassman, John E. Rolph, Laura P. Petersen, Melissa A. Bradley, and Richard L. Kravitz, "Physician's Personal Malpractice Experiences Are Not Related to Defensive Clinical Practices," *Journal of Health Politics, Policy and Law* 21, no. 2 (1996): 219–241.

12. This special economic character of the "trust" relationship with doctors has long been noted and is discussed in Adam Smith's seminal 1776 treatise, *The Wealth of Nations.*

13. Michael C. Jensen and William H. Meckling, "Agency Costs in the Firm" and "Theory of the Firm: Managerial Behavior, Agency Costs and Ownership Structure," *Journal of Financial Economics* 3, no. 4 (1976): 305–360. The extensive economic analysis of agency has focused primarily on the manager of a firm who makes decisions on behalf of shareholders. Many of these models are applicable, but because medical outcomes are not as readily measured as the profits of a firm, and because death has even more moral overtones than bankruptcy, the doctor–patient bond has important aspects above and beyond those that characterize the relationships of owner-to-shareholder or supervisor-to-employee. See the books by Gawande and Millenson in Suggestions for Further Reading, and see Mark V. Pauly, "Taxation, Health Insurance, and Market Failure in the Medical Economy," *Journal of Economic Literature* 24, no. 2 (1986): 629–675; Robert L. Kane and Matthew Maciejewski, "The Relationship of Patient Satisfaction with Care and Clinical Outcomes," *Medical Care* 35, no. 7 (1997): 714–730.

14. Kenneth J. Arrow, "Uncertainty and the Welfare Economics of Medical Care," *American Economic Review* 53, no. 3 (1963): 941–973.

15. To give a guarantee means to provide a contract stipulating what you will receive if something goes wrong (replace the item, give money back, etc.). What would a "medical guarantee" look like? The broken transmission of a car can be repaired for $700, making money a fully satisfactory replacement. There is no such replacement for health or the pain of disease. Even if we could agree on a monetary amount, it would be different for every illness,

different for every person, and different even if it was the same person and illness at a later time of life. There is no way to write a satisfactory contract in advance, hence the need for a substitute form of commercial relationship.

16. Richard Shryock, *Medical Licensing in America, 1650–1965* (Baltimore: Johns Hopkins University Press, 1967).

17. Elton Rayack, *Professional Power and American Medicine: The Economics of the American Medical Association* (Cleveland, Ohio: World Publishing, 1967).

18. U.S. Bureau of Labor Statistics, *Occupational Outlook,* BLS Bulletin 2450 (Washington, D.C.: U.S. Government Printing Office, 1994).

19. Formal licensure actions against physicians are infrequent and are usually for misconduct (drug abuse, fraud, sexual advances) rather than poor quality of care, which has led some observers to conclude that the institution of licensure was never intended to improve quality. However, note that revoking of a driver's license is similarly rare. The quality of daily driving is measured by a 15-minute test when a person is first licensed, but not thereafter, and revocation of drivers' licenses reflects a similar pattern of egregious personal flaws rather than the traits associated with quality (vision, eye–hand coordination, etc.).

20. Eliot Freidson, *Professional Dominance: The Social Structure of Medical Care* (New York: Atherton, 1970); and *Professional Powers: A Study in the Institutionalization of Formal Knowledge* (Chicago: University of Chicago Press, 1986).

21. Unfortunately, the desire to maintain the value of physician licensure also provides an incentive to cover up cases of poor quality. Admitting that some licensed physicians were actually bad doctors would reduce demand and thus diminish the value of all licenses. Therefore, sometimes physicians act to protect their own by hiding evidence of malpractice or other failures even when they strongly disapprove and could get rid of the offender.

22. John Duffy, *From Humors to Medical Science: A History of American Medicine* (Urbana: University of Illinois Press, 1993).

23. *A Consumer Guide to Coronary Artery Bypass Graft Surgery,* Vol. IV, 1993 Data. PHC4 (Harrisburg: Pennsylvania Health Care Cost Containment Council, 1995).

CHAPTER 7

MEDICAL EDUCATION, ORGANIZATION, AND BUSINESS PRACTICES

QUESTIONS

1. Who controls the supply of physicians: the government or the American Medical Association (AMA)?
2. Are doctors more or less productive than they were twenty years ago?
3. Why do patients in Boston undergo more surgeries than patients in San Francisco?
4. Why are there more foreign doctors practicing in the United States than U.S. doctors practicing overseas if the needs are much greater there?
5. Can medical groups advertise to attract more patients and increase market power? Are bigger practices more efficient?
6. Is price discrimination legal? Why are some patients charged more for the same service? Why and how are doctors giving discounts on fees?
7. Do physicians trade patients? Are payments between doctors for referrals legal, ethical, or efficient?
8. Are chiropractors a substitute for physicians, or are they a complement?
9. Who sets the standards of practice to guide clinical decisions?

7.1 MEDICAL EDUCATION

A select and hard-working group of 17,500 students will graduate with doctor of medicine (MD) degrees from one of 127 U.S. medical schools this year.[1] For most of them it will be the middle of an arduous process that has taken over most of their lives since high school, and it will forever change the way they view the world and how the world views them. Many first thought about becoming doctors in elementary school, but some decided after pursuing other careers. All had to take premed courses in chemistry, biology, and physics and did rather well on average—almost half of them had an A average as undergraduates (grade point average (GPA) of 3.6 or higher). Getting into medical school was serious business that took substantial effort, and many applied to 10 or more schools. Much of the selection, however, was self-selection. Weaker students generally chose not to apply. Less than half of the applicants to medical school were rejected. Of those who were admitted, 98 percent chose to enroll, and of those, 95 percent will graduate, almost all of whom will then enter a hospital-based residency training program lasting three years or more before becoming generalist family physicians or specialists in one of the other 22 recognized areas of medical practice eligible for board certification.

Although much has been made of the cost of medical education, most of that cost is borne indirectly by the government and the health insurance system. Just 4 percent of medical school costs are covered by tuition payments from students, whereas 46 percent comes from patient fees, 30 percent from research, and 20 percent from government appropriations and gifts.[2] Although tuition might run as high as $50,000 per year and most medical students (83 percent) are left with debts from student loans when they graduate, the amount of those loans (which average about $110,000) is not very large in relation to the income a physician can expect: less than 1 percent of lifetime earnings.[3] Far more onerous than the monetary obligations are the years of toil spent in learning the practice of medicine.

7.2 THE ORIGINS OF LICENSURE AND LINKAGE TO MEDICAL EDUCATION

At the time of the American Revolution, there were about 3,500 established medical practitioners in what was to become the United States, but only 400 had received any formal training and fewer than 200 held degrees. The ability to read and quote some Latin and serving an apprenticeship were considered sufficient qualifications for hanging out a shingle and calling oneself a doctor. As late as 1830, the University of Virginia provided all its students with instruction in medicine. Yet before 1900, there was little scientific basis for the way most doctors practiced medicine, and indeed the treatments prescribed were about as likely to harm health as to improve it. Because there was really no benefit from seeing a trained professional, there was no support for restricting the practice of medicine through licensure. Although state medical associations repeatedly pushed for licensure and were sometimes temporarily successful, the lack of public benefit doomed such efforts. In New Jersey, licensure laws were passed and then repealed at least 16 times between 1800 and 1900.[4] In other states, licensure laws were on the books but did not mean much because they were not enforced.

Two major technological breakthroughs radically changed the nature of medicine: anesthesiology (pain killing) and antisepsis (germ killing). Although surgery had been practiced since the dawn of humankind, the lack of anesthesia meant that most operations could last only a few minutes, and even then many patients went into shock and died. The other problem was postsurgical infection, which claimed almost as many lives as the injuries that were treated. Very few of the hundreds of thousands of soldiers who died during the Civil War were actually killed in battle; most died in hospitals days or weeks later. Today, most of those wounded soldiers could easily be saved. Anesthesia and antiseptics changed surgery from a last resort for the desperate patient who would otherwise die into a routine procedure used in the treatment of many diseases. The fact that 20th-century surgery was more effective also paradoxically increased the risks. Patients who never before would have considered letting themselves be cut open went under the knife willingly.

Anesthesia, antiseptics, and a host of other scientific breakthroughs changed the promise, and the politics, of medicine. There was no longer any question that doctors must be educated and examined before they were allowed to practice. The Flexner Report of 1910 to the Carnegie Commission, which was supported by the AMA, called for the closure of all medical schools that did not require an undergraduate college degree for admission and provide laboratory training in biology and chemistry, clinical internships, and full-time faculty members. These standards, first viewed as utopian, were implemented with increasing force over the next three decades.

Legal control over physicians resides with state licensure boards, yet supply is actually determined by control over the number of students allowed to enter medical school (and the number of foreign medical graduates allowed to come to the United States for training, who often stay to practice). Unlike law school, in which many students fail to graduate, or graduate and fail the bar exam, or pass the bar exam and cannot find a job, almost all medical students graduate and practice medicine. There are exams in school and afterward, but almost everyone passes, and the limitation of numbers is sufficient to ensure that everyone who wants to can find a position practicing medicine. By the end of the Depression, the old laissez-faire system of unregulated physician practice with open entry had been entirely replaced by a modern system of medical licensure, with control over supply resting in the hands of the medical schools (which, in turn, were largely controlled by the joint AMA and Association of American Medical Colleges [AAMC] Committee on Medical Education).

A major practical difficulty in implementing licensure was how to handle all the existing physicians then in practice who had not received such an education. Although many were poorly trained and lacked ability, others were good physicians who had the respect of their communities and their colleagues. In order to allow these experienced doctors to continue to practice while upgrading standards for new entrants to the profession, they were "**grandfathered**" in. That is, a doctor could become licensed either by graduating from an acceptable medical school or by being an accepted member of the county medical society. Over time, the more highly qualified new graduates would replace the older cohort of non-university physicians. Analyzed in terms of property rights, the existing physicians owned the rights to vote on standards. It would not be in their self-interest to vote for higher standards that would put them out of a job, yet a higher quality standard would increase demand and benefit all physicians. The grandfather clause allowed them to reap the rewards from licensure reform and in a sense became a form of payment for their property: control over the future of the profession. As usual, all parties, including the incumbents, must be made better off for a successful political exchange to occur.

AMA Controls over Physician Supply, 1930–1965

With reform curtailing new entrants and forcing unqualified older practitioners out of business, physician supply declined steadily from its 1900 level of 1.73 MDs per 1,000 population to 1.33 MDs per 1,000 population in 1930 (Figure 7.1). The supply of physicians held constant at this level for the next 35 years. Yet improvements in medicine greatly increased public demand, as did the rise in personal income over these four decades. With supply constant and demand increasing, earnings of physicians rose, as depicted in Figure 6.3. Concern was voiced that not enough physicians were available and that a shortage had arisen.[5]

There are several ways this shortage could have been rectified. The steep price rise that did occur held quantity demanded in check and made physicians happy, but it did little for the public. Supply could have been expanded by increasing the productivity of physicians, changing the organization of medical practice, and using more ancillary health workers; some illnesses could have been treated by physician substitutes such as doctors of osteopathy (DOs) or chiropractors; or physicians could have been imported from overseas. These alternatives would have undercut organized medicine's control over physician supply and incomes and were strongly resisted by the AMA. Productivity improvements and lower prices were most strongly identified with prepaid group practices such as the Kaiser Health Plan in California and the Group Health Association in Washington, D.C. (see Chapters 5 and 12). Concerted opposition by local medical societies led to the expulsion of group practice doctors and an obstinate denial of hospital privileges to physicians who were clearly qualified by education and experience.[6] In 1941, the Washington, D.C., Medical Society and the AMA were indicted, found guilty, and fined by the U.S. Department of Justice for having conspired to monopolize trade in physician services. This is but one of many in a string of cases across the country that left group practices bruised and hampered, but alive. Relations slowly improved, but opposition to prepaid group practice did not end until the 1970s.

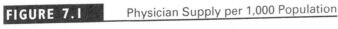

FIGURE 7.1 Physician Supply per 1,000 Population

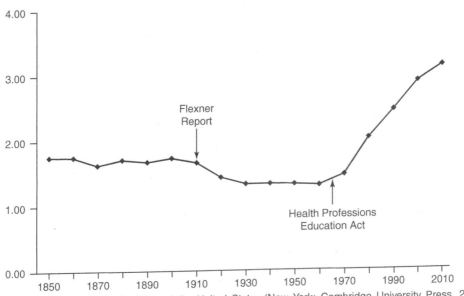

Source: U.S. Historical Statistics of the United States (New York: Cambridge University Press, 2000) and other census publications.

The response of organized medicine to substitute providers took two forms: co-opting the competition and all-out war. DOs emphasized spinal manipulation in addition to standard medical practices and formed a separate type of care in 1900 with their own DO hospitals, but they carried out many of the same Flexnerian educational reforms in those transitional years. Over time, MD and DO cooperation increased through sharing of hospital privileges, enrollment in each other's residency programs, and formation of joint political and social groups.[7] DOs were tolerated by the AMA and ultimately brought into the fold as slightly less polished MDs. Today, the differences between an MD and a DO degree are almost nonexistent, except that DOs are more likely to be general practitioners and do not control any of the high-prestige medical schools. In many states a single licensure board covers both types of physicians, and in California the MD and DO societies merged in 1961, although separate boards were later reestablished. Until about 1990, the number of DOs relative to MDs remained roughly constant at around 5 percent, and hence osteopathy had become more a partner to the AMA in controlling supply rather than a competitive threat.

Chiropractors, who often rely exclusively on spinal manipulation to treat disease and still train some practitioners in for-profit schools, have been severely and relentlessly attacked by the AMA.[8] Licensure acts explicitly exclude chiropractors from the practice of medicine, and this opposition has not changed even though the AMA has not been able to ban chiropractic practice, or indeed to prevent some of its own members from referring patients to chiropractors. Although some of the AMA opposition to chiropractic care is based on the lack of scientific foundation for manipulative treatments, much of it is motivated by economic concerns.

Breaking the Contract: The Great Medical Student Expansion of 1970–1980

Under the control of the AMA and the medical schools, enough new MDs and DOs were being produced to keep pace with the growth in the U.S. population (about 1 percent a year), but not with the increase in demand due to improved technology or higher disposable incomes. As the benefits of modern medicine became more evident, access to care was increasingly seen as a necessity in the rising American standard of living, one that workers had already paid for through their health insurance premiums. The constraints on supply caused longer waits for an appointment, less time for a patient to talk with an increasingly rushed physician, fewer old-style general practitioners willing to make house calls, and other deteriorations in service. The public was unhappy, and the politicians, who now provided most of the financing for medical schools, were willing to do something to redress the imbalance.

In essence, frustration with the inaction of the AMA led the government to unilaterally disrupt the old system. Congress passed the Health Professions Educational Assistance Act of 1963, forcing medical schools to admit more students and allowing more foreign physicians to immigrate to the United States. In response to the act and subsequent amendments, physician supply rose steadily to 1.61 physicians per 1,000 population in 1970, 2.02 in 1980, 2.44 in 1990, and 3.12 in 2010, more than twice the level of supply that prevailed from 1930 through 1965 (see Figure 7.1 and Figure 7.2). The number of entering students almost doubled in 10 years, from 8,759 in 1965 to 15,351 in 1975. The government used two methods to bring about this increase.[9] First, it built more medical schools. Second, it offered additional funding on the condition that existing schools increase the number of students enrolled by at least 5 percent each year. By this time, federal and state funding accounted for 63 percent of medical school financing; hence, the schools were not in a good position to resist, even if they had wanted to. At the same time, changes in immigration rules were made to favor "shortage" occupations, including physicians. Foreign graduates made up just 6 percent of all physicians in practice in 1960, but by 1965 that fraction had doubled to 12 percent and further increased to 17 percent in 1970 and 20 percent in 1980.

FIGURE 7.2   Additions to U.S. Physician Supply, 1950–2010

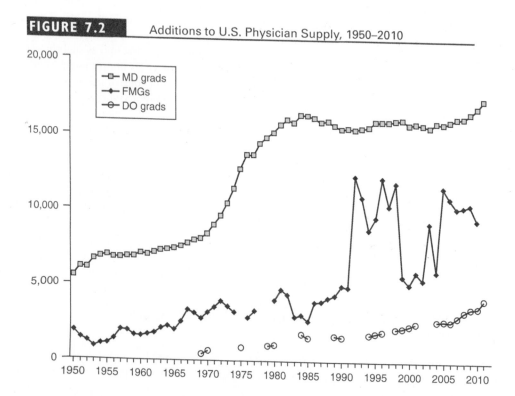

Building Pressure: Fixed Domestic Graduation Rates, 1980–2010

As the number of residents in training grew rapidly during the 1970s, it began to seem as though there were already plenty of physicians. The AMA complained loudly about a potential surplus, commissioning several studies to show that the United States was training an excess of physicians and that foreign graduates were no longer needed. These arguments were successful in helping the profession reestablish control over supply, and by 1980 the tide of public opinion had turned. The 1981 Report of the Graduate Medical Education National Advisory Committee, widely known as the GMENAC Report, projected a growing surplus, raising the possibility that in the future some physicians would face unemployment.[10] The flow of foreign graduates had already been severely restricted by changes in immigration law included in the Health Professions Educational Assistance Act of 1976. Moves were now made to reduce the rate of growth in the number of U.S. physicians. No more new schools were to be built. Class sizes were fixed at the current level.

The number of first-year MD students peaked at 17,268 in 1981 and was held below that number until 2005, then rose to 19,230 in 2011. There has been a growing recognition that instead of a surplus, a future shortage of physicians could occur.[11] Because the number of U.S. medical graduates has not kept pace with the growth in U.S. population, much less the growth in technology and incomes that raised effective demand, all the expansion in supply over the last 20 years has had to come from three other sources: the delayed effect of the 1965–1975 "physician boom," increased immigration of non-U.S. physicians, and increased production of non-MD physicians.

7.3   ADJUSTING PHYSICIAN SUPPLY

The Flow of New Entrants and the Stock of Physicians

Although the number of students entering medical school jumped by 50 percent between 1968 and 1973, this had no immediate effect on physician supply because these extra students were still in school for four years. Even then, the sudden increase in the number of new MDs caused only a gradual rise in the supply of physicians. To see why, it is necessary to trace the life cycle of work, distinguishing the stock of physicians (the number available at any point in time) from the flow of entrants and retirees into and out of the labor force. Suppose that the average physician began to practice at age 33 and retired at age 66. If the same number of physicians started work each year and retired after 33 years, 1/33, or 3 percent, of all the physicians in practice would leave each year and another 3 percent would join. The number of physicians in practice (the physician stock) would stay the same from year to year in this steady state. What would happen if the nation decided to double the physician supply by doubling the number of new graduates each year? In 33 years there would be twice as many, or 100 percent more, practicing physicians, but in the first year there would only be 3 percent more. The number of new additions would be twice as much as before, or $2 \times 3\% = 6\%$ of the total, and the retirements would be the same, 3 percent, so that net growth would be 3 percent in the first year, 6 percent after two years, 9 percent after three years, and so on. The actual response would be even slower, because there is a lag of eight years from the time new students are admitted until they complete their residencies and become practicing physicians. The full effects of the 1965–1975 "doctor boom" (and subsequent bust) will not be fully realized until this cohort of new physicians has moved through the professional ranks and completed their work lives, some time between the years 2000 and 2025 (see Figure 7.3). The 2005 increase in first-year enrollment creates an uptick in the number of MD graduates in 2009, and this crop of new doctors will continue to move through the system until 2050.

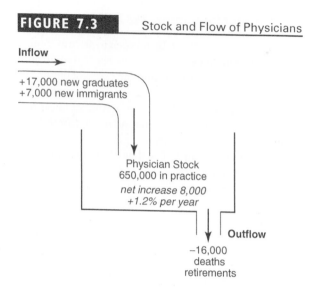

FIGURE 7.3   Stock and Flow of Physicians

Immigration of International Medical Graduates

The number of foreign medical graduates practicing in the United States doubled in just three years, from 15,154 in 1960 to 30,925 in 1963, with 15,000 more arriving in the next four years. By 1980 there were 97,726 international medical graduates (IMGs) practicing in the United States, 20 percent of the total physician supply. Despite continued restrictions on immigration, the number of IMGs doubled from 1980 to 2000 and now constitute 26 percent of practicing physicians.[12] Although the number of IMGs entering U.S. residency training programs has leveled off at around 6,000 per year since 1995, the effects of the entry bulge from 1988 to 1995 will continue to expand this component of physician supply for decades to come.

Growth in Non-MD Physicians

Although smaller in number, the growth in non-MD physicians (primarily DOs) has been even more dramatic. In 1970, some 12,600 DOs constituted just 4 percent of the total physician supply. Whereas the number of MD graduates was essentially held constant at 17,000 from 1980 to 2000, the number of DO graduates jumped from 1,059 to 2,304.[13] The number of schools of osteopathy rose from 14 to 19, class size continued to increase, and DOs constituted an ever-larger fraction of the U.S. medical graduates entering residency programs.

Balancing Supply and Incomes: Tracing the Past and Projecting the Future

The development of scientific medicine created the need for a new type of doctor in the 20th century, and the history of physician supply and licensure must be interpreted in that context. To raise the quality of the individuals in the profession (as well as their prestige and incomes), the reforms envisioned by AMA leaders and the Flexner Report required that most of the inadequately trained practitioners be forced out, thus reducing physician supply from 1900 to 1930. From then until 1965, the number of new MDs graduating each year was held steady at about 4 percent of the total physician stock, numbers just sufficient to offset the 3 percent who retired each year and a 1 percent growth in the U.S. population, so that the physician-to-population ratio remained constant at about 133 per 10,000.

For a professional thinking technically in terms of medical "need" (a specific, fixed number of physicians required to treat a given number of illnesses), a constant physician-to-population ratio was sufficient to meet demand. From an economic perspective emphasizing responsiveness to prices and incomes, it is clear how inadequate both the concept and the numbers used by the medical profession were. Changing expectations, new technology, and a rising standard of living meant that demand was increasing, and the 1 percent growth in physicians set to match the 1 percent increase in population was not enough to forestall market stress, public dissatisfaction, and growing perceptions of a shortage.

What evidence does the market provide about whether too many or too few physicians were trained or allowed to immigrate? Pent-up demand kept physician incomes from falling during the 1970s as supply rose. Although real earnings dipped in 1985, and again during 1989–1990, physicians have done much better than the average American worker over the last 20 years. Groups that had to make an extra effort to enter the profession (IMGs, DOs) clearly found it worthwhile to do so and pushed for access in record numbers. Such effort and expansion in auxiliary sources indicates that demand was growing faster than regular domestic supply. However, fewer college students were applying to medical schools. About 2 percent of those admitted to medical school did not attend. Although this fraction refusing the opportunity of a medical education was still quite small, it was fourfold above the rate between 1975 and 1985, when just 0.5 percent of those offered a place in medical school turned it down.

Although projecting the future is always to some extent speculative, it is possible to give a reasonable assessment of the economic situation and prospects of physicians from these trends.[14] Becoming a doctor still offers above-average rates of return on post-college education (see Chapter 12). However, the very high earnings growth that physicians enjoyed during the 1960s and 1970s was a temporary historical aberration, brought about by rapid growth in demand owing to new technology in the context of fixed supply. In the future, doctors will have high, but not such extraordinarily high, earnings. Although they still will do much better than most graduates from other fields, new physicians will face more competition as they enter the market, and thus they will be more likely to become employees holding salaried jobs and to hold on to such positions for longer during their careers. The few who become truly wealthy will be those who have worked their way up the ladder in large health care organizations or who have taken substantial risks as entrepreneurs.

7.4 GROUP PRACTICE: HOW ORGANIZATION AND TECHNOLOGY AFFECT TRANSACTIONS

Physicians who join together in groups have higher net earnings than those who practice alone: $201,000 for solo doctors compared with $255,000 for those in two-physician partnerships, $288,000 for those in three-physician groups, and more than $300,000 for those in larger groups (see Table 6.3). Physicians in group practices usually have better lifestyles: more interaction with colleagues, more support services, and fewer nights spent handling emergencies.[15] Economists must ascertain which factors lead to greater efficiency and hence higher incomes for group practice and, conversely, which factors limit the attractiveness of groups so that one third of all physicians still choose to practice alone. There are fundamentally three ways that group practices serve to increase net income:

- Economies of scale raise the productivity of inputs, and hence lower costs.
- Added market power brings in greater revenues.
- Sharing spreads risk.

What does it mean to have **economies of scale** that make larger practices more efficient in the use of inputs? To a physician owner, it could mean either (a) that the cost of inputs required to produce a given amount of output has been reduced or (b) that the output in visits per hour of physician time has been increased. Analysis of group practice expenditures shows that some of both occurs.[16] Equipment and office space comes in discrete units and therefore is inefficiently used in small practices. An x-ray machine that can handle 10,000 patients might cost only 50 percent more than one that can handle 2,000, and even the smaller one is often idle for a doctor practicing alone. A large group can match equipment needs to the total patient volume of the group as a whole, and thereby achieve economies of scale. Similarly, each physician might need from one to four exam rooms at a time to maximize patient flow and from two to six assistants. A solo doctor will compromise by having an office with three exam rooms and four assistants, and thus sometimes the ancillary inputs will be overcrowded and limit productivity, while at other times they sit idle and waste money. A group can plan for an average, because it is unlikely that all the physicians will be busy or inactive at the same time, and thus achieve a better match. Office rent takes up 12 percent of the gross revenues of solo practices, 10 percent of two-physician partnerships, and only 7 percent of large group practices.

On the other hand, labor costs and full-time equivalent (FTE) employees per physician increase as practice size increases. A large group can allow for more specialization in the use of labor, so that a group of 10 physicians can have a laboratory technician, billing specialist, receptionist, intake nurse, exam room assistant, and so on, whereas a solo practice must make do with a general-purpose medical assistant or nurse. Increasing the productivity of an input can either decrease or increase its share of total expenditures depending on the elasticity of

COMPARATIVE ADVANTAGE AND PHYSICIAN ASSISTANTS

The principle that people and firms should produce the things at which they are relatively more efficient and use others to produce the things at which they are relatively less efficient is known as **comparative advantage**. There are gains from trade when relative costs differ, even if one party is better at everything. That is why investment bankers let someone else balance their checkbooks, great artists let helpers fill in the background scenery, great athletes let someone else play on punt returns, and even countries for which production of everything is inefficient export some goods to get the things they are most inefficient at producing. It makes sense to trade even when you can produce the item for less cost, if doing so frees up time and resources that can be used more valuably elsewhere.

For example, suppose that a physician takes 15 minutes to do an intake examination and 5 minutes to do a follow-up. The physician assistant (PA) takes 40 minutes to do an intake examination and 30 minutes to do a follow-up. Even though the PA is less efficient at both tasks, the medical group will use the principle of comparative advantage and make the PAs do intakes, not follow-ups. Why? Because in eight hours a PA could do 12 intakes, freeing up three hours of physician time to do high-value surgery, while having the PA do 16 follow-ups would free up just 1 hour and 20 minutes of physician time. It is not the "cost" of using the PA to provide services that matters, it is the value of the additional services that the physician can provide. Trade should follow the course of comparative advantage, even though absolute productivity will determine rewards: The physician will earn more per hour than the PA.

It is worth noting how the principle of comparative advantage can work against some of the human traits we value in doctors. Both nurses and doctors can listen and show compassion, and spending more time yields better results. However, the physician can accomplish more high-tech diagnostic procedures per hour than the nurse and will tend to specialize in that direction, at the expense of listening. Even if we tell our doctors that we want them to spend more time with us and they are very good at listening, they are apt to hire assistants to do so because their comparative advantage lies in the application of medical technology.[17]

substitution with other inputs. (Although increased productivity means that the same amount of output could be produced with less input, the fact that the input has become so much more productive might make the group shift to use more and more of it; computers are a good example.) Office space apparently cannot be substituted for physician time; thus, as it becomes more productive per square foot it takes up a smaller fraction of total practice expenditures. Ancillary labor can be substituted for physician time, and as this labor becomes more productive, physicians use more employees rather than fewer. It is worth paying for more assistants to save the physicians' time because their net profit per hour of work increases.

Risk sharing across the members of the group also creates economies of scale. Just as random variation in the number of exam rooms required by each doctor can be averaged out in a large group, so can other revenues and expenses, so that the group can collectively enjoy a smoother and more certain income stream. Perhaps even more important, the emergency calls that interrupt the home life of every doctor are much less disruptive when combined and redistributed in a group. A solo practitioner must be "on call" every night or find someone else who is willing to cover. On Sunday, one emergency call could interrupt a football game, and there might be no more calls until a sleep-shattering call at 3 A.M. For a group, it is usual for each doctor to accept all the calls for a single day. The group doctor might handle seven emergencies on a Sunday but know that Friday night and Saturday are free, because any patients who need assistance then will be handled by one of the partners. The burden of emergencies is not the time spent in caring for patients but the uneven spacing. This is the risk that is shared, and thus effectively reduced, in a group.

Because it is obviously so much more efficient for a doctor to handle 10 patients in one night than one to three patients each night per week, why don't solo doctors contract with each other to do just that? For that matter, why can't independent physicians arrange to share office space or nurses? To some extent they do, and to that extent they start to become a group. As the contracts and sharing become more complete and cover more aspects of practice, the doctors who trade with each other become a single firm—that is, a group practice. However, it is difficult to share. All the doctors must agree to standardize certain practices, coordinate efforts, pick a leader, accept the leader's ruling on disputes among them, and so on—in short, to be managed. It means being an employee or partner rather than the boss. Management is costly, and good physician managers, like all good managers, are rare and valuable commodities. Some studies of physician productivity overestimated economies of scale because they did not account for the time physicians must spend in management and how that management time increases as the size of the practice increases.[18] For some physicians, it is cheaper (and more fun) to put up with some inefficiencies and lack of specialized inputs to be their own bosses and not have to listen to, or give orders to, anyone else.

Contracting between many parties and managing larger operations create the costs that limit the attractiveness of group practice. Transaction costs are also the source of the economies of scale in marketing and revenue generation, which are often more important than production cost economies. Consider what happens when a successful older doctor combines his practice with that of a younger physician who is just starting out. The older physician has too many patients and must turn some away or provide poor service. The young physician has too few patients and must spend hours waiting for people to show up or moonlighting as an employee in a hospital emergency department. By combining their practices, the successful doctor is, in effect, selling some patients to the younger doctor in return for a part of the younger doctor's income. For such a transfer to occur, patients must be convinced that the junior doctor is as good as the senior one. The senior doctor guarantees the quality of the junior doctor by the act of forming a partnership. In effect, the senior doctor is saying, "I trust this doctor; so should you." Transfer is also facilitated by arranging for the junior partner to take a disproportionate share of night emergencies, the new patients who show up at the door for the first time, and those who do not want to wait weeks to see the senior partner.

It is the patient's concerns about quality and trust that make the doctor–patient relationship special and that makes it hard to obtain economies of scale by treating patients en masse. For a group to act as a collective, the guarantee of quality must extend to all the physicians in it. Just as all licensed physicians benefit from monitoring the quality of care provided by the profession and eliminating or reforming bad doctors, a medical group practice benefits from increased demand to the extent that it can closely monitor and control the quality of all its members.[19] The Mayo Clinic is an example of a medical group practice that acts as a brand-name firm. It gains a marketing and revenue advantage from being perceived as a group with identifiable quality rather than just a random collection of individual physicians who happen to work in the same building.[20]

7.5 KICKBACKS, SELF-DEALING, AND SIDE PAYMENTS

"And if a doctor shall cheat his patient by overcharging for medicaments, then shall a finger of his left hand be cut off."
— *Code of Hammurabi, 2300* B.C.

From the beginning, the AMA code of medical ethics has dealt with economic issues, rightfully noting that doctors must put the health of patients above profits if people are to trust them. The agency relationship is most threatened in day-to-day business by the practice of paying "referral fees" or **kickbacks**. The agent is supposed to be, and is, paid for acting in the principal's (the patient's) best interest. When doctors accept a fee for referring patients to one hospital rather than another, or for giving a surgical case to Dr. B instead of Dr. A, they may be tempted to go with the one who will pay them the most, not the one who will provide the best care. In ordinary business dealings, such a payment would be termed a bribe or a kickback. Corporate purchasing agents are sometimes caught accepting presents or kickbacks from suppliers in return for steering business their way. For suppliers to pay for business is not bad: they can give rebates or provide customer treats or price discounts. The problem is the distortion caused by directing a payment to the agent who is supposed to be making an objective choice, rather than the principal, who is supposed to get the benefits of any discounts. Before medicine became established as a profession, such practices were common. Surgeons in the large cities would advertise in rural newspapers their willingness to pay $100 or more for each case sent to them. Although such behavior seems unthinkable now, kickbacks keep cropping up. What was once the largest chain of psychiatric hospitals was investigated and convicted for paying physicians and social workers who sent in clients. The kickback scheme had become so well established that there was a standard going rate of $70 for each patient day.[21]

Why do kickbacks continue to occur if everyone knows that they are bad and they are condemned by all the official governing organizations? They continue because an agent's control over who gets the business is valuable property. To not make use of that value—that is, to act ethically and follow professional standards that put the interests of patients first—forces a doctor to put aside his or her own narrow self-interest. In the short run, it is easy to profit by betraying a trust to make a dollar. The violator hopes not to get caught. Even if an unethical physician does get caught, much of the punishment actually falls on other doctors because the profession as a whole gets blamed for a lack of standards and suffers from a reduced demand and falling prices for services. Trust and agency build professional value, and taking a kickback is one way for a member to steal part of that value, benefiting personally while harming others.

One of the major activities of physicians is prescribing drugs. If drug companies made payments to physicians, those dollars could distort the physicians' choices on behalf of their patients, perhaps by prescribing a drug that is less effective or one that is effective but three times as expensive as all the substitute drugs that would work just as well.[22] An even more difficult problem arises when the physician is not only prescribing the drug but also selling it. Knowing that the patient is in pain and trusts the physician, physicians could fatten their profit margins by overcharging for drugs. That such a problem is not new is evidenced by the quote from the code of Hammurabi at the beginning of this section. The potential for abuse is so high that physicians in this country have been legally prohibited from selling drugs or owning pharmacies since 1934. Even a pharmacy in a medical clinic must be run as a separate business to avoid conflicts of interest. In Japan, where no such law exists, the government sets price controls to keep physicians from overcharging, but that does not stop them from overprescribing. General-practice physicians in Japan get about a third of their net income from sales of pharmacy items, and their patients are prescribed twice as many drugs as similar patients in the United States.

In the quote from the code of Hammurabi, the prohibition is on overcharging for *medication*. Why isn't overcharging for service similarly condemned? The issue with kickbacks is not price, it is deceit. If Dr. Andrews says, "I am better than the others, and I want $20 more for each visit," that is her privilege. Patients can agree or go somewhere else. There is no fraud. To prescribe a drug and accept a $20 rebate from the manufacturer, or to send a surgical case to Dr. Jones knowing that he will send a case of wine in return, is fraud. The patient is unknowingly paying and has an agent whose decisions may be influenced by kickbacks rather than the patient's welfare. The patient going to Dr. Andrews, and *unaware that Dr. Andrews has any business arrangement with another doctor*, has a right to expect Dr. Andrews to objectively choose the surgeon who is best and to negotiate the lowest price.

As medicine has become more complex, with more transactions involved in each episode of patient care, it has become even more difficult to avoid conflicts of interest. Of particular concern in recent years have been incidences in which for-profit companies providing ancillary services (e.g., diagnostic radiology, home intravenous therapy) offer physicians "investments" in these businesses in return for sending patients.[23] So many such abuses took place that in 1976 federal anti-kickback laws were passed prohibiting any Medicare or Medicaid payment from companies to physicians based on the volume of patient referrals. The 1989 "Stark law" (named after its sponsor, U.S. Representative Fortney Stark of California) banned physicians from referring patients to clinical laboratories in which they have a financial interest. The 1993 "Stark II" law widened the ban to prohibit self-referrals to hospitals or radiology laboratories in which physicians are invested. The law also prohibits bonus plans within group practices based on the volume of laboratory referrals. Only a minority (less than 10 percent) of physicians invest in businesses that raise conflict of interest issues from self-referral, and only a few engage in profiteering at the expense of the government and patients.[24] Yet the actions of these few are so troubling to a public already dismayed over the high cost of health care that it is likely that further restrictions will be placed on independent diagnostic and therapeutic facilities owned by physicians.

7.6   PRICE DISCRIMINATION

One of the characteristics of the medical markets first noted by economists was that different patients pay different prices for the same service.[25] Some price differences are attributable to differences in cost or value (e.g., surgery by an experienced board-certified specialist versus a new resident still in training, midnight treatment in the emergency department versus a routine visit to the doctor's office). However, even after these factors are taken into account, there is still a sizable and systematic variation in charges. It is often noted that people who are well insured or have high incomes pay more, laboratory and other small-ticket items are overpriced, and services for which patients can "shop around" (e.g., eye exams, normal births, physical therapy) show less price variation than emergency medical care where immediate treatment is required.

A major reason for **price discrimination**, charging different prices for the same service to different types of patients or patients in different types of care, is that it increases total revenue. The change in revenue, marginal revenue, depends on price elasticity as well as price (see Section 2.3). More formally,

$$\text{Marginal Revenue} = \text{Price}(1 + 1/\text{Elasticity})$$

To maximize revenues when providing two different types of care, physicians should charge different prices even if their costs are the same for each service, and they should *charge a higher price where demand is least price sensitive* (i.e., where price elasticity, which is always negative, is smaller in magnitude). Conversely, where demand is very price sensitive, a reduction in price will bring in many more patients and increase revenues (see Figure 7.4). Pain, fear of dying, and wealth all serve to reduce price sensitivity. However, the most important factor making medical consumers less price sensitive is insurance (see Figure 7.5). Therefore, we would generally expect physicians to charge more for services that are more fully covered by insurance, are more life-threatening, are more painful, and for which patients have the least ability to shop around. Some ancillary services (lab tests, x-rays, sonograms) are not very price sensitive, even when insurance coverage is incomplete, because they are considered secondary and inevitable by-products, and thus they rarely receive the kind of scrutiny given an operation or other major expense.[26]

There is an important empirical discrepancy at odds with the revenue-maximization model of physician price discrimination: The lower price is sometimes clearly below the cost of providing the service (sometimes care is even free), and therefore it must decrease rather than increase the physician's income. Indeed, when queried about differential pricing, some physicians respond angrily to the suggestion that they are maximizing profits and assert that they act from a benevolent impulse, charging high prices to those who can afford to pay (or are well insured) so that they can take care of the destitute. Under closer examination, however, it

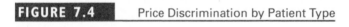

FIGURE 7.4   Price Discrimination by Patient Type

Price

To increase profits, raise prices where demand is inelastic, and lower prices where demand is elastic.

Price-sensitive patients

Patients not sensitive to price

Quantity

FIGURE 7.5   Price Discrimination by Insurance Status

becomes evident that there is a mixture of motivations that includes both charity and higher incomes in a blend that is not always clearly separable. Charging students less helps out a group that is usually poor and might not get care if they had to pay full price, and it brings in more revenue for exactly the same reason. (Why do you think movie theaters and airlines give student discounts? Is it a charitable impulse or a smart business practice to raise revenues because they know students have little discretionary money and wouldn't come to the theater or fly as often otherwise?) Price discrimination is pervasive in medicine and well accepted by patients, the government, and insurance companies. Yet if two people come into a shop and one is charged twice as much for oil, food, or rent, the person charged extra will complain or threaten to sue. The unusual willingness of people to accept or even praise price discrimination in medicine is one of the factors that has convinced economists that health care markets differ in significant ways from markets for most other goods and services.

7.7   PRACTICE VARIATIONS

The agency relationship arises because the patient trusts the physician to do what is right. What happens when the physician confronts a lack of information or when medical science provides no clear guidelines on what to do? The professional concept of "need," which assumes there is a right way to treat an illness and hence no necessity for examining trade-offs among costly alternatives, falters if the clinical pathway becomes ambiguous. The fact that some medical practices have been widely used with confidence, only to be later discarded as ineffective or harmful, fosters some doubts about the infallibility of medicine.

In a 1934 study, the American Child Health Association chose 1,000 schoolchildren to be examined by physicians to determine whether or not they should have their tonsils removed.[27] Six hundred children had already had the procedure. The remaining 400 were examined, and the physicians recommended that 45 percent of them have a tonsillectomy. Then the 220 not recommended for surgery in the first round were examined by another group of physicians, who recommended that 46 percent of them have their tonsils out. A third exam by another set of physicians on the 118 who were left resulted in recommendations that 44 percent have their tonsils removed. After these three examinations, only 65 of the original 1,000 children were not recommended for a tonsillectomy! From this study, the experimenters concluded that the decision about whether a child needed a tonsillectomy was not primarily based on signs or symptoms or any objective evidence, but on a generally held opinion among the doctors consulted that they should give tonsillectomies to one-third to one-half of all the children they treated in that age range.

Today, tonsillectomy is a much less commonly performed procedure, in part because of these pioneering epidemiologic experiments (epidemiology is the study of the distribution of diseases in populations, applying statistical methods to groups rather than studying individual patients). However, the insights regarding the range of uncertainty in common diagnoses were essentially ignored during the glory years of medicine after World War II, when it seemed that science could diagnose and cure every ailment. This optimistic conviction that medical advances would be continuous and consistently beneficial faded as the Vietnam War, an oil crisis, and rising environmental concerns led to a more cautious and critical assessment of technology.

In what was then (in 1973) a little-noticed study, John Wennberg and colleagues found that the rates of many common types of surgery varied widely across counties in Vermont, with differences as large as six-fold, which were not explainable by differences in insurance, availability of hospitals, or illness rates.[28] For tonsillectomies, the rate varied from as few as 8 per 10,000 to as many as 60 per 10,000. In a subsequent study, Wennberg found that the people of Boston, Massachusetts, had more hospital beds, had more employees per bed, and paid 87 percent more on average for hospital care than the people of New Haven, Connecticut, yet in both cities the average health statistics were about the same and most people received high-quality medical care, with many patients treated in academic medical schools. Interestingly, Wennberg found that whereas the overall rate of surgery was higher in Boston, for certain conditions the rate of surgery was instead significantly higher in New Haven. Thus, it is not simply a question of more or less, but of a large degree of unexplainable variation (see Figure 7.6).

This phenomenon of **practice variation** or **small-area variation** has been confirmed by a number of researchers. It suggests that there is a large element of ambiguity that can make widely different treatment choices constitute acceptable medical practice. Conditions in which indications are not so clear, or for which there are good alternative forms of treatment, show large variations (e.g., knee replacement, spinal surgery for back pain, tonsillectomy, treatment of psychosespsychosis). However, for conditions in which there are clear indications and a generally accepted treatment, the range of variation is much smaller (e.g., hernia repair, open-heart surgery, lung resection). Work is now under way to develop more formal clinical pathways, sets of instructions developed by medical professionals based on verified results of scientifically validated studies. These **clinical pathways** suggest how a particular illness should be managed, including which tests to perform, which medications to give, how long to wait for symptoms to improve before surgery, and so on. Many doctors denigrate such efforts as "cookbook medicine," but others recognize that clinical pathways, although not able to replace the physician's personal judgment, can help make treatment more efficient.

What is important to recognize is that repeated demonstrations of wide variations in practice patterns have called into question the role of the individual doctor as final arbiter of right and wrong treatments. Impetus has been given to health policy promoting **evidence-based medicine**, which relies on the results of carefully constructed clinical studies with verifiable costs and outcomes of care, rather than accepting current practices as a standard or relying on the opinions expressed by professional associations.

Small-area variation is one form of **population medicine** that uses groups rather than individual patients to define quality of care.[29] Although long used in public health (see Chapter 14), it is only with the spread of managed-care contracting for large numbers of people that

FIGURE 7.6   Variation in Age-Adjusted Rates of Hospitalization for Different Diagnoses and Procedures

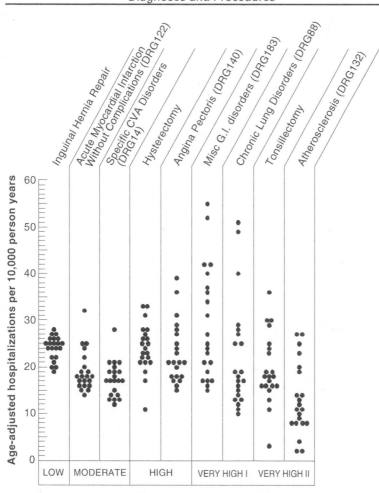

Each dot represents one hospital market area.

Source: J. Wennberg, K. McPherson, and P. Caper, *New England Journal of Medicine* 311 (1984): 298.

population medicine has become recognized as a valuable tool for assessing the quality of physician practice. As hospitals become integrated into health care systems to organize and better manage the care they provide to the community, decisions regarding treatment will be shaped more by analysis of statistics on large numbers of patients and will be less dependent on the experience of a single physician.[30]

7.8   INSURANCE, PRICE COMPETITION, AND THE STRUCTURE OF MEDICAL MARKETS

The effects of medical uncertainty, agency, and insurance are combined in the health care system so that prices are almost uniquely *un*important for consumer behavior or well-being. Licensure and other monitoring procedures try to guarantee that any doctor available to serve

---

UNCERTAINTY REGARDING HORMONE REPLACEMENT THERAPY

For many years, estrogen and progestin were routinely prescribed for postmenopausal women to replace hormones their bodies could no longer produce in quantity. Clinical judgment suggested that such hormone replacement therapy reduced the risks of heart disease, stroke, and osteoporosis that accompanied aging. Observational studies indicated that risk reductions on the order of 40 percent to 50 percent could be obtained, but there were no randomized studies that established the magnitude of effect with certainty.

The Women's Health Initiative was begun in 1991, and it eventually screened 373,092 women for participation. Of these, 16,608 were enrolled in clinical trials and randomized to receive either hormones or a placebo (inert pill). Participants were to be followed and repeatedly assessed medically for 8.5 years. However, the trial was stopped after only five years of observation because there were excess deaths and adverse events among the group receiving the hormones. The negative impact was small but conclusively demonstrated. Hormone replacement therapy did not help overall and on average probably harmed those who received it.

No single physician, or group of physicians practicing together, would ever have been able to see these effects. Among 8,000 women over five years, there were approximately six excess heart attack fatalities and three excess stroke deaths, an annualized difference of only 0.01 percent. Only statistical methods and rigorously planned, carefully recorded observations of thousands of patients at many hospitals and clinics can distinguish effects such as these. In retrospect, the reliance placed on individual judgment and clinical experience resulted in many useless or harmful treatments.[31]

---

you will provide excellent treatment using up-to-date technology, and insurance takes away the impact of cost and any incentive to spend time comparison shopping. Consider how unusual this market is. For cars, clothing, and housing, one expects that better quality will cost more and that only the wealthy will buy the superior brands. Not so for hospitals or surgery. It all costs the same more or less: a small copayment, a deductible, or nothing. In picking a movie or a pair of shoes, consumers assume that they will suffer the consequences of some inevitable bad and poorly informed choices on their part. Not in medical care. It is the doctor's fault, not mine, if the treatment does not fit or does not work properly. Nowhere else is price so irrelevant. Surgeons don't even list their fees, much less put up sale signs offering 40 percent off to increase business. If you buy expensive clothes, you will have to give up your expensive car, or your new apartment, or your tuition for graduate school. However, a person can get the best medical care in the world and walk out with their checkbook balance nearly unaffected.

NO MORE DR. WELBY

Marcus Welby, MD, was one of the most popular shows on the ABC network from 1969 to 1976. Like the earlier Dr. Kildare (played by Joel McCrea in 1937 and Richard Chamberlain in the 1960s), the noble, warm, and caring physician played by Robert Young was everyone's ideal of what a doctor should be. However, like the wise dad Young played in *Father Knows Best,* the character of Marcus Welby was a Hollywood fiction that pleased audiences because it conformed to an ideal rather than to reality. When Robert Young died at the age of 91 in 1997, the era of happy TV families and kindly doctors who acted solely out of altruism had already passed.[32]

Dr. Jones for eight years, he's made a bundle off of me, and my arthritis isn't any better."

At the urging of the mayor, Dr. Jones and Rodrigo get together to talk about the problem. Afterward, each has a much different point of view. Rodrigo states, "Dr. Jones is an honest and hardworking doctor who has the best interests of the community at heart. He actually loses money taking care of Chicanos and should be paid more. I will work with him in every case I can." Dr. Jones says, "Rodrigo is an exceptionally talented young man who knows more than any layperson, and even some doctors I have met, about the practice of medicine. We are in complete agreement about the tremendous need for better medical care in Calexico and will work together to solve this problem. Many Chicano patients who cannot afford to see me on a regular basis can be treated just as well by Rodrigo after I have done any initial diagnosis and evaluation, and I will send them to him. Together we can provide better medical care for all."

Explain why this togetherness occurred among two people, each of whom had claimed the previous night that the other was a killer. In your answer, assume that each was motivated solely by economic considerations. Why does Rodrigo say that Dr. Jones should raise his prices?

C. One year later, Dr. Jones announces, "Working with Rodrigo has opened my eyes to the plight of Chicanos and the reluctance of Anglos to accept them as equal members of society. Furthermore, as I become older I face the inevitable diminution of my ability to meet the needs of our community, and as a doctor I face the responsibility of ensuring that Calexico can continue to receive good medical care. Therefore, I have formed La Raza de Calexico Scholarship Fund. Rodrigo will work as a staff member at my clinic part time while he completes college and his medical education. He will, of course, continue to help the Chicanos who have always come to him, but he will also treat Anglo patients. This exceptional person should not work as a field hand when he can so ably act to meet the medical needs of all citizens in Calexico. We have just signed a contract that will make him my junior partner the day he graduates from medical school and that will turn over my full practice to him when I retire." *Given that both of them had a good deal with their cooperative arrangement, why take this further step?*

D. In 1994 Rodrigo said, "I can only be grateful to Dr. Jones and his unselfish commitment to helping Chicanos like myself." In 2000, after graduating from medical school, he condemns Dr. Jones as "a racist exploiter who sought to take advantage of me and the whole Chicano community to help himself alone" and seeks to void the 1994 contract and have Dr. Jones expelled from the county medical society. *Why would he do that?*

ENDNOTES

1. Enrollments and other data are taken from the annual "Medical Education" issue of *Journal of the American Medical Association.*
2. J. Ganem, J. Krakower, and R. Beran, "Review of U.S. Medical School Finances, 1993–1994," *Journal of the American Medical Association,* 274, no. 9 (1995): 723–730; Sherry A. Gleid, Ashwin Prabhu, Norman Edelman, "The Cost of Primary Care Doctors," NBER working paper #14568, December 2008.
3. American Association of Medical Colleges, *AAMC Data Book 2002,* tables E1, E4. It is worth noting that whereas the average doctor younger than 35 years was at least $200,000 in debt, just 10 percent of that debt was for student loans, and 90 percent was for home mortgage, indicating that tuition was not financially burdensome relative to current and expected income; see Lawrence Farber, "How Financially Secure Are Young Doctors?" *Medical Economics* 75, no. 16 (August 24 1998): 34–43.

4. Richard Shryock, *Medical Licensing in America, 1650–1965* (Baltimore: Johns Hopkins University Press, 1967); Rosemary Stevens, *American Medicine and the Public Interest* (New Haven: Yale University Press, 1971).

5. Rashi Fein, *The Doctor Shortage: An Economic Diagnosis* (Washington, D.C.: Brookings Institution, 1967).

6. Edward Berkowitz and Wendy Wolf, *Group Health Association: A Portrait of a Health Maintenance Organization* (Philadelphia: Temple University Press, 1988).

7. Erwin Blackstone, "The AMA and the Osteopaths: A Study of the Power of Organized Medicine," *Antitrust Bulletin* (Summer 1977); Jeff Forster, "Remember When Osteopathy Was Called a Cult?" *Medical Economics* 75, no. 8 (April 27 1998): 220.

8. Elton Rayack, "The Physicians Service Industry," in Walter Adams, ed., *The Structure of American Industry*, 5th edition (New York: Macmillan, 1982), 407–408.

9. U.S. Department of Health and Human Services, *Fifth Report to the President and Congress on the Status of Health Personnel in the United States* (Washington, D.C.: U.S. Government Printing Office, 1984).

10. U.S. Department of Health and Human Services, Office of Graduate Medical Education, *Report of the Graduate Medical Education National Advisory Committee to the Secretary, DHHS*. Pub. No. 81–651 (Washington, D.C.: U.S. Government Printing Office, 1981). This became widely known as the "GMENAC Report."

11. Richard A. Cooper, Thomas E. Getzen, Heather J. McKee, and Prakash Laud, "Economic and Demographic Trends Signal an Impending Physician Shortage," Health Affairs 21, no. 1 (2002): 1140–1154.

12. American Medical Association, *Physician Characteristics and Distribution in the U.S., 2002–2003* (Chicago: American Medical Association, 2004).

13. Health, United States, 2002, Tables 103, 104 (www.cdc.gov/nchs); Peter Hilsenrath and Fernando Wilson, "Osteopathic Medicine and Physician Supply in the United States," *Journal of Health Care Finance* 35, no. 1 (2008): 34–43.

14. Richard A. Cooper, Thomas E. Getzen, Heather J. McKee, and Prakash Laud, "Economic and Demographic Trends Signal an Impending Physician Shortage," *Health Affairs* 21, no. 1 (2002): 1140–1154; Richard Cooper, Thomas Getzen, and Prakash Laud, "Economic Expansion Is a Major Determinant of Physician Supply and Utilization," *Health Services Research* 38, no. 2 (2003): 675–696.

15. Frederick Wolinsky and William Marder, *The Organization of Medical Practice and the Practice of Medicine* (Ann Arbor: Health Administration Press, 1985). James Rebitzer and Mark Vortuba, "Organizational Economics and Physician Practices." NBER working paper #17535, October 2011.

16. Uwe Reinhardt, *Physician Productivity and the Demand for Health Manpower* (Cambridge, Mass.: Ballinger, 1974).

17. R. A. Cooper et al., "Current and Projected Workforce of Nonphysician Clinicians," *Journal of the American Medical Association* 280, no. 9 (1988): 788–794; B. G. Druss et al., "Trends in Care by Nonphysician Clinicians in the United States," *New England Journal of Medicine* 348, no. 2 (2003): 130–137.

18. Joseph Newhouse, *The Economics of Medical Care* (Reading, Mass.: Addison-Wesley, 1978), 40.

19. Thomas Getzen, "A 'Brand Name' Firm Theory of Medical Group Practice," *Journal of Industrial Economics* 33, no. 2 (1984): 199–215.

20. Helen Clapesattle, *The Doctors Mayo* (Minneapolis: University of Minnesota Press, 1941).

21. Sandy Lutz, "Troubled Times for Psych Hospitals," *Modern Healthcare* 21, no. 50 (1991): 26–27, 30–33; and "NME Totals Costs of Psych Woes," *Modern Healthcare* 23, no. 43 (2006): 20.

22. Troyen A. Brennan et al., "Health Industry Practices That Create Conflicts of Interest," *Journal of the American Medical Association* 295, no. 4 (2006): 429–433.

23. Jean M. Mitchell and Jonathan H. Sunshine, "Consequences of Physician's Ownership of Health Care Facilities—Joint Ventures in Radiology," *New England Journal of Medicine* 327, no. 21 (1992): 1497–1501. D. R. Hughes, M. Bhargavan, and J. H. Sunshine, "Imaging Self-Referral Associated with Higher Costs and Limited Impact on Duration of Illness," *Health Affairs* 29, no. 12 (2010): 2244–2251; Laurence H. Baker, "Acquisition of MRI Equipment by Doctors Drives up Imaging Use and Spending." *Health Affairs* 29, no. 12 (2010): 2252–2259.

24. Physicians are allowed to buy stocks and make other forms of investments in laboratories, hospitals, and medical businesses, but they cannot be partners or get special treatment different from nonphysicians who are not in a position to refer patients. See Bruce J. Hillman and Jeff Goldsmith, "Imaging: The Self-Referral Boom and the Ongoing Search for Effective Policies to Contain It," *Health Affairs* 29, no. 12 (2010): 2231–2236.

25. Reuben Kessel, "Price Discrimination in Medicine," *Journal of Law and Economics* 1, no. 2 (1958): 20–53.

26. The same process of overcharging for less price-sensitive ancillary items is found when purchasing an automobile, as the dealer puts a larger mark-up on radios, air bags, floor mats, and so on.

27. American Child Health Association, *Physical Defects: The Pathway to Correction* (New York: American Child Health Association, 1934), 80–96, as cited in David Eddy, "Variations in Physician Practice: The Role of Uncertainty," *Health Affairs* 3, no. 2 (1984): 74–89.

28. John Wennberg, J. L. Freeman, and W. J. Culp, "Are Hospital Services Rationed in New Haven or Over-Utilised in Boston?" *Lancet* 329, no. 8543 (1987): 1185–1188; John Wennberg, Klim McPherson, and Philip Caper, "Will

Payment Based on Diagnosis-Related Groups Control Hospital Costs?" *New England Journal of Medicine* 311, no. 5 (1984): 295–303.

29. David Kindig, *Purchasing Population Health: Paying for Results* (Ann Arbor: University of Michigan Press, 1997).

30. Charles Phelps, "Information Diffusion and Best Practice Adoption," in A. J. Culyer and J. P. Newhouse, *Handbook of Health Economics* (Amsterdam: Elsevier, 2000), 223–264.

31. Writing Group for the Women's Health Initiative Investigators, "Risks and Benefits of Estrogen Plus Progestin in Healthy Post-menopausal Women," *Journal of the American Medical Association* 288, no. 3 (2002): 321–333, http://jama.ama-assn.org/issues/v288n3/fpdf/joc21036.pdf.

32. David Dranove, *From Marcus Welby to Managed Care, The Economic Evolution of American Health Care* (Princeton: Princeton University Press, 2000). Of interest to a health economist, the title of the first Dr. Kildare movie was *Interns Can't Take Money.* The young Dr. Kildare saves the life of a gangster, but as a doctor in training, he is not allowed to be paid for his services. The gangster, not bound by social rules, gives him a small fortune ($1,000), which the impoverished young doctor, acting nobly, returns.

33. Randall Cebul et al., "Unhealthy Insurance Markets: Search Frictions and the Cost and Quality of Health Insurance," *American Economic Review* 101, no. 5 (2011): 1842–1871. Hanming Fang and Alessandro Gavazza, "Dynamic Inefficiencies in an Employment–Based Health Insurance System: Theory and Evidence," *American Economic Review* 101, no. 7 (2011): 3047–3077.

CHAPTER **8**

HOSPITALS

QUESTIONS

1. How do hospitals get paid? What do they pay for?
2. Does it make a difference to hospitals that 95 percent of their funds come from third-party insurance rather than patients?
3. Why don't philanthropists donate as much to hospitals as they used to?
4. Who pays for medical research?
5. Does cost-shifting help the poor or the rich?
6. Does reimbursement increase employment? Does it drive up costs?
7. Who owns a nonprofit hospital?
8. Are hospitals charitable institutions or instruments of corporate control?

8.1 FROM CHARITABLE INSTITUTIONS TO CORPORATE CHAINS: DEVELOPMENT OF THE MODERN HOSPITAL

The hospital as an institution for the care of the sick has a long and noble history. During the 20th century, the hospital became the dominant organizational force in health care and the biggest user of health care funds. As the 21st century proceeds, hospitals are being replaced or transformed into larger and more complex "health systems" that encompass different modes of care (inpatient, ambulatory centers, home health, nursing homes) spanning multiple sites.[1]

As long as people have gotten sick, society has needed a place to care for them, both to provide special support and to isolate the ill from the rest of the community. In prescientific times, cure was often identified with casting out evil, and hospitals were religious structures. In classical Greece (600 B.C. to A.D. 1), temples known as *asclepia* took in the sick, especially those who were poor and lacked resources to be cared for at home.[2] Cities used taxes to support hospitals and dispensaries staffed by physicians, who also received fees from those who could afford to pay. The Romans, who created their large-scale hierarchical organizations to rule a vast empire, found it necessary to provide hospitals for the slaves and gladiators who served on plantations or in the military, respectively. The word "hospital" was first used in the 12th century to refer to a facility run by the church that housed and cared for the sick, the disabled, and the insane and provided lodging for pilgrims and other travelers, orphans, and the poor. Only those who had no homes stayed in hospitals, because everyone else, even if ill, preferred to remain with their families.

Economic changes and the great epidemics that came with the expansion of trade greatly increased the need for institutional care. By the end of the 13th century, 19,000 hospitals were scattered across Europe. The shift from religious care to scientific cures took place gradually over the next 600 years, but they came even more rapidly toward the end of the 19th century. Florence Nightingale's work with injured and sick British soldiers during the Crimean War

172

became the basis for her two books, *Notes on Hospitals* (1858) and *Notes on Nursing* (1859), which significantly changed the shape of the hospital and are still influential today.[3]

Hospitals were founded in 1527 in Mexico and 1635 in Canada, but it was not until 1751 that a hospital was founded in the American colonies. The Pennsylvania Hospital, still a major hospital today, was created by a bill passed in the Assembly with the support of Benjamin Franklin, which obligated the governor to provide £2,000 to match £2,000 in public donations for construction.[4] Philadelphia already had an almshouse and quarantine hospitals (temporary housing for sailors and others with contagious diseases), but the new building was slated to be a grander and more permanent edifice that would promote science as well as provide care. The six physicians who worked twice a week without pay were selected because they were outstanding and were mostly trained abroad. Other notable early American hospitals were the New York hospital chartered by King George III in 1771 to provide care for the sick poor and instruction to medical students of the Columbia Medical School, and the Massachusetts General Hospital, built in 1821 at a cost of more than $100,000, an imposing structure superior to the European hospitals of that time and the first to have indoor plumbing. American hospitals were based on the model of the British and Continental voluntary hospitals. However, the American hospitals were more likely to have paying patients who tended to be charged extra to subsidize care for the poor.[5]

These three important hospitals still exist, but the economics of hospital operations have changed drastically. In the 18th and 19th centuries, most funding came from donations, with patient fees playing a minor role, and insurance reimbursement was nonexistent. The major category of expenditure was food, and the work of the staff was supplemented by making patients labor alongside employees cleaning, cooking, and nursing. Today "hotel costs" (room, meals) account for less than 10 percent of hospital expenditures, and it is impossible to imagine making patients work alongside doctors and nurses. The colonial hospitals were similar to many modern hospitals in that they were nonprofit institutions run by volunteer governing boards, with medical care directed and conducted by physician staff members who were not paid by the hospital but who were in private practice as independent businesses in the community.

The development of the modern hospital, like the development of medical specialties, was driven by the creation of new technology. With anesthesia and antiseptics making safe surgery possible, a clean and controlled operating suite with skilled assistants became a necessity. The discovery of x-rays made it necessary to acquire access to radiographic equipment. Advances in clinical pathology and chemistry made the laboratory vital for diagnosis. Major capital investment was required to obtain access to all these new technologies. A solo physician practicing alone could not make full use of this new equipment or manage all the specialized technicians who operated it. It was necessary to bring all the patients of many physicians together under one roof, to obtain funding and make effective use of the new technology, and to hire a manager to coordinate the efforts of medical and ancillary staff.

An organizational revolution had to take place.[6] Within the custodial institutions that had existed for centuries serving the disabled poor there arose a new type of hospital, a modern organization with sophisticated and expensive equipment to provide scientific cures where middle-class patients wanted to be treated and were willing to pay. The large and uncertain monetary requirements caused a corresponding financial revolution (insurance reimbursement), which further increased demand and made possible the massive flow of funds required to support a technologically sophisticated system of intensive care costing thousands of dollars for each patient.

8.2 HOSPITAL FINANCING: REVENUES

From the founding of the Pennsylvania Hospital in 1751 until the beginnings of Blue Cross in 1929, the primary source of hospital funding was philanthropy from the community, supplemented by patient fees. Since 1940, hospital revenues have grown rapidly, but philanthropy and patient fees have decreased drastically as a percentage of the total. Now the largest sources of payment are Medicare, which provides government funding for the 60 percent of patient days used by the elderly, and health insurance firms shopping for low prices and good information systems to control costs. Around 1960, the dominant payers were nonprofit Blue Cross plans. At that time, these plans were affiliated with various hospital associations. They were designed to reimburse the full cost of patient care, thus allowing hospitals to break even while taking care of the indigent and undertaking whichever new treatments, diagnostic technology, or research they wanted. By 1995, several Blue Cross plans had fallen into bankruptcy. The survivors all started managed care plans to compete with (or complement) their traditional insurance plans. Some, such as the giant Blue Cross of California, have turned themselves into billion-dollar private for-profit firms.[7]

A new financing system had to be created and re-created again and again to provide all the new technology and services that Americans wanted. By 2010, 250 times more money was transferred from the pockets of the public into hospital expenses than had been paid at the end of World War II, with an average increase of more than 10 percent a year. Revenue growth slowed substantially in the mid 1990s as managed care took hold, with an increasing share of revenues coming from outpatient services or new business ventures (ambulance, nutrition counseling, home health care). Since 2000, revenue growth has once again accelerated. In 2009, the average community hospital's revenues were around $138 million, receiving more than $8,000 for each patient admitted. About 41 percent of revenues came from ambulatory outpatient services. Table 8.1 lists the current sources of hospital revenues.[8]

TABLE 8.1	Hospital Characteristics
Total number of hospitals	5,795
Community hospitals	5,008
Average number of beds	161
Occupancy rate	66%
Admissions per 100 population	11.6
Average length of stay	5.4 days
Emergency department visits per day	70
Outpatient visits per day	270
Number of employees	936
Number of RNs	253
Average cost per inpatient day	$1,396
Average cost per outpatient visit	$419
Percentage of revenues from outpatients	41%
Average cost per adjusted patient day	$1,853
Revenue per hospital	$138 million
Average profit margin	5.2%
Sources of Funds	
Patients self-pay	3%
Private insurance	35%
Philanthropy, other private	5%
Medicare	28%
Medicaid	20%
Other government	9%
	100 %
Uses of Funds	
Labor	53%
Professional fees	5%
Supplies, other	34%
Depreciation and interest	8%
	100 %

Source: American Hospital Association, *Hospital Statistics 2011*, Table 3.

The first thing to note from Table 8.1 is that it is unlikely and implausible that hospital behavior will be significantly shaped by consumers' decisions based on prices. In this environment more than 95 percent of revenues come from someone other than the recipient of services.[9] The second important fact to note is that the "someone else" is likely to be the government, which accounts for almost 60 percent of all revenues. The next thing to realize is that these are complex contracts for hundreds of thousands, even millions of dollars. Although we talk about "patient revenues" or the "price" of a laboratory test, to actually bring in revenues a hospital chief financial officer (CFO) has to enter an intricate legal relationship with Medicare or a joint venture with a group of radiologists or has to structure a risk-sharing arrangement with a consortium of community physicians. Such deals are quite different from retail sales added up at the cash register.

Sources of Revenues

Although a complete picture of hospital revenues is beyond the scope of this book (and indeed beyond the grasp of most economists and accountants and even experienced hospital financial managers—the details, exceptions, exclusions, covenants, and formulas go on forever), an overview of the major ways that revenues flow into hospitals is helpful in grasping the financial incentives they face (see box "Major Types of Hospital Reimbursement").

MAJOR TYPES OF HOSPITAL REIMBURSEMENT

- Philanthropy and grants
- Global budgets
- Charges
- Per diem
- Cost reimbursement DRGs (per admission)
- Capitation
- Managed care contracts

Philanthropy and Grants   Grants are funds that are donated for a specific purpose: to conduct cancer research, build a new operating pavilion, provide outreach programs for prenatal care, and so on. Donors want to make sure that funds are used for the purpose intended, but there is little direct pressure to compete on price or to control costs. The program director spends the budget and, if sufficiently good results are achieved in public-relations terms, another grant usually will be forthcoming sometime in the future. This revenue flows from the donor's belief that the task facing the hospital is important and socially valuable. It is not provided to make profits or even necessarily to show measurable effects. All nonprofit organizations must begin with a charitable grant. Tax appropriations are a form of grant, with the donor being the government. Tax breaks in the form of relief from property taxes and user fees are even more important to many hospitals these days and have become increasingly controversial.[10]

Global Budgets   A hospital operating under a global budget is getting a grant for all its costs. This form of payment is typical for state mental hospitals, military hospitals, and hospitals run by the Department of Veterans Affairs and other government entities, as well as a few specialized private institutions. Because a global budget is fixed, there are few incentives either to attract more patients or to reduce costs. In Canada, England, and much of the developed world outside the United States, global budgets are the most common form of hospital payment.

Charges   Hospital charges are known as "list prices" in most industries. A hospital, like a flower shop, can set its charges at whatever level it likes. It is rare for a patient, or an insurance company, to actually pay what is "charged." However, these paper charges often form the basis for reimbursement under a system of "discounted charges" (e.g., 60 percent of list price) or under a cost-reimbursement system that will be described shortly.

Per Diem   Latin for "per day," per diem payments were common when hospitals originated and are increasingly favored in managed care contracts today. Originally, per diems were charges set by the hospital, and they usually exceeded costs to help subsidize nonpaying patients. Today per diems are often negotiated with managed-care firms under very competitive conditions and are sometimes set below average costs per day in order for a hospital to maintain or increase its market share.

Cost Reimbursement   Cost reimbursement sets the payment level equal to the hospital's audited costs. "Days" and "discharges" are poor measures of the hospital's "product" because they do not account for variations in quality, severity of illness, or use of new technology. Because the hospital's output is so difficult to define and measure, it may be more equi- table and easier to reimburse for incurred costs rather than try to set appropriate prices. The Blue Cross (BC) plans, organized under the aegis of the American Hospital Association, wrote manuals describing how nonprofit hospitals can break even by setting charges to cover costs (including costs for treating nonpaying patients and setting aside money for a prudent reserve) and designed a method of cost reimbursement to break even. This method is known as **ratio of cost to charges applied to charges** (**RCCAC**). The RCCAC method is complex in practice but simple in concept: Estimate the cost per dollar billed in each department (Emer- gency, Laboratory, OR, Oncology) and then apply that to all of the bills paid by each type of insurance (Blue Cross, Medicare, Medicaid, etc.) so as to send each insurer one big bill at the end of the year.

When Medicare was created in 1965, it adopted the RCCAC methodology; therefore, this form of cost reimbursement became the dominant method by which funds flowed into hospitals from the 1960s until the mid-1980s. The RCCAC methodology is still used to determine most hospital unit costs today. The RCCAC is calculated separately for each revenue-producing hospital department using this formula:

$$\text{RCCAC Method } BC\ Payment = \frac{\text{Total Department Costs}_{all\ payers}}{\text{Total Department Charges}_{all\ payers}} \times BC\ Charges$$

Thus, if radiology costs are $6 million and total charges to all payers (i.e., for every insurance company and self-paying patient) are $10 million, the cost-to-charges ratio would be 0.60, and if BC patients have a total of $3 million in charges, BC would send the hospital a check for .60 × $3 million = $1.8 million as payment for its share of the costs. Although the reimbursement calculation uses charges, the amount paid does not depend on the level of charges. If the hospital doubles its charges (to $20 million), its ratio of cost-to-charges is cut in half (to 0.30), and even though the BC charges are doubled (to $6 million), the reimbursement stays the same.

The complicated RCCAC formula is needed because costs must be divided among different payers who are responsible for the costs of different patients. If there were only one payer, it would pay all costs, and cost reimbursement would be like an open-ended grant. With many payers some way must be found to allocate the costs across patients, and the RCCAC method uses the hospital's billed charges to do so. The method worked very well for a number of years to reimburse hospitals for all their costs. Indeed, it worked so well that costs rose explosively and cutbacks are now needed to reduce employee health benefits costs and government budget deficits (see Section 9.6 and Chapter 17).

Diagnostically Related Groups   Diagnostically related group (DRG) payments are fixed payments made based on the patient's diagnosis at discharge. DRG payments cover the complete hospital stay, including all ancillary services (but not surgery and other physician fees). To create this prospective payment system for Medicare payments, the government split all illnesses into 473 DRGs and estimated the cost per case within each group (similar to the resource-based relative value scale [RBRVS] payment system for physician services discussed in Section 6.1). Adjustments are made for these factors: local wages in the area in which the hospital is located, extremely long or short stays, hospitals with large teaching programs, and hospitals with a large percentage of indigent patients. In essence, DRGs are administered prices set by the government at what the government believes is a fair rate.[11] It is called a prospective payment system because the DRG rates are set in advance, unlike the previous retrospective cost reimbursement payments that were continually adjusted to match any change in costs so that the final amount was never set until long after the year ended.

Capitation   Capitation means payment "per person," so that, for example, a hospital would get paid $120 per month for each person within a group (covered by the plan), and the payment would remain the same amount regardless of how many patients were admitted from the group or how many days they stayed in the hospital (see Chapter 5). Capitation is a relatively rare form of payment for hospitals, because a large and well-defined number of patients must be pooled to reduce risks and make actuarial projections. Once an organization agrees to accept payment on a capitation basis, it in effect becomes a risk-bearing insurer. Usually, when it is said that a hospital is setting up a capitation arrangement, what is really meant is that some larger organization, such as the corporation that controls a number of hospitals, is creating an insurance company and health maintenance organization (HMO) to provide services on a capitated basis. Once the contract extends to multiple institutions and different kinds of care, the hospital becomes a "health system" rather than a traditional community hospital.

CASE RATES ADJUSTED FOR SPECIAL SITUATIONS*

Case-mix classification systems are used to determine the amounts that Medicare pays for the hospital inpatient care its beneficiaries receive. These systems include diagnosis-related groups (DRGs) for acute care hospitals, case-mix groups (CMGs) for inpatient rehabilitation facilities (IRFs), and long-term care (LTC) DRGs (LTC-DRGs) for long-term care hospitals (LTCHs). Payment rates are established prospectively and are expressed on a case or discharge basis, depending primarily on the diagnoses, procedures, and other clinical indicators for each patient. To avoid overpayments that can promote early discharge and underpayments that can jeopardize access, Medicare pays additional or reduced amounts in the following situations:

- Short-stay outliers
- Transfers and readmissions
- Patients who die
- High-cost outliers

(Continued)

CASE RATES ADJUSTED FOR SPECIAL SITUATIONS (CONTINUED)

The total net payment for these situations is budget-neutral—that is, the net amount for these situations translates into a corresponding decrease in the amount available for care rendered under all other circumstances.

Short-Stay Outliers

Some patients have significantly shorter stays than average for their case-mix group. Typically, a short stay costs remarkably less than the corresponding case rate. If the full rate were paid, hospitals would have financial incentives to discharge patients prematurely and would strongly prefer patients who could be discharged quickly to other care settings. In general, Medicare relies on per diem methods to reimburse short stays to align costs and payments more closely. An extra amount may be paid for the first day to acknowledge the disproportionately higher costs associated with the earliest portion of the stay.

For example, for LTCH patients staying no more than five-sixths of the *geometric* average length of stay for the appropriate LTC-DRG, the payment amount equals the lowest of: (1) 120 percent of the estimated cost of the case, (2) 120 percent of the LTC-DRG per diem rate multiplied by the patient's length of stay, or (3) the full LTC-DRG rate. The closer the stay is to the threshold, the more likely the full rate will be the lowest of the three amounts.

For IRF patients who are discharged within three days after being hospitalized, Medicare pays a CMG rate established specifically for short-stay patients. This rate equals about 17 percent of the amount paid for the typical long-stay patient who receives a full course of treatment.

Transfers and Readmissions

A patient may be discharged to another care setting and subsequently readmitted to the discharging hospital. If the intervening period is relatively short and two separate case rates were paid (one each for the discharge and readmission), hospitals would have financial incentives to shift patients around solely to maximize net income. The incentives would be especially alluring if the discharging and receiving facilities were under common ownership or located on the same campus. Medicare makes reduced payments to dilute these incentives.

For instance, if an LTCH patient is discharged to an acute care hospital and readmitted to the discharging hospital within nine days, the discharge and readmission is defined as one stay and one LTC-DRG rate is paid to the discharging hospital. The threshold is 27 days for IRFs and 45 days for skilled nursing facilities. In addition, there is a 5 percent cap on the proportion of Medicare patients that hospitals within hospitals, distinct-part skilled nursing facilities, and other co-located facilities may discharge and readmit annually. If the cap is exceeded, each corresponding onsite discharge and readmission is paid as one discharge, including those occurring before the cap was surpassed.

Medicare also pays a reduced amount for an IRF patient whose length of stay exceeds three days but is below the average for his or her CMG and who is discharged to another rehabilitation facility. The reduction assumes that care in one inpatient setting is substituted for care in another inpatient setting. No reduction applies, however, if a patient is discharged to a home health agency on the assumption that this pattern represents a normal progression of care. Payment is based on a per diem rate that includes an extra 50 percent for the first day. Thus, if a patient stays six days and the applicable per diem rate is $900, the payment would be $5,850 = (6 \times \$900) + (0.50 \times \$900)$.

(Continued)

CASE RATES ADJUSTED FOR SPECIAL SITUATIONS (CONTINUED)

Patients transferred between acute care hospitals are paid for similarly. Medicare pays the transferring hospital on a per diem basis up to the full DRG rate, whereas the receiving hospital that ultimately discharges the patient is paid the full DRG rate. For 10 specific DRGs, an acute care hospital is paid on a per diem basis up to the full DRG rate for Medicare patients who are transferred to a skilled nursing facility or other post–acute-care setting, including an extra amount for the first hospital day.

Patients Who Die

A reduced amount is paid for certain patients who die while hospitalized. For IRFs, there are four distinct CMGs for Medicare patients who stay longer than three days but die before treatment is completed. The case rate varies with the patient's length of stay and whether he or she was hospitalized for an orthopedic condition. Similarly, Medicare pays acute-care hospitals a distinct case rate for neonates who die before discharge or who are transferred to another facility.

High-Cost Outliers

Additional payments are made for Medicare patients who are extraordinarily costly to treat. The extra amount is determined by multiplying the excess of the estimated cost of treating the patient over a cost threshold by a marginal cost factor. The cost of treating the patient is estimated by multiplying the amount billed for covered services by the facility's cost-to-charges ratio. The threshold equals the DRG rate plus a predetermined "fixed-loss" amount (e.g., $24,450 for LTCHs and $33,560 for acute care hospitals for fiscal year 2003), which reflects the loss a hospital incurs before outlier payments begin. The marginal cost factor is generally 80 percent. Thus, if a hospital's cost-to-charge ratio is 65 percent and billed charges equal $80,000, the estimated cost would be $52,000 = $80,000 × 0.65. If the cost outlier threshold is $42,000, the outlier payment would be $8,000 = 0.80 × ($52,000 − $42,000). If the DRG rate is $23,000, the total payment would be $31,000 = $23,000 + $8,000.

*This box on case rate adjustment was prepared by Paul L. Grimaldi, Ph.D., health finance consultant and lecturer, © 2003.

Managed-Care Contracts   Blue Cross and most private insurance companies have shifted to managed-care contracts with hospitals (see Chapter 5). In these arrangements, payment is usually made on the basis of per diems, discounted charges, or a negotiated fee schedule. The crucial difference that sets managed-care contracts apart from cost reimbursement or payment of charges is the role of the care manager. Rather than just paying the bills, the insurance company has a specialized **utilization review** (UR) nurse or physician critically examine each case to determine, for example, whether hospitalization was justified, a lower-cost alternative (such as outpatient surgery) was available, and adequate documentation was provided for all laboratory tests. By negotiating discounts, discouraging use, and denying payment for disallowed or undocumented charges, managed-care firms can usually obtain medical care for their clients at a lower cost than traditional indemnity or cost-reimbursement insurers and therefore are taking over the market. Being constantly questioned and audited has not been easy or pleasant for the doctors who admit patients or for those working in hospital financial departments. Patients also dislike having to justify and obtain approval for every additional service or extra day in the hospital, but they are willing to put up with it if premiums are sufficiently reduced.

8.3   HOSPITAL FINANCING: EXPENSES

Hospitals are personal care institutions, and labor accounts for the bulk of their costs. Surgery and many other physician services are paid for separately (as they were in 1750) and therefore not included in the hospital budget. Some physicians are employees of the hospital, but the services of contracted pathologists, radiologists, emergency doctors, hospitalists, and primary care practioners often show up under the category "professional fees." It might be thought that the acquisition of lithotripters, magnetic resonance imaging (MRI) scanners, and other expensive medical technology would make "equipment" a large category, yet the wages of the skilled people required to operate each new piece of equipment usually runs two or three times the cost of the machinery itself. Much of the category "other" takes the form of services and thus also involves labor hired in the local market. When payroll, professional fees, and local services are added together, about 75 percent of a hospital's costs are labor. This fact makes it politically difficult to cut costs, since the only way to do so is to cut people, by reducing wages or laying off employees. Energy, raw materials, and other goods traded in competitive national and international markets are relatively unimportant in the hospital budget. Access to capital, however, has significantly shaped the growth of health care systems (see Chapter 12).

8.4   FINANCIAL MANAGEMENT AND COST SHIFTING

Revenues must exceed expenses for an organization to survive, but there is no reason that the individuals for whom expenditures are incurred must be the same as the individuals from whom revenues are obtained. Whereas individual matching of benefits and payments is common in most consumer markets, in health care this almost never takes place. For the early hospitals, donations by the wealthy members of the community and general tax funds (paid mostly by landowners) were used to provide services to the sick and to poor people with disabilities. Funding and benefits were matched at the level of the community, not the individual. It was considered fair that those who benefited most from the economy should give the most to help those in need. Paying patients who could afford hospitalization were usually charged a bit extra to help support the hospital's charitable mission. In effect, the excess of charges above costs constituted a "hospital tax" on the working-class and upper-class people who happened to get sick.

When hospitals took care of the poor who could not help themselves, it was obvious and necessary that the burden of financing would fall primarily on a different group of people who did have money: philanthropists and taxpayers. As technology advanced and hospital services became more desirable to all people, it was inevitable that there would be a great increase in hospital expenditures and that there would be more overlap between the people who paid and the people who received care. Insurance, pooling funds from the many so that a few could receive care, was a significant extension of financing that furthered the ability of the market to transfer the burden of payment away from the individual who was sick. One of the expenses that was factored into private insurance premiums was charity care; thus, insured patients were also paying for those who had no insurance.

The process of using revenues from one group of clients to subsidize another group is known in health care as **cost shifting**. Under philanthropic funding, all revenues are cost shifted—they are intended as donations to benefit others, not the giver. With insurance and cost reimbursement, the flows are more complex, but it is clear that somebody else is paying for the nonpaying patients (bad debt, charity care) since they do not bring any revenues into the hospital. Several other functions, such as medical education, research, and community outreach, are usually supported through cost shifting because they bring in very little revenue, certainly less than what they cost to provide.

Cost shifting has always existed, but the extensive and sophisticated form found today probably has its origins in the need for hospitals to perform more and more autopsies as surgery became common in the early 20th century. Even though vital to maintaining and improving the quality of medical care, autopsies obviously could not be billed to the patient. Clinical pathologists found it easy to support this scientific need by charging separately for laboratory tests that previously had been included as part of the regular hospital per diem for services. Billing for lab tests met with so little resistance that charges were pushed up and up, and by the 1970s it was not uncommon for a lab to charge ten times what a test cost and to be a major source of excess revenues for subsidizing other parts of the hospital, such as the emergency department, which was a chronic loser.

Research programs must conduct extensive tests, keep patients in the hospital for extra days, and perform experimental surgeries that might turn out to be totally useless to perfect techniques and make new discoveries. Because these bills are paid just like any other patient care, research costs are shifted to the insurance company. Also, the bill for a day in the intensive care unit (ICU) is based on the average; thus, the easy cases (which actually cost less) provide an implicit subsidy for the complex cases and research. Medical education is expensive and is usually conducted along with the research that keeps faculties on the cutting edge. Teaching salaries and research equipment are included when calculating the basis for cost reimbursement. Cost per day in a major university hospital is often two to three times that in a small community hospital. Because insurance pays whether the patient gets a broken arm fixed in a local hospital at $1,100 or a university hospital at $3,600, insurance is paying for most research and educational expense—or actually the employees from whose paychecks the insurance premiums are taken are truly the ones paying.[12]

Cost shifting and cross subsidies are pervasive and long-standing features of medical care reimbursement. In general, hospitals have had public support for taking revenues from a variety of sources and using them to fund not just basic care but also outreach to indigent people, community prevention programs, research, teaching, and other activities that were seen as being in the public interest. However, decades of rising costs, incomprehensible billing, and meaningless prices, combined with organizational infighting among payers and providers, has left the public confused and ever more resistant to spending. These forces led to the rise of managed care and are now getting stronger, reflected in strident calls for transparency and regulation of billing. The American public is in the process of giving up on the old system of financing, but it has not yet been able to find and agree on a new one.[13]

Distortions in pricing are not just confusing, they create unintended consequences. By limiting its services to those that are overpriced, and not providing the services that are more costly and need subsidy, a hospital can reap extraordinary profits and is said to be is **cream skimming**. Ambulatory surgery centers, independent diagnostic clinics, and orthopedic, cardiac, and other specialty units are able to maintain margins well in excess of most community hospitals.[14] While tradition and expressions of polite disapproval were able to limit the extent to which profits were drained from the system by cream skimming before the 1970s, today's fiscally challenged and starkly competitive environment has made it impossible to do so.

8.5   HOW DO HOSPITALS COMPETE?

The flow of revenues into a hospital follows the flow of patients. In some cases, such as emergency department or outpatient clinic visits, patients themselves decide where to go, and for these types of care, hospitals compete directly by trying to attract patients. However, for most care the decision regarding hospitalization is made by the physician. The agency relationship changes the nature of the transaction, so that the patient follows the advice of the physician and therefore the hospitals compete for doctors. If the ability to decide on hospitalization is taken out of the doctor's hands by the insurance company, as it sometimes is under managed care (see Chapter 5), then hospitals must compete for contracts and appeal to payers, which usually forces a hospital to put more emphasis on lowering prices. The important point is that the hospital must compete for the contracting party that has the power to make the revenues come to them, not necessarily for the patient.

Competing for Patients

The types of care for which patients make their own decisions are those in which they are able to judge important aspects of quality and in which they pay a large share of cost directly out of their own pockets. Maternity care is a good example. Many mothers want to have their babies close to home, have strong preferences regarding patient services (natural childbirth, religious orientation, attitude of staff), and can get good information for comparing hospitals by talking to other mothers in the neighborhood. Because the need for care is known months in advance, potential parents can do the kind of comparison shopping that is impossible to do after accidents or heart attacks. Also, the fact that births are expected means that they are not "risks" in the insurance sense and therefore often are reimbursed on a shared or fixed-price basis that leaves much of the marginal cost to the parents. For these reasons, hospitals must actively compete for patients on the basis of price and service. Casual investigation reveals a number of special deals, from free baby clothes, gourmet meals, and a postpartum vacation to cut-rate "fixed-price packages," not unlike the competition for selling cars and houses. Outpatient clinics, where patients are more likely to self-refer and where cost sharing is usually higher, also use marketing strategies such as nice waiting rooms, receptionists who call to make or remind patients about appointments, free transportation to the clinic, and deductible or copayment waivers. The rise of "preferred provider" plans (see Chapter 5) that provide full coverage only for a limited group of hospitals has also increased the importance of direct marketing to patients.

Increasing competition by making more information on price and quality available to patients has generated considerable interest. However, most of the "report card" efforts directed at consumers have shown little impact. Indeed, it appears that patients are more sensitive to superficial differences in amenities (good food, attentive staff, pleasant surroundings) than to significant differences in mortality rates, surgical qualifications, or charges.[15]

Competing for Physicians

The agency relationship and control over admissions means that most hospital competition is over doctors rather than over patients. An increasing number of doctors have become salaried employees in recent years, and more than half of all large medical groups are owned by hospital health systems, but a majority of physicians and specialty practices are still independent. Another visible sign of the competition to gain the loyalty (and patient referrals) of physicians are recruitment incentives. Income guarantees (e.g., if you come to hospital X, and your income in the first year is less than $125,000, we will make up the difference), relocation assistance, and promises of referrals from other doctors on the medical staff are common contractual provisions, especially in rural areas. Sometimes there is even a "signing bonus" similar to what a professional athlete might receive. As Mark Pauly's "doctor's workshop" model suggests, hospitals also compete by helping physicians earn more money in their private practices by providing free or subsidized office space; providing secretarial, phone, and billing services; setting aside 10 beds for nephrology or another specialty so that the specialist will always be able to admit a patient; and so on.[16]

Reducing practice costs or work effort is a limited competitive tool. Far more important is that the hospital help a physician build his or her practice through the hospital's reputation for quality and the technological sophistication of services offered.[17] A cardiologist is able to attract more patients if he or she is the only cardiologist in town who has access to a catheterization lab that does stents or percutaneous transluminal coronary angioplasty (PTCA). In some instances, such competition can lead to a sort of "**medical arms race**," in which nearby hospitals each try to be the first with the most and respond strategically. For example, if one hospital gets an MRI scanner, the other one gets one that is bigger; if one gets a lithotripter, the other gets one that has more settings and finer resolution; and so on. It is possible that competing on the basis of which hospital has the most new technology can lead to inefficiencies and escalating costs, with the two scanners and two lithotripters empty half the time because there are only enough patients in the market to keep one piece of equipment operating at full capacity.

This points out one of the major problems of hospital markets structured on the basis of competing for physicians to increase patient flow. A hospital has an incentive to subsidize office space to attract physicians but not to reduce charges to patients, change billing practices, or make trade-offs that lead to overall reductions in the cost of medical care. The competition for physicians does not necessarily push hospitals toward an efficient use of inputs or mix of services.

Competing for Contracts

The scale on which medical practice is conducted is increasing. When organized on the basis of atomistic transactions between individuals, the choice of hospital falls to the doctors acting as agents for the patients under their care. However, it has become more and more common for a payer to make contracts directly with hospitals, negotiating a fixed or discounted price, and limiting patients to hospitals with which the payer has a contract. Payers can direct patient flow even when contracts are not fully binding. Although Medicare has a contract with every hospital, it allows heart transplants only in certain approved facilities, and in a request for proposals to become an approved provider, price is a factor. Health maintenance organizations (HMOs) can be even more aggressive, sometimes threatening to transfer a large group of patients to a rival facility unless negotiations result in a substantial discount or making approval conditional on assurances that the HMO will receive the lowest price the hospital gives to any contractor.

Although managed-care contracting at this level is a relatively recent development, structurally it bears a resemblance to the original social contract between the hospital and the community and to the agreements under which hospitals receive tax subsidies and other favorable treatment from the government. In each of these contracts, there are two parties: the hospital and a representative of consumers as a group (community, insurance plan, taxpayers). Such large-scale arrangements are inevitably less accommodating to the needs of individual patients and the professional autonomy of physicians. However, any attempt to implement public accountability and successful cost control involves compromises. Trade-offs are necessary in any system that takes its broader social responsibilities seriously and are the core concept for creating economic efficiency in health care (see Table 8.2).

TABLE 8.2	Competition between Hospitals
Hospitals Compete for	**On the Basis of Quality and**
Patients	Amenities, out-of-pocket payments
Doctors	Salary, technology, assistance
Contracts	Price, information systems

Measuring Competitive Success

How can it be determined which hospitals are more successful in the competition for patients? A firm that has failed by going out of business is clearly not successful, and economists have used "survivor analysis" to measure competitive success by counting the number of new entrants or exits (bankruptcy, takeover) within different categories. Survivor analysis has been used to show that hospitals with fewer than 100 or more than 500 beds appear to be inefficient and less able to compete.[18] Such analysis has also shown that for-profit hospitals are not necessarily more efficient or better competitors than nonprofits (the number of for-profit hospitals has fluctuated, but these hospitals accounted for around 10 percent to 20 percent of total bed supply throughout the 20th century, indicating competitive performance that is about average). A hospital that has grown relative to its competitors is clearly more successful, and such traditional measures as total assets, market share, and geographic spread have been used as indicators.

With 90 percent of hospitals operated by either voluntary (charitable and/or religious) or government organizations, profits are less useful as a measure of success than they are in other industries. However, the excess of revenues over expenditures is available to fund growth and is necessary to avoid bankruptcy, and thus it can be a useful indicator. Today's successful institutions are those that acquire others to create health systems, while the losers are those that get swallowed up and lose their identity (see Chapter 12). Strong earnings and large financial reserves clearly provide a competitive advantage in the current environment, with health systems trying to increase market share, expand geographically, and maintain a full line of services through acquisitions. Almost all of the small hospitals that "join" systems are forced to do so by competitive forces rather than by choice.

What has proved almost impossible to measure is the success of a hospital in achieving its goals as a provider of health care to the community. Although charity care, participation in outreach programs, and mortality rates are often monitored and commented on, there is general agreement that these are incomplete and inadequate measures at best, and are often misleading. Attempts are being made to assess community benefit in more comprehensive and objective ways, but there is as yet no reason to believe that these will be any more convincing than previous efforts.[19] Economists and other policy makers are in the awkward position of recognizing that they know which dimensions are most important (quality, compassion, technological advances), but they do not know how to gauge them numerically or even how to make a fair comparison between hospitals.

Measuring the Competitiveness of Markets

Competition can be a significant factor in forcing hospitals to become more efficient and provide better services.[20] However, a single hospital in a rural area or a chain that controls almost all the hospitals in an urban market is not constrained by competition. The potential loss of consumer welfare because of a merger or acquisition that reduces the amount of competition is the central concern of the Federal Trade Commission (FTC) and a source of much litigation under antitrust law. This litigation provides many consulting projects for economists called in to testify as expert witnesses on how competitive a particular market is or will be.

Competition is usually measured by the number of hospitals or concentration of market share in a geographic area (e.g., within a 15-mile radius; within a city, county, or metropolitan statistical area) or by the overlap between hospital services (how many patients use several hospitals). Although the complexities of antitrust law and the economic assessment of competition policy are beyond the scope of this text, it is worth noting that all hospitals are multiproduct firms. The relevant market for services such as liver transplantation, residential psychiatric care, and abortion, therefore, covers a large area because patients are willing to travel hundreds of miles for treatment, whereas the market for other services such as kidney dialysis, outpatient psychiatry, and prenatal care depend on patients living nearby and hence is much smaller. After decades of being exempt or ignored, hospitals have come under increasing scrutiny by the FTC, and antitrust enforcement is now considered an important alternative to regulation as a means of controlling costs.

8.6   ORGANIZATION: WHO CONTROLS THE HOSPITAL AND FOR WHAT ENDS?

Hospitals differ from the standard textbook model of the firm in three significant ways:

- Patients do not pay because of insurance or charity.
- Ownership is usually unclear because of nonprofit voluntary or governmental organization.
- Medical care is largely controlled by doctors, who neither pay nor receive any money from the hospital and therefore have no direct connection from a financial perspective.

Doctors are neither customers nor employees nor owners, but in practice they are the dominant voice in hospital operations; therefore, they sometimes look like they are all three. This structure—combining power, money, and service with no direct line of control or financial accountability—is a unique form of economic organization that makes it difficult to model or predict the behavior of hospitals. A hospital does not do anything without directions from a physician; only physicians are allowed to admit patients, perform surgery, or prescribe drugs. The hospital organizes a medical staff, but some claim that the reality is the other way around: that the medical staff organizes a hospital as its workshop. This is the basis of Mark Pauly's model of the hospital as the doctor's workshop, which hypothesizes that the hospital will behave to maximize the profits of the doctors who are on staff, rather than to maximize the profits of the organization (see Chapter 6).[21]

Joseph Newhouse has pointed out that hospitals are nonprofit organizations with no owners who can claim the profits, and he suggests that hospitals and other nonprofit organizations are run for the benefit of managers.[22] Managers want their hospitals to be the biggest and the best, which, not incidentally, justifies the highest managerial salaries and hence maximizes some combination of quantity and quality of services rather than profits or doctors' incomes. Employees are also important stakeholders, but because their importance derives from being input suppliers, their influence in hospitals is not much different from their influence in other organizations.

Most hospital mission statements claim that their primary concern is patient care, yet this sort of general assertion does not address the method by which prices are set, the trade-off between one group of patients and another (e.g., surgery or immunization, abortion or family-planning clinics), or the trade-offs between employees and doctors. The American Hospital Association maintains that hospitals are, in essence, public institutions whose purpose is to benefit the community. From a financing perspective, this makes sense, because most of the capital investment in a voluntary hospital comes from the community in the form of charitable donations and taxes. The problem is: How is community benefit defined and who, exactly, exercises control?[23] The board, although in theory representing the community, is often deferential to the medical staff and depends on the information provided by the administration to make decisions (see box "Who Gets the Profits from a Nonprofit Hospital?").

Who Gets the Profits from a Nonprofit Hospital?

Doctors?
Administrators?
Employees?
Patients?
Community?

Despite a considerable amount of theoretical and empirical work by economists and a clear recognition that insurance, nonprofit status, and medical control over admissions and treatment make hospitals different, no truly satisfactory theory of the hospital as a distinct type of organization has been developed. Research has shown that nonprofit hospitals are more likely to serve the urban poor and provide unprofitable services (immunization, pre-natal care, emergency department, drug detoxification), whereas for-profits are more likely to charge higher prices, locate facilities in growing suburbs where patients have higher incomes and better insurance, and emphasize high-margin procedures (diagnostic radiology, invasive cardiology).[24]

However, the differences are usually small. One possible reason is that competition and the pressure to survive forces a hospital to maximize revenues and minimize costs much like a for-profit firm. The greater the amount of debt, the more pressure a hospital faces, and any deviation from profit-maximizing behavior becomes a threat to survival. The lack of substantial differences might also result from social expectations that force for-profit hospitals to meet the standards of community benefit and medical professionalism to attract patients. An area with mostly nonprofit hospitals seems to have for-profits behaving more like nonprofits, and conversely in an area dominated by for-profit hospitals the nonprofits appear more overtly commercial.

Although all general acute hospitals seem to behave in similar ways, it is possible to discern a continuum, with for-profits at one end being more aggressive and quick to respond to incentives, government hospitals at the other end being a bit more inflexible and committed to public service, and voluntary nonprofits occupying the broad middle ground. The large hospitals that do most of the teaching and research are almost always nonprofit institutions. The range of behavior resulting from differences in hospital ownership category is fairly narrow, and it is outweighed by differences related to mission, size, teaching status, and local factors.

SUGGESTIONS FOR FURTHER READING

American Hospital Association, *Hospital Statistics and Hospital Guide* is published annually.

David M. Cutler, ed., *The Changing Hospital Industry: Comparing Not-for-Profit and For-Profit Institutions* (Chicago: University of Chicago Press, 2000).

Modern Healthcare and *Hospitals and Health Networks* are biweekly magazines covering the hospital industry in depth.

Rosemary Stevens, *In Sickness and In Wealth: American Hospitals in the Twentieth Century* (New York: Basic Books, 1989).

SUMMARY

1.   The Pennsylvania Hospital, founded in 1751, was the first hospital in the United States. Like most **early hospitals**, it was **funded primarily by charitable donations and government** tax appropriations and **housed the sick and poor** people with disabilities, although some paying patients were admitted.

2.   The development of **new technology** created the need for a central facility where the **capital cost** of equipment could be shared by many doctors and where dangerous surgical procedures could be performed in a more controlled and supportive environment.

3.   More than **95 percent of all hospital revenues come from third parties,** and more than half come from government through the Medicare and Medicaid programs. Patients pay so little of the hospital bill that **charges are almost irrelevant in decision making.** Cost-based reimbursement using the RCCAC (ratio-of-cost-to-charges-applied-to-charges) formula developed by Blue Cross plans under the aegis of the American Hospital Association was the major form of payment from 1965 to 1985. Since then the prospective DRG per-case payments and a variety of managed managed-care plans have become the main sources of revenues. Approximately one-third of hospital revenues come from outpatient services, and an increasing amount comes from home health, long-term care, and other related services.

4.   Hospitals obtain revenues in a variety of ways, including **philanthropy** and grants, **global budgets,** billed **charges,** per-day (**per diem**) payments, **DRG** per-case payments, **cost reimbursement,** and **managed-care** contracts.

5.   **Labor** is the largest category of health care expenditure. When employees of local service firms are included, personnel accounts for more than 75 percent of a hospital's costs. Therefore, the only way to cut costs is to reduce wages or reduce employment, neither of which is politically popular. **Doctors are usually independent contractors** paid separately by the patient and thus do not show up as a large item on hospital budgets, even though they play a dominant role in providing and directing care.

6.   **Cost shifting** is the process of charging one group (e.g., commercially insured patients) more to cover the loss due to undercharging another group (indigent patients, Medicaid). The pervasiveness of cost shifting and insurance coverage gave financial managers far more room to raise revenues as a means of supporting the hospital and little incentive to find efficiencies that would reduce costs. **Cream skimming** is the action of taking on only the profitable patients for whom services are priced considerably above unit costs, while avoiding the loss-making patients with heavy care needs. Changes in Medicare reimbursement and the advent of managed-care firms that shop to obtain hospital services at the lowest possible price have eroded the ability of hospitals to cross subsidize and have made it difficult to support research, teaching, and charity care.

7.   **Hospitals compete for physicians,** because physicians control the flow of patients (and hence, revenues). Unlike most businesses, hospitals do not compete directly for "customers" because their customers do not pay their own bills and do not make their own choices, but are directed by physicians who act as their agents. Only for some patient-initiated or relatively uninsured services is direct competition important for patients (plastic surgery, childbirth). Larger scale and cost pressures are causing hospitals to compete for contracts, trying to attract employees, HMOs, or insurance companies directly. To do so, they must compete more and more on the basis of price rather than quality.

8.   Hospitals differ from most firms in that they are largely paid for by third parties, are often **nonprofit organizations** directed by volunteer boards rather than owners and **dominated by doctors** who are often **independent professionals** working for themselves with no direct financial ties to the hospital. Despite much research and lots of theoretical expectations, there appear to be only slight differences among voluntary not-for-profit, government, and private for-profit hospitals. In general, for-profits appear to be somewhat less likely to take on charity care, research, teaching, and outreach and tend to react more quickly to changes in reimbursement regulations, with government

hospitals at the other extreme and voluntary hospitals falling in the middle, but most differences are small and occur only occasionally.

PROBLEMS

1. {*industrial organization*} Which technological, organizational, and financial innovations caused the rise of hospitals in the 20th century?

2. {*incidence*} Who pays for most of the care in hospitals? Are the people who pay the bills the same as the people who receive the care?

3. {*flow of funds*} Which input accounts for the largest portion of hospital costs? Which input is responsible for most of the growth in hospital cost per patient day?

4. {*payment methodology*} Both Hospital A and Hospital B are paid by Medicare using the DRG methodology. Assume that the reimbursement for the average Medicare patient (case weight of 1.0) is $2,600. Hospital A has an average case-mix index of 1.32 and admits 24 patients who stay in the hospital a total of 192 days, whereas Hospital B has an average case-mix index of 0.95 and admits 35 patients who stay in the hospital a total of 238 days. Which hospital gets paid more? Which hospital gets paid more per case? Which hospital gets paid more per diem? Which hospital gets paid more for an appendectomy (case weight of 0.85)?

5. {*flow of funds*} Over the past 100 years, the major source of hospital revenues has changed three times. Name these types of payments, and explain why each one gave way to the next.

6. {*payment*} If a hospital decides to raise prices because it needs more money, what effect does this have on the following:
   a. Patients who pay their own bills
   b. Patients whose bills are paid by an insurance company
   c. Hospitals with insurance contracts that reimburse on the basis of costs
   d. Hospitals with previously negotiated per-diem contracts with HMOs

7. {*cost shifting*} Is the mark-up (ratio of prices to direct per-unit costs) relatively constant across different types of hospitals? Are mark-ups the same for different services or departments within a hospital?

8. {*cost shifting*} How do hospitals pay for medical research?

9. {*ownership*} Are doctors usually employees, owners, or managers of hospitals?

10. {*ownership*} Who owns most hospitals? Who gets the profit when a nonprofit hospital makes money? Can nonprofit hospitals be bought and sold?

11. {*competition*} Wills Eye Hospital in Philadelphia is a 114-bed hospital specializing in ophthalmologic surgery. Whom do you think competes with Wills Eye?

12. {*competition*} Describe the factors you would expect to be most important in competition for patients for each of the following services. For which services is price more important? Location? Quality? Would hospitals compete for patients or for doctors?
    a. Heart transplants
    b. Maternity
    c. Immunization
    d. Depression
    e. Chemotherapy

    f. Plastic surgery

    g. AIDS

13. {*cost shifting*} What does it mean for Medicare to act as a "prudent buyer" of hospital services? Does doing so strengthen or weaken Medicare as a social insurance program?

14. {*cost shifting*} What adjustments would a hospital have to make if it began to serve a larger number of indigent patients? Would most of the adjustments come on the revenue side or the expenditure side?

15. {*cost shifting*} Who benefits from cost shifting: the poor or the rich? Do any health care workers benefit from cost shifting?

ENDNOTES

1. Paul Starr, *The Social Transformation of American Medicine* (New York: Basic Books, 1992); Rosemary Stevens, *In Sickness and in Wealth: American Hospitals in the Twentieth Century* (New York: Basic Books, 1989).
2. George Rosen, *A History of Public Health* (New York: MD Publications, 1958).
3. Florence Nightingale, *Notes on Nursing: What It Is, and What It Is Not* (New York: Appleton-Century, 1938).
4. Charles Lawrence, *History of the Philadelphia Almshouses and Hospitals from the Beginning of the Eighteenth to the Ending of the Nineteenth Centuries* (Philadelphia: C. Lawrence, 1905).
5. Marshall K. Raffel and Norma K. Raffel, *The U.S. Health System: Origins and Functions,* 4th ed. (Albany: Delmar, 1994).
6. An illustrative case study is found in the history of the Mayo clinic. See Helen Clapesattle, *The Doctors Mayo* (Minneapolis: University of Minnesota Press, 1941); Gunther W. Nagel, *The Mayo Legacy* (Springfield, Ill.: Charles C Thomas, 1966); and compare with an annual report of the Mayo Clinic (now operating in Arizona and Florida as well as Minnesota) in the 1990s.
7. J. Hermann, "Blue Cross of California Goes for the Gold—Wellpoint Health Networks," *Health Systems Review* 26, no. 3 (1993): 14–19; T. Kertesz, "California Blue Cross Tries Again With Bigger Foundation Plan," *Modern Healthcare* 25, no. 16 (1995): 2–3, 1995.
8. American Hospital Association, *Hospital Statistics* (Chicago: American Hospital Association, 2002).
9. Prices paid by patients are even less important than Table 8.2 would suggest, because much of the 3 percent is actually deductibles, copayments, and other charges that are in effect insurance premiums or taxes and not directly related to the prices of the services chosen.
10. Some legislators argue that hospitals are no longer providing the charitable public services for which they were founded and hence do not deserve help, and that public funds should be redirected toward community programs or inner-city hospitals. The city of Philadelphia, for example, has forced local hospitals to pay millions of dollars under its PILOTs/SILOTs program (Payments/Services In Lieu of Taxes). A hospital is assessed an amount equal to its tax liability, and then it must document provision of services provided without compensation of an equal amount or pay the city the difference.
11. State Medicaid plans used the DRG system but generally paid few dollars for each patient. In time, this underpayment led to complaints and a series of lawsuits. Temple University Hospital sued the state of Pennsylvania under the Boren Amendment to the Social Security Act, which obligated states to make payments sufficient to cover the cost of efficiently provided services. The hospital eventually won, creating a precedent that hospitals around the country quickly followed (and that forced state budgets into deficits). Hence, although in concept a charge system gives all the power to the seller, and an administered price system (like DRGs) gives all the power to the buyer, in reality both sides are at least to some extent constrained by the political process and public opinion.
12. A. Dobson, J. DaVanzo, and N. Sen, "The Cost-Shift Payment Hydraulic: Foundation, History and Implications," *Health Affairs* 25, no. 1 (2006): 22–33.
13. Henry J. Aaron and Robert D. Reischauer, "The Medicare Reform Debate: What Is the Next Step?" *Health Affairs* 14, no. 4 (1995): 8–30.
14. Melanie Evans, "Juggling the Lineup: Seeking Better Financial Results, Providers Change Services," *Modern Healthcare* 42, no. 3 (2012): 6–17; M. R. Plotzke and C. Courtemanche, "Does Procedure Profitability Impact Whether an Outpatient Surgery Procedure is Performed at an Ambulatory Surgery Center or Hospital?" *Health Economics* 20, no. 7 (2011): 817–830.
15. Dana Goldman and John Romley, "Hospitals as Hotels: The Role of Patient Amenities in Hospital Demand," NBER working paper #14619, December 2008; Mark W. Legnini et al., "Where Does Performance Measurement Go from Here?" *Health Affairs* 19, no. 3 (2000): 173–177; P. S. Romano and H. Zhou, "Do Well-Publicized Risk-Adjusted Outcomes Reports Affect Hospital Volume?" *Medical Care* 42, no. 4 (2004): 367–377; Michael Rothberg

et al., "Choosing the Best Hospital: The Limitations of Public Quality Reporting," *Health Affairs* 276): 1680–1687, 2008.

16. Mark Pauly and Michael Redisch, "The Not-for-Profit Hospital as a Physicians Cooperative," *American Economic Review* 63, no. 1 (1973): 87–99; Mark V. Pauly, *The Doctor's Workshop* (Philadelphia: University of Pennsylvania Press, 1980).

17. H. Luft, J. Robinson, D. Garnick, S. Maerki, and S. McPhee, "The Role of Specialized Clinical Services in the Competition Among Hospitals," *Inquiry* 23, no. 1 (1986): 83–94.

18. Carson W. Bays, "The Determinants of Hospital Size: A Survivor Analysis," *Applied Economics* 18, no. 4 (1986): 359–377.

19. Robert Sigmond and J. David Seay, "Community Benefit Standards for Hospitals: Perception and Performance," *Frontiers of Health Services Management* Spring 1989.

20. Jean M. Abraham, Martin S. Gaynor, and William B. Vogt, "Entry and Competition in Local Hospital Markets," NBER working paper #11649, September 2005.

21. Mark V. Pauly, *Doctors and Their Workshops: Economic Models of Physician Behavior* (Chicago: University of Chicago Press, 1980).

22. Joseph Newhouse, "How Do Hospitals Make Choices?" in *The Economics of Medical Care* (Reading, Mass.: Addison-Wesley, 1978), 68–73.

23. Robert Sigmond and J. D. Seay, "Community Benefit Standards for Hospitals: Perceptions and Performance," in "The Future of Tax-Exempt Status for Hospitals," *Frontiers of Health Services Management* Spring 1989.

24. E. R. Becker and Frank Sloan, "Hospital Ownership and Performance," *Economic Inquiry* 23, no. 1 (1985): 21–36; 33–44; Mark Schlesinger, Theodore Marmor, and R. Smithey, "Non-Profit and For-Profit Medical Care," *Journal of Health Politics, Policy and Law* 12, no. 3 (1987): 427–457; Sujoy Chakravarty, Martin Gaynor, Steven Klepper, and William B. Vogt, "Does the Profit Motive Make Jack Nimble? Ownership Form and the Evolution of the U.S. Hospital Industry," NBER working paper #11705, October 2005; Jill R. Horwitz and Austin Nichols, "What Do Nonprofits Maximize? Nonprofit Hospital Service Provision and Market Ownership Mix," NBER working paper #13246, July 2007; Jill Horwitz, "Making Profits and Providing Care: Comparing Nonprofit, For-Profit and Government Hospitals," *Health Affairs* 24, no. 3 (2005): 790–801; J. Silverman and J. Skinner, "Medicare Upcoding and Hospital Ownership," *Journal of Health Economics* 23, no. 2 (2004): 369–389; Hsien-Ming Lien, Shin-Yi Chou, and Jin-Tan Liu, "Hospital Ownership and Performance: Evidence from Stoke and Cardiac Treatment in Taiwan," *Journal of Health Economics* 27, no. 5 (2008): 1208–1223.

CHAPTER 9

MANAGEMENT AND REGULATION OF HOSPITAL COSTS

QUESTIONS

1. Why do some hospitals cost more than others?
2. Why is a hospital bill so hard to understand? Why doesn't a hospital just post a list of prices like most businesses?
3. The number of patients and the number of days each patient spends in the hospital has gone down. Why have hospital costs continued to increase faster than other health care costs?
4. Are large hospitals expensive because they suffer from diseconomies of scale or because they admit the most difficult-to-treat patients?
5. Why would a hospital want to buy a new magnetic resonance imaging (MRI) scanner if it expects the MRI to be busy only half the time and the hospital next door already has such a machine?
6. Will computers and other new technology improve efficiency and hence reduce costs, or will they improve quality and raise costs?
7. Has regulation cut costs or cut competition?

9.1 WHY DO SOME HOSPITALS COST MORE THAN OTHERS?

The cost of a day in the hospital can be as little as $400 or more than $4,500. Which factors could account for such a wide variation? It is not surprising if a day in the hospital costs $4,500 for a critically wounded trauma patient in an intensive care unit (ICU) and just $400 for a patient resting after breaking a leg while skiing.[1] The ICU patient is much sicker and requires more complex services. It is also understandable that staying in one of the nation's top research and teaching hospitals under the care of famous doctors can cost more than staying in a small rural facility with limited equipment and staff.[2] The hospital bill can be a misleading guide to costs. One hospital might charge more but give every patient a discount while another sticks to list prices. One hospital could charge $400 for the bed, with extra charges for medication, laboratory tests, physical therapy, and so on, while another hospital charges $900 for the bed and all other services, making it less expensive (see the box "Reasons for Differences in Hospital Costs").

REASONS FOR DIFFERENCES IN HOSPITAL COSTS

Severity of patient's illness

Quality of care

Intensity of services (e.g., number of nursing hours or lab tests)

Cost shifting to pay for research and teaching

Differences in billing

Prices of labor and other inputs

Efficiency

It is often assumed that a hospital with a lower cost per patient day is more efficient, but such a conclusion is only justified if the comparison hospital provides the same services to similar patients under similar conditions. Unless this *ceteris paribus* (all other things constant) assumption is valid, which it rarely is, efforts must be made to adjust for all the other factors listed in the box "Reasons for Differences in Hospital Costs" to compare costs. Of course, patients and their insurance companies prefer a cheaper stay in the hospital to a more expensive stay if all other factors are constant. If not, the more relevant question is: Is a hospital that costs 10 percent more (or 20 percent, or 400 percent) really worth that much more? Although this relative value question is more meaningful, it is also much more difficult to answer, and the answer depends on the patient's values as well as calculations of technical efficiency. Therefore, it is useful to look first at the simpler and more standard question of variations in costs for the same unit of service.

9.2   HOW MANAGEMENT CONTROLS COSTS

Short-Run versus Long-Run Cost Functions

What can management do to change the costs of production? If a hospital receives fewer admissions than expected this morning and wants to reduce its costs by the afternoon, not much can be done. People have already shown up for work, meals have been prepared, ambulances and wheelchair transport have been arranged, and so on. *In the short run almost all costs are fixed.* Thus any reduction in the number of patients will cause the average cost per patient to be higher than usual. If the reduction in admissions continues and management is given enough time to respond, the hospital could shut down a wing, refrain from hiring, and perhaps lay off some employees. This is but one case demonstrating the general rule that as more time is allowed for adjustment, more changes can be made, and as more changes are made, costs per unit become lower.

In the very long run, almost all costs become variable. The director can train new management, hire clinical staff, rewrite treatment protocols, replace the existing building with a new one, pave some grounds for parking, and even move the facility to a more accessible site near a freeway. This ability to plan and choose the optimal scale and combination of inputs allows management to minimize the costs of production for any desired level of output. If management expects to average only 100 patients per day, it would build a smaller hospital, hire fewer people, and incur lower fixed costs. If management expects 175 patients a day, it would build a medium-sized hospital. If 300 patients a day are expected, management would

FIGURE 9.1   Cost per Unit Varies with Plant Size

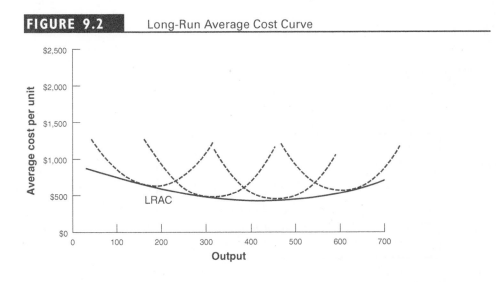

build a large hospital with a dedicated computer system, pneumatic transport tubes to speed laboratory samples between floors, and other equipment (Figure 9.1).

For any expected level of output, management would choose a building size and number of permanent employees that would minimize costs. In geometric terms, the long-run average cost curve (LRAC) is an envelope that traces a minimum, just touching all the possible short-run average cost curves (SRAC), as shown in Figure 9.2. No SRAC can fall below the LRAC because if a short-run cost function with lower costs exists, management would choose that production configuration instead and incorporate it into the long-run function. Whether a particular cost is fixed or variable is determined by the time frame for decision making. Decisions regarding temporary agency nurses can be made on a day-to-day basis and thus are fixed for only 24 hours or so. Permanent employees take a while to train or to terminate when they are no longer needed, and thus they are fixed for at least several months. Reducing the number of

FIGURE 9.2   Long-Run Average Cost Curve

vice presidents is so traumatic that it can take several years. Construction is a fixed cost once completed, but it is a variable cost during the planning stage.

Uncertainty and Budgeting

A director must deal with two kinds of variation in the level of output: foreseeable and unknown. Expansion to accommodate a growing population in the suburbs, eliminating maternity beds in response to declining fertility, and opening a cardiac rehabilitation unit to serve an aging community are all examples of foreseeable long-run changes. The lower number of hospital admissions on Saturday and Sunday, on Christmas and New Year's day, and during August are examples of foreseeable short-run changes. Adjustment to foreseeable changes can be planned in advance. For example, hiring and training can be accomplished efficiently over a reasonable period of time, and space and building modifications can be accomplished on a schedule, so that the path and pace of adjustment reflect conscious decisions by management to minimize costs.

Random variations, on the other hand, must be accommodated in the operations of the organization but are not known in advance. For example, there may be 16 surgeries on Monday, 12 on Tuesday, 22 on Wednesday, 13 on Thursday, 18 on Friday, and 15 on Saturday, and there may be twice as much work for the admitting office to do on Wednesday as on Tuesday with the same amount of staff and equipment. Staff members are likely to do only what is necessary on a particular day, and perhaps even work late, while putting off until the next day some routine tasks, such as filing charts, checking documentation, and entering data into forms. Long-run unknown changes in output might occur because a new factory is built nearby, resulting in many new families moving to the area, an epidemic such as AIDS increases the demand for care, or a competing hospital is built and reduces demand. Such major changes often force a hospital to change its long-run strategy (see Figure 9.3).

How do managers control costs? Primarily through the use of a budget, a plan stated in dollars.[3] A budget that does not change with volume is called a **fixed budget** (also known as a standard budget), and a budget that changes with volume is called a **flexible budget**. Typically, a hospital or medical group practice creates an **operating budget** that projects all anticipated expenses for the next year. For example, if labor expenses rose 7 percent in 2001 and 9 percent in 2002, management might project an increase of 8 percent in labor costs for 2003. Managers usually define short-run changes as those that occur during the current budget period. Long-run changes and plans are incorporated in a **strategic budget** (also known as a **long-run capital budget**) that focuses on trends in the number of patients and capital renovations and expansions (new buildings and equipment, adding partners). These budgets often are accompanied by financial projections, or **pro forma financial statements** of incomes, assets,

FIGURE 9.3   How Organizations Deal with Change

	Planned (known)	Random (uncertain)
Short Run	Scheduling Weekly budget Part-timers	Overtime, temps Inventory Maintain excess capacity
Long Run	Capital budgeting Change plant size Facility conversion	Hold financial reserves Encroachment by or on competitors Bankruptcy

and fund balances for a period of three, five, or even twenty years in summary format. Only infrequently are detailed budgets prepared for more than one year in advance. Most managers define *long-run* changes as those that occur more than one year in the future, but some managers designate changes that occur during the next two to five years as *intermediate-run* changes. In any such analysis the terms are relative, making definitions somewhat arbitrary. The important points to gain from economic theory are that short-run adjustment is always more costly than long-run adjustment and that as the time perspective changes, so does the focus of management attention on cost control.

Known short-run variations are dealt with by making limited changes in the number of staff scheduled. For example, fewer nurses work on Sundays and at 3:00 A.M. However, the percentage change in staff is less than the percentage change in patient load, because all units must still have a head nurse, technical support, and so on, even though they are only partially full. Changes in plant capacity are prohibitively expensive in the short run. Although 50 beds may be empty in the hospital on Sunday night, not all of them would be in unit 7-East. To close that unit down, many patients would have to be transferred out of that unit on Sunday and transferred back in on Monday when patient occupancy increased again. The savings from not having a head nurse on 7-East on Sunday would be more than offset by all the transfers; thus, it would actually cost more to shut down one unit for the sake of "efficiency." Therefore, most units are underutilized on weekends and most staff members usually have an easy day.

A *known long-run change,* such as a declining trend in admissions due to the closure of a local manufacturing plant, calls for a permanent reduction in capacity. Unit 7-East can be converted into storage or nursing home beds, or it can be leased to a group of physical therapists. Furthermore, staffing should be reduced proportionate to the long-run decline in patients, so that every employee carries a regular workload, rather than making partial staff adjustments on nights and weekends.

Random short-run fluctuations are dealt with primarily by building in some excess reserve capacity, making the staff work faster or slower, and allocating less immediate tasks to the slower days. Suppose that the number of surgeries are as suggested earlier: 16 on Monday, 12 on Tuesday, 22 on Wednesday, 13 on Thursday, 18 on Friday, and 15 on Saturday. The manager does not care about the cost of care on Monday or Tuesday but wants to minimize the cost for the week as a whole. There is no reason to reprimand a manager for having too many nurses on duty on Thursday, because there was no way to tell whether admissions would be light until the shift started. Also, although management might be able to get staff members to work extra hard and put in overtime on Wednesday to accommodate the influx of patients, they will not stay if they are abused with continual overloads. They will quit and go to work at another hospital, raising labor costs at the first hospital, because the manager would have to use temporary employees and retrain new staff members frequently. If the hospital has a range of 10 to 25 admissions per day, with an average of 16, it can staff for 16 admissions plus a bit of reserve. However, if another hospital had less random variation and always had 14 to 18 admissions per day, it could match staffing more exactly to the number of patients, would need less reserve capacity, and would have a lower average cost per unit for the same average number of patients. This is only one example of the general principle that dealing with uncertainty is costly, and the greater the range of uncertainty, the greater the cost.

Unforeseen long-run changes in output really provide the test of the organization's ability to control costs. Here, tactical attention to detail is not enough: The hospital must make a strategic gamble based on a specific expectation of the future (e.g., population will grow older and increase demand, or people will move to Florida, reducing demand; a major competitor will go bankrupt, giving the hospital a great opportunity, or perhaps the competitor will go all out trying to survive by stealing the hospital's patients). The hospital could build in flexibility by making investments to cover both alternatives, but it would then incur higher costs per unit regardless of which alternative happens.

9.3   CONFLICT BETWEEN ECONOMIC THEORY AND ACCOUNTING MEASURES OF PER UNIT COST

Timing

In Table 9.1, the cost per surgical operation is examined from two perspectives: direct accounting costs and a full economic cost that includes the hidden cost of dealing with disruptions (staff burnout, mistakes, overtime). In this example, the budgeted fixed costs are $5,000 per day and the variable costs are $300 per operation. The direct cost on Monday, when the expected number of patients (16) are operated on, is $5,000 + (16 × $300) = $9,800; therefore, the cost per operation is $9,800 ÷ 16 = $613. On Wednesday, if more patients (22) were operated on than the staff expected, the calculated average cost per operation is $11,600 ÷ 22 = $527. It appears that the hospital benefited from its mistake in planning for too small a number of patients. Why not increase the advantage by planning for only 15 operations instead of 16? Everyone would work even harder and faster, and if that is not good enough, the hospital could just plan for 12 or 10 or 6 operations and keep pushing the staff to become more and more efficient.

Taking the example to an extreme highlights the flaw in the reasoning. The accounting measure does not accurately capture all costs. Let's consider what really happens. To work so hard on Wednesday, the staff must put off some of their routine tasks until Thursday, and they also expect extra consideration from management on Friday when they ask to go home early. Once these costs of catching up afterward are factored in, the surge of patients on Wednesday is seen to have been very costly, not cheap. If everything went according to plan, 16 operations each day would cost $9,800, for an average cost per operation of $613. Yet extra operations mean disrupting the plan. To accommodate the costs of making sudden adjustments, an "adjustment cost" must be added (here hypothetically assumed to be proportional to the square of the measured deviation [*actual vs. expected*] operations). For deviating from the plan by one operation, the added cost of adjustment is $100; for two, $400; for three, $900; and so on.[4] The actual economic costs (with adjustments) are $15,200 for 22 operations, an average of $681 per operation rather than $613. Of course, it would be cheaper if a hospital could get patients to come in at evenly spaced intervals, exactly 16 each day, all between the hours of 9:00 A.M. and 4:00 P.M. so that workload could be exactly matched to staff and equipment. Yet illness does not go according to plan, and the flow of admissions is never smooth. Health care managers

TABLE 9.1   Accounting versus Economic Cost per Unit with Short-Run Fluctuations

Day	Surgeries	Direct Cost ($)	Accounting Cost per Operation ($)	Adjustment Cost ($)	Total Cost ($)	Economic "Cost" per Operation (AC curve) ($)
Monday	16	9,800	613	—	9,800	613
Tuesday	12	8,600	717	1,600	10,200	850
Wednesday	22	11,600	527	3,600	15,200	691
Thursday	13	8,900	685	900	9,800	754
Friday	18	10,400	578	400	10,800	600
Saturday	15	9,500	633	100	9,600	640
Average	16	9,800	613	—	10,900	681

Note: Accounting costs per surgery are lower for days with many surgeries, even though economic costs are higher. In this hypothetical example, a hospital has planned for 16 surgeries each day and has fixed costs of $5,000 plus $300 per surgery. Deviations from the plan disrupt operations, reducing efficiency by a cost of $100 × (deviation squared) (i.e., being 1 surgery above or below the planned amount reduces efficiency by $100, 2 surgeries off by $400, 3 by $900, and so on).

have learned that such disruptions are costly and that every deviation from the planned level of operation raises costs.

In accountants' terms, the per unit cost in row three of Table 9.1 is calculated on a cash basis (when spent), rather than allocating costs to different days on an accrual basis (when actually earned or obligated). In practice, accrual and all other adjustments made to the cost accounting system are inevitably incomplete and imperfect. The advantage of using economic theory is that the contradiction of the general principle—short-run costs must logically always exceed long-run costs—lets us know immediately that something was wrong with the analysis and that these cost-accounting figures, no matter how precise they might have seemed, did not reflect reality. It also explains why the budgeted $613 per operation was less than the actual expenses of $681: Random fluctuations forced the payment of overtime, hiring of temps, rush ordering of exhausted supplies, and all other daily crises that managers are hired to work out.

Careful examination of Table 9.1 shows that cost per operation was not minimized on Monday, when the expected number of patients were operated on, but that the cost per operation was actually lower on Friday, when more than the expected number patients came in, even after including adjustment costs (see Figure 9.4). Why is it not more efficient to increase output or downsize the facility so that the lowest cost per unit comes at the expected level of output? The reason is that the manager must minimize not the cost on the day when output hits the expected level but the average cost per unit over all the days, with their randomly varying levels of output. If the average number of operations had been 18 instead of 16, 24 operations might have occurred on the heavy Wednesday, exceeding capacity limits so greatly that an additional $2,800 in costs would have been incurred. Having extra reserve capacity is expensive, but not as expensive as not having it when you need it.

In general, managers need to be able to accommodate the usual fluctuations in volume without major disruptions—to have flexibility that minimizes cost over a range. It is possible to have a highly routine production process that is very efficient at a set level of output but would become very inefficient if it had to be speeded up or slowed down. Such fixed-output mass production can work well for manufacturing cars or light bulbs, but it is not well adapted to services such as medical care, where constant adjustments and varying demand are the norm. Managers are willing to pay a bit extra in fixed costs to increase flexibility (see Figure 9.5). Building a facility that is very efficient when exactly the expected number of patients shows up, but that cannot easily accommodate changes in the level of demand (represented by the dark line), is less efficient in the long run than a more flexible facility (represented by the dashed line) that has slightly higher costs at the expected level of output but is able to maintain average costs per unit at a low level over a wider range.

FIGURE 9.4   Accounting versus Economic Costs

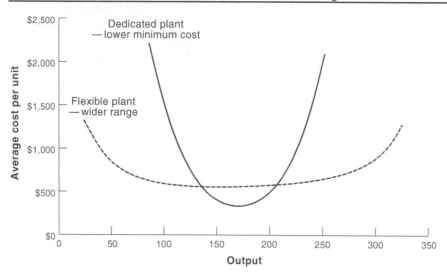

FIGURE 9.5   A Specialized Plant Has Lower Cost within a Narrow Range, but the Flexible Plant Has Wider Range

Whose Costs?

The displacement of costs in time is only one accounting mistake that can be made. Attempts to increase efficiency lead to many management practices that are clearly wrong yet persist for years because of an inability to count all costs. For example, many public clinics provide services free to indigent patients. They try hard to produce these services at the lowest cost to maximize the number of clients they can serve (and to keep taxes down). One way public clinics produce services at lower costs is to bring patients in early and keep them waiting so that the doctor's flow of work is never delayed because a patient is late or an appointment is broken. Such "block booking" or "clinic appointments" maximize the number of patients that can be seen by the physician, but they make patients unhappy because they have to spend many hours waiting. If the cost of the patient's time is included, it becomes apparent that block booking is not efficient; it only seems so because the clinic budget counts only direct costs.

How can economists tell that block booking is inefficient? Because if block booking were truly efficient, some paying patients would choose to patronize doctors who block booked, putting up with extra long waits to save a little money (i.e., choosing to pay $30 for a block-booked visit rather than $35 for care by appointment). The fact that doctors cannot attract patients by block booking demonstrates that the extra patient waiting time is more valuable than the small $5 savings in the doctor's time. Indigent patients are forced to accept block booking: either they must put up with inefficiency because they cannot obtain the convenience of an appointment by paying just the marginal $5 cost differential or they must forgo free care entirely and pay the whole $35 private market price to obtain care by appointment. One might argue that the indigent patient has a lower cost of time and thus is more willing to put up with longer waits than most paying patients. However, the fact that even physicians in low-income neighborhoods have to provide appointments suggests that it is the large gap between marginal amenity cost ($5) and average per visit cost ($35), not lower value per hour of patient time, that allows free clinics to continue block booking.

Time, pain, and other nonmarket costs borne by patients do not show up on the hospital bill. Yet it is precisely these issues—suffering, fear of death, a need for caring and respect—that distinguish the economics of medical care. These intangible issues are one reason this textbook began with a broader perspective on optimization using the techniques of cost-benefit analysis (Chapter 3) rather than a narrow look at minimizing cash outlays. Some of the common mistakes made in accounting for the true costs of medical care are as follows:

- Provider costs are misallocated (displaced in time, overhead, or wrong department).
- Patient costs are not counted (wait time, transportation, family care).
- Emotional costs are not counted (pride, fear, pain, lack of respect).

9.4 ECONOMIES OF SCALE

Hospitals exist to allow a large number of doctors to share expensive capital equipment and cooperate in the care of many patients. Because many of these costs are fixed, hospitals should show economies of scale (i.e., average cost per patient-day falling as more patients are treated).[5] It appears that basic hospital services for routine care are most efficiently delivered when they are organized and staffed in units of 20 to 40 beds, usually known as a floor or wing. The need to accommodate random fluctuations in the number of admissions and to preserve a buffer of empty beds for emergencies creates economies of scale. Admissions to a 40-bed hospital might fluctuate by 10; therefore only 30 beds could be occupied on average. In a 400-bed hospital, excess admissions to one unit are likely to offset a lack of admissions in another; therefore, the overall fluctuation might be 25, which is larger in absolute numbers but much smaller as a percentage. Thus percentage occupancy rates can be higher, and per-unit costs can be lower, in a large facility that is more able to smooth out patient flow. The greater division of labor in a large hospital that allows staff to become more specialized and efficient at a particular function also creates economies of scale.

There is good evidence that economies of scale are important in hospital services. Hospitals with fewer than 100 beds are usually too small to offer a full range of services; are unable to fully utilize operating suites, computed tomography (CT) scanners, and other diagnostic equipment; and cannot allow staff to specialize. Very small hospitals clearly have higher costs per day, although this is somewhat obscured because they tend to offer fewer expensive and technologically advanced services. A better indication that hospitals with fewer than 100 beds suffer from a lack of economies of scale is that a disproportionate number of them have gone bankrupt or been absorbed by larger institutions over the past 20 years. Only in rural areas have small general hospitals been able to thrive, and even there numbers are falling as better highways and helicopter transport have reduced the time required to travel to large urban medical centers.

Diseconomies of scale arise from the difficulties of coordinating and managing larger institutions. Relatively few hospitals have more than 500 beds, evidence that costly administrative and transportation difficulties arise when this number of beds is exceeded. Patients increasingly complain about "getting lost in the system" and being part of a "factory" rather than a caring institution. Table 9.2 shows that cost per day rises long before the 500-bed size limit is reached. How can such large hospitals continue to exist in a competitive environment?

TABLE 9.2

Average Cost per Adjusted Patient-Day by Hospital Size

Number of Beds	Average Cost ($)
6–24	1,536
25–49	1,432
50–99	1,161
100–199	1,476
200–299	1,832
300–399	1,963
400–499	2,214
500 or more	2,358

Source: American Hospital Association, *Hospital Statistics 2011*, Table 2.

The Hospital Is a Multiproduct Firm

Hospitals are complex institutions, and different parts of a hospital actually produce very different products. The "average" is made up of units for routine care along with some very specialized units, such as heart transplant, oncology, and respiratory intensive care. Although it might take only 20 beds to create an efficient sized cardiac-care unit, only a large hospital has enough cardiac admissions to fill such a specialized unit. Most 400-bed university hospitals are, in fact, composites, with perhaps 100 beds providing general care, with 20 dedicated to oncology, 15 to nephrology and kidney transplant, 20 to cardiology, 40 to pediatrics, and so on. Thus, although the efficient size of a unit that produces one product is just 20 beds, the more specialized types of care a hospital provides, the larger it must be to reach efficient scale. Indeed, a hospital large enough to provide heart transplants and nuclear medicine efficiently is too large to produce routine care for broken bones and pneumonia, and therefore suffers from diseconomies of scale with regard to these less specialized services.

One solution to the conflict between economies and diseconomies of scale is to treat patients who have uncomplicated illnesses at local community hospitals of relatively modest size (100 to 150 beds) with few specialized services and to refer patients whose treatment demands sophisticated technology and expertise to large "tertiary" institutions usually affiliated with universities. However, just as increasing hospital size causes diseconomies of scale by making management communication and coordination more difficult, so too does the process of transferring patients back and forth between community and specialty hospitals. The savings from triaging patients so that their illnesses are treated in the most efficient sized hospital are to some extent offset and eventually reversed by the increase in the number of transfers required, because each transfer requires some extra documentation, management oversight, duplication of tests, and so on.

Contracting Out

Some services show economies of scale even at sizes far larger than any hospital in existence. Laboratory testing, for example, has become so automated that costs are minimized in facilities that process hundreds of thousands of tests per day. The cost of equipment, information systems, and technical expertise that constitute a good laboratory is largely a fixed cost; therefore, overhead per unit continues to decline even when millions of samples are being processed. To take advantage of such economies of scale, many hospitals are contracting out such services. Rather than having their own laboratories for conducting routine tests, they use a reference laboratory that services hundreds of hospitals. Food services, security, and even emergency departments are now contracted out to allow hospitals access to economies of scale through contractual relationships.

9.5   QUALITY AND COST

Technology: Cutting Costs or Enhancing Quality?

What does it mean when someone says that technological improvements have made the production process better? It can mean that the identical product can now be produced at a lower cost per unit. It can also mean that a better product can be produced, regardless of cost. Medicine has been dominated by the latter type of technological change. The tremendous value of any increase in cure rates is one factor biasing researchers toward discoveries that have the effect of increasing costs. Yet quality enhancements have occurred rapidly in other areas of technology, such as computing, while still reducing unit costs. Why have such developments been so notably absent in medicine? Quite simply, it has been much more profitable to discover a new cure than to find a method to cut costs.

Insurance and cost reimbursement virtually eliminated price competition in hospital care. Without it, there was no incentive for research laboratories to seek innovations that reduced costs or for hospitals to switch to cheaper versions of existing equipment. The process of trading off a small reduction in speed or accuracy for a large reduction in price that occurs in most markets has rarely taken place in health care.

Improved Efficiency May Raise Total Spending

It is important to recognize that improved production efficiency always causes the "real" cost function to fall, even though the amount spent and cost per unit can rise because making quality and quantity more available and affordable can make people spend more. This is illustrated in Table 9.3. Suppose, for example, that in 1980 a person had a heart attack (myocardial infarction, or MI) and faced the choice of (a) taking medication that cost $150 and gave a 30 percent chance of having a fatal MI within five years (70 percent mortality) or (b) undergoing a new, experimental operation costing $25,000 that gave a slightly better chance of survival, with 68 percent mortality. It would be rational for one to take the medication rather than to give up $24,850 additional dollars for such a slight improvement in one's chances. Let's also suppose that in 2010, much better medication more than doubled the chance of survival, with only 29 percent mortality, and cost only $75. In addition, research and practice improved surgery to the point where it had only a 14 percent five-year mortality and a reduced cost of $15,000. The 2010 option of giving up $14,925 to cut the risk of dying in half is very attractive. Thus, even though technological advances reduced the cost of both options, the amount spent on medical care would rise. Improvements in medical production frequently create this type of response. Even though 1980s medicine can be produced now for less than it cost in 1980, patients choose to spend more to get high-quality modern medicine that would have been impossible or prohibitively expensive to obtain in 1980.

Quality costs money, and the drive for higher quality is one of the defining characteristics of modern medicine. Although we cannot always agree on what quality is, we know that more quality is always preferred to less and that the cost–quality trade-off is usually more important in understanding the economics of medical practice than the cost–volume trade-off. Before making a comparison on the basis of cost per unit, it is first necessary to ask, "What is the product?" If the product is defined as "a day in the hospital," a top-flight research center may seem very expensive. If the product is "an increase in my chance of survival to age 75," the same institution's $2,500 per day charges might seem like a bargain.

TABLE 9.3	Total Spending Can Rise Even as Greater Efficiency Reduces Costs per Unit
1980	**2010**
Medication cost $150 　Post-MI mortality = 70%	Medication cost $75 　Post-MI mortality = 29%
Surgery cost $25,000 　Post-MI mortality = 68%	Surgery cost $15,000 　Post-MI mortality = 14%
Decision: 　Take medication for $150	Decision: 　Have surgery for $15,000

9.6   HOSPITAL CHARGES, COSTS, AND PRICES: CONFUSION AND CHAOS

It is often assumed that there is some relationship between hospital prices and costs. There is, sort of. In total, the revenues a hospital receives are within a few percentage points of the total costs. However, for any single item, the amount paid may be less than cost, more than cost, or a thousand times cost (the famous $25 aspirin). A patient who is insured might pay more, or less, than a patient without insurance. Almost certainly, a hospital providing the same service to two patients rarely (if ever) receives the same payment if the patients have different insurance plans, and the amount each patient has to pay out-of-pocket will bear almost no relationship to costs. Table 9.4 and Table 9.5 illustrate some of the wide variations in prices for relatively standard services.[6]

TABLE 9.4   State Variations in Payments to Five Different Hospitals by One Insurance Company

Hospital	Appendectomy ($)		Coronary Artery Bypass Graft ($)	
	California	New Jersey	California	New Jersey
A	1,800	2,708	33,000	26,342
B	2,900	3,320	54,600	34,277
C	4,700	3,412	64,500	36,792
D	9,500	3,524	72,300	37,019
E	13,700	4,230	99,800	45,343

Although Table 9.5 deals only with diagnostic imaging, similarly wide variations are observed for outpatient visits and inpatient surgery. The GAO contacted 19 hospitals to determine the price of knee replacement surgery, and most of them asked for information that most consumers would not have, such as the exact list of CPT (current procedure terminology) codes, the model of artificial joint to be implanted, type of anesthesia, and amount of time used in the operating room.[7] Only seven of the hospitals provided any type of price information, and they usually gave a range, such as between $32,974 and $100,676, or an average such as $82,390, and these were all based on billed charges and did not reflect what would typically be paid by an insurer or by the patient out-of-pocket.

TABLE 9.5   National Range of Insurance Payments for Diagnostic Imaging

Range	Midwest	Southwest	Southeast	Northeast
Digital Screening Mammogram				
Low	$ 160	$ 150	$ 180	$ 190
High	$ 270	$ 260	$ 550	$ 330
Scan of Pelvis with Contrast				
Low	$ 240	$ 230	$ 350	$ 475
High	$ 530	$1,800	$1,800	$1,550
PET Scan, Base of Skull to Mid-thigh				
Low	$1,400	$1,240	$2,500	$3,500
High	$2,500	$3,000	$3,500	$4,800

Chargemaster and Negotiated Fees

To cut through this confusion it helps to remember than almost all hospital revenues come from third parties, not patients, and are parts of complicated group contracts, not regular retail transactions. Each hospital creates a **chargemaster** listing charges for every kind of service. This was once a thick book specifying a charge for each of several hundred items, but now it is usually an array in a database with tens of thousands of items cross referenced by clinical and financial codes so that it can be more easily used and modified. An uninsured person would, in principle, be liable for the full charges for all services rendered, but in practice such patients usually pay little or nothing (bad debt) because they are uninsured.[8] A typical third-party contract bargains over some items that are expensive (heart transplant, hip replacement) or frequently used (ambulatory visit, routine ED, maternity) and then specifies a percentage of charges (say, 75 percent or 30 percent, depending on overall markup and bargaining power) for everything else, commonly referred to as *discounted fees.*[9]

Cost Finding: Gross Revenues and the RCCAC

The audited financial report offers a precise and public measure of the total charges for all of the services provided and billed by a hospital during the year (gross revenues), of the amount actually received in payments (net revenues), and of the total costs. Dividing (total charges ÷ total cost) gives a good estimate of the average overall markup. For example, 1.50 would imply that on average items were marked up by 50 percent, and 4.00 would imply that sum of all charges would be four times total costs, or an average markup of 300 percent. Reversing this division yields the cost-to-charge ratio used in the RCCAC reimbursement method (see section 8.2). If total charges are four times total costs, then on average the cost of all items is about 25 percent of the listed charge (ratio of cost to charges = .25). Similarly, dividing (net revenues ÷ gross revenues) gives an estimate of the average discount from charges. So long as the cost-to-charge ratio is less than the discount, the hospital is in the black. Thus hospital A with a cost-to-charge ratio of 25 percent that discounts to 30 percent of charges receives the difference as profit, exactly the same operating margin as hospital B with a ratio of 50 percent that discounts to 60 percent of charges.

This simple calculation works fine on average, and it is the source of almost all estimates of the "cost" of each hospital service, but the logic is flawed and circular. The cost estimate depends on the listed charge and the ratio, and may have nothing to do with any economic concept of cost for any specific service or item. If a nephrology visit has a list charge of $250 and a neurology visit has a list charge of $125, then this cost-finding procedure puts forth an estimate that the cost per visit in nephrology is twice as much, even if those visits take half the time, use less equipment and fewer supplies, and were conducted by a clinician paid less per hour. The disconnect between the available estimates (charges, approximate ratio) and any economic concept of cost (marginal, total, or average; see Chapter 3) is there even before any of a host of other accounting problems are considered: overhead allocation, technological change, cost shifting, indexing, taxes, or the distorted prices of stents, hip joints, and fees for licensed professionals. Why would the hospital, or the *Wall Street Journal,* use such an estimate? Primarily because they have nothing better and because it has become standard industry practice.

Medicare as a Standard for Pricing

Medicare has become the largest source of hospital payments, and its reimbursements for each item of service are made public and are much more stable and reliable than a hospital charge-master. Therefore it is not surprising that Medicare charges have become a common standard for third-party contracts, which often specify payment as 80 percent or 115 percent of Medicare. Furthermore, because almost all hospitals are legally required to file a "Medicare cost report" that allows calculation of RCCAC ratios by department, it is easy to calculate an estimated cost for each service item in a hospital by multiplying the relevant Medicare charge by the hospital's departmental RCCAC ratio. However, Medicare charges, like those in the chargemaster, are often arbitrary or based on outdated technology, and thus the cost-finding is again an exercise in circular logic. Furthermore, even within the heavily regulated Medicare system, there are substantial differences in payment across hospitals. Although the basic hospital payment is fixed by diagnosis (DRG; see Section 8.2) and hence essentially the same for any hospital performing a hip replacement (approximately $11,300 per case), a study determined that the variations in re-admissions ($582 to $1,052), post-discharge care ($3,840 to $9,725), and physician services ($2,056 to $2,651) were substantial.[10] Although the spread of payments is much smaller than for private insurance, it is still a lot to have within the heavily regulated and uniform Medicare system that deliberately removes the ability of hospitals to manipulate charges.

There are a host of reasons that what is paid for care varies across hospitals, and cost is only one of them (see box "Reasons Charges (and Amounts Paid) Vary Among Hospitals"). Unlike the competitive market discussed in Chapters 1 and 2, there really isn't anything like a normal "price" for most medical care. Some items have meaningful prices related to cost, but they are things like generic drugs (see Chapter 11), goods that are bought and sold like cereal in a supermarket, and hence they barely resemble the usual medical transaction involving doctor and patient in a relationship of trust where money is rarely acknowledged much less discussed or compared.

REASONS CHARGES (AND AMOUNTS PAID) VARY AMONG HOSPITALS

Costs are different.

A strategic choice has been made to mark up one item more (less) than another.

There is a larger or smaller overall markup (RCCCAC, ratio of gross to net revenues).

Overhead is put in different places.

Charges are set at different times using different standards and technologies.

Insurance plans differ.

Just because … since few people know or care anyway.

Most hospital revenues come from complex third-party group contracts and cannot validly be separated into discrete items. Hospitals are concerned mainly with the difference between total revenues and total costs, not the pricing of each service. Insurance companies are similarly focused. Both have an interest in keeping payment details hidden from the public and each other, lest government move to adjust and reduce profit margins or a competitor gain an advantage. Comparison shopping by patients is usually not possible, and revenue competition more often leads to cost shifting than to efficient use of resources. Once the link between payment and receipt of services is broken by insurance, there is little reason to put it back together or analyze what it might have been. Hospital price transparency is elusive and probably always will be. To find real solutions to rising health care costs and unaffordable health insurance premiums, it will eventually be necessary to deal with the complex reality of health care systems as they are today rather than the illusion of hospital prices suddenly made transparent and meaningful.

9.7 CONTROLLING HOSPITAL COSTS THROUGH REGULATION

Hospital costs have risen steadily throughout the post World War II era, from $9 per day in 1946 to $74 in 1970, then rising 300 percent in the next 10 years to $244 in 1980, to $682 in 1990, $1,148 in 2000, and more than $1,800 today.[11] Hospital costs have grown 9 percent a year over the past 50 years. Even after adjusting for inflation, the increase in cost per day is still an astounding 1,750 percent from 1950 to 2009 (an average of 5 percent above inflation each year). By and large, the public has wanted the additional care and new technology and has not been displeased with the billions of dollars expended. However, after the passage of Medicare and Medicaid in 1965, costs became a problem for public policy for two reasons: The influx of government money caused costs to rise much more rapidly than before and the costs were now being paid by the government (i.e., taxpayers) rather than the mutually agreed-upon private transactions of individuals or employer-paid insurance, and thus caused state and federal budget deficits (see Table 9.6 and Figure 9.6).

In the immediate postwar period, the Hill–Burton Act of 1946 funded the building of more hospitals, and the Health Professions Educational Assistance Act of 1963 increased the number of doctors. The early 1960s were boom years when it seemed that the economy would continue to grow robustly "forever." This desire to continue spending enabled Congress to create Medicare and Medicaid as entitlement programs in 1965. However, by 1975, the United States was trapped in a global recession, federal and state expenditures had escalated far beyond even the most outlandish budget projections, and the need for cost-cutting was clear. It was thought that system efficiencies could be generated through better planning and therefore a number of initiatives were funded to promote "regional medical programs" and create planning boards for oversight. Evaluations showing that planning alone could not affect costs, and the obvious excess capacity created by the Hill–Burton construction boom led to the idea

TABLE 9.6   Hospital Costs per Patient-Day, 1950–2009

Year	Cost per Day	Cost per Day in 2009 Dollars
1946	$ 9	$ 76
1950	14	106
1955	21	139
1960	29	173
1965	40	222
1970	74	332
1975	134	438
1980	245	563
1985	460	819
1990	687	1,043
1991	752	1,103
1992	820	1,175
1993	880	1,233
1994	931	1,278
1995	968	1,302
1996	1,006	1,327
1997	1,033	1,339
1998	1,067	1,368
1999	1,103	1,394
2000	1,149	1,421
2001	1,217	1,472
2002	1,290	1,535
2003	1,379	1,607
2004	1,450	1,644
2005	1,522	1,670
2006	1,612	1,713
2007	1,696	1,752
2008	1,782	1,801
2009	1,853	1,853

Hospital cost per adjusted patient day in nominal current dollars and inflation adjusted to 2009 dollars using GDP deflator.
Source: American Hospital Association.

FIGURE 9.6	Hospital Costs per Patient-Day 1950–2009

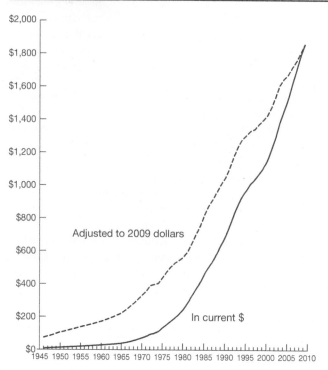

that a forced reduction in the growth of hospital beds could reduce the rate of growth in hospital costs.

Certificate-of-need (CON) legislation required that a planning body conduct a study and approve any capital project that would increase the number of hospital beds in the region.[12] In an insightful study of the economics of hospital regulation, David Salkever and Thomas Bice showed that although CON legislation reduced the number of new beds built, hospitals increased the amount of capital equipment for each bed; thus, capital spending continued to rise at the same rate.[13] In discussing their findings, Salkever and Bice argued that "CON regulation is like pushing on a balloon": forcing costs down in one dimension caused them to bulge in another dimension. Similar dynamics have been demonstrated in other studies of many regulatory initiatives over the years; the type of cost subject to regulation declines, but any savings are negated by an overflow in another area so that total health care costs are unchanged (see box "Types of Regulation to Control Hospital Costs").

TYPES OF REGULATION TO CONTROL HOSPITAL COSTS

Certificate of need (CON)

Utilization review (UR, PSRO)

Budgetary review

Price controls (ESPN)

Administered prices (DRGs, PPS, BBA)

An unintended side effect of CON and most other regulations is that they create barriers that make it harder for new organizations to enter the market, thus protecting existing hospitals and retarding the evolution of the health care system toward more efficient configurations. Studies of CONs in operation confirmed the economists' version of the golden rule ("Them that has the gold makes the rules"). Almost every well-established, wealthy, and politically connected hospital that applied for certification eventually got it, while denials fell disproportionately on outsiders that threatened the status quo or weaker institutions that lacked a constituency (see discussion of CONs in Chapter 10, Section 4). The death knell for CONs came in the form of a Supreme Court ruling that discriminatory reimbursement of a hospital chain that refused to apply for a CON (which the chain knew would be denied because of opposition from existing local hospitals) constituted an illegal restraint of trade under antitrust laws and harmed consumers by restricting competition.

The attempt to impose controls over other dimensions moved on to utilization review (UR), a process to eliminate unnecessary surgery and other services by having a panel of doctors and nurses in a professional standards review organization (PSRO) review patients' charts to find cases of inappropriate care. The PSRO or other agency would be empowered to order the doctor to change improper behavior and, failing that, to deny payment. In practice, the process proved cumbersome and ineffective, although the current managed-care review, which does appear to work better (see Chapter 5), developed from the experience with UR.

Rapid inflation and an unwillingness to accept the lessons of history led the Nixon administration to impose **price controls** in 1971. Although removed for most sectors of the economy in 1973, they were maintained in hospitals for an extra year. Rate setting through **budgetary review** was a much more labor-intensive process, involving the line-by-line examination of spending plans. A notable example was the legislation passed in the state of Washington in 1973 when a severe local recession crimped the state's ability to raise tax revenues. The legislation lasted, albeit in weaker and weaker form, for 10 years.

Perhaps the most far-reaching cost-control regulation was the replacement of Medicare's open-ended system of retrospective cost reimbursement by the **prospective payment system (PPS)** in 1984, in which **diagnostically related groups (DRGs)** were used for setting federally administered prices per discharge covering the entire patient stay. However, the demonstrable reductions in cost per inpatient admission were more than offset by rapid increases in outpatient charges; therefore, overall Medicare costs continued to rise as rapidly as before—another example of a regulation pushing on one side of the balloon.

The **Balanced Budget Act of 1997 (BBA)** was much more successful in cutting costs, at least in the short run. It directly reduced Medicare payments to physicians, hospitals, and home health agencies, set a "sustainable growth rate" formula that linked the allowable growth in total physician reimbursement to the annual rate of growth in GDP, reduced payments for graduate medical education, created the expert Medicare Payment Advisory Commission (MedPAC), to recommend the update factor (annual base payment increase percentage) for hospitals, allowed HMOs to compete for Medicare beneficiaries through the "Medicare+Choice" program, and established a prospective payment system for home health benefits. Home health, which had been the most rapidly growing part of Medicare, fell from $14 billion in 1996 to $8 billion in 1999.[14] Altogether, these reductions were able to save more than $100 billion over five years. However, as the curbs put in place by BBA really began to bite, protests from hospitals and physician groups grew louder and politicians more sympathetic. By early 2003, a consensus had arisen that some release from the stringent constraints imposed on Medicare payment increases would be implemented soon. Since then, Medicare costs have again risen rapidly (home health expenditures are now above $32 billion), as have federal and state budget deficits.

The experience with CONs, price controls, state rate regulation, and PPS shows that whatever successes might be attributed to cost-control regulation have been limited and short lived.[15] The failure of regular market competition or government price regulation to control costs should not come as a surprise, because the central difficulty in medical care transactions is the inability to specify what the product is. Special market adaptations, such as nonprofit status and the agency relationships between physicians and patients, are signals that any attempts to set prices or to quantify quality and other important attributes are likely to be exercises in futility. A government official in a state capital, or in Washington, D.C., is not going to be able to write a detailed contract in advance to purchase something that the participants have trouble measuring even after the fact (e.g., how good the obstetrical care really was for a low-birthweight baby left with disabilities). It would be easy to cut spending on Medicare and Medicaid in a number of ways (set global budget caps, eliminate services, deny eligibility), but there is not sufficient public consensus or political willpower to do so. The implementation of the 2010 Affordable Care Act (Obamacare; see Chapter 17) might bring some relief, but the macroeconomic cost pressures we examine in Chapters 13 to 18 will eventually force the public to face these hard choices—and force politicians to deal with the fallout.

SUGGESTIONS FOR FURTHER READING

Healthcare Financial Management, a monthly journal of the Healthcare Financial Management Association (www.HFMA.org).

U.S. Government Accountability Office, *Health Care Price Transparency: Meaningful Price Information is Difficult for Consumers to Obtain Prior to Receiving Care.* GAO-11-791 (Washington DC, September 11, 2011).

William O. Cleverley and Andrew E. Cameron, *Essentials of Health Care Finance,* 5th ed. (Gaithersburg, Md.: Aspen, 2002).

Steven A. Finkler and David M. Ward, *Cost Accounting for Health Care Organizations,* 2nd ed. (Gaithersburg, Md.: Aspen, 1999).

Uwe Reinhardt, "The Many Different Prices Paid To Providers And The Flawed Theory Of Cost Shifting." *Health Affairs* 30, no. 11 (2011): 2125–2133.

SUMMARY

1. Managers plan to produce efficiently and any deviation from the plan (more or fewer patients, shifting wage rates) tends to increase average cost per unit, particularly in the short run. Because management can more fully adapt operations over the long run, the short-run average cost curve always lies at or above the long-run average cost curve. The primary way **managers control hospital costs is through the budget process**. Often extra capacity and flexibility is built in so that uncertainty and changes are not so difficult to deal with.

2. **Economies of scale** are said to exist when increasing the level of output causes the average cost per unit to fall. Gains from the **specialization of labor and spreading the fixed costs of capital equipment** over more volume are the major factors creating economies of scale. **Diseconomies of scale**, in which rising costs per unit eventually set in, are primarily due to the **difficulty of managing and coordinating larger operations**. Hospitals appear to show economies of scale up to a size of about 120 beds and diseconomies of scale after reaching a size of about 500 beds. For simple services, small hospitals appear to be relatively efficient, but only a large hospital has enough patients of a particular type (e.g., brain cancer) to run a specialized service at an efficient volume. Thus, a hospital may be both too big to deliver some services efficiently and too small to deliver others efficiently.

3. **Cost per day in the hospital varies for many reasons** such as differences in quality and type of services offered, cost shifting to pay for research and teaching, billing practices, severity of patient illness, prices of labor and other inputs, and differences in production efficiency. **Hospitals are multiproduct firms** providing many types of care, hence comparisons of cost per day or per case may not be very meaningful indicators of how efficiently a hospital is producing care.

4. **Accounting costs often do not measure true economic costs**. A larger-than-expected number of patients can make average costs appear lower, but actually the overcrowding and staff stress tend to increase costs. Patient time, pain, and worry are other costs often not counted.

5. **Technology** has tended to increase total spending in health care because generous insurance payments and cost reimbursement have given little incentive to develop cost-reducing techniques or to give up a little quality for a large reduction in cost. An increase in capability to improve health often makes more spending worthwhile.

6. Effective **price competition has never really developed for hospital services**, mainly because insurance breaks the link between payment and use so that there **are no real market prices** that would drive patients toward lower-cost providers. Transactions are not transparent, each patient yields different revenue, and listed **charges** are often wildly different from what the insurance company or the patient pays.

7. **Regulation** has shifted cost from one part of health care to another (pushing on a balloon), but has not succeeded in controlling total costs overall. CON regulations to control construction and prospective price setting (PPS, DRGs) have forced hospitals to respond in a number of ways, but total spending has continued to soar. Government is financially responsible for most of a hospital's patients (66 percent of inpatient days are paid for by Medicare and Medicaid) but is unable or unwilling to pay the price, forcing the health care system toward a crisis point. The cost shifting under which the rich cared for the poor and the healthy contributed to pay for the sick has begun to crack under the strain of unequal payments and a burgeoning federal deficit.

PROBLEMS

1. {*economies of scale*} What major factors create economies of scale in hospitals? Diseconomies of scale? Are most hospitals of optimal size, too small, or too large?

2. {*case mix, cost shifting*} Why do university teaching hospitals cost so much more per day of care than local community hospitals?

3. {*economies of scale*} Misericordia Hospital had a 20 percent increase in admissions from 1995 to 2000. Total patient care costs went from $50 million to $61 million. Does Misericordia show evidence of economies of scale or diseconomies of scale? Could other factors besides the number of admissions affect the costs of care?

4. {*economies of scale*} The number of patients at Harbordale Hospital increased from 120 to 144 from Monday to Tuesday. The hospital's costs increased $720,000 to $722,000 as temporary nurses were called in to deal with the heavy patient load. Does Harbordale Hospital show economies or diseconomies of scale? Which hospital is better managed for cost control: Harbordale or Misericordia (in Problem 3)? Which is more costly, short-run adjustment between Monday and Tuesday or long-run adjustment between 1995 and 2000?

5. {*marginal cost, accounting*} What is the cost of an extra admission to a hospital? Does it make a difference whether the admission is for an emergency service or for a scheduled service? Who bears the costs of additional emergency admission? Is there any difference in who bears the cost of a 50 percent increase in emergency room admission in the short run and the long run?

6. {*compensation*} Should hospital managers be rewarded for dealing with random fluctuations in demand or for dealing with planned changes in demand?

7. {*efficiency, case mix*} Costs per day are usually lower in community hospitals than in university hospitals. Does this mean that transferring patients from university hospitals to community hospitals would increase efficiency?

8. {*substitution*} Why do people spend so long waiting to be treated in an emergency department? Would it be more efficient if there were sufficient doctors available so that people could be treated right away?

9. {*economies of scale, discrimination*} Many rural counties have fewer hospital beds than urban and suburban counties, even when rural counties experience more accidents and injuries for which immediate access to care is crucial. Does this disparity indicate systematic discrimination against rural counties?

10. {*transaction costs*} Why would a hospital that just expanded its home health care agency to service the patients of other hospitals in the region close down its clinical laboratory and purchase lab services from a neighboring hospital?

11. {*quality*} Why have quality improvements in health care caused costs to rise, while quality improvements in computers have caused costs to fall?

12. {*technological change*} Automation has vastly increased the efficiency and accuracy of laboratory testing. The cost per test has fallen by more than 75 percent in many cases. Do you think that the total cost of laboratory testing has fallen by more or less than 75 percent? Why?

13. {*price controls*} What would you expect to be the effect of a set of regulations limiting hospital revenues to an increase of 1 percent a year on the following?
    a. Number of nurses hired
    b. Number of doctors
    c. Quality of care
    d. Advertising budgets
    e. Emergency room staffing
    f. New construction
    g. Depreciation

    Would there be a difference if the regulation applied to just one hospital rather than to all hospitals? Would there be a difference between short-run and long-run effects?

14. {*regulation*} CON regulation effectively limited the number of new hospital beds constructed in a region. Who would favor CONs? Who would be against CONs? When hospitals in a state with CON regulation renovate old buildings, would you expect the cost per bed to be more or less than in a state without CON regulation?

ENDNOTES

1. E. R. Becker and B. Steinwald, "The Determinants of Hospital Case-Mix Complexity," *Health Services Research* 16, no. 1 (1981): 439–458.
2. Frank Sloan, Roger Feldman, and Bruce Steinwald, "The Effects of Teaching on Hospital Costs," *Journal of Health Economics* 2, no. 1 (1983): 1–28; Howard Berman and Louis Weeks, *The Financial Management of Hospitals,* 5th edition (Ann Arbor: Health Administration Press, 1990).
3. Howard Berman and Louis Weeks, *The Financial Management of Hospitals,* 5th Edition, (Ann Arbor: Health Administration Press, 1990).
4. The adjustment calculation used here is arbitrary and is intended for illustrative purposes only rather than as an estimation of actual cost penalties. The important point is that being over or under the optimal level of planned output causes a disproportionate increase in per-unit costs.
5. T. W. Granneman, R. S. Brown, and M. V. Pauly, "Estimating Hospital Costs: A Multiple-Output Analysis," *Journal of Health Economics* 5, no. 2 (1986): 107–127; T. G. Cowing, A. G. Holtman, and S. Powers, "Hospital

Cost Analysis: A Survey and Evaluation of Recent Studies," *Advances in Health Economics and Health Services Research* 4 (1983): 257–303.

6. Uwe Reinhardt, "The Many Different Prices Paid To Providers And The Flawed Theory Of Cost Shifting," *Health Affairs* 30, no. 11 (2011): 2125–2133. "Shopping Around for Surgery," *The Economist*, February 4, 2012, 70. Kelly Kennedy, "Health Care Cost Vary Widely, Study Shows," *USA Today*, July 1, 2011; ChangeHealthcare, Healthcare Transparency Index: Q2 2011 Report: Diagnostic Imaging. http://www.changehealthcare.com/hcti/index.html, accessed June 12, 2012.

7. U.S. Government Accountability Office, *Health Care Price Transparency: Meaningful Price Information is Difficult for Consumers to Obtain Prior to Receiving Care.* GAO-11-791 (Washington DC: Government Accountability Office, 2011).

8. In practice most patients without insurance who run up thousands of dollars in hospital bills simply walk out the door. However, the full amount is a real debt and if that uninsured patient has a job, or cares about their credit rating, it matters. Of course the hospital never expects to receive that much, but the bill can still be sent to a collection agency, and the person's wages can be garnisheed. Because charges are usually way above what the hospital would normally receive for the services, almost any hospital billing office approached by the patient will gladly settle for a fraction of the amount billed (suggestion: start by explaining the situation and offering to pay what Medicaid would, or maybe $50 a month). See also Glen Melnick Katya Fonkych, "Hospital Pricing and the Uninsured: Do the Uninsured Pay Higher Prices?" *Health Affairs* 27, no. 2 (2010): w116–w112.

9. While unusual, such pricing on the basis of entirely arbitrary fees is hardly rare. Many used bookstores individually price only a few items and sell the rest at 30 percent or 50 percent of the list price. Bulk resalers of returned clothing may use similar "percentage of of marked sale price" methods to move large quantities of merchandise without having to re-price each item. For a more extended discussion of the vagaries of hospital pricing and charges, see C. P. Tompkins, S. H. Altman, and E. Eilat, "The Precarious Pricing System for Hospital for Hospital Services," *Health Affairs* 25, no. 1 (2006, 2008): 45–56.

10. David C. Miller et al., "Large Variations in Medicare Payments for Surgery Highlight Savings Potential From Bundled Payment Systems," *Health Affairs* 30, no. 11 (2011): 2017–2115.

11. American Hospital Association, *Hospital Statistics* (Chicago: American Hospital Association, various years).

12. CON, UR, PSROs, DRGs, and other regulations have all taken many different forms in different state or national programs over time. The brief discussion here refers to general conclusions about that type of regulation, rather than any particular specific program. The interested reader should consult one of the many comprehensive reviews that have been written, such as those in Paul Joskow, *Controlling Hospital Costs: The Role of Government Regulation* (Cambridge, Mass.: MIT Press, 1981); D. Abernathy and D. A. Pearson, *Regulating Hospital Costs: The Development of Public Policy* (Ann Arbor: Health Administration Press, 1979); or the relevant chapters of Michael Rosko and Robert W. Broyles, *The Economics of Health Care: A Reference Handbook* (New York: Greenwood Press, 1988); or Sherman Folland, Allen Goodman, and Miron Stano, *The Economics of Health and Health Care*, 5th ed. (New York: Prentice Hall, 2006).

13. David Salkever and Thomas Bice, *Hospital Certificate-of-Need Controls: Impact on Investment, Costs and Use* (Washington, D.C.: American Enterprise Institute, 1979).

14. Nelda McCall et al., "Medicare Home Health Before and After the BBS," *Health Affairs* 20, no. 3 (2001): 189–198; Charles N. Kahn and Hanns Kuttner, "Budget Bills and Medicare Policy: The Politics of the BBA," *Health Affairs* 18, no. 1 (1999): 37–47.

15. David Dranove and Kenneth Cone, "Do State Rate-Setting Regulations Really Lower Hospital Expenses?" *Journal of Health Economics* 4, no. 2 (1985): 159–165; C. L. Eby and D. Cohodes, "What Do We Know About Rate-Setting?" *Journal of Health Politics, Policy and Law* 10, no. 2 (1985): 299–327.

CHAPTER 10

LONG-TERM CARE

QUESTIONS

1. Do the elderly pay to be cured, or to be cared for?

2. Who provides most long-term care for the disabled elderly? Who is the largest insurer?

3. As people live longer, does that mean that they are healthier and thus spend less on medical care, or more disabled and spend more?

4. What do nursing home owners compete for? Do they want patients who are more sick or less sick?

5. How can substituting nursing homes for hospitals increase the total cost of care if the cost per day is lower at nursing homes?

6. Have government payments and regulations raised or lowered the quality of care?

7. How can Medicaid payments create an excess and a shortage of patients at the same time?

8. Do certificate-of-need (CON) rules reduce costs or reduce access?

Of the $231 billion paid for **long-term care** (**LTC**) in 2012, most was spent for institutional services in nursing homes. Yet for every person in a nursing home, there are two or more equally disabled people living in the community who are cared for by family and friends. Hence, more care comes from unpaid labor and acts of obligation and love than from patient fees or third-party payments.[1] LTC revolves around care rather than cure, around quality of life rather than treatment of disease. LTC needs are defined by a person's ability to function, the ability to conduct activities of daily living. Most LTC patients continue to require assistance for the rest of their lives. Food, housing, comfort, and social relationships are more important than diagnostic tests and surgical procedures. Although doctors, hospitals, nurses, drugs, and all the other elements of modern medicine are employed in LTC, they are actively involved in only a small portion of the care that patients receive. LTC is not "medical" in the same way that most acute care is. These differences—long-term chronic disabilities rather than short-term diseases capable of being cured, predominantly human caring rather than medical science, and a reliance on unpaid acts of love and obligation rather than services purchased in the market— tend to make LTC transactions somewhat different from acute medical care transactions and from the ordinary two-party transactions for most economic goods and services.

The challenge of meeting both medical and social needs has left LTC public policy in a confused state, with legislators uncertain about which aspects of care should be funded through social welfare programs and which should be funded as part of the health care system. The response to people with chronic illness and disability is an LTC system in which boundaries are often unclear and many fundamental issues are unresolved. This chapter presents a few aspects of the many and multifaceted economic entities that make up the fragmented LTC sector.

10.1   DEVELOPMENT OF THE LONG-TERM CARE MARKET

The original hospitals were LTC facilities. They served destitute patients who could not work and could no longer live at home. Most people had family members who took care of them at home when they became sick, old, or infirm, and the wealthy called upon the services of paid home nurses; therefore, only a small group of disabled and indigent paupers were forced to reside in hospitals. After the scientific revolutions of the 19th century, curative medicine was increasingly separated from caring for the disabled. By the start of World War II, the distinction between acute medical care and LTC was clearly demarcated in the minds of the public and in the flow of funds. It was hoped that poorhouses and "almshouse hospitality" would disappear as infectious diseases were cured and the desperately poor were elevated by a rising economy.

To a large extent, sanitation and Social Security did cause the old system to fade, but some problems were troublingly persistent. No cure was found for mental illness, and more people were confined to state hospitals. These institutions made limited attempts at cure, often serving more to relieve the community of a burden rather than to improve the patients' quality of life. Rising incomes meant that fewer and fewer elderly people were left truly destitute, but there were always some who had no friends, no family, and no place to go except to a county "home" once they could no longer work. Although people with severe mental illness and homeless elderly people had persistent needs, these groups were a small part of the population and were almost ignored in planning for the overall health care system. In 1940, nursing home expenditures constituted less than 1 percent of the nation's total health spending.

The number of elderly people rose rapidly in the postwar era, from 10 million in 1940 to 42 million in 2012. This burgeoning group of elderly Americans is relatively healthy thanks to years of good nutrition and sanitation, and they are relatively wealthy thanks to pensions and years of saving. After the 1960s, a sizable population could look forward to living for many years after working, with no need to depend on their children for financial support. This emerging group of retirees constituted a distinct market. They wanted to enjoy their "golden years" and often looked to each other for social activity. Retirement communities sprang up in Florida, California, and Arizona that catered to this growing group of middle-class elderly people. Retirement communities were specially designed to appeal to the elderly, featuring single-story dwellings without steps; limited traffic; and social centers for bridge games, dancing, and crafts. Many of these communities discouraged or excluded families with children. This market response to the special needs of the elderly occurred without any reference to medicine or LTC.

Nursing home patients constituted another small group within the elderly population that was destined to grow rapidly during the postwar era. The fraction of total health expenditures devoted to nursing homes, which was less than 1 percent in 1940, more than doubled by 1950, doubled again by 1960, and nearly doubled again by 1970, but it was increasingly constrained after that (see Table 10.1). The fraction of total health spending devoted to nursing homes

TABLE 10.1		Changes in the Long-Term Care Market			
Year	Persons aged 65+	% of population	Nursing home $ (millions)	% of total health $	Home health $	% of total health $
1940	9,540,000	7.2%	$ 28	0.7%	—	—
1950	12,400,000	8.1%	$ 178	1.5%	—	—
1960	16,600,000	9.2%	$ 980	3.6%	$ 37	0.1%
1970	20,100,000	9.8%	$ 4,867	6.5%	$ 143	0.2%
1980	25,710,000	11.3%	$ 19,989	8.0%	$ 1,347	0.5%
1990	30,390,000	12.2%	$ 54,810	7.9%	$11,056	1.2%
2000	34,778,000	12.6%	$ 92,947	7.1%	$32,426	2.4%
2010	40,268,000	13.0%	$143,077	5.5%	$70,172	2.7%

peaked at 8 percent around 1980 and has fallen steadily since then, while the number of active retirees living in segregated housing with special amenities continues to soar. Distinguishing the active senior citizens from the institutionalized patients is easy at the extremes, but there is a range in-between for which neat separation is impossible. The simple dichotomy of "at home" versus "in a nursing home" has been replaced by a range of organizational settings, from high-intensity facilities that are almost like hospitals, to a variety of intermediate care and assisted-living facilities, to houses identical to those occupied by young families. The picture is further clouded by the provision of visiting nurse services, home intravenous (IV) and physical therapy, hospice care, and other supplemental services that make it possible to deliver a wide range of care in the homes where people live before they become disabled.

Although some disabled younger people receive LTC, the majority of people who receive LTC are older than 65 years, and the rate of institutionalization increases with advancing age (Table 10.2). Residents in nursing homes are disproportionately female (74 percent) and poor. Older men who are disabled are more likely to be married and hence receive assistance from a spouse or adult child. Traditionally, care of disabled elders has been provided by adult daughters, who were expected to take on the task of caring for one or more parents or parents-in-law after their own children were raised. This informal system was adequate in the 1950s, when most women married and had children early and did not have careers. Now that the majority of women are in the labor force, and childbearing is delayed so that children often do not leave home until their mothers are their fifties, finding time to care for a 78-year-old parent is much more difficult. The "shadow price" (forgone wage opportunity) of unpaid middle-aged women has become much greater. At the same time, demand has risen. In the immediate postwar 1950s era, fewer parents lived past age 70. In addition, families were larger; therefore, middle-aged women were likely to have several sisters to help share the burden. As family size shrank and longevity increased, there were more elderly disabled parents per potential caregiver daughter. The stress and family complications became greater. As the supply of unpaid labor fell and demand rose, what formerly had been care provided within the household became care purchased in the marketplace.[2]

TABLE 10.2

Percentage of Population in a Nursing Home, by Age

Age (Years)	Percentage
<65	0.1
65–74	0.9
75–84	3.6
85+	13.9

Source: CDC, NCHS, 2004 National Nursing Home Survey (2010).

The services provided by family members are invisible in the national income (gross domestic product [GDP]) accounts: No one is billed, no one is paid, and from one point of view, no transaction has taken place. Yet from another point of view, one that predates the existence of money, the obligations of parents to care for children, of neighbors to care for the sick, and of any person present to ease the pain of dying are fundamental transactions that define society. In LTC, the boundary between market and nonmarket activities is blurred. The fact that nursing home admissions or expenditures double does not mean that twice as many disabled people are getting care or that they are getting more or better services. Some of that increase is simply the movement from the realm of household production and family obligation into monetarized commerce.

10.2 AGE AND HEALTH CARE SPENDING

It is widely assumed that aging increases the need for, and the use of, medical services. This assumption, at least in its simplest form, is not well supported. As an economist, you would quickly point out the constraints imposed by a limited life span. Treating disease in a patient who is expected to die of other causes within five years is less valuable than treating a young

TABLE 10.3   Per Capita Personal Health Expenditures* by Age Group, 1953–2004

Population	1953	1963	1970	1977	1987	1996	2000	2004
All persons	$69	$143	$291	$616	$1,664	$3,153	$3,803	$5,276
<65 years	$65	127	234	452	1,088	2,115	2,650	3,953
Age 65 and older	$109	299	809	1,962	5,830	10,285	11,778	14,797
Ratio >65 to <65	1.7	2.4	3.5	4.3	5.4	4.9	4.4	3.7

*In nominal current dollars.
Sources: Cutler and Meara, 1997, 2004; Hartman, 2009.

patient likely to live another 50 years. When scarce medical resources have to be allocated, most people, even the elderly, support favoring the young. Scarcity imposes another constraint that can limit use: elderly people who cannot afford care. In 1953, older people in the United States spent about 1.7 times as much ($109 versus $65) on medical care as the middle-aged.[3] This is more, but not a lot more. With the advent of Medicare, older people spent more than three times as much on medical care as those younger than 65 years in 1970 and five times as much in 1987, then dropping to less than four times as much in 2004 (see Table 10.3 and Figure 10.1).[4] So much more money is spent on medical care for the elderly today than 50 years ago because the system has made more money available, not because today's elderly are sicker. Comparisons made with other countries confirm that income and insurance, not aging, have caused expenditures to rise.[5]

Close examination of the data shows that today's elderly are healthier and less likely to be disabled than in prior years. Much of the growth in spending has been for the oldest old and for LTC rather than for curative medicine or surgery.[6] The data suggest that the number of elderly is growing and cumulative disability is increasing but that health status at age 65,

FIGURE 10.1   Health Care Spending Ratio: Old vs. Average vs. Young, 1953–2004

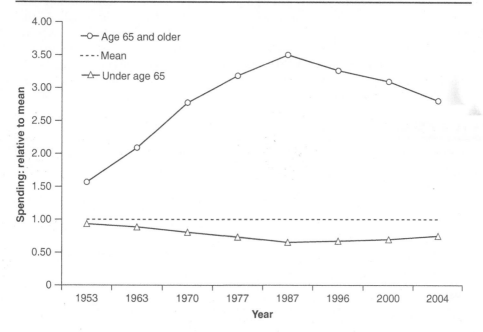

at age 75, and even at age 85 is markedly improving. Spending on medical care is significantly higher for the last year of life, but that final year, by definition, only occurs once in each lifetime. Furthermore, heroic efforts to save life that seem necessary at age 30, and perhaps justified at age 70, look intrusive and wasteful at age 90. Thus, the actual pattern of spending for medical intervention peaks at about age 75 and begins to decline after that as family and physicians become more willing to accept the dictates of nature. Total health spending continues to rise with advancing age mostly because more is spent for nursing home, hospice, home health, and related supportive care.

10.3 DEFINING LTC: TYPES OF CARE

A person's potential need for LTC can be analyzed as occurring in three dimensions: physical illness (medical diagnoses), functional disability (ability to perform activities of daily living (ADLs) and instrumental activities of daily living (IADLs), and psycho-socio-economic deficits (mental status and family support); see Tables 10.4 and 10.5. LTC can be provided either at home or in an institutional setting. Institutional settings can be ranked by the intensity of medical intervention: acute hospitals, long-term hospitals providing rehabilitation and psychiatric treatment, nursing homes (skilled, intermediate), assisted living, board-and-care homes, or continuing care retirement communities (CCRCs). Placement depends on the interaction among medical, social, economic, and functional needs rather than any single dimension. A postoperative patient who only needs regular bathing and hourly medication could be cared for at home if there is sufficient support from the family. A patient without actively involved family members may be a candidate for nursing home placement, and if there are no available nursing home beds, the patient might continue to stay in the hospital for many days.[7]

Home health care is growing rapidly in two different directions.[8] On the one hand, medical treatments that used to be performed in the hospital are being performed in the patient's home, paralleling the trend away from the hospital evidenced by shorter lengths of stay, the growth of ambulatory surgery, and the development of outpatient rehabilitation. For home medical care to be effective, the physician and nurse must be able to count on a high degree of family support to assist in monitoring the patient, administering medication, and performing basic nursing functions such as feeding, bathing, and changing clothes. On the other hand, personal home care is provided to otherwise healthy but homebound individuals whose lack of relatives at home is compensated for by having unskilled aides do ordinary cleaning, cooking, and other household tasks. Meals on Wheels, a publicly funded program that delivers hot meals to the homebound, is a good example. Although the services are quite different, the terminology and

TABLE 10.4 Dimensions of Long-Term Care Need

Type of Care	Medical Need	Functional Need	Social Need
Acute hospital	********	—	—
Rehab hospital	***	***	—
Nursing home	*	********	********
Hospice	*	—	***
CCRC	—	—	*
Skilled home care	********	***	*
Personal home care	*	***	***
Family or community	*	*	*

******** High
*** Medium
* Low
— Varies or not applicable

TABLE 10.5	Activities of Daily Living (ADL) Evaluation Form

For each area of functioning listed below, check the description that applies.*

Bathing: Either sponge bath, tub bath, or shower

☐	☐	☐
Receives no assistance (gets in and out of tub by self if tub is usual means of bathing)	Receives assistance in bathing only one part of the body (such as the back or a leg)	Receives assistance in bathing more than one part of the body (or not bathed)

Dressing: Gets clothes from closets and drawers, including underclothes and outer garments, and uses fasteners (including braces, if worn)

☐	☐	☐
Gets clothes and gets completely dressed without assistance	Gets clothes and gets dressed without assistance except for assistance in tying shoes	Receives assistance in getting clothes or in getting dressed, or stays partly or completely undressed

Toileting: Going to the "toilet room" for bowel and urine elimination; cleaning self after elimination and arranging clothes

☐	☐	☐
Goes to "toilet room," cleans self, and arranges clothes without assistance (may use object for support such as cane, walker, or wheelchair)	Receives assistance in going to "toilet room" or in cleansing self or in arranging clothes after elimination or in use of night bed pan or commode	Doesn't go to room termed "toilet" for the elimination process

Transfer

☐	☐	☐
Moves in and out of bed as well as in and out of chair without assistance	Moves in and out of bed or chair with assistance	Doesn't get out of bed

Continence

☐	☐	☐
Controls urination and bowel movement completely by self	Has occasional "accidents"	Supervision helps keep urine or bowel control; catheter is used or is incontinent

Feeding

☐	☐	☐
Feeds self without assistance	Feeds self except for getting assistance in cutting meat or buttering bread	Receives assistance in feeding or is fed partly or completely by using tubes or intravenous fluids

* The word *assistance* means supervision, direction, or personal assistance.

Source: Adapted from Katz et al., "Studies of Illness in the Aged. The Index of ADL: A Standardized Measure of Biological and Psychosocial Function," *Journal of the American Medical Association* 185 (1963): 94ff.

provision can become confusing, because a single provider might do both. A visiting nurse could stop at one house to change an IV antibiotic and proceed to the next house where the only service provided is to help someone into a wheelchair.

A person who has good friends, good health, and no functional limitations can have an active life in the community. As elderly people begin to need more care and protection, their likelihood of being placed in a nursing home depends most of all on the presence of social support. For example, most married people with Alzheimer's disease can continue to live at home and be cared for by their spouses at least through the early phases of the disease. Those who have children, but no spouse, are less likely to be able to remain at home, and those with no family nearby are likely to be institutionalized. The extent of disability is the second most important factor. Eventually, almost every family who cares for a person with Alzheimer's becomes overwhelmed by the necessity to provide constant attention, as well as by the pain and alienation of caring for someone who might not know or appreciate any of the things being done. Mental dysfunction is a significant cause in more than half of all LTC institutionalizations. Medical needs, although often critical in precipitating a crisis, are relatively less important than social, housing, and functional needs in determining the use of LTC.

TABLE 10.6

Breakdown of Nursing Home Costs

Cost	Percentage
Physician Services	1%
RNs (estimated)	8%
Other Wages & Salaries	46%
Employee Benefits	11%
Food	4%
Drugs	3%
Other Supplies	6%
Contract Services	8%
Utilities	2%
Equipment	2%
Interest	4%
Depreciation	4%
Rent, etc.	1%

Source: CMS National Nursing Home Input Price Index Market Basket, 2005 http://www.cms.hhs.gov/Medicare ProgramRatesStats/downloads/ mktbskt-snf.pdf.

The goal of acute care is to increase the level of functioning and reduce the risk of dying. In contrast, most LTC is supportive. Attempts are made to slow the patient's decline and stabilize functioning, but only rarely is an attempt made to achieve a definitive cure, and it is expected that the person will remain dependent. Because acute medical care is focused on cure, the quality of the meals, the room, and social functions are incidentals and contribute little to the total cost of a hospital stay. Most of the cost of LTC, on the other hand, is for helping people with their daily lives, not for providing treatment. Drugs are supposed to help the patient get through the day, not to get better, and curative procedures account for a relatively minor fraction of total expenditures. A physician might show up at a nursing home only once a month. In studies of nursing home costs, physician services account for only 1 percent of costs, whereas wages, salaries, and benefits, mostly for unskilled labor, account for 66 percent. A breakdown of nursing home inputs by category (Table 10.6) shows that most LTC expenses result from providing supported living rather than medical care.

10.4 MEDICAID: NURSING HOMES AS A TWO-PART MARKET

The nursing home market was radically transformed, almost created anew, by the passage of Medicare, Title XVII, and Medicaid, Title XIX, of the Social Security Amendments of 1965. When Medicare was drafted to provide health insurance for the elderly, Medicaid was somewhat of an afterthought. Medicare explicitly did not pay for the kind of supportive care provided by most nursing homes.[9] It was presumed that housing, nutrition, and personal assistance were individual or family responsibilities. Inability to provide for oneself indicated a need for charity or welfare assistance, not medical insurance.[10] Originally, Medicaid was intended mostly to expand and consolidate insurance coverage of medical services for indigent women and children who received Aid to Families with Dependent Children.

Because it was directed toward a dependent indigent population, Medicaid did pay for social support such as that provided in nursing homes. Therefore, elderly people who were

FIGURE 10.2   Nursing Home Sources and Uses of Funds

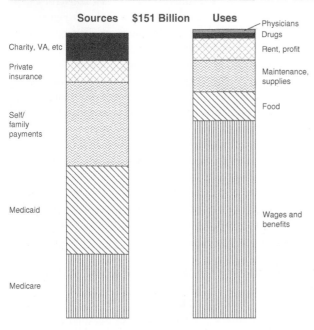

poor, or who became poor after spending down or giving away their savings, could obtain government insurance payments for institutional LTC. Soon Medicaid was funneling billions of dollars each year into nursing homes. Medicaid now accounts for 31 percent of total nursing home funding, with Medicare paying 22 percent (mostly for skilled medical nursing care and therapy), as illustrated in Figure 10.2. Medicaid is a joint state and federal program, with poor states getting as much as 80 percent of their total Medicaid funding from the federal government, whereas wealthy states get only 50 percent. States are required to cover basic medical services for people who are on public assistance and/or meet federal poverty definitions, but states have discretion to increase benefits and eligibility above these limits. (Please note that any brief description of Medicaid must be qualified, because there are more than fifty state Medicaid payment systems with numerous clauses, exceptions, and special programs.)

Although nursing homes were only a minor consideration in the creation of the Medicaid program, LTC payments soon soared out of control, more than doubling every five years. Governors and state budget officials discovered that Medicaid, even with federal matching funds, was an onerous financial burden. In most years since 1965, Medicaid has been the most rapidly growing category of state spending. The surge of Medicaid money into what had been a tiny market caused a rapid increase in prices and a shortage of spaces for millions of new patients. As prices rose, state financial burdens increased. Any new nursing homes built were quickly filled with more of the waiting Medicaid-eligible people, adding millions to state budget outlays.

States responded to this financial drain in two ways: capping the price they would pay for each day of nursing home care and halting the construction of new nursing homes. The methods of price control varied, but usually regulations were based on costs incurred or on a set percentage increase over prior years (see Section 10.5). Control over the number of beds was established by requiring nursing home owners to obtain a certificate of need (CON) before building or expanding facilities (see Section 10.4 and the discussion of hospital CONs in Section 9.6).

With these two moves—price controls and capacity constraints—government created a unique market for nursing home beds. This market's distinctive feature is a constant excess demand, but it is an excess of below-market-price Medicaid patients only. Consider Figure 10.3. On the upper-left side is private market demand, with a normal, downward-sloping demand schedule. The upper-right panel shows Medicaid demand. Because price is fixed by government regulation, there is no change in price as quantity increases; therefore, the demand curve is a right angle. Nursing homes can get as many patients they want at the state-regulated price, until there are no more Medicaid-eligible patients in the area. The lower-left panel shows the combined private and Medicaid demand. Only private-pay patients can be served above the fixed Medicaid price; thus, the initial portion of the demand curve is composed solely of private patients and is downward sloping. Once the Medicaid price is reached, the demand curve flattens out, because the nursing home can get more patients without reducing price. If a nursing home became too large, it would eventually exhaust the excess Medicaid demand and have to attract additional private patients with even lower prices, as shown by the bottom third, downward-sloping segment. Increasing the number of beds sufficient to force nursing home owners to dip into the demand of those only willing to pay an amount less than Medicaid pays is usually unintentional, because expansion typically ceases before all Medicaid patients are served.

The two-part market faced by the nursing home owner is shown in more detail in the lower-right panel of Figure 10.3.[11] The vertical line represents the total bed capacity of the nursing home, the maximum number of patients that can be cared for. To maximize profits, the owner first sets a price for private-pay patients, P_{pp}, that maximizes the total amount of excess revenues above the Medicaid rate (i.e., the dashed rectangle: $Q_{pp} \times (P_{pp} - P_{Medicaid})$). The owner then fills the remaining beds from the waiting list of Medicaid patients who pay the state-regulated price $P_{Medicaid}$ (the shaded rectangle: $(Q_{max} - Q_{pp}) \times P_{Medicaid}$).

The two-part market structure causes nursing home utilization to have an unusual U-shaped relationship to income. Although most normal goods show demand steadily rising as income rises, in this market utilization is high at low incomes (where patients readily qualify for Medicaid), drops for middle incomes (where lack of coverage reduces demand), and rises at high incomes (where wealthy people can afford $80,000 or more per year for care).

The real world is, of course, more complicated than the straight lines drawn in Figure 10.3. Many nursing homes only admit private-pay patients. Many patients come into a nursing home with considerable assets, but over the years they **spend down** all their savings by paying for care, and only then do they become poor enough to be eligible for Medicaid (a common guideline is less than $2,000 in financial assets and $564 per month in income for a single person).[12] There are stories of couples becoming divorced solely to allow the spouse who is disabled to qualify for Medicaid so that the one who is still living at home can keep the savings accounts. Elderly couples are protected to some extent by federal guidelines that allow the spouse at home to keep the house, car, and some additional assets. Elderly single people may give their assets to their children in anticipation of entering a nursing home. This must be planned with care, however, because most states include recently transferred assets as part of personal funds to be used before Medicaid reimbursement is allowed. Families that would never consider "going on welfare" use asset transfers to make aging parents dependent on state funds as indigents.

With 50 percent of all nursing home bills paid for by Medicaid, the conclusion that many middle-class and wealthy people are benefiting from a program designed for the poor is inescapable.[13] The fact that a certain amount of subterfuge is required ("convenience" divorces, paper-only transfers of ownership of cars and land, "giving" to children money that the parent still controls) only makes this process more distasteful and morally undermining.[14] Medicaid is an entrenched part of the nursing home market, but it is not well liked by taxpayers or beneficiaries, and it is difficult to justify Medicaid as being either equitable or ethical.

FIGURE 10.3   Two-Part Nursing Home Market

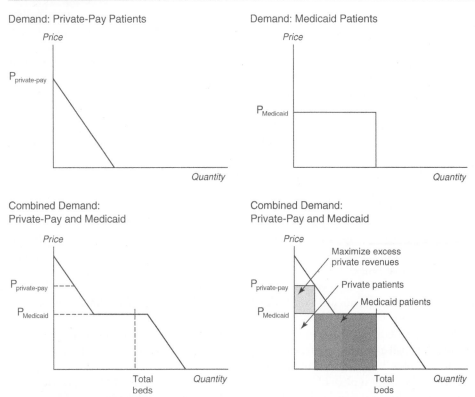

10.5   CERTIFICATE OF NEED: WHOSE NEEDS?

It is important to understand the implications of regulatory constraints on the LTC market and to examine whose interests are served by creating a situation of chronic excess demand in which frail and sick patients must wait months for a bed. For example, the surge of Medicaid money into nursing home care after 1965 meant that there would be a shortage of beds for the years it would take until the market could catch up. In addition, imposing a construction moratorium through the CON process increased the shortage and made it permanent.

Money and Quality

It would seem that pushing more money into nursing homes during the late 1960s would have improved the quality of care provided. However, for perfectly rational economic reasons, conditions actually became worse in many nursing homes. For instance, a nursing home owner does not choose furniture or service based on what can be afforded but on what will maximize profits. With a long line of Medicaid patients waiting to get in, it was not necessary to keep up the appearance of the nursing home to attract new patients, nor was it necessary to provide good nursing service or good food to keep patients there. Because every bed was always filled from the waiting list, profits were maximized by reducing costs (e.g., providing fewer hours of nursing, employing less-skilled nurses, making fewer repairs, providing less maintenance). The flood of Medicaid money washed away any incentive to provide high-quality care to attract more patients.

Competing for Certificates of Need, Not for Patients

With chronic excess demand guaranteeing full occupancy from the first day, new nursing homes were sure money-makers. If placed in nice locations to attract a sizable share of private-pay patients, even more money could be made. CON regulations slowed, but did not entirely stop, the construction of new nursing homes. Since a CON was required, what would determine who could build these facilities and where would they be placed? State officials faced a dilemma. If the nursing home was built in a nice area, it would generate higher profits and would not cost the state as much money, because only a few beds would be taken by Medicaid patients. On the other hand, placing a nursing home in a poorer area of high need would do more to relieve the shortage of Medicaid beds but would cost the state more money. The conflict between patient needs and state budget pressures made it necessary to compromise. It is unlikely that CON regulation actually did much to change or improve the location of new nursing home beds.

Who Gets to Build?   Certainly the state might favor faith-based groups that donated money to help care for patients. Being political, however, the state might favor nursing home owners who donated money to help elect a congressperson or senator. With chronic excess demand, the CON itself became valuable property. In effect, one could "buy" patients by obtaining a CON from the government. Once a nursing home owner had a CON, the supply of Medicaid patients was assured, and the owner would not have to do any marketing or make any quality improvements to attract patients. Competition was thus shifted away from the market into the political regulatory arena.

Windfall profits accrued to anyone who was able to obtain a CON for new construction or who already owned a nursing home. However, this does not mean that the next owner would make excess profits. When the facility was sold, the new owner had to pay for the building and implicitly for the CON, a piece of paper whose value was roughly equal to the expected future profits of the facility. The new owner, after paying $10 million for a $5 million building to get the CON, would have high fixed costs and would find it hard to make a profit unless he or she reduced operating costs and hence reduced quality.

Who Pays?   CON restrictions succeeded in reducing state Medicaid budgets and providing excess profits to nursing home owners. The question then became: if both owners and regulators benefited, who got hurt? The answer is that patients and their families paid, directly or indirectly, to generate those financial gains. Without competition among nursing homes, patients were often forced to take whichever bed they could get. Instead of conducting market research to meet patient needs, nursing home operators sensibly devoted their dollars to lobbying for continued regulation. Restrictions on supply also meant higher prices for private-pay patients. The biggest cost of CON regulation is all the hours of unpaid labor and disruption imposed on families who could not get their loved ones into a needed nursing home bed or who had to wait months to do so. In the highest need category (people with dementia, people with multiple impairments in performing ADLs), more than 90 percent are in nursing homes in states where there is no shortage of beds, but only 50 percent of similarly impaired patients are in nursing homes in states that continue to impose tight limits on bed supply.[15] What happens to the other 40 percent? Who cares for them and at what personal sacrifice? Just because family labor and unnecessary declines in quality of life are not charged for in the market does not make them less costly.

Evidence on the Effects of Certificates of Need

The primary purpose of a CON from the beginning has been to limit the growth of states' Medicaid expenditures. The crisis atmosphere generated after Medicaid suddenly flooded the market has eased over time, and the reflexive need to use regulations to impose order on a market out of control faded. The shortage of beds created by restricting supply became more of an issue. Long waiting lists and the protests of families whose lives were disrupted by having to provide unpaid caregiving put pressure on states to relax or eliminate their CON rules. The differences between states that have continued to use CONs and those that have stopped illustrate some of the effects of artificial controls on supply. The length of time a patient has to wait for a bed has fallen in states where the CON requirement has been repealed. Also, the large disparity in waiting time between private-pay and Medicaid patients has been reduced or eliminated as shortages have disappeared.

It often has been assumed that nursing homes with a high percentage of Medicaid patients are less successful in attracting private-pay patients and are thus of lower-than-average quality. A study comparing states with and without CON requirements showed that higher percentages of Medicaid reimbursement were indeed associated with lower quality in states where CON regulations caused a chronic shortage of beds.[16] However, this was not the case in the states without CON regulations. As free entry made more beds available, nursing homes had to compete for Medicaid patients by providing better quality. Since 1990, the supply situation has continued to ease, and more and more states show declines in occupancy. With empty beds, competition for all types of patients has intensified.

10.6   COST CONTROL BY SUBSTITUTION

The lack of extra payment for patients who need extra care might mean that they cannot be transferred to a nursing home and hence must remain in a high-cost acute care hospital bed for additional **administratively necessary days** (**ANDs**). It seems obvious that total costs could be reduced by moving patients from a hospital bed ($1,600 per day) to a cheaper nursing home bed ($150 per day) to receive care. Indeed, some hospitals have purchased nursing homes just to make it easier to discharge their post–acute-care patients. Yet opportunities for system-wide savings are often passed up because different parties are paying different bills. For instance, Medicare (federal) pays most hospital bills, whereas Medicaid (state) pays most nursing home bills. A state may be unwilling to pay for additional nursing home days, even though each additional hospital day is much more expensive, because the cost of hospital days is borne by the federal government rather than the state.

A larger and more general problem in trying to use service substitution to reduce costs is controlling who gets the additional days of nursing home care. Increased bed supply and changes in reimbursement that make it easier to transfer patients from hospitals to nursing homes also make it easier for new patients to obtain care. The extra costs from providing care to these new patients tends to outweigh the savings obtained by switching some patients from hospitals to nursing homes. A large experiment that attempted to demonstrate cost savings by using social workers to channel patients at high risk for repeat hospitalization into less expensive forms of care ended up with higher total costs.[17] The channeling project was not able to generate savings because only a few hospitalizations could be avoided and so many people not previously hospitalized got placed in nursing homes. The additional "low cost" services outweighed the few "expensive" hospital days avoided.

It was similarly thought that expanded home health care and ambulatory surgery could save money for Medicare by reducing hospitalization. Part A (hospital) expenses have indeed declined in recent years, but Part B (professional services) expenses have increased by a much greater amount. For example, cataract surgery, IV antibiotics, and physical therapy are cheaper when performed on an outpatient basis, but once the need for a hospital admission was eliminated, so many new patients utilized these services that the total cost of treatment more than doubled. Attempts to reduce nursing home costs through expanded substitution of home health and hospice services have also led to disappointing results.

10.7   CASE-MIX REIMBURSEMENT

Even with an adequate supply of beds, the fact that the state pays only a single fixed rate per day for nursing home care means that some patients may be denied care. A patient who is very sick or whose disruptive mental condition requires frequent attention costs more than a patient who is healthy and lucid. With revenue per day fixed, a nursing home can increase profits by accepting only less costly patients who need very little care. To provide nursing homes with incentives to admit more severely ill patients, some states have developed **case-mix reimbursement** systems that increase payments based on an index of need. Whereas the starting point for acute medical case-mix reimbursement is the diagnosis (see Section 8.2 for a discussion of diagnostically related group [DRG] reimbursement in hospitals), in LTC the starting point is the patient's level of functioning. Most commonly, this is measured in terms of the number of ADLs for which the individual needs assistance (dressing, grooming, bathing, eating, mobility, transferring, walking, toileting; see Table 10.5) as well as the level of assistance required.[18] In New York state, the association between number of **ADL**s and cost of care was used to create a number of **resource utilization groups** (**RUGs**).

The U.S. General Accounting Office (now the Government Accountability Office) issued a report in 1990 showing that the problem that "heavy care" patients have in obtaining a nursing home bed is substantially reduced in states with systems that adjust reimbursement according to case mix. However, the adjustment is always imperfect, and even with differential payment rates, nursing homes can find it profitable to accept some patients while turning others away. Minnesota created a system with eleven levels of reimbursement from A (patients with zero to three ADLs and no special problems) to K (patients with seven or eight ADLs who require special nursing). To the extent that differences in payment rate correctly adjust for differences in cost, a nursing home would have no reason to selectively admit one group rather than another. However, researchers at the University of Minnesota estimated that categories H and J were significantly overcompensated, and categories C and F were significantly undercompensated.[19] The total number of days of care remained basically the same from for the first five years of the case-mix reimbursement system, but nursing homes admitted more patients in the overcompensated categories over time and admitted fewer patients in the undercompensated categories. Even though some of the change might have been due to gaming of the regulatory system by reclassifying patients into more profitable categories, part of the change appears to have been a result of selective admissions policies. The lesson of this study is that nursing homes, even nonprofit nursing homes, respond to any remaining inaccuracies in case-mix reimbursement.

HOW MANY VISITS? GAMING THE MEDICARE PAYMENT SYSTEM

In 2010, the *Wall Street Journal* published an investigative article suggesting that four publicly traded home health firms appeared to show unusual patterns in the number of therapy visits that would have the effect of increasing their Medicare reimbursements.[20] A follow-up report by the U.S. Senate Finance Committee staff in 2011 concluded that these four companies "*encouraged therapists to target the most profitable number of therapy visits, even when patient need alone may not have justified such patterns.*"

The Balanced Budget Act of 1997 changed Medicare home health payments, replacing cost reimbursement with a single payment for each 60-day period. The amount of payment

(Continued)

HOW MANY VISITS? GAMING THE MEDICARE PAYMENT SYSTEM (CONTINUED)

depends upon which of the 80 case-mix adjusted home health resource groups the patient was classified into based on clinical (eight criteria), functional (five criteria), and service utilization (two criteria) factors. The two utilization criteria were "hospital discharge within last 14 days" and "more or less than 10 therapy visits." Analysis of Medicare records showed that payment for patients with 1 to 9 visits averaged about $1,900, and payment for those with 10 to 15 visits averaged $4,400. Medicare officials recognized that simple visit counts were subject to manipulation, but they wanted to make sure that home health companies did not skimp by providing too few. What developed over time is the pattern seen in Figure 10.4: The companies seemed to push the number of visits just enough to meet the criteria for higher payment.

FIGURE 10.4   Unusual Distribution of Home Health Therapy Visits, 2007

Source: U.S. Senate Finance Committee: *Staff Report on Home Health and the Medicare Therapy Threshold*, Sept. 2011

Furthermore, the investigators found company emails actively encouraging managers to meet the 10-visit threshold, pressuring clinicians to "maximize reimbursements" and pointing out how small changes in visit patterns could add hundreds of thousands or even millions of dollars to company profits. When Medicare subsequently changed the classification system in 2008 to one with three utilization levels (6, 14, and 20 visits) and 153 categories, the number of patients having exactly 10 visits immediately fell. Although no official sanctions have been applied since these investigative reports appeared, Medicare has begun to develop a new case-mix adjustment system that will no longer use visit counts, the four companies' market value has precipitously declined, and their bond ratings have been revised downward.

Sources: Barbara Martinez, "Home Care Yields Medicare Bounty," *Wall Street Journal*, April 26 2010; U.S. Senate Finance Committee, *Staff Report on Home Health And the Medicare Therapy Threshold* (Washington, D.C.: U.S. Government Printing Office, 2011).

10.8   LONG-TERM CARE INSURANCE

Is Long-Term Care "Medical"?

The Medicare program is immensely popular (and immensely expensive) because it serves every elderly person regardless of need and therefore provides an upper-middle-class standard of care to all by using taxpayers' money. Attempts to forge an equally popular LTC insurance program have failed. Although numerous cultural and political factors are involved, a major reason is that most of the features that characterize medical care (randomly occurring illness, reliance on physicians when quality can be a life-and-death issue, rapid technological innovation) are missing in LTC. Instead, much of the cost of LTC is for housing, food, social amenities—things normally identified as personal responsibilities or lifestyle choices rather than medical care. The boundaries between medical care, social services, and living expenses often become ambiguous. Distinctions between professional services and unpaid family help are often similarly unclear. The divergence between medical care and LTC suggests that the types of health insurance financing developed for medical care might not be appropriate for financing the costs of assisted daily living characteristic of most LTC.

What difference does it make whether LTC is called *medical* or not? In a word: money. Distinguishing services as *medical* makes it more likely that they will be covered by insurance, more likely that the people providing services will be licensed, and more likely that quality will be regulated and that choices by consumers in the marketplace will be supplanted by professional standards. LTC has more in common with social insurance programs such as disability, workers' compensation, pensions, and Social Security than it does with medicine. Yet the tremendous cost of expanding entitlements and the lack of taxpayer support has caused many advocates to try to find ways to "medicalize" LTC to increase the flow of funds to professionals and institutions. Hospice care is purely palliative; it is not intended to rehabilitate or cure but only to ease pain and help with adjustment to dying. Since it is not "medically necessary" and therefore does not meet the regular criterion for coverage, special legislation was required to get Medicare to pay for this form of LTC as a benefit.

Although most medical care is paid for through third-party insurance, private LTC insurance did not even come into existence until the 1980s and still pays for less than 4 percent of nursing home and home health care bills. There are several major reasons LTC insurance is not as attractive to consumers as insurance for acute medical care, which are summarized in box "Reasons that Long-Term Care Insurance Is Not Popular".[21] The incidence of disability requiring LTC is not so much random as delayed. If we live long enough, almost all of us will need some form of LTC. Yet if we wait until age 70 to purchase LTC insurance the premiums will be very high because the likelihood of needing that insurance is so great. A more prudent

---

REASONS THAT LONG-TERM CARE INSURANCE IS NOT POPULAR

Incidence of LTC is less random than acute illness.

- Insurance must be purchased so far in advance of anticipated need that savings become a good alternative to insurance.
- Medicaid is always there, providing a stop-loss against large expenditures.
- To get benefits paid, the purchaser must often be admitted to a nursing home. Unlike treatment for acute illness, that person would rather not be admitted for care, but instead stay at home.
- Benefits mostly reduce expenditures by heirs and Medicaid, rather than helping the patients who pay the premiums.

course would be to plan in advance. However, people who purchase LTC insurance at age 40 will have to wait many years to obtain benefits. Financially, they might do almost as well if they put aside savings to be used for LTC if the need arises, letting interest accrue over the intervening years. In addition, people might die without entering a nursing home, and hence the money used for LTC premiums could instead be passed on to their heirs. If one did end up needing a lot of LTC and ran out of savings, there would always be Medicaid to fall back on. Why should people pay premiums for 30 years when the government would pay if they really needed help?

A final barrier to LTC insurance is the nature of the benefit: payment for a nursing home stay. Unlike payment for acute medical treatment, which is expected to improve health or reduce the risk of premature death, payment for nursing home care just makes it easier to be taken from home and be placed in an institution. It is hard to get excited about paying thousands of dollars to merely slow the rate of decline and extend the number of years spent living with disability. On reflection, it becomes clear that the greatest beneficiaries of LTC insurance are not the patients but their children and the Medicaid program. Children benefit because they might find it easier to send a disabled parent to a nursing home if the charges are paid for by insurance. In addition, children protect their inheritance by having the risk of caring for a disabled parent insured. Medicaid also benefits because nursing home charges are paid for by premiums rather than state and federal tax monies. Expansion of private LTC insurance will be limited until (a) benefits are modified so that they help patients continue to live at home rather than making it easier to be admitted to a nursing home; (b) payments are made in advance with favorable tax treatment by employers, as is the case with most group medical insurance; and (c) policies are coordinated with Medicaid so that they yield financial benefits to patients, their spouses, and heirs, instead of offsetting government expenditures. Even so, LTC insurance might remain unpopular. It is noteworthy that the first element of the Affordable Care Act of 2010 to be repealed was the Community Living Assistance Services and Support program (CLASS Act), which would have provided government subsidies for private LTC insurance.

10.9   RETIREMENT, ASSISTED LIVING, AND THE WEALTHY ELDERLY

Elderly people with enough money to afford LTC insurance have not been particularly interested in purchasing it. However, the wealthy elderly have flocked to retirement communities and other market alternatives. Among the most successful have been **assisted-living** facilities, life care communities, or **continuing-care retirement communities** (CCRCs). These residential developments combine elements of housing and managed care financing of LTC in a retirement community, guaranteeing people a pleasant place to live and nursing care for the remainder of their lives.[22] In most retirement communities, new entrants (usually married couples in their 70s or 80s) pay a substantial fixed fee upon entry ($75,000 to $375,000) for their apartments and then a monthly fee ($1,200 to $6,000 a month) for maintenance, housekeeping, social services, and some or all meals. Home health nurses are provided when needed. As a person becomes disabled, he or she can enter a nursing home on the premises. Residents do not own their apartments, but they do have the right to live in them until they die or are admitted to the nursing facility. Major advantages of CCRCs are the controlled environment geared toward the elderly, the possibilities of creating a new circle of friends even as health declines, and the ability to continue seeing these friends daily even after entering the nursing facility. CCRCs range from modestly nice to quite luxurious. The nursing facilities tend to be less institutional than those in most nursing homes. Even severely impaired people may still have table linens, candles with dinner, and a homelike atmosphere.

The large entry fee and sizable monthly payments generate two problems: the possibility of bankruptcy or fraud on the part of the owner and lack of affordability. The first CCRCs depended almost entirely on entry fees and had very low monthly rates. Many were "sponsored" but not financially supported by religious denominations. After taking the up-front fee (sometimes, the entire savings and estate of the couple), CCRCs were obligated to provide care for life. The facilities ought to have invested the money wisely so that interest income could have been used to pay for maintenance and nursing home care. Unfortunately, the actuarial estimates were often quite far from the mark. Financial projections assumed that apartments could be turned over and resold every 10 years or so, but the people who chose to enter lived much longer than usual for their ages (a form of adverse selection). In many cases, the husband began to need nursing home care (which cost extra) while the wife continued to live for many years (occupying a large apartment that could not be resold). Some religious leaders were uncomfortable about raising monthly fees when millions of dollars in investments were in the bank, even though the future obligations for nursing home care and maintenance were greater than what could be covered by the interest. Necessary financial reserves were depleted over time when monthly rates were not raised promptly.

These factors alone would have been sufficient to cause problems, but they were compounded in case after case when unscrupulous CCRC operators paid themselves excessive sales fees or salaries or simply embezzled funds. Immediately after a facility opened, there would be millions of dollars in entry fees in the bank. The loss or mismanagement of these funds would not become evident until years later, when buildings needed repair or residents needed nursing home care. By then, the money was sometimes literally out of the country.

Numerous reforms have been instituted to maintain the financial integrity of CCRCs. Now, if a religious denomination agrees to sponsor a facility, it must legally guarantee future expenses. Reserves must be routinely reported, and financial viability, including coverage of medical and nursing home expenses, must be demonstrated. The risky "pay everything up front" financing has been supplanted so that more costs are covered by monthly fees, and often the nursing home care component is paid for separately and subject to standard underwriting practices (e.g., waiting periods, extra fees, exclusions for those entering with preexisting conditions such as cancer or Alzheimer's disease).

More and more elderly people can afford the cost of entering a CCRC. Definitions of "wealthy" are to some extent always subjective, but by any measure, the wealth of the elderly has risen dramatically both in absolute terms and relative to the wealth of the younger population. In the 1950s, many elderly were poor, still struggling with the aftermath of the Depression. In contrast, young families faced bright economic prospects, and relatively few children lived in poverty. By 1990, Social Security, marital patterns, and other factors had reversed the incidence of poverty. The elderly were much better off than their children. Favorable tax and transfer treatment, along with years of savings, have made people 65 to 74 the wealthiest group in America, with a net worth of $1,015,200 in 2007, and people 55 to 64 almost equal in net worth at $935,800 (see Table 10.7).[23] This does not mean, however, that there are no subgroups

TABLE 10.7	Average Income and Wealth for Different Age Categories			
	Income		Wealth	
Age Category (Years)	**Median**	**Average**	**Median**	**Average**
All families	$47,300	$84,300	$120,300	$556,300
Under 35	37,400	51,700	11,800	106,000
35 to 44	56,600	83,700	86,600	325,600
45 to 54	64,200	112,400	182,500	661,200
55 to 64	54,600	111,200	253,700	935,800
65 to 74	39,000	92,400	239,400	1,015,200
75 and older	22,800	45,700	213,500	638,200

Source: Survey of Consumer Finances, Federal Reserve Bulletin (February 2009): A1-35.

of the elderly with high poverty rates (the single black elderly are notably poor, as are the oldest old, people older than 85 years), but it does mean that many can afford to buy care and protection in the market using their own substantial assets rather than depending on government programs. Married couples reaching age 65 have higher average incomes than the rest of the population and twice as many financial assets. At least half of them can readily afford a CCRC or other market-based LTC financing mechanism. Public protection of the poor will always be necessary. What is important to change is the perception that all or even most of the elderly are "poor."

The market for supportive services among the elderly is affected not only by demand but also by supply. In this regard, it is important to remember that most care is actually provided by unpaid family and friends. Estimates by Darius Lakdawalla and Tomas Philipson suggest that the increase in the number of healthy older people able to care for others, and particularly the increase in the percentage of the elderly who are male (and thus likely to be married to the more numerous females), will reduce the number of elderly people placed in institutions.[24] It is the lack of someone at home to care for the person, not just disability, that drives up the rate of nursing home admissions.

10.10   FINANCIAL REIMBURSEMENT CYCLES

Having reviewed the economics of payers and providers in Chapters 4 through 10, it is appropriate to reflect on a recurrent cycle of scarcity, generosity, and abuse that occurs in the financing of medical services. This is well illustrated by home health care, which just moved through a surge of uncontrolled spending and is now being restrained. There are typically four stages of reimbursement (see box "Stages in the Reimbursement Cycle"), beginning with charitable assistance, moving through cost reimbursement and complex administered price systems, and ending with firm controls over total budgets. This extended cycle is seen in the development of financing for hospitals, ambulatory surgery, nursing homes and, more recently, home health care. Before the spread of insurance coverage, most medical organizations were nonprofit and the need for more services (and more funding) was broadly recognized. Requests for payment were based on trust. It was assumed that the fees were less than the cost of care or that any excess was being used to subsidize needy people. The amount of funding was limited primarily by the availability of donors. For home health care, this situation held for a number of years. The dominant providers were community and regional visiting nurse services, charitable agencies that employed salaried nurses to visit the disabled homebound. Home health care was a minor and unprofitable niche within the health care system, accounting for less than 0.3 percent of national medical expenditures.

STAGES IN THE REIMBURSEMENT CYCLE

Stage 1	**"What you ask for":** Trusting charity providers
Stage 2	**Cost reimbursement:** Leads to expansion, manipulation of cost reports
Stage 3	**Complex administered prices:** Prospective payment systems put in place to reduce costs get gamed by providers seeking even more reimbursement
Stage 4	**Global budget control:** Set reimbursement increases to match increases in resource funding base
Stage 5	**Start over:** Entrepreneurs and investors move on to a new area

As the length of stay in hospitals began to shorten, patients were discharged "quicker and sicker," raising the need for skilled assistance at home. Reimbursement on the traditional "what you ask for" basis was made, mostly to visiting nurse services. Soon, Medicare was paying 25 to 30 percent of the bills, with Medicaid picking up another 5 to 10 percent. Entrepreneurs spotted a new guaranteed stream of funding and developed for-profit businesses that were tightly managed, paid nurses well (and made them see more patients per hour), and raised charges to build the bottom line and expand rapidly. By 1980, home health care had become a $2 billion business, accounting for about 1 percent of total health expenditures, rising to $12 billion (1.7 percent of national health expenditures) in 1990.

The second stage of the reimbursement cycle commences when the payer attempts to replace traditional fees with a more precise determination of what services actually cost. This impulse is driven by two opposing claims: (1) from the providers, that the existing payments are not sufficient to cover their costs and will not allow expansion to provide services to all patients who need care, and (2) from the payers, a suspicion that fees are too large and provide excess profits and incentive to create new providers where none are needed. So begins the debate and the implementation of reimbursement based on costs rather than fees.

Cost reimbursement appears simple—and then the accountants move in. What exactly is "cost" anyway? Shouldn't owners be paid for the use of their buildings and other capital rather than only for operating expenses? Isn't it important to pay owners extra to ensure that patients who are more difficult to treat (those with dementia or AIDS) are able to obtain service? Shouldn't every new home health care agency that opens receive enough cost reimbursement to make sure that it stays in operation? Although these positions are defensible, such cost reimbursement is much different from the way capital markets respond to investors opening new restaurants and predictably leads to a massive increase in capacity. The facile comment regarding accountants should not be taken as disparaging. The accountants who work for health care providers are doing their jobs, which in this situation is to maximize reimbursement so that providers can grow and do more. Over time, the accounting system becomes more highly regulated and more complex but no more satisfactory. No matter how costs are counted, there always will be disputes (overtime wages, capital arbitrage, sunk costs) and continual expansion (because more costs mean more reimbursement). Eventually, the cost-reimbursement system becomes unsustainable, and the era of cost control arrives. For home health care, this turning point was reached in the early 1990s. Within five years, home health expenditures more than doubled, reaching $32 billion and taking more than 3 percent of all health spending.

After the pathologies of open-ended cost reimbursement have become apparent, attempts are made to set payment limits in advance, usually based on an objective indicator such as diagnosis. This method was adopted by hospitals (via DRGs), physicians (via the resource-based relative value scale, RBRVS), and nursing homes (via RUGS). These payments were more difficult to arrange in home health care because the extent of disability and social isolation, not medical need, drives care. Also, unlike surgery or nursing home admission, home health visits were actively welcomed by the homebound elderly and even by elderly people who just needed someone to change their sheets, make a meal, and chat for a while. In some cases, agencies appear to have driven demand by calling elderly patients and asking "Would you like someone to visit you at home? Medicare will pay for it." Abuse of the system became rampant. Payments, which rose 17 percent a year from 1980 to 1989, rose by 40 percent in 1990, 35 percent in 1991, and 37 percent in 1992. This exploitation of the system was unsustainable and led to the inevitable retrenchment with multimillion dollar lawsuits for fraudulent billing and improper referrals.[25] Several years were required to bring the system under control. In 1996, Medicare and Medicaid were still paying $20 billion for home health care, more than half of all home health care expenses. Whereas Medicaid expenditures continued to rise slightly, by 2000 Medicare had cut payments by 50 percent to just $9 billion. Forcing patients and private insurance to pay directly for more visits restored some balance to the system.

October 2000 marked the implementation of the newest Medicare home health financing reform, a fixed predetermined payment rate per 60-day episode.[26] The payment rate depends on an assessment of the patient's overall need for care as classified into one of 80 home health resource groups (HHRGs). Doctors must certify (and recertify) a patient as qualifying for care when the first visit is made, but the number of visits made within a 60-day episode has no effect on total payments. It appears that home health care reimbursement has entered the third stage of the reimbursement cycle, because it is semi-fixed and largely divorced from the cost-accounting procedures of providers. Growth has moderated and home health is now held below 3 percent of national health expenditures.

The endpoint of cost control comes when the payer decides to match payments to the availability of funding, not to the number of patients or visits or to diagnoses. This has already happened for Medicare payment of physicians under the rubric of the sustainable growth rate (SGR), a mechanism for linking the increase in total payments each year to the increase in gross domestic product (and hence to the tax revenues available). Such a rigid and mechanical approach to funding brings its own problems, leading to further amendments, enlargements, reforms, and revolutions. In this regard, it is not so much the end as the start of a new cycle.

What is important in this discussion is not the specifics of home health care or federal payment regulations, but the fact that the *financial reimbursement cycle* is repeated over and over again as a strategic game between payers and providers in different contexts: hospitals, physicians, nursing homes, home health. One side wants to control costs, while the other side wants to increase revenues. The rules are not abstract truths or arbitrary legal dictums written in stone but are themselves part of the game. Recently, inpatient rehabilitation facilities (IRFs) implemented an IRF PPS system for rehabilitation of hip replacements, stroke, etc. and joined the group of medical providers passing through the cycle.[27] Expanded funding in a new area, such as home health care, inevitably means excesses and a certain amount of fraud. Hospices for care of the dying, which were almost entirely small local charitable endeavors just a few decades ago, now provide care to more than 1.5 million patients a year (42 percent of all deaths) and have 89 percent of the bills paid by Medicare.[28] Now more than 50 percent of hospices are for-profit firms, and often belong to national corporate chains. Reports of fraud and false billing are being reported in the press. Such excesses will, to a greater or lesser extent, be corrected over time.

SUGGESTIONS FOR FURTHER READING

National Institutes of Health National Institute on Aging (www.nih.nia.gov).

AARP (www.aarp.org).

National Center for Health Statistics, Trends in Health and Aging, (http://www.cdc.gov/nchs/).

C. Caffrey, M. Sengupta, A. Moss, L. Harris-Kojetin, and R. Valverde, "Home Health Care and Discharged Hospice Care Patients: United States, 2000 and 2007," *National Health Statistics Reports* no 38. (Hyattsville, MD: National Center for Health Statistics, 2011).

National Hospice and Palliative Care Organization, NHPCO Facts and Figures <www.nhcpo.org>

Karen Buhler-Wilkerson. "Care of the Chronically Ill at Home: An Unresolved Dilemma in Health Policy for the United States," *Millbank Quarterly* 85, no. 4 (2007): 611-639.

Connie J. Evashwick, ed. *The Continuum of Long-Term Care* (Albany, N.Y.: Delmar Publishers, 2005). Micah Hartman et al., "U.S. Health Spending by Age," *Health Affairs* 27, no. 1 (2008): w1–w12.

Darius Lakdawalla and Tomas Philipson, "The Rise in Old-Age Longevity and the Market for Long-Term Care," *American Economic Review* 92, no. 1 (2002): 295–306.

HS Kaye, C Harrington, and MP LaPlante, "Long-Term Care: Who Gets it, Who Provides It, Who Pays, and How Much?" *Health Affairs* 29, no. 1 (2010): 11-21.

SUMMARY

1. Most LTC expenditures are for nursing home care, but most care of the disabled elderly is **provided by unpaid family members** and friends.

2. As the number of elderly rose and the **shadow price of labor** by adult daughters increased, more and more LTC was shifted from unpaid household production to commercial market purchases of care.

3. Nursing home economics is dominated by a **split two-part market**. Private-pay patients tend to pay more and sometimes receive better care. Medicaid patients must demonstrate to the state that they qualify by being poor. The state pays their bills but will not pay as much; therefore, there is a chronic excess of Medicaid patients trying to get into beds that nursing home owners would prefer to fill with private-pay patients.

4. CON **regulations** were intended to slow down the construction of new nursing homes after the passage of Medicaid in 1965 greatly increased demand and hence the tax burden on the states. CON requirements have exacerbated the shortage of nursing homes and caused patients to wait months for a bed. **Competing for CONs** has helped regulators and nursing home owners, but it has not helped the patients who are forced to wait months for a bed or accept substandard care.

5. In a shortage situation, patients most in need of nursing home care are more likely to be denied a bed because their care tends to be more costly. To alleviate this problem, some states have replaced the flat-rate per diem with a rate that is **case-mix adjusted** for differences in need. Such systems help match reimbursement with cost, but they can never be perfect.

6. **Substituting** lower-cost LTC for hospital care (or home health care for nursing home care) sounds good, but it usually increases total system costs because so many new patients are brought in.

7. LTC primarily provides assistance to people with disabilities to help them perform activities of daily living, and financing is appropriately done through social insurance. "**Medicalizing**" LTC enables providers to tap new sources of funding, allows workers to justify licensure, probably increases quality, and clearly increases total costs.

8. It has become clear that **increases in income and insurance**, not increases in disease and disability, **have allowed medical care expenditures to rise**. The cost of medical care for the elderly is now five times higher than the cost of medical care for the middle-aged, whereas in 1950 the cost of medical care for the elderly was less than two times the cost of medical care for the middle-aged.

9. People in the United States are living longer. Although this means that there will be more and **more elderly people**, the average person aged 75 **will be healthier**, more likely to live at home, and more likely to be able to care for a spouse or friend so that he or she too can live at home rather than being admitted to a nursing home.

10. Payment for home health care, like that of most other medical services, proceeded through a *financial reimbursement cycle* with four stages:

    a. **Fees** paid to trusted voluntary organizations

    b. **Cost reimbursements**

    c. Complex **administered prices**

    d. Total cost control through global **budgets** adjusted to match growth in GDP.

    This reimbursement cycle is driven by the strategic behavior of providers who push the boundaries and game the system to maximize revenues.

PROBLEMS

1. {*market size*} How much is the average cost per day of a nursing home stay? On a typical day in the United States, are there more patients in hospitals or in nursing homes? Which type of care is growing more rapidly? What is the most rapidly growing form of LTC?

2. {*incidence, social insurance*} Who provides most of the care for elderly people who need assistance with the daily tasks of living? How do these helpers get paid?

3. {*case-mix selection*} Does the administrator of a hospital want to admit patients who are more sick than average or less sick than average? Does the administrator of an LTC facility want to admit patients who are sicker than average or healthier than average? Why do LTC administrators face financial incentives that are different from those that hospital administrators face?

4. {*competition*} Hospitals compete for doctors and the newest technology. How do nursing homes compete? Does price play more or less of a role? What about technology?

5. {*supply controls*} Draw a set of supply and demand diagrams illustrating how CON legislation could cause waiting lists and increase the price of care.

6. {*labor markets*} Several major trends have characterized labor markets in the United States over the past 80 years: Wages have increased, life expectancy has increased, and women's participation in the labor force has increased. Discuss how each of these has affected the market for LTC services. Which has been more important in determining the shape of LTC markets: changes in labor market factors or changes in medical technology?

7. {*substitution*} Use supply and demand diagrams to show what would happen if additional LTC insurance allowed more substitution of nursing home care for hospital care. According to your diagram, do LTC expenditures increase or decrease? Do hospital expenditures increase or decrease? Do total expenditures (LTC + hospital) increase or decrease?

8. {*rent seeking* } If there is competition for CONs, what is the price of a CON? Who gets paid? Is the CON worth more than is paid for it? If so, who obtains these gains from trade?

9. {*shortages, discrimination*} Would a shortage of beds created by regulation make it easier or more difficult for a nursing home administrator to racially discriminate among patients for admission? Draw supply and demand graphs to illustrate.

10. {*risk*} Are the risks in LTC insurance different from the risks in hospital insurance?

11. {*substitution*} Does the federal and state-funded Medicaid program expand or contract the market for private LTC insurance? Who would benefit from a federal subsidy of private LTC insurance plans?

12. {*productivity, outcomes*} To measure the productivity of medical care, economists attempt to measure outcomes of treatment: increases in longevity, fewer sick days, increased earnings. Which measures would you use to compare the productivity of two nursing homes?

13. {*Medicaid, two-part market, tax incidence*} If you were elderly, would you be in favor of or against a proposal to increase the amount paid per day under Medicaid? Which factors would your response depend on?

14. {*management, vertical integration*} In what ways is a CCRC like an HMO? In what ways is a CCRC different? Are payments made on a similar or different basis? Which is more subject to adverse selection? To moral hazard? Which relies more on gatekeepers? On financial incentives to physicians?

15. { *incidence* } Which socioeconomic groups in the United States benefit most from extensive government funding of LTC? Is the flow of funds progressive or regressive?

16. { *risk aversion, Medigap insurance* } Virtually all elderly people in the United States qualify for Medicare. Almost 70 percent also purchase Medigap insurance, which covers copayments, deductibles, and often home health care and pharmaceuticals. Which insurance, Medicare or Medigap, provides the largest "welfare gain from risk pooling" (see Chapters 4 and 5). Does Medigap insurance increase or decrease the cost of Medicare?

ENDNOTES

1. Peter S. Arno, Carol Levine, and Margaret M. Memmott, "The Economic Value of Informal Caregiving," *Health Affairs* 18, no. 2 (1999): 182–188. France Weaver et al, "Proximity to Death and Participation in the Long-Term Care Market," *Health Economics* 18, no. 8 (2009): 867-883.
2. A. E. Benjamin, "An Historical Perspective on Home Care," *Milbank Quarterly* 71, no. 1 (1993): 129–166.
3. David M. Cutler and Ellen Meara, "The Medical Costs of the Young and Old: A Forty-Year Perspective," National Bureau of Economic Research Working Paper #6114, Cambridge, Mass. (July 1997).
4. The relative reduction since 1987 is even more pronounced among the oldest old aged 85+, who spent 6.9 times as much in 1987 but just 5.7 times as much in 2004. See Micah Hartman et al., "U.S. Health Spending by Age," *Health Affairs* 27, no. 1 (2008): w1–w12; James Lubitz et al., "Three Decades of Health Care Use By the Elderly, 1965–1998," *Health Affairs* 20, no. 2 (2001): 19–21.
5. Thomas E. Getzen, "Population Aging and the Growth of Health Expenditures," *Journal of Gerontology: Social Sciences* 47, no. 3 (1992): S98–S104.
6. Brenda C. Spillman and James Lubitz, "The Effect of Longevity on Spending for Acute and Long-Term Care," *New England Journal of Medicine* 342, no. 19 (2000): 1409–1415.
7. Robert L. Kane, Joseph G. Ouslander, and Itamar B. Abras, *Essentials of Clinical Geriatrics* (New York: McGraw-Hill, 1989), 30–44.
8. Susan Hughes, "Home Health Care," in Connie J. Evashwick, ed., *The Continuum of Long-Term Care* (Albany, N.Y.: Delmar Publishers, 1996), 61–81. H. S. Kaye, C. Harrington, and M. P. LaPlante, "Long-Term Care: Who Provides It, Who Gets it, Who Pays, and How Much?" *Health Affairs* 29, no. 1 (2010): 11-21.
9. Brian Burwell, William H. Crown, Carol O'Shaunessy, and Richard Price, "Financing Long-Term Care," in Connie Evashwick, ed., *The Continuum of Long-Term Care* (Albany, N.Y.: Delmar Publishers, 1996), 199.
10. William Aaronson, "Financing the Continuum of Care: A Disintegrating Past and an Integrating Future," in Connie Evashwick, ed., *The Continuum of Long-Term Care* (Albany, N.Y.: Delmar Publishers, 1996), 225.
11. William P. Scanlon, "A Theory of the Nursing Home Market," *Inquiry* 17, no. 1 (1980): 25–41.
12. Korbin Liu, Pamela Doty, and Kenneth Manton, "Medicaid Spend-Down in Nursing Homes," *The Gerontologist* 30, no. 10 (1990): 7; H. Temkin-Greener, M. Meiner, E. Petty, and J. Szydlowski, "Spending Down to Medicaid in the Nursing Home and in the Community," *Medical Care* 31, no. 8 (1993): 663–679.
13. Brian Burwell, *Middle-Class Welfare: Medicaid Estate Planning for Long-Term Care Coverage* (Lexington, Mass.: Systemetrics, 1991).
14. S. Moses, "The Fallacy of Impoverishment," *The Gerontologist* 30, no. 1 (1990): 21–25.
15. U.S. General Accounting Office, *Nursing Homes: Admission Problems for Medicaid Recipients and Attempts to Solve Them*, GAO Report #GAO/HRD-90-135 (Washington, D.C.: U.S. Government Printing Office, 1990).
16. John Nyman, "The Demand for Nursing Home Care," *Journal of Health Economics* 8, no. 2 (1989), 209-232; and "Excess Demand, the Percentage of Nursing Home Patients, and the Quality of Nursing Home Care," *Journal of Human Resources* 23, no. 1 (1988): 76–92.
17. P. Kemper, "The Evaluation of the National Long-Term Care Demonstration," *Health Services Research* 23, no. 1 special issue (1988).
18. S. Katz, A. B. Ford, R. W. Moskowitz, B. A. Jackson, and M. W. Jaffee, "Studies of Illness in the Aged. The Index of ADL: A Standardized Measure of Biological and Psychosocial Function," *Journal of the American Medical Association* 185, no. 12 (1963): 914-919.
19. J. A. Nyman and R. A. Connor, "Do Case-Mix Adjusted Nursing Home Reimbursements Actually Reflect Costs? Minnesota's Experience," *Journal of Health Economics* 13, no. 2 (1994): 145–162.
20. Barbara Martinez, "Home Care Yields Medicare Bounty," *Wall Street Journal,* April 26 2010; US Senate Finance Committee, *Staff Report on Home Health And the Medicare Therapy Threshold* (Washington, D.C.: U.S. Government Printing Office, 2011).
21. M. V. Pauly "Rational Non-purchase of Long-Term-Care Insurance." *Journal of Political Economy* 98, no. 1 (1990): 153-168; AT Cramer, GA Jensen, "Why Don't People Buy Long-Term-Care Insurance?" *Journal of Gerontology:*

Social Sciences 61, no. 4 (2006): S185-S193. Rebecca Vesely. "Heading for the Exit: Turmoil Hits Long-Term-Care Insurance Companies," *Modern Healthcare* (November 29, 2010): 32.

22. H. S. Ruchlin, "Continuing Care Retirement Communities: An Analysis of Financial Viability and Health Care Coverage," *The Gerontologist* 28, no. 2 (1989): 156–162; David G. Stevenson and David Grabowski, "Sizing up the Market for Assisted Living" *Health Affairs* 29, no. 1 (2010): 35-43.

23. B. K. Bucks, A. B. Kennickell, T. L. Mach, and K. B. Moore, "Changes in U.S. Family Finances from 2004 to 2007: Evidence from the Survey of Consumer Finances," *Federal Reserve Bulletin* (2008): A8–A38. http://www.federalreserve.gov/pubs/bulletin/.

24. Darius Lakdawalla and Tomas Philipson, "The Rise in Old-Age Longevity and the Market for Long-Term Care," *American Economic Review* 92, no. 1 (2002): 295–306.

25. George Anders and Laurie McGinley, "How Do You Tame a Wild U.S. Program? Slowly and Reluctantly. Medicare Home Health Visits Are a Boon for Entrepreneurs; Costs Explode 30% a Year," *Wall Street Journal,* March 6, 1996, p A1ff.

26. Paul L. Grimaldi, "Medicare's New Home Health Prospective Payment System Explained," *Health Care Financial Management* 54, no. 11 (2000): 46–56.

27. Nereraj Sood, Melinda Buntin, Jose Escarce, "Does How Much and How You Pay Matter? Evidence from the Inpatient Rehabilitation Care Prospective Payment System," *Journal of Health Economics* 27, no. 4 (2008): 1046–1059.

28. National Hospice and Palliative Care Organization. *NHPCO Facts and Figures, 2012.* EY Park-Lee and FH Decker, "Comparison of Home Health and Hospice Care Agencies by Organizational Characteristics and Services Provided: US 2007," *National Health Statistics Reports* #30, November 9, 2010. Staff Report, "FBI Arrests 5 Nurses in $9.3 Million Hospice Fraud," *Philadelphia Inquirer,* March 23, 2012. JE Perry and RC Stone, "In the Business of Dying: Questioning the Commercialization of Hospice," *Journal of Law, Medicine and Ethics* (Summer 2011): 224-234. Peter Waldman, "Aided By Referral Bonuses, Hospice Industry Blooms," Bloomberg News published in *The Washington Post/Bloomberg,* December 17, 2011.

CHAPTER 11

PHARMACEUTICALS

QUESTIONS

1. Which are more important in the pharmaceutical industry: fixed costs or variable costs?
2. How many drugs do Americans take? Who pays for them?
3. What events led to the regulation of prescription drugs by the Food and Drug Administration (FDA)?
4. Are patents a cost or an asset?
5. Why is so much more spent on marketing drugs than on marketing surgery or psychotherapy?
6. How profitable is the drug industry?
7. Do patents raise or lower the productivity of research?
8. Do generic drugs replace or compete with brand-name drugs?
9. How are prescription costs "managed" by insurance companies?
10. What are the major costs in developing a new drug?

In any given week, more than 80 percent of U.S. adults use some form of medication, with 50 percent taking a drug prescribed by a doctor.[1] Twelve prescriptions per year are filled for the average American. It is this "ethical" prescription pharmaceutical market that we examine in this chapter. Sales of creams, ointments, vitamins, herbal supplements, headache pills, digestive aids, and other over-the-counter (OTC) medications, which can be obtained without a prescription, amount to around $50 billion—a large sum, but only a fraction of the $290 billion spent on prescription drugs in 2010.[2] The cost structure (large sunk costs for research, development, and marketing, then very low variable cost per pill no matter how high the price) makes the economics of pharmaceuticals dramatically different from most medical care and more like software, books, DVDs, and other "information goods." Pharmaceuticals can be easily packaged, stored, and shipped overseas, which is a primary reason that this part of health production is truly international. U.S. companies make more than a third of their sales overseas, and several major U.S. suppliers are based in Europe and Asia (see "Pharmaceuticals" in Chapter 17).

Pharmaceuticals make up 10 percent of national health expenditures but are a much larger part of the free cash flow in health care. The reason is that the industry is so concentrated and profitable—consisting of a dozen companies earning billions of dollars. With many prices far above marginal cost, drug companies are vulnerable to criticism, and repeated calls have been made for price controls. However, it is evident even to critics that pharmaceuticals have been one of the major technological success stories of the 20th century, with new drugs extending life span and productivity at much lower cost than surgery and hospitalization. The profits earned by shareholders, while perhaps excessive in some cases, have been the incentive for expanding corporate research and development (R&D), which has increased from $2 billion in 1980 to $67 billion in 2010. The gains in health directly attributable to profit-driven pharmaceutical innovation are collectively worth far more than all sunk costs and shareholder dividends.

11.1   PHARMACEUTICAL REVENUES: SOURCES OF FINANCING

As with all health care services, funding for pharmaceutical products comes from a variety of sources, including patients, employers and private insurance, and federal and state governments (see Table 11.1). The process of obtaining a drug begins with the patient visiting a physician. After making a diagnosis, the physician might give the patient a prescription for a specific drug and directions for its use. Although all drugs are approved for sale by the **Food and Drug Administration (FDA)** based on specific indications, physicians may prescribe drugs as they think appropriate. When writing a prescription, physicians stipulate name and dosage but do not have to specify diagnosis. Hence the drug may be used "off-label" for unendorsed ailments. The prescription may be written using the generic scientific name of the drug or a brand name made up by the manufacturer that first patented the drug.

The patient usually takes the prescription to the local pharmacy, where a licensed pharmacist fills the prescription. Pharmacists provide additional information about how to take the drug and its potential side effects. If the drug has been in use for a long time, the original patent period might have expired and there is apt to be a chemically and biologically equivalent FDA-approved **generic drug** that is cheaper than the original brand-name version. The pharmacist usually substitutes the cheaper version unless the prescription explicitly requires the brand name (78 percent of all prescriptions were filled with generics in 2010, but generics cost so much less that they took just 20 percent of dollars spent). The average prescription has a retail cost of about $72: $138 for brand names and $35 for generics (Table 11.2).[3]

In 1970, 82 percent of all drug costs were paid by patients out of pocket. The little bit of drug insurance that was available operated retrospectively through "major medical" benefits, requiring the patient to submit bills and wait for payment, or through government programs for the indigent. This situation was totally reversed by 2012, when only 18 percent of prescription costs were paid out of pocket. Shifting payments to insurance and providing a "drug card" that could be used at the local pharmacy required the development of a new form of contractual intermediary: the **pharmacy benefit manager (PBM),** which took care of all claims and rebates that had to be processed. PBMs expanded rapidly and were responsible for most prescriptions filled in 2012.

Most patients have insurance and pay only the copayment, which currently averages $5 to $10 for generics and $20 to $45 for brand names. Some insurance plans require the patient to pay a percentage of the price (coinsurance) rather than a specified amount, and other insurance plans require the patient to pay in full when the prescription is filled and send a copy of the

TABLE 11.1	Sources of Funds for Pharmaceuticals Products
2012 Total	$918 per person, 10% of national health expenditures
Out of pocket	18%
Private insurance	44%
Medicare	25%
Medicaid	8%
Other public programs	5%

Source: CMS National Health Account Projections.

TABLE 11.2	Pharmaceutical Sales, R&D, and Profits			
Major Pharmaceuticals Manufacturers	**Revenues ($ millions, 2010)**	**U.S. Sales**	*Profit*	**A Major Drug**
Abbot	$35,166		*$4,626*	Humira
Amgen	15,053	12,700	*4,627*	Epogen
AstraZeneca	33,981	18,300	*8,053*	Nexium
Bristol-Myers/Squibb	19,484		*3,102*	Abilify
Eli Lilly	23,076	14,300	*5,069*	Cymbalta
Endo	1,716		*259*	Percodan
GlaxoSmithKline	44,460	13,600	*2,515*	Advair
Hoffman-LaRoche	51,000	13,800	*18,000*	Avastin
Johnson & Johnson	61,587	12,900	*13,334*	Tylenol
Merck	45,987	18,800	*861*	Singulair
Mylan	5,451		*345*	*Generics*
Novartis	50,624	15,700	*9,794*	Gleevec
Pfizer	67,791	26,000	*8,266*	Lipitor
Pudu Pharma	(privately held)			Oxycontin
Teva Pharmaceuticals	16,121	13,700	*3,331*	*generics*
Watson (generics)	3,567		*116*	*generics*
Total sales	$856,000	307,400		
generics	$231,000	$42,000		
R&D Expenditures	$67,400	$50,000		

Source: Standard & Poors Industry Profile, Pharmaceuticals, 2010, IMS Institute 2010, PhRMA Profile 1011.

bill for full or partial reimbursement later. These alternatives are more confusing and more cumbersome, which is one reason the market has shifted over time to the copayment system run by carve-out managed-care organizations, the PBMs. PBMs are subcontractors used by insurance companies to develop benefit plans, administer claims, and manage relationships with pharmaceutical companies (manufacturers) and retail pharmacies that operate behind the scenes and so are mostly invisible to patients. PBMs do not have any direct control over physicians' prescribing behavior. However, by creating a formulary (list of preferred drugs) and setting differential copayments (see the discussion of three-tiered benefits in Section 5.5), PBMs indirectly influence physicians' choices through patients' pocketbooks. In addition, PBMs have become sophisticated about calling physicians and suggesting product substitutions.

Inpatient Pharmaceuticals

The process of receiving a drug as an inpatient in a hospital differs significantly from the process used for outpatients. Again, it begins with a physician writing a prescription, but the prescription goes directly to the hospital pharmacy. The prescription is filled by the staff pharmacist and administered to the patient by the nursing staff. All medications are carefully noted on the patient's hospital chart.

Payment for an inpatient's drug depends on how the hospital is reimbursed for its services. Under Medicare, the hospital receives a flat, fixed payment based on patient diagnosis and the average cost of treating a patient with that diagnosis (DRG, as described in Section 8.2). A component of this payment is based on average drug utilization, but the hospital does not receive payment linked directly to drug utilization. A number of states have adopted all-payer DRG reimbursements that extend this form of payment to all patients. If the hospital is being paid on a per diem rate, average drug utilization generally is incorporated into the daily rate. Again, the hospital does not receive any payment directly associated with drug utilization. Only in cases where the hospital is paid on a "charges" basis is drug utilization itemized and billed directly to the patient or third-party payer. Thus the hospital usually bears the cost of paying for the drugs used there.

Because hospitals often bear the price of the drugs they administer to patients, they have a strong financial incentive to minimize the overall pharmaceutical budget. In pursuit of this objective, hospitals will establish their own formulary of drugs they keep in stock and from which physicians may prescribe. By negotiating with pharmaceutical companies over including particular drugs in the formulary, hospitals are able to use their market power to obtain discounts on drugs that have close competitors. However, a hospital must balance these economic decisions against antagonizing the physicians on the hospital medical staff, on whom the hospital must rely for admissions.

11.2 USES OF FUNDS

When a person goes to a local pharmacy to fill a prescription, the retailer gets 15 to 25 percent of the $72 (average price) total to cover the costs of labor, overhead, and profit.[4] Most of the remainder, 70 to 80 percent, goes to the pharmaceutical company that manufactured the drug. A small amount, 3 or 4 percent, goes to a wholesaler that obtains drugs from many manufacturers and then warehouses and delivers them to a variety of retail pharmacies. The flow of funds is complicated because most payments come from insurance companies (which must be compensated for risk bearing) and go through PBMs (which must get compensated for claims processing and negotiating), and the PBMs then receive "rebates" from the manufacturers, part of which are passed back to insurers. This flow of funds also depends in large part upon the negotiating power of each party. A diagram of this flow is presented in Figure 11.1, which has been simplified to reduce clutter and make the flow of funds more understandable. In addition, the amounts are approximate because only partial or incomplete survey estimates are available for many aspects of the industry. Patients using their own money are not involved in this complex set of transfers—and they lose! Patients without insurance pay list rather than discounted prices, which are 5 to 45 percent higher than what HMOs, insurance companies, and Medicaid plans pay for the identical prescription filled at the same pharmacy.[5]

Retail Pharmacies

There are 55,000 local pharmacies, with more than half in three large chains (CVS, Walgreens, and Rite-Aid).[6] Increased competitive pressure and the need for sophisticated information systems for insurance billing, ordering, marketing to consumers, and preventing drug interactions have caused the number of independent pharmacies to fall and an increasing number of them to be located in chain stores. Patients who have chronic illnesses and take large quantities of medicines on a continuing basis have increasingly turned to mail-order and Internet pharmacies with even lower prices and distribution costs. Mail order now accounts for more than 20 percent of retail drug sales. Most independent retail pharmacies purchase inventories from wholesalers that buy both generic and brand-name drugs from the manufacturers. Because of the many drugs available, most local pharmacies do not carry a large inventory of each drug but rely on computerized inventory systems to get daily deliveries from the wholesaler. Wholesalers and pharmacists usually cannot switch patients from one product to another (except for generic products). As a result, they are unable to exert market power against the manufacturer but instead must pay the full list price of the drug, often called the **average wholesale price** (**AWP**). Hospitals purchasing drugs for inpatient use might buy directly from the manufacturers, but they usually purchase from wholesalers.

FIGURE 11.1   Flow of Pharmaceutical Funds

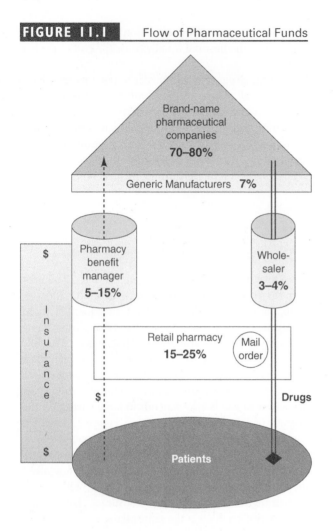

Wholesalers

Three companies (McKesson, Cardinal, and AmerisourceBergen) account for more than 80 percent of the wholesaling business. Their jobs are limited to warehousing and distribution; they play no role in the acquisition of patients or insurance financing. Thus, the physical movement of drugs—buying and selling on the wholesale side—is totally separate from the complex flow of funds on the patient/retail side. Because it has no effect on payments and moving drugs is cheap, wholesalers account for only a small fraction of total costs despite the large volume of items being shipped around.

Insurance Companies and PBMs

The financial side of the pharmaceutical business is made up of insurance companies and PBMs, some of which are not entirely distinguishable from one another because large insurers (such as Aetna, CIGNA, Wellpoint) have their own PBMs. Managed care has had a major impact on the way the pharmaceutical industry conducts business. PBMs consolidate the purchasing power of multiple insurance companies and employer health benefits plans covering millions of people, and thus they can force manufacturers to give sizable discounts. The big PBMs (Medco, Argus, Express Scripts, CVS/Caremark) have a majority of the business and are relatively independent, although they have equity ties to insurance entities, to pharmaceutical manufacturers, and to retail chains. Most of the total pharmaceutical dollars now flow through PBMs, leaving perhaps one-sixth still flowing through unmanaged insurance payment systems.

The PBM gets fees from the insurance company for handling claims (and is sometimes even a capitated, risk-bearing provider of benefits), but it gets most of its funding from pharmaceutical manufacturer discounts paid back as "rebates." Although the prescription passes through the wholesaler at list (AWP) price with a retail markup, the PBM negotiates with the manufacturer, and a rebate of 5 to 15 percent is paid directly to the PBM. Medicaid gets a special superdiscount of 15.1 percent based on the best available price given to any nongovernment buyer, which returned $5 billion to state budgets in 2002.[7] The fact that aggregate purchasing power is exercised in the form of mandatory rebates rather than price discounts makes the flow of funds obscure and hard to track, especially because some of the rebates get passed on the insurers and other parties. These hidden transfers make it difficult to determine exactly who gets what in dollar terms.[8] Health insurance premiums paid by employers and patients include prescription coverage, but the amount attributable to pharmaceuticals (with or without overhead) cannot be determined without using a set of arbitrary allocations. Thus, the percentages in Figure 11.1 should be considered approximations rather than exact measures.

Pharmaceutical Firms

About $290 billion dollars in 2012 went to the pharmaceutical manufacturing companies, accounting for the bulk (80 percent) of all drug costs. The top brand name blockbuster drugs (e.g., Lipitor, Zocor, Prevacid, Procrit, Plavix, Advair, Epogen, Nexium, Zoloft, Zyprexa) have more than $3 billion in annual sales, and a single drug can make or break a company (see Table 11.2). The largest pharmaceutical companies (Merck, Johnson & Johnson, Pfizer, GlaxoSmithKline) each have more than $30 billion in sales, and the top ten pharmaceutical companies account for 60 percent of all prescription dollars.[9] Conversely, although generics account for 75 percent of all prescription volume and are four of the ten most commonly prescribed drugs in terms of units, they account for only 21 percent of total sales in dollars.

TABLE 11.3	
Uses of Funds for Pharmaceutical Products	
Cost of goods	30%
Research & development	13%
Sales, marketing, admin	31%
Taxes	6%
Net income	20%

Source: CMS Health Care Industry Update—Pharmaceuticals, 2003.

The funds that flow into pharmaceutical firms are used for research and development (R&D), marketing, and profits to a significantly greater degree than is common in other industries (Table 11.3). Manufacturing the drugs takes about one quarter of pharmaceutical companies' resources. Most studies have shown that there are constant returns to scale in the manufacturing of pharmaceutical products; that is, the average manufacturing cost is independent of the amount produced. In part this is because most drugs are manufactured in small batches rather than in a continual process. Production in small batches is a result of the need to maintain high quality standards. Although large batches are generally more economical to manufacture, there may be a greater variance in the quality of the product and a greater chance that some of the units will have either too much or too little of the active ingredients. With pharmaceutical products, such deviations could be deadly, hence small manufacturing batches are the norm. However, the initial development of the sophisticated extraction and production process is itself very costly and constitutes a large fixed (sunk) cost, which gives rise to economies of scale.

Advertising and promotional activities account for 20 to 35 percent of the pharmaceutical dollar. These activities primarily consist of detailing, sampling, and journal advertising. Of these, detailing and sampling are the most important. Detailing involves a representative of the pharmaceutical firm calling on an individual physician. During this meeting, the representative discusses one or two products with the physician. For each drug discussed, the representative gives the physician the results of recent tests, explains how the drug works and what the potential side effects are, and discusses the advantages of this drug over competitors' drugs. The representative might give the physician literature on the drug, as well as free samples to pass on to patients. In addition, the detailer answers questions the physician might have about the drug or its use. The information presented and literature given to the physician must meet strict FDA guidelines. Empirical studies have shown that detailing can have a large impact on a physician's prescribing behavior and on the elasticity of demand for individual products. As a result of these studies, a number of politicians have charged that the promotional activities of the industry are wasteful and excessive and have called for increased regulation of the industry. Whether such actions are justified, and their overall social impact, are the subject of ongoing research and debate.

R&D expenditures account for 10 to 25 percent of the total pharmaceutical dollar and are best seen as (risky) investments in intangible capital (possible patents; see Chapter 12). Current cash flows are the result of past R&D expenditures. Future cash flows are the primary incentive for corporate R&D (see Chapter 12). Profits account for 10 to 25 percent of the pharmaceutical dollar. Pharmaceutical firms are consistently ranked among the most profitable by *Fortune* magazine and have been for many years. In 2009, average profitability was reported as 19 percent of sales, whereas median profitability of all industries was reported at 3.3 percent.[10]

Cost Structure

The *economics of the pharmaceutical industry are dominated by fixed costs.* Discovery, R&D, regulatory approval, and market introduction all are sunk costs when the first pill is sold. The cost of manufacturing an additional unit is a fraction of the price, usually less than 20 percent, and sometimes amounts to mere pennies on the dollar. After fixed costs are recovered, each additional unit sold is almost pure profit. This makes it worthwhile to put millions, even billions, into marketing. The pharmaceutical industry is an exemplar of the postmodern information economy, where a label is worth much more than the cost of the product on which it is placed. Other industries in which most costs are fixed, such as information technology (software, websites), media (movies, CDs, books), and luxury goods (clothes, perfume) tend to use mega-marketing techniques for the same reason—the gross margins (revenue less variable cost) are so attractive.

Such a disproportionate cost structure does not apply to the other parts of the pharmacy industry: retail drug stores, wholesalers, insurance companies, and PBMs. Although there are some economies of scale, costs rise almost proportionately (perhaps 80 percent) with volume. Because there are substantial incremental variable costs per unit, it is not worth pushing so hard for more sales or putting so much money into marketing. Hence, behavior in these parts of the industry resembles that of more traditional manufacturing and retail firms.

11.3 HISTORY AND REGULATION OF PHARMACEUTICALS

The pharmaceutical industry has existed in its current form since the 1930s. Before then, local pharmacists (or chemists) mixed potions and elixirs from bulk chemicals using either standardized formulas or their own concoctions. Today, the modern U.S. pharmaceutical industry comprises more than 1,200 firms that produce a wide range of products for treating and preventing disease, although the industry is dominated by a much smaller number (about 20) of very large firms. The pharmaceutical industry has drawn considerable attention for its pricing and promotional policies. Some politicians have alleged that the industry charges excessive prices and spends too much money promoting products to physicians. These allegations have resulted in calls to regulate prices in the pharmaceutical industry.

Regulation of the pharmaceutical industry and its products evolved during the 20th century in response to increased potency, effectiveness, and toxicity of drugs. Until the late 1800s, most "pharmaceutical preparations" had an immediate effect of making the patient feel better, although in most instances they did little to cure the underlying disease. This meant that patients could directly evaluate the benefits of the drug and did not need extensive guidance from health care professionals in choosing which products to use.

The first "modern" pharmaceutical product, diphtheria antitoxin, was developed in the 1890s and dramatically reduced the incidence of diphtheria. However, because this new drug did not have an immediate effect on the patient (it prevented the person from becoming sick), it was much more difficult for the patient to evaluate the drug's benefit. (Would he or she have gotten sick without the drug?) Also, although the benefits were not readily apparent to the patient, some of the dangerous side effects were all too obvious. Hence health care professionals with specialized knowledge about drugs became more involved in helping patients decide which products to use.

The first regulation of pharmaceutical products was the Biologics Control Act of 1902. This legislation was a direct response to a contaminated batch of diphtheria antitoxin that fatally infected 13 children. The incident contributed to overall concerns about the safety of the food and drug supply that were being raised in the popular press and in books, such as Upton Sinclair's *The Jungle*. These events were quickly followed by the passage of the Pure Food and Drug Act of 1906. Although the act focused primarily on the food supply, it required drug manufacturers to provide adequate labeling. Manufacturers either had to use a standardized formula for making the product or provide a complete list of their product's contents.

These companies were not producing pharmaceuticals the way today's integrated firms do. Mostly, they were producing bulk and specialty chemicals for sale to packaging firms and local pharmacies. They were contract producers, with firms providing similar lists of products and competing on the basis of price and service, not science.[11] Moreover, despite the production of many "drugs," few diseases could actually be cured or controlled by drugs. The 1902 and 1906 acts reduced the number of competitors, making the remaining firms larger and more profitable. Then the start of World War I brought an unexpected and inadvertent windfall. Germany, at that time the leader in chemical and pharmaceutical research, held most scientific and process patents. U.S. firms paid license fees for use of these patents but rarely did their own research. When the United States entered the war against Germany, the existing patents were voided or transferred to U.S. firms, and the production of specialty chemicals greatly increased (because obviously the nation could not depend on an enemy to provide medications).

U.S. firms came out of the war flush with profits, with a portfolio of patents taken from German firms such as Bayer and IG Farben, and vastly increased technological capabilities. During the 1920s and 1930s, pharmaceutical firms built a new strategy, forging alliances with physicians and being identified with "ethical" (prescribed) medications rather than industrial chemical suppliers and secret tonics for home use.[12] Previously, most drug profits had come from tonics and "patent medicines" (which did not have patents) using secret formulas (usually heavy on alcohol and opiates) with fancy names (Lydia's Little Liquid Drops, Dr. Johnson's Miracle Feelgood) marketed directly to people at medicine shows held in rural areas or general stores in town. After 1940, profits increasingly came from purified medicines with listed ingredients made at pharmaceutical companies under strict supervision and prescribed and administered by doctors.

In 1931, the regulatory aspects of the federal Bureau of Chemistry became known as the FDA, which today is responsible for evaluating new products and overseeing their manufacture (see Table 11.4). In this era before antibiotics, the discovery of broad-spectrum sulfa drugs was a major breakthrough. Although saving many lives, they also precipitated a major public disaster.

TABLE 11.4	Major Legislation Affecting Pharmaceuticals
1902	Biologics Control Act
1906	Pure Food and Drug Act
1938	Food, Drugs, and Cosmetics Act
1962	Harris-Kefauver Drug Act Amendments
1984	Hatch-Waxman Drug Price Competition and Patent Restoration Act
1992	Prescription Drug User Fee Act
2001	TRIPS: Agreement on Trade-Related Aspects of Intellectual Property Rights (World Trade Organization)

Produced as a yellow powder, sulfa was awkward to ingest in large quantities. The Massengill Company decided to provide a liquid formulation, but the powder would not dissolve in water or alcohol. Eventually the company produced Elixir Sulfanilamide by dissolving sulfa in ethylene glycol. This solvent, commonly referred to as antifreeze, is quite poisonous. In 1937 more than a hundred people who drank the new product convulsed from pain and suffered agonizing deaths. Outraged, the public called for sanctions but could find no law the company had broken. Massengill, an old and proud company, was mortified and anxious to make amends. Killing people with a toxic product was not yet against the law; therefore, the company pled guilty to "mislabeling" (technically "elixir" was supposed to mean "in alcohol") and paid a fine of $26,100, the largest such fine ever paid up to that time. Reaction to the incident led to major legislation.[13]

The Food, Drug, and Cosmetics Act of 1938 had several important provisions. First, it required preregistration of all new drugs with the FDA, giving the agency the opportunity to test the drug before marketing. The act also gave the FDA the mandate of preventing unsafe drugs from *entering* the market. The new law, however, specifically excluded drugs that were administered by "trained professionals" for testing purposes. Second, it increased the amount of information that had to be included on the label of any drug sold without a prescription. This information included statements of recommended uses and potential dangers. Drugs sold "by prescription only" were not held to these same labeling standards.

Through these labeling provisions, the Food, Drug, and Cosmetics Act created the first real distinction between prescription and over-the-counter (OTC) drugs. Although previously any non-narcotic could be sold as either prescription or OTC, after 1938 nearly all new drugs were classified as prescription only. This was an unintended effect of the law; the original intent was not to restrict self-medication but simply to place the use of the most dangerous drugs under professional supervision. However manufacturers soon realized that *restricting sales of a product to prescription only reduced the elasticity of demand,* because the physician writing the prescription was not directly paying for the drug and the patient paying for the drug rarely challenged the physician's authority. The lower price elasticity allowed the firm to charge a higher price because the patient and pharmacist could not substitute a cheaper product once the prescription was written. Moreover, requiring a prescription gave the appearance that the drug was more potent or effective. Finally, the medical profession strongly supported these restrictions. In part this was because the profession benefited indirectly (increased demand) by forcing patients to see a physician before receiving a drug for treatment.

During the 1940s, three key changes dramatically altered the pharmaceutical industry. First, new techniques for discovering and isolating potentially beneficial substances were developed in the process of discovering streptomycin. Second, the U.S. Patent Office ruled that the chemical modifications made to streptomycin, which enabled it to be isolated and purified, created a new product. The process that developed this product as well as the product itself were deemed patentable. Third, instead of licensing patents to competitors, as had been done in the past, pharmaceutical firms began to exercise their patent rights to control the production, distribution, and price of the product. Together, these changes ushered in the era of the modern pharmaceutical firm. These firms are R&D driven and use patents to maintain prices above short-run marginal cost and reap the rewards of R&D activities.

The 1950s and early 1960s represented a heyday of drug development, as one firm after another introduced "wonder drugs." Many states passed antisubstitution laws, which further reduced the elasticity of demand by requiring pharmacists to fill prescriptions as written rather than substituting cheaper generic products. However, questions began to arise about the effectiveness of some of these new drugs and if the prices were too high. In 1959, Senator Estes Kefauver's Antitrust and Monopoly Subcommittee began hearings on whether too many drugs that were minor variations of existing drugs were being introduced to extend the patent life of a product line, a concern that has a familiar ring today. However, it was the thalidomide incident in 1961–1962 that triggered passage of the 1962 Harris-Kefauver Drug Amendments and brought this heyday of drug development to a screeching halt.

Thalidomide was a drug used to treat nausea during pregnancy. Although it had not yet received FDA approval, it was being widely distributed to physicians for "experimental purposes" when it was discovered that it caused major birth defects in some babies born to women who had taken the drug. This inflamed fears that drug companies, in their rush to market new drugs and earn large profits, were "egregiously exposing humans to potentially harmful drugs during clinical trials."[14] Congress passed legislation that greatly increased the burden on pharmaceutical firms not only to show that their products were safe but also to show that they were effective when used in the manner directed. In addition, the testing procedures used to establish these results were put under the oversight of the FDA. The 1962 amendments also required pharmaceutical firms to follow "good manufacturing and laboratory practices" as defined by the FDA and gave the FDA the authority to inspect manufacturing plants. Finally, the 1962 amendments extended these testing requirements to both generic (identical) and similar (me-too) drugs. The new rules dramatically increased the length of time required to develop a new drug, from an average of 35 months in 1960 to 145 months in 1980, and also greatly increased costs. As a result, the rate of new drug introductions slowed, falling from 255 in the five prior years to just 20 per year afterward. The amendments also had a chilling effect on the introduction of generic products, because manufacturers of generics now had to duplicate all the research done by the pioneering firm to gain approval, whereas previously these drugs could avoid premarket testing through certification from the FDA that they were chemically identical and equivalent in effect.

In 1984, Congress passed the Drug Price Competition and Patent Term Restoration Act (known as the Hatch-Waxman Act after its sponsors), which attempted to remedy some of the problems created by the 1962 amendments. First, the act established the Abbreviated New Drug Application (ANDA), which allowed a generic manufacturer to show that its drug was "bioequivalent" to the pioneer manufacturer's product rather than repeating all the safety and efficacy studies. Since 1984, hundreds of products have been introduced under the ANDA provisions. Second, the act established a formula for increasing the patent life of a new product to restore some of the time (up to five years) lost during to the premarket regulatory process. The 1997 FDA Modernization Act made a number of changes to speed the approval of new drugs. It also allowed seriously ill patients easier access to experimental compounds, provided new incentives for development of pediatric medicines, and expanded the ability of pharmaceutical companies to provide information about off-label (unapproved) uses of drugs.

The World Trade Organization (WTO) brought drug patents into the global trading system through the Agreement on Trade-Related Aspects of Intellectual Property Rights (TRIPS) adopted at the November 2001 meeting in Doha, Qatar. The TRIPS agreement establishes minimum international obligations, including a patent term of 20 years and a period of exclusivity for clinical data. This agreement has been adopted by 140 countries and represents a major step forward. In negotiations, exceptions were provided to allow countries to take special measures to protect public health, thus creating special mechanisms to provide AIDS medications to developing countries at low cost.

Regulation of the pharmaceutical industry has evolved over the past hundred years by responding to the perceived needs for consumer protection and industry development, attempting to balance the benefits and costs of regulation. What began as a requirement for adequate labeling, ensuring that the public was protected from adulterated or misrepresented products, grew into a system in which consumers no longer make choices about the drugs they receive but rely on their physicians (and sometimes even third-party payers) to make these choices for them. Along the way, the entire industry was transformed from one that simply manufactured bulk products to one that spent $41 billion dollars actively searching for new products in 2011.

11.4   RESEARCH AND DEVELOPMENT

The pharmaceutical industry consists of many small companies, each producing only one or two products, and about 20 large global corporations that have broader product lines. Even in the largest corporations, however, one or two blockbuster drugs with sales in the billions of dollars bring in most of the revenue. The success or failure of even a single product could mean the success or failure of the corporation. As a result, new product launches and R&D drive competition. Development cost ranges from $150 million to $1.5 billion and can take more than 10 years. Once drugs are developed, patents are used to protect the new drug from competition. Patents give the innovator the exclusive right to manufacture and sell that product, once approved, for up to 22 years from the time of discovery. Pharmaceutical firms spent an amount equal to 17.7 percent of sales on R&D in 2001, more than four times the 4 percent of sales spent by the average nonpharmaceutical firm and significantly more than the 11.9 percent pharmaceutical companies spent on R&D in 1980.[15] To understand competition in this industry, one must be familiar with the R&D process.

There are six distinct steps in R&D, with the pharmaceutical company making decisions on whether to continue the project or abandon it at each step. The first step is the **discovery/ synthesis stage**, reflecting two very different approaches to new drug development. In discovery, natural chemical compounds having desirable properties are isolated from biological samples. Alternatively, in synthesis, a new synthetic compound is created in the laboratory based on the results of previous research or computer models. Once a new compound has been isolated, regardless of its source, it is generally immediately patented and then screened for pharmacologic activity and toxicity, first in vitro (i.e., in test tubes with tissue cultures) and then in animals. This **preclinical phase** can take up to three years, and literally thousands of compounds are examined and rejected for each one that moves on to the next stage of testing.

Once a promising compound has been found, the firm files an **Investigational New Drug (IND)** application with the FDA and, unless the application is rejected, the firm can begin testing in humans within 30 days of filing the application. There were 602 commercial INDs filed in 2010, somewhat below the average for the previous decade.[16]

Clinical trials (i.e., human testing) are generally conducted in three distinct phases (see Figure 11.2). **Phase I** testing is usually performed on a small number of healthy patients, although cancer drugs are typically tested on patients who are terminally ill because a high level of toxicity is generally necessary to kill the cancer cells. The objective of these studies is to obtain preliminary information on the toxicity and tolerable dosage range in humans. Generally, the drug is given sequentially to sets of three patients at each dosage level until a preset toxicity threshold is crossed (the acceptable toxicity level depends greatly on the nature of the disease the drug is intended to treat and the availability of alternative therapies) or until a predetermined dose is reached. During Phase I trials, data are also collected on the drug's

| **FIGURE 11.2** | Stages of Drug Testing |

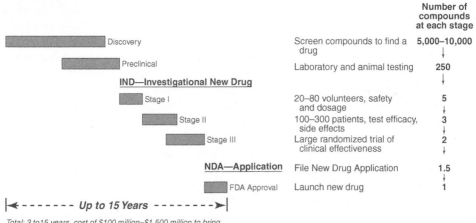

		Number of compounds at each stage
Discovery	Screen compounds to find a drug	5,000–10,000
Preclinical	Laboratory and animal testing	250
IND—Investigational New Drug		
Stage I	20–80 volunteers, safety and dosage	5
Stage II	100–300 patients, test efficacy, side effects	3
Stage III	Large randomized trial of clinical effectiveness	2
NDA—Application	File New Drug Application	1.5
FDA Approval	Launch new drug	1

|◄ - - - - - - - **Up to 15 Years** - - - - - - - ►|

Total: 3 to15 years, cost of $100 million–$1,500 million to bring one new drug to market.

absorption, its metabolic effects, and how the body eliminates the drug. These trials generally last one to two years. Although signs of efficacy are always encouraging, they are not necessary for moving on to the Phase II trials because the sample size is so small.

In **Phase II**, the drug is administered to a limited number of patients whom the drug is intended to benefit (generally 30–300 patients). The first evidence of efficacy is obtained at this stage, even though the general focus of the trial is still on safety. The trial also begins to examine the cumulative effects of the drug. On average, these trials last two to three years. If the safety profile continues to look good and there are signs of beneficial effects, the drug is moved into the final stage of human testing.

The final stage of clinical testing, the **Phase III** trials, are intended to establish the efficacy claims of the manufacturer. Large samples, commonly thousands of patients, are exposed to the new drug. Often, these trials are double blind, where neither the patient nor the treating physician knows whether a specific patient is taking the experimental drug or the control drug (perhaps a placebo). In addition to looking for evidence of efficacy, researchers continue to look at the safety profile of the drug and begin to look for potential adverse reactions to the drug.[17] To obtain information on the long-term effects of the drug, these Phase III clinical trials last an average of nearly three years.

When the clinical trials are under way, pharmaceutical firms typically continue their long-term animal testing, looking for possible adverse genetic and/or reproductive effects. Once the firm believes that it has sufficient information to show that the product is both safe and effective, it files a **New Drug Application (NDA)** with the FDA. Once the NDA is filed, the FDA has 60 days to determine whether there is sufficient information in the NDA for the agency to conduct a substantive review. Although the FDA is supposed to render a decision within six months, the Office of Technology Assessment estimated that for drugs approved in 1990, the average time from application to approval was nearly 30 months. Part of this delay was the result of additional testing required by the FDA before granting approval. A section of the FDA Modernization Act of 1997 extended the 1993 Prescription Drug User Fee Act, allowing the FDA to charge companies for applications and to use the money (more than $100 million per year) to hire extra personnel. This reduced the time required for approval to 16 months.

On average, only one out of five drugs for which an IND is filed with the FDA ultimately obtains FDA approval for use. As a result of the lengthy testing and approval process, a total of more than 10 years generally elapses from the time the firm first began spending money on researching a new product until a successful drug is introduced to the market. Because of this lengthy period of time, it is very important to take into account (capitalize) the opportunity cost of money. In perhaps the most comprehensive analysis to date, DiMasi and colleagues estimated direct out-of-pocket costs to pharmaceutical firms averaged $403 million, and when capitalized to present value at the point of market approval averaged $802 million (in year 2000 pretax dollars).[18] This figure includes the cost of projects abandoned along the way. Thus, every drug reaching the market represents a substantial investment of at-risk resources the firm made in many possible drugs in the hope that one would be approved and provide large profits many years later. Other research has estimated that just one out of five drugs approved has sufficient sales to cover the cost of R&D.[19]

A portfolio of patents, and the creativity and expertise of the scientists who generated them, are major assets to the pharmaceutical firm. Mergers are often carried out to obtain a set of patents, to fill out a product line, or to create synergies in research. Whereas marketing benefits from increased size, it appears that economies of scale and scope are quite limited in research.[20] Indeed, some of the most innovative work is performed in small boutique biotech firms with a few scientists moonlighting from university laboratories.

11.5   PHARMACOECONOMICS AND TECHNOLOGY ASSESSMENT

Are new drugs worth the high prices drug companies charge to cover their R&D and marketing costs? Drug discovery in general is obviously beneficial, but should we really pay $2 per pill (or $250 or $1,500 per prescription) for a particular drug? Could the company get by with charging only $1.50 per pill? Conversely, from the company's point of view, since blockbuster drugs are rare and must cover the cost of many failed R&D efforts, could the company reasonably charge $2.50 per pill? An entire discipline with its own scientific journals, conferences, and university professorships has developed to answer these questions. Known variously as **pharmacoeconomics**, disease management, outcomes research, and health technology assessment, this discipline attempts to determine the following:

- How much of a gain in health (outcome) will this drug provide?
- How much will people value that gain?
- Do other drugs provide similar effectiveness in treating this disease?
- How many people will benefit from this drug?
- Will some people benefit more than others?
- Will some people value the drug more than others?

A number of countries with national health systems have gone beyond asking questions and have empanelled experts to help the government make decisions about pharmaceutical reimbursement. Leading the field is the UK's National Institute for Clinical Effectiveness (NICE).[21] Established in 1999, NICE convenes groups of experts on request from the Department of Health to examine specific illness or therapies, then reviews medical studies and models costs and benefits to determine clinical effectiveness. Once the review is complete, a report is issued that is instrumental in determining payment policies. Other official review agencies include the Australian Pharmaceutical Benefits Advisory Committee (PBAC), Canadian Agency for Drugs and Technology in Health (CATH), and German Institute for Quality and Efficiency in Health Care (IQWIG). A drug may be approved at full price, considered so ineffective that it should not be reimbursed at all, sent out for further review, or placed in some intermediate category. For example, a *reference price* may be set that is equal to the current price of an equivalent drug already being used for that disease.

Even in the United States, where administrative pharmaceutical price controls do not exist, drug companies have found it useful to employ health economists to estimate the potential size of the market for a new drug and to create an economic justification to help sell the drug to price-conscious buyers with limited budgets (Medicaid, hospital pharmacies, and increasingly, PBMs) and to follow the activities of NICE and other national advisory bodies. Indeed, so many economists are now looking at the value of drugs that some doctors and pharmacists think that this is all there is to health economics, and some use the term "health economics" as a synonym for pharmacy value studies without considering all the other issues covered in the chapters of this textbook.

Most health economists in pharmaceutical companies are employed in the marketing department. Even though committed to objective social and medical science, their job is to sell drugs and to help the company sell the largest amount of drugs at the highest price possible (actually, to maximize the present value of future cash flows, which is a bit more complex). To obtain greater expertise and credibility, corporate health economists often work with or fund studies conducted at universities. However, as most economists would predict, studies funded by pharmaceutical companies are consistently more favorable to the products of those companies (and unfavorable to competitors) than those done independently, leading to increased calls that all conflicts of interest be publicly identified.[22] It is not realistic to expect that funding will have no effect on judgment, even for scientists.

11.6   INDUSTRY STRUCTURE AND COMPETITION

The market for pharmaceutical products can be divided into three segments based on the type of buyer: **individual** patients, **group** purchasers (hospitals, PBMs), and **government**. Competition for sales differs significantly across these segments. In the traditional retail market, physicians prescribe drugs and consumers and insurers pay for them. Because these actions are separate, individual patients have little influence over what the physician prescribes and, as a result, this market segment is not very price sensitive. Competition takes place among products on the basis of product quality, detailing to physicians, and sometimes direct advertising to consumers to get them to ask physicians for a specific brand name drug. **Detailing** is a form of marketing that is unique to the pharmaceutical industry. A salesperson, or detailer, provides a physician with detailed information on the approved uses of a product. Even though much of the demand for a drug may be for treating a disease for which the drug is not yet (or ever) approved by the FDA, detailers are prohibited from discussing such **off-label** uses of the product.[23] Studies have consistently shown that detailers greatly influence a physician's choice of drugs. Moreover, once a physician becomes familiar with a particular product, its method of action, and its potential side effects, he or she may be reluctant to try a new product unless it offers either a substantial advantage in efficacy or a decrease in side effects. Price tends not to be an important criterion for consumers. Because competition in this market is usually based on product quality, effectiveness, and detailing rather than price, generics have not been able gain as much ground as in the group or government markets.

The growth, and most of the change, has come in the managed segment. PBMs and hospitals paying directly for drugs can influence the purchase of drugs and can bargain effectively for discounts and rebates. These bulk purchasers are the ones most interested in and able to assess price and cost-effectiveness, and are where generics have had the greatest impact. When the patent expired on Eli Lilly's blockbuster drug Prozac, 70 percent of prescriptions were switched to generic substitutes within a single month, and prices eventually dropped to one-fifth the earlier level.[24] Most large pharmaceutical companies have developed sales, marketing, and research groups aimed at addressing the concerns of the managed market and provide extensive pharmacoeconomic studies to support their products.

To date, government purchasers have chosen not to fully exercise their **monopsony** market power on a drug-by-drug basis. Medicare part D explicitly disallows governmental price negotiations, and Medicaid has adopted a standardized discount policy that pharmaceutical firms can either accept or reject. Under this policy, the government is rebated an amount equal to 15.1 percent of the average wholesale price for Medicaid purchases, or equal to the best deal given by the drug company on a particular product. Similar provisions have been established for other government contracts. In exchange for agreeing to these discounts, Medicaid agreed not to establish restrictive formularies. Thus, although pharmaceutical firms must cut prices to sell in this market, they are essentially free to detail physicians on their products and do not face stiff competition from generics.

STRATEGIC PROTECTION OF PATENTS … AND PROFITS

Sales of Lipitor (*atorvastatin*) exceeded $7 billion in 2010, more than any other drug. The loss of patent protection in 2011 loomed as a major threat to profits, even for the largest pharmaceutical company in the world, Pfizer. Under the Waxman Act, the first generic producer would obtain 6 months' exclusivity as an incentive to enter the market. Back in 2000, many blockbuster drugs had partially deflected this strategy through "pay-for-delay," literally paying the first generic manufacturer a few million (or tens or hundreds of millions of dollars) to hold back production so that the brand name product could continue to sell at a monopoly price for that six months. The Federal Trade Commission brought action in numerous cases during 2000–2006 so that courts became increasingly skeptical and hostile to this tactic, with some holding that such contracts were *per se* illegal.[25] However, legal "workarounds" subsequently increased the number of patent litigation settlements that linked delays in generic production to compensation from the brand manufacturer from 0 in 2004 to 19 in 2009.

The first generic competitor for Lipitor was to be produced by Ranbaxy, but they faced major pressure in the courts and regulatory proceedings that delayed introduction of their version from June 2010 to November 2010. When they did get to market, Ranbaxy found that Pfizer had cut a deal with another generic company, Watson Pharmaceuticals, to produce an "authorized copycat" (in return for which Pfizer received 70 percent of Watson's revenues) and had also reduced the price of Lipitor while continuing to promote it heavily. In addition, Pfizer gave out special discount cards that allowed consumers to obtain a month's supply of brand name Lipitor with a copay of just $4, equal to or lower than most generic copays. These strategic moves to undercut Ranbaxy and retain market share were unusually aggressive, so much so that at least one major PBM, Express Scripts, advised all the health plans it works with not to accept the Pfizer deals for Lipitor.

It is still too early to tell how effective this strategic defense of Lipitor will be, but the initial indicators are not promising. Pfizer's behavior has been criticized as anticompetitive and harmful to health care cost control in the *New England Journal of Medicine*, the *New York Times*, and other newspapers. More significantly, Lipitor's share of the market has fallen by two-thirds after just two months, a decline somewhat more rapid than the average brand name losing patent over the last five years.[26]

Value, Cost, and Marketing

The structure of the pharmaceutical industry is dictated by a single fact: the large and important costs are all sunk costs. The value of a drug depends on how useful it is in treating disease, not how many years it took to conduct clinical trials or perfect the production process, or on the number of failed projects the company had to fund in order to get a winner. Research and testing to bring the pill to market costs so much more than manufacturing that there is essentially no rational connection between price and cost, however measured. Instead, value and price depend on therapeutic effectiveness.[27]

Medical "value" is worthless economically unless potential buyers know how effective a drug is. Treatment capability must be turned into effective demand. This means marketing. Given the large gross margin (profit per unit) caused by the combination of high sunk research costs and low per-unit variable production costs, it is inevitable that marketing will be much more important and expensive than physical distribution—as it is for products with a similar cost structure, such as software, movies, music, and perfume. Most drug marketing is directed toward doctors, because they are the ones who write prescriptions. For each practicing physician, pharmaceutical companies spent more than $2,500 on meals, events, and scientific meetings (some conducted in very nice resorts).[28] Spending on personal visits by industry representatives and free samples was more than $10,000 per doctor. The size of the expenditure on marketing indicates how valuable the power to influence doctors is in terms of company profits.

Marketing creates additional divergence between price and "unit cost" because the value of each pill increases as it becomes better and better known as a brand-name drug. Although clinical value might not depend on marketing, economic value does. Once the drug is launched in the market, any distinction between the value added from increased therapeutic effectiveness and the value added from increased marketing is not meaningful. (How much of a blockbuster movie's profits are derived from star power? From plot? From the cool 30-second trailer that drew everyone into standing in line to see it the first weekend?) Even the drastic difference in price between brand name and generic versions (20, 40, 50, or even 80 percent) probably underestimates the value added by marketing. Perfectly good drugs have languished almost unused for years because they were not being advertised and detailed to doctors.

Once marketing launches a drug, the brand name is worth something even if the drug has been superseded by superior competitors (similar to the way old sports stars still get used to sell athletic shoes). The brand-name version often continues to sell at the old high price even after the patent has expired in order to capture the consumer surplus of customers who are not price sensitive. Also, competition from generic manufacturers has created incentives for research-based, brand-name companies to introduce and subsequently patent minor changes in their most important products. These changes might include introducing a sustained release or once-a-day formulation, or changing the route of administration from injection to inhaler or pill. AstraZeneca made such an effort to shift users of Prilosec, its blockbuster antiulcer drug, to a new improved version, Nexium, which retained the distinctive purple coloration of the original and incorporated minor modifications protected by new patents to limit the impact from generic competitors.

The Prilosec/Nexium example illustrates an important aspect of the pharmaceutical market: Competition is between treatments for a specific disease (in this case, ulcers). Most drugs do not compete with one another because they are used for different illnesses. The real market is "treatments for disease X" and thus is much narrower than "all prescription drugs." Firms focus their research and marketing efforts on a particular set of diseases (cardiovascular, neurological, gastric), making the effective market share (and market power) of the top firm, or top three firms, more concentrated than it appears to be when reviewing industry-wide statistics.

The Role of Middlemen: Distribution versus Marketing

Wholesalers distribute drugs. They buy in bulk from pharmaceutical manufacturers and distribute on demand to retail pharmacies and hospitals. The customer is not involved in this back-office physical distribution network, and it is a commodity business with low margins. Conversely, the PBM never touches the physical product, but it controls the flow of customers and money, and for performing this market aggregating function, it is paid handsomely. The essential element here is control. Assume that a drug cures a horrible disease and thus is worth more than $1,000 to the patient, but production cost is only $1. This difference is up for grabs. If there is lots of competition, prices might get forced down toward $1.50, providing just enough for the costs of manufacture, distribution, and a small profit. If patents or market power keep competition out, then profits of $100 or $500 or even $999 per customer are possible. It is *that* possibility that makes marketing so valuable.

Consider how different the case of diamonds is. The product itself (not the label) is valuable; therefore, anyone involved in transport and transfer must be trustworthy and highly compensated: It is worth a lot of money to keep from losing a few diamonds. Jewelry stores can advise, but they cannot prescribe, 2 carats, extremely fine yellow-white, or Lucida cut. Hence the diamond market is almost the opposite of the pharmaceutical market; wholesaling and physical distribution are relatively profitable, while marketing is not because intense competition keeps jewelry store margins close to the cost of operations.

The essential question is control—who "owns" the business. To a large extent, the business of patients is controlled (owned) by the doctors who write the prescriptions for them. However, these doctors are prohibited by law and ethics from taking any of that $999 in surplus value. If there is only one treatment for an illness and it is protected by a patent, the company with the patent in effect "owns" the business. The main question becomes how much business (total sales) there will be. A company will detail doctors to push them to prescribe more, but it does not have to worry about competing drugs. If there are two or more treatments for an illness, the situation becomes more complex. In theory, the choice should be made by the patient, balancing therapeutic effectiveness, cost, and side effects. In that case, marketing focuses directly on the patient (**direct-to-consumer** (**DTC**) advertising). However, patients often do not have enough information or confidence to make complex choices and tend to rely on their doctors to advise them. Thus, the marketing effort (detailing, scientific meetings at nice resorts) is directed at the doctor.

STEPPING UP IN PRICE: PROVIGIL TO NUVIGIL

Provigil is a drug used to treat narcolepsy. Although only a modest seller ($950 million in 2008) it accounts for almost half the total sales of Cephalon, the company that makes it. Provigil went off patent and became subject to generic competition in 2012. To meet that challenge, the company brought out a longer-acting version, Nuvigil, which has a patent that extends to 2023. To switch consumers to the new drug rather than losing them to cheaper generic competition, Cephalon followed a strategy of aggressive price increases. The price per pill for Provigil stayed relatively steady around $5.00 after the drug's introduction in 1999 until being bumped above $6.00 in 2004 and to $8.71 in 2008.[29] Cephalon stated to investors that it planned to keep pushing the price upward to generate extra revenues (see Chapter 2 for discussion of *long-run* versus *short-run price elasticity* and *marginal revenue*) so that the new branded substitute could be priced significantly lower on a per-dose basis when it was introduced in 2010, thus gathering a dedicated block of users before generic competition could come in.

Patients who take the drug for its official FDA-approved uses and have health insurance did not experience much of the price increases, but Provigil is often taken off-label as a "lifestyle" drug to help patients stay awake during work or leisure activities rather than for diagnosed narcolepsy or related conditions (Cephalon agreed to pay a fine of $444 million in September 2008 to settle federal and state allegations that it illegally promoted off-label uses). Optional lifestyle use is not medically necessary, and hence even though a patient has obtained a prescription from a doctor, the bills are not covered by insurance. For patients without insurance, or for the many who use Provigil off-label, the price increases are substantial.

Insurance companies pay for most drugs, and they may be able to induce some patients to switch from treatment B to treatment A by making the copayment for B much larger. The insurance company might even insist that it will provide reimbursement for drug A, and only A, if that drug is chemically equivalent to B. In this case, the insurer and PBM capture some of the surplus. Notice how little market power and how little excess profit the pharmacy is able to get. Even though pharmacies are the point of contact where the patient obtains the drug, they have to fill the prescription as written by the doctor or as modified by the insurer (generic substitution, tiered copayments) and are not allowed to try to shift patients from A to B. Pharmacies are almost as neutral and powerless as wholesalers—they simply distribute pills from the manufacturer to the patient. It is much more difficult and costly at the individual retail end, which is why retail accounts for 15 to 25 percent of costs and wholesale only 3 to 4 percent, but there is not a lot of excess profit to be obtained here. Actually, one of the most lucrative parts of the retail pharmacy business is all the other stuff (candy, bandages) that pharmacies sell at above-average markups to people who come in to fill their prescriptions. That is, the pharmacy does not "own" the prescription business (because there are so many retail pharmacy competitors and wholesale prices are fixed), but it does own the idle shopping time of the patient who is waiting to have his or her prescription filled—and can exploit that to sell high-markup magazines, mints, and other items.

Research Productivity

Research is a sunk cost for drugs already on the market. These drugs would still be manufactured even if prices were reduced to the level of marginal cost, but then no new research would be undertaken. The high prices are the incentives for investing millions of dollars in the hope of making a discovery. Almost every economist and politician accepts this simple premise connecting research expenditures and innovation to the promise of future profits. However, some issues remain. How much profit is necessary to provide an incentive? If a company can make $1 billion on a new drug at a price of $30, will allowing the company to make $2 billion at a price of $60 double the productivity of its research labs—or increase it only by 10 percent? Although there is no question that higher profits lead to more research, the magnitude of the gains and the real importance to patients is still an open and relevant issue.

Research indicates that increases and decreases in R&D funding are more tied to short-run changes in past profits than to the changes in expected future profits as theory would predict.[30] More disturbing, it is not clear whether more R&D spending leads to the development of more innovative new drugs. Much of the expenditure goes for imitative "me-too" drugs to fight off the competitive threat from generics and chemically related drugs that other companies have made sufficiently different (by adding some side molecules or by using a new production process) to engineer around existing patents and claim their own brand names. Whereas 46 percent of all new drug approvals in 1991 were for new molecular entities (NMEs), by 2001 only 35 percent of approvals were for new molecules. Furthermore, only seven of these 24 NMEs were ranked by the FDA as priority drugs promising important advances entitled to expedited review, compared with 19 in 1999.[31] During the 1990s, research spending grew from $10 billion to $30 billion, yet the number of important new drugs brought to market fell, and the number of INDs submitted by pharmaceutical companies to the FDA declined from 2,116 to 1,872.

CLARITIN: DIRECT-TO-CONSUMER ADVERTISING, OVER-THE-COUNTER MEDICATION, AND PRICING

Claritin had a tortuous transition from laboratory to market. Schering-Plough submitted a new drug application (NDA) for the compound (scientific name, loratadine) in 1980, but

(Continued)

CLARITIN: DIRECT-TO-CONSUMER ADVERTISING, OVER-THE-COUNTER MEDICATION, AND PRICING (CONTINUED)

it did not obtain approval until 1993, by which time there were only five years left on the basic patent.[32] The FDA felt little pressure to approve what was classified as a me-too drug that promised little clinical advance over existing prescription and OTC antihistamine remedies for allergy and hay fever. However, when FDA rules regarding **direct-to-consumers** (**DTC**) advertising were relaxed in 1997, Schering-Plough spent $322 million promoting Claritin to the public. Ads featuring clear skies and happy faces (with pollen-carrying flowers in the background) were seen on TV shows, billboards, bus stops, and leaflets handed out on street corners. Sales of Claritin ballooned to more than $2.6 billion in 2000.

In clinical trials, 46 percent of allergy sufferers showed improvement with Claritin, compared with 35 percent who showed improvement when given a placebo. Tests indicated that Schering-Plough's old drug, Chlor-Trimeton, now sold cheaply over the counter, was equally or perhaps more effective in relieving symptoms, and it might not have been much more sleep-inducing when used in a low dose. Was it really worth paying six times as much for the new version? The question rarely arose because prescriptions were covered by insurance.

Wellpoint, a large health insurance company, sued in 1998 to force Claritin and similar allergy drugs to be sold over the counter without prescription, claiming that they clearly were safer than the existing OTC medications such as Chlor-Trimeton. If Claritin were declared safe enough to be used without a prescription, then it would no longer qualify for insurance reimbursement, consumers would have to pay out of pocket, and demand would become much more price sensitive. Despite concerted efforts by Schering-Plough and other pharmaceutical firms, the insurance companies made a persuasive case. In November 2002 the FDA approved Claritin for OTC use. Schering-Plough's stock dropped precipitously as the price of Claritin had to be cut, and cut again, to compete in the more wide-open OTC market, and as Johnson & Johnson and Wyeth geared up production of generic versions of loratadine to sell at less than $20.

Since then, trends have not improved and may have worsened, despite massive increases in R&D funding. The number of new drug approvals by the FDA has steadily fallen from 39 in 1997 to 27 in 2000 and down to just 21 in 2010 while the R&D cost per new drug doubled. The *Wall Street Journal,* Standard and Poor's industry surveys, *Modern Healthcare* magazine, and most reputable analysts agree that the major financial problem facing the industry is a lack of important new drugs in the pipeline. More than 15 years of increased R&D spending have not provided impressive results, making it hard to argue that having a bit more profit to pour into laboratories would make a big difference in the rate of therapeutic advances or drug discovery.

It may be that research productivity is in a stage of secular decline. Some analysts suggest that "discovery" methods have been played out, with most significant compounds already investigated and under patent, so that any surge of new drugs will have to come from "synthesis" and rational drug design, perhaps following from the increased understanding of fundamental disease processes brought about by deciphering the human genome. There is great hope for "precision" medicine personalized to the body chemistry of the individual.[33] Most analysts opine that a real therapeutic benefit from such breakthroughs is at least 10 (maybe 15, 25, or 35?) years in the future. Someday there will be designer drugs customized for each patient—not one pill for high cholesterol and another for gastric reflux, but one pill for the current health condition (and preventive needs) of Mr. ABC at age 36, who has decided to run a marathon and move to Tampa. The gains from that set of advances will be amazing—and a long time in coming.

SUGGESTIONS FOR FURTHER READING

Geeta Anand, "Support System: Through Charities, Drug Makers Help People—and Themselves," *Wall Street Journal,* December 1, 2005: 1.

Stirling Bryan, Jestyn Williams, and Shirley McIver, "Seeing the NICE Side of Cost-Effectiveness Analysis: A Qualitative Investigation of the Use of CEA in NICE Technology Appraisals," *Health Economics* 16, no. 2 (2007): 179–193.

Iain M. Cockburn and Rebecca M. Henderson, "Scale and Scope in Drug Development: Unpack the Advantages of Size in Pharmaceutical Research," *Journal of Health Economics* 20, no. 6 (2001): 1003–1057.

Daniel McFadden, "Free Markets and Fettered Consumers," *American Economic Review* 96, no. 1 (2006): 5–29.

Reza Mirnezami et al. "Preparing for Precision Medicine," *New England Journal of Medicine* 366, no. 6 (2012):489–491.

NICE: National Institute for Clinical Effectiveness http://www.nice.org.uk

Kaiser Family Foundation, *Prescription Drug Trends,* www.kff.org

Standard & Poor's Industry Surveys—Healthcare: Pharmaceuticals, December 2011. Standard & Poor's, www.standardandpoors.com

2011 Profile, PhRMA (Pharmaceutical Research and Manufacturers of America), www.phrma. org

SUMMARY

1. The average American fills 12 prescriptions a year. Pharmaceuticals were a **$290 billion industry** in 2012, for which government (41 percent) and private insurance (40 percent) paid most of the bills. Of all the funds flowing in, about 70 percent go to pharmaceutical companies, 20 percent to retail pharmacies, and 10 percent to PBMs and insurers, much of that in the form of rebates from manufacturers.

2. Once an industry that made most of its profits from household potions and elixirs, the pharmaceutical industry has been revolutionized by **science, regulation**, and **insurance**. Pharmacology is among the most successful of technologies, having greatly improved human welfare and generated enormous profits: 18.7 percent of sales in 2001, more than any other industry in the Fortune 500. A single successful drug can earn more than $5 billion in a year and make or break the company.

3. **R&D** of new products is a risky, lengthy, and costly process. Only one in a thousand compounds initially studied eventually makes it to the market. On average, the time from discovery to successful market introduction is more than 10 years, at a total cost of $800 million. The most costly parts of the process are the clinical trials needed to establish safety and efficacy claims, which can take up to five years and involve thousands of patients.

4. **Patent protection** means that the price of a drug is determined by its value to consumers, not the cost of production. The hope of making large profits from discovering the next blockbuster product keeps pharmaceutical firms investing in R&D and fuels progress in the pharmaceutical industry.

5. The **dominant** economic feature of the pharmaceutical industry is the large **sunk costs**, first for R&D and then for the physician detailing and marketing blitz required to launch sales. The marginal cost of producing additional pills is small; therefore most of the price is pure profit once these large fixed costs are covered. The ability to control the flow of funds determines who will hold onto most of these profits; the brand-name manufacturer with a patent, the generic competitor, the government, the physician, the PBM, the insurance company, or the patient.

6. **Generics** (chemically identical compounds made by other firms) have increased in importance since the legal changes in 1984 enabled easier approval. Generic drugs sell for

much less than branded products ($25 versus $75) and have been increasingly successful as the **price-sensitive** managed-care PBM market has grown.

7.   Pharmaceutical manufacturers have begun to respond to changes in their markets brought about by managed care and generic competition. These changes include the use of discounts, development of **pharmacoeconomics** and disease management, and the development of various forms of risk-sharing contracts.

PROBLEMS

1.   {*value*} What determines the price of a drug?

2.   {*economic structure*} Why are fixed costs more important for pharmaceuticals than physical therapy? How does this affect marketing expenditures?

3.   {*regulation*} What events led to the formation of the FDA? Does regulation change because of successes or because of failures?

4.   {*dynamic efficiency*} Do patents raise or lower the productivity of research?

5.   {*incentives*} How are prescription costs "managed" by insurance companies?

6.   {*flow of funds*} What fraction of the total cost of pharmaceuticals is paid for directly by patients? Does this mean that price is more, or less, important than for other types of medical care?

7.   {*research, incidence*} How is most pharmaceutical research paid for? What is the most costly aspect of pharmaceutical research?

8.   {*market segmentation*} How many distinct market segments exist in the pharmaceutical industry? How do these segments differ?

9.   {*competition*} On what basis do pharmaceutical firms compete in each market segment? Is price a more important factor for the choice of which doctor to see or for which drug is prescribed?

10.   {*insurance coverage*} The major form of health insurance coverage for the elderly is Medicare, and the elderly are much heavier users of pharmaceuticals than other groups. It would seem reasonable to expect that Medicare is the largest source of payment for drugs. Is it?

11.   {*marginal costs, revenues*} Do hospitals have more of an incentive to control the costs of surgical implants, anesthesiologists' fees, or pharmaceuticals? In which case do they bear the highest fraction of marginal cost? In which case do they receive the highest fraction of marginal revenue?

12.   {*patents*} How would a change in the length of the patent period affect the structure of the pharmaceutical industry?

13.   {*competition*} Marketing accounts for a much larger portion of the cost of pharmaceuticals than the cost of other forms of care. Why? To whom are most pharmaceutical marketing efforts targeted?

14.   {*capital investment*} If $50 million is invested in a drug that subsequently fails to gain approval from the FDA, what is the rate of return on this investment? Are pharmaceutical firms more, or less, capital intensive than hospitals? Than doctor's office practices?

15.   {*antitrust*} Because FDA regulations limit the entry of new drugs into the market, do they constitute an "unfair restraint of trade" that reduces competition and raises prices to consumers?

16. {*price elasticity*} When a brand-name drug loses patent protection after 17 years and competing generic products enter the market, will the price of the brand-name drug increase or decrease? (*Hint:* What changes occur in the brand-name drug's demand curve?)

17. {*risk*} Which form of investment is more risky: developing a new drug or building a new nursing home? Which type of publicly traded for-profit firm would you expect to show greater variability in earnings, a pharmaceutical firm or a nursing home chain? (*Hint:* See Chapter 12).

ENDNOTES

1. David W. Kaufman et al., "Recent Patterns of Medication Use in the Ambulatory Adult Population of the United States," *Journal of the American Medical Association* 287, no. 3 (2002): 337–344. IMS Institute for Health Informatics, *Use of Medicines in the United States,* www.ims.com.
2. "Drugs," *The Economist,* June 3, 2000: 106.
3. Kaiser Family Foundation, *Prescription Drug Trends,* May 2010. (www.kff.org).
4. Kaiser Family Foundation, *Prescription Drug Trends,* 2000, Exhibit 3.2.
5. John K. Iglehart, "Medicare and Prescription Drugs," *New England Journal of Medicine* 344, no. 13 (2001): 1010–1015; *Prescription Drug Trends 2000,* Exhibit 1.4.
6. IMS Institute for Health Informatics, "The Use of Medicines in the United States." www.ims.com. Pembroke Consulting, "Pharmacy Market Share 2011." www.pembrokeconsulting.com.
7. Kaiser Family Foundation, *Prescription Drug Trends,* May 2011.
8. Ernst Berndt, "Pricing and Reimbursement in U.S. Pharmaceutical Markets," NBER working paper #16297, August 2010; David McCann, "Drug Companies May Win This Drug War: Express Scripts and Walgreen," *CFO Magazine,* March 2012: 27.
9. *Standard & Poor's Industry Surveys—Healthcare: Pharmaceuticals,* December 2011, Standard & Poor's (www.standardandpoors.com).
10. "Industry Rankings," *Fortune,* April 15, 2011, www.money.cnn.com/fortune/
11. Jonathan Leibenau, *Medical Science and Medical Industry: The Formation of the American Pharmaceutical Industry* (London: Macmillan, 1987), 34: 79.
12. Edward Kremers and George Urdang, *History of Pharmacy,* 2nd ed. (Philadelphia: Lippincott, 1951).
13. Peter Temin, *Taking Your Medicine: Drug Regulation in the U.S.* (Boston: Harvard University Press, 1980).
14. S. Peltzman, "An Evaluation of Consumer Protection Legislation: The 1962 Drug Amendments," *Journal of Political Economy* 81, no. 5 (1973): 1050–1051.
15. *Standard & Poor's Industry Surveys: Health–Pharmaceuticals,* December 2011, Standard & Poor's (www.standardandpoors.com).
16. PhRMA, *Pharmaceutical Industry Profile 2011,* www.phrma.org.; *Standard & Poor's Industry Surveys: Health–Pharmaceuticals,* December 2011, Standard & Poor's (www.standardandpoors.com); FDA, "NMEs Approved by CDER 2006-2010" www.FDA.gov
17. Despite the relatively large sample sizes, many important adverse reactions can be missed during the Phase III studies because they have a low probability of occurring. For example, a 1:10,000 adverse reaction causing death could easily go unnoticed in a Phase III trial on several thousand patients, even though it could cause 30,000 deaths if the drug were released to all 300 million citizens. As a result, when a new drug is released, the FDA requires the pharmaceutical firm to conduct extensive postmarketing surveillance for any adverse reactions and to immediately report all deaths of people taking the drug, regardless of whether there appears to be a direct link between the death and the drug use.
18. JA Vernon, JH Golec, J DiMasi, "Drug Development Costs When Financial Risk is Measured using the Fama-French Three-Factor Model," *Health Economics* 19, no. 8 (2010):1002–1005; CP Adams V Brannter, "Spending on New Drug Development," *Health Economics* 19, no. 2 (2010):130–142; J. A. DiMasi, R. W. Hansen, H. G. Grabowski, and L. Lasagna, "The Price of Innovation: New Estimates of Drug Development Costs," *Journal of Health Economics* 22, (2003): 151–185.
19. Henry J. Grabowski and John Vernon, "A New Look at the Returns and Risks to Pharmaceutical R&D," *Management Science* 36, no. 7 (1990): 804–821.
20. Iain M. Cockburn and Rebecca M. Henderson, "Scale and Scope in Drug Development: Unpack the Advantages of Size in Pharmaceutical Research," *Journal of Health Economics* 20(6): 1033–1057, 2001.
21. Stirling Byan, Jestyn Williams, and Shirley McIver, "Seeing the NICE Side of Cost-Effectiveness Analysis: A Qualitative Investigation of the Use of CEA in NICE Technology Appraisals," *Health Economics* 16, no. 2 (2007): 179–193.

22. Niteesh K. Choudhry, Henry Thomas Stelfox, and Allan S. Detsky, "Relationships Between Authors of Clinical Practice Guidelines and the Pharmaceutical Industry," *Journal of the American Medical Association* 287, no. 5 (2002): 612–617; H. T. Stelfox, G. Chua, K. O'Rourke, A. S. Detsky, "Conflict of Interest in the Debate Over Calcium Channel Antagonists," *New England Journal of Medicine* 338, no. 2 (1998): 101–106; F. Davidoff et al., "Sponsorship, Authorship, and Accountability," *Journal of the American Medical Association* 286, no. 10 (2001): 1232–1234.

23. As discussed earlier, although a product is approved by the Food and Drug Administration for a specific use or indication and some drugs have multiple indications, physicians are permitted to prescribe the product as they see fit. At the same time, physicians and drug companies are always exploring potentially new (or related) uses for the drug. The results of these studies are often published in the literature long before a new indication is obtained from the FDA. As a result of these publications, many drugs are prescribed for conditions outside of their indications. This practice is called off-label prescribing.

24. Ernst Berndt and Murray Aitken, "Brand Loyalty, Generic Entry and Price Competition in Pharmaceuticals in the Quarter Century After the 1984 Waxman-Hatch Legislation," NBER working paper #16431, October 2010: IMS, "The Use of Medicines in the US: Review of 2010." www.IMS.com.

25. U.S. Federal Trade Commission, *Pay-For-Delay: How Drug Company Pay-Offs Cost Consumers Billions.* January 2010, www.FTC.gov

26. C. A. Jackevicius, M. M. Chou, J. S. Ross, et al., "Generic Atorvastatin and Health Care Costs," *New England Journal of Medicine* 366, no. 3 (2011): 201–204; Drug Channels, "Is Pfizer's Lipitor Strategy Working?" www.drugchannels.net, January 2012; "Generics Take Toll on Pfizer, Lilly Profits," *Chicago Tribune,* January 31, 2012. "Cliffhanger: Big Pharma Struggles to Protect its Blockbusters as They Lose Patent Protection," *The Economist,* December 3 2011: 76. Note: As of July 2012, Pfizer appeared to have discontinued its efforts to protect the "Lipitor" brand and accepted that atorvastatin had become a generic.

27. Ernst Berndt, "Pricing and Reimbursement in US Pharmaceutical Markets," NBER working paper #16297, August 2010. Z. John Lu and William S. Comanor, "Strategic Pricing of New Pharmaceuticals," *Review of Economics and Statistics* 80, no. 1 (2002): 108–118.

28. Scott Hensley, "AMA, Prescription Drug Makers Agree Ethics Policy Needs Better Implementation," *Wall Street Journal,* January 21, 2002.

29. Jonathan D. Rockoff, "How a Drug Maker Tries to Outwit Generics," *Wall Street Journal,* November 17, 2008.

30. F. M. Scherer, "The Link Between Gross Profitability and Pharmaceutical R&D Spending," *Health Affairs* 20, no. 5 (2001): 216–221.

31. See note 16.

32. Stephen S. Hall, "The Claritin Effect: Prescription for Profit," *New York Times* Magazine Section, March 11, 2001: 40 ff.; Laura Benko, "Ugly Wait at the Counter: Insurer Pushes to Make Allergy Drugs Nonprescription," *Modern Healthcare,* August 6, 2001: 22–23; Cynthia A. Jackevicius et al., "Use of Ezetimibe in the U.S. and Canada," *New England Journal of Medicine* 358, no. 17 (2008): 1819–1828. Dharval Dave and Henry Saffer, "The Impact of Direct-To-Consumer Advertising on Pharmaceutical Prices and Demand," NBER working paper #15969, May 2010.

33. R. Mirnezami, J. Nicholson, A. Darzi, "Preparing for Precision Medicine," *New England Journal of Medicine* 366, no. 6 (2012):489–491.

CHAPTER 12

FINANCING AND OWNERSHIP OF HEALTH CARE PROVIDERS

QUESTIONS

1. How much is a year of medical education worth?

2. Which faces greater risk of bankruptcy: a nursing home company or a pharmaceutical company? Which has the more diversified "portfolio" of assets?

3. What are the major financial risks facing an insurance company?

4. Does financial innovation in health care improve productivity and consumer welfare the way technological innovation does?

5. Do changes in Medicare change the value of hospitals? Do they change the value of the hospitals' bonds?

6. Is an insurance company more concerned about fixed capital or working capital? Does this make it easier or harder to finance rapid growth?

7. Why did hospitals borrow so much and load up their balance sheets with debt during the 1980s?

8. Who owns a nonprofit hospital? Who gets the profits?

The previous chapter (Pharmaceuticals) reported an estimate of $1.2 billion for the cost of each new drug researched, tested, and approved by the FDA. It might have surprised you that half of that cost was indirect, the opportunity cost of the money invested. How can it cost an extra $600 million for financing? Because the $600 million for clinical testing and other direct costs had to be paid in advance, over *many years*, and to cover the cost of many failures. Investors only invested because they hoped that they *might* be successful and double their money. This chapter briefly reviews how **time** and **risk**, the core elements of finance, are used to calculate the opportunity cost of capital, rate of return, value, stock price, and so on. These basic finance tools are then used to analyze some aspects of medicine (physician education, nursing homes, biotech). That raises the question of why so many health care organizations are nonprofit and how they differ from for-profit corporations such as a pharmaceutical firms. Concepts of ownership and agency illustrate how profit or nonprofit status can affect efficiency, expansion, and scope of hospitals, nursing homes, or medical education.

12.1 WHAT IS FINANCING?

For any for-profit or nonprofit organization, whether in health care, farming, or computer services, the total inflow of money must exceed the cumulative outflow or the organization ceases to exist. The funds can come in the form of loans, gifts, equity capital, sales, or reimbursements, but if the amount that has gone out ever exceeds the amount that has come in, the organization can no longer pay its bills and bankruptcy occurs. This poses significant issues at each point in the life cycle of an organization from beginning to end:

- **Start-up** financing must come from somewhere before operations can begin.
- **Regular operations** must generate funds: Revenues must be greater than expenses.
- **Ending residual** funds (or debts) must be transferred or cleared.

The three elements are interrelated but distinct. Corporate finance textbooks deal more with the start-up (debt and equity) and ending residual (mergers and acquisitions, bankruptcy) phases but do not say much about ordinary business operations. In contrast, health officials often talk about financing as if it were only a matter of getting the operating revenues to stay above expenses and usually leave start-up and ending issues aside. The CFO (chief financial officer) of an organization must deal with both, although the relative allocation of effort differs markedly across industries.[1] In a public health center, the CFO spends most of his or her time on transactions: filing for reimbursement, negotiating rates, paying bills, and overseeing all of the daily operational tasks common to the accounting department. A real estate CFO only occasionally thinks about how rents are collected or utility bills are paid but focuses constantly on buying and selling properties, the interest rates on loans, and the ability to raise equity capital by selling shares in the market.

Physicians might or might not think of their careers in financial terms. People are often attracted to medicine at an early age and consider it a job in which they can help people, deal with the latest scientific advances, and not worry too much about money. On the other hand, aspiring doctors also know that medical school takes a long time, costs a lot, and provides better than average incomes. Junior physicians worry about paying back school loans and how difficult it is to start a practice, so many of them work on salary for a clinic or a hospital for a while to accumulate funds. Conversely, senior physicians are often trying to extract capitalized value from their successful practices and patient goodwill as they get older and no longer want to work so many hours.

In medicine, unlike real estate or banking, finance is not the main interest. Yet without financing a doctor cannot set up a practice or keep the door open any easier than a bank or shopping mall can. The development of financial institutions and intermediaries such as guaranteed loans, tax-exempt municipal bonds, insurance and reinsurance, and the use of venture capital to finance biotechnology research has been crucial to the growth of modern medicine. Careful review of a few simple financial terms and equations can help us understand certain aspects of the practice of medicine. Students wanting more background than can be provided in this very brief review should consult one of the standard finance texts such as Brealey and Myers's *Principles of Corporate Finance* or Louis Gapenski's *Understanding Health Care Finance*.

12.2 VALUE AND RATE OF RETURN

The Time Value of Money

Is it worthwhile to spend all those years studying hard and paying a high tuition in order to become a doctor? As economists, we have to conclude from the fact that people choose to do so that it must seem worthwhile to them, but that is also true of people who study poetry or art history or who take a few dance lessons or join a gym just to look better. What about in strictly financial terms, leaving aside all of the other considerations (which may be more important but can here usefully be ignored)? Most people think that becoming a doctor is financially worthwhile because physician incomes are higher than average ($200,000 versus $42,000), but a number of other factors must be accounted for even in a strictly financial analysis: tuition paid, long hours, years of unpaid study and practice, the fact that medical students are above-average to begin with and would probably earn more anyway, the chance of flunking out or graduating and being hit by a bus two weeks later, and so on. To begin, it is helpful to start with a simple example: A hypothetical therapist who is graduating in May with a BS and will earn $40,000, but could spend the extra year at school necessary to obtain an MS in order to earn a higher annual salary of $46,000. Is this worthwhile? More specifically, what is the rate of return on the MS degree compared to the BS?

To get the higher salary, the therapist will have to give up working for a year (opportunity cost) but will gain a higher salary ($46,000 − $40,000). The approximate rate of return is found by considering "gains" divided by "costs."

$$(\text{approximate}) \text{ Rate of Return} = \text{Gains} \div \text{Costs} = \$6,000/\$40,000 = 0.15 \text{ or } 15\%$$

Another way of stating this is to say that if one put $40,000 in an investment paying a 15 percent rate of return, then one would receive $6,000 each year. This is an approximation with many simplifying assumptions to make the calculation easy: the cost of tuition, the work may be harder, earnings will not last forever but only until age 60 or 70, taxes will take part of the raise and so on. Nonetheless, it is a pretty good first approximation.

Interest Rates and Present Value

If the therapist put $40,000 in a bank account with a 6 percent annualized rate of interest, at the end of the year the balance would be ($40,000) × (1.06) = $42,400. After five years, it would be $40,000 × (1.06) × (1.06) × (1.06) × (1.06) × (1.06) = $53,529. Repeat multiplication or compounding means that the five-year return is not five times 6 percent (that would be 30 percent) but actually 1.3382 times the original amount, or 33.82 percent.

In finance class, you probably learned that getting $53,529 five years from now (the future value) was equivalent to getting $40,000 today if the interest rate is 6 percent. Stated succinctly, the **present value** of $53,529 in five years at 6 percent is $40,000. This means that the present value of a single dollar received in five years (at 6 percent interest) is $40,000/$53,529 = $0.75 (more precisely, $0.747258), which is equivalent to 1/1.3382 or 1 divided by 1.06 five times. The present value of each dollar next year at 8 percent is $1/1.08 = $0.9259, and the present value of each dollar in five years at 8 percent is (letting you do the division five times on your own calculator) $0.68. The present value of each dollar received 40 years from now at 8 percent is less than $0.05, which is why we often ignore the financial consequences of money far into the future.

Note, however, that the present value of a dollar received in 40 years evaluated at 6 percent is more than twice as large ($0.09722), and at 3 percent it is substantially larger ($0.3066). At the 15 percent rate of return the therapist is getting on his education, the present value of a dollar in 40 years is less than one-half penny ($0.00373)—so one could say that from a financial point of view, if rates are that high, things happening 40 years from now only matter 1/300th as much as they do today.

The discount (reduction in value) is obviously less if the waiting period is shorter. Thus although the present value of a dollar received in 40 years at 6 percent is $0.10, for a wait of 10 years the value of a dollar has fallen only to $0.55. Differences in interest rates matter more the longer the period. The difference between 6 percent and 8 percent is large in 40 years and gigantic after a century. The difference between annual rates of 6 percent and 15 percent is substantial even over a single year, but it might not make much difference to someone borrowing money for just a week or two.

Which rate should be used to calculate present value? It depends (see your finance textbook for more discussion). The "appropriate" rate of return for a month is different from the rate for a year, the rate for a month with 28 days is different from the rate for a month with 31 days, and it might also vary from one year to the next. The present value is determined by applying the appropriate discount for each period. For example, if the interest rate in the first year is 6 percent, then 15 percent in the second year, and 8 percent in the third year, the present value is $1 \div [(1.06) \times (1.15) \times (1.08)] = \$0.7596$ today for each dollar received in three years.

What is the gain from obtaining an MS degree described above worth? Cash flows that are the same in each period (\$6,000) and last forever are called a **perpetuity**, and if the same interest rate is used for discounting each period, a single equation links present value, annual payment, and interest rate.

Present Value of a Perpetuity = (\$ amount)/(interest rate) = $\$6,000/0.15 = \$40,000$

This is just a formal restatement of the remark made above, "If one put \$40,000 in an investment paying a 15 percent rate of return, then one would receive \$6,000 each year." But is 15 percent the appropriate rate of return? If instead of getting an education, one put money in a bank at 6 percent, it would take $\$6,000 \div 0.06 = \$100,000$ on deposit to earn \$6,000 each year. Is the value of an extra \$6,000 per year in salary worth \$40,000 or \$100,000? How can the therapist correctly evaluate the financial impact of going to school relative to alternative investments of his time?

IRR: The Internal Rate of Return

The first calculation in the example above told us that spending a year getting an MS provides approximately a 15 percent rate of return, which seems substantially better than the 6 percent return the bank would provide if he spent the year working and deposited all paychecks into a savings account. Comparisons based on rates of return are often used by financial analysts because they are quick and easy to understand, and they also avoid the forced choice of one (or two or three) interest rates for discounting to find present value. Such calculations are called the *internal rate of return* (IRR) because they require that the analyst know only the cash flows of the project itself and not external considerations such as the market interest rate(s), what the potential risks are, future tax rates, and other factors affecting the decision as to which discount rate might be appropriate. IRR calculations are more objective and purely financial because they stay away from judgments and external considerations. For any given set of cash flows, every financial analyst would calculate the same IRR. If asked to determine "true" value, each would have to apply external assumptions, and to the extent that those analysts' assumptions varied, so would their estimates of value.

The calculation of IRR is easy for a perpetuity, but if the cash flows are not the same in each period (and in most business they are not), there is no simple formula to determine IRR. Fortunately we have computers with spreadsheets, and we can make use of the more general definition of IRR as the interest rate that, when used to discount a set of cash flows, makes the net present value neither positive nor negative but just equal to 0.

Internal Rate of Return = *the interest rate at which Net Present Value = 0*

For the typical project that requires initial investment to gain future rewards, if the first interest rate assumption makes the PV > 0 (positive), then keep raising the interest rate in the spreadsheet until PV = 0. If the initial interest rate estimate makes PV negative, then reduce the interest rate. There are several problems at the end of the chapter to give you practice in finding IRRs. For now, consider the simple example used above with investment of $40,000 and returns of $6,000 each year. A discount rate of 12 percent yields an estimated value $6,000 ÷ 0.12 or $50,000 minus the ($40,000) initial cost and thus a positive NPV. A discount rate of 18 percent yields $6,000 ÷ 0.18 or $33,333 minus ($40,000) and thus a negative NPV. At 15 percent the estimated value of $40,000 minus the ($40,000) initial cost makes NPV = 0, so 15 percent is the correct rate of return. By a similar process of trial and error using the NPV timeline spreadsheet, we could determine that the IRR for the investment in the MS degree taking account of tuition at $12,000 (half of which is paid back by the therapist's employer after three years on the job), books costing $500, and the fact that he is already 40 years old and expects to spend only another 18 years working, not forever, is 11 percent.

SPREADSHEET TIMELINE FOR NPV AND INTERNAL RATE OF RETURN

Calculating net present value was a laborious task before spreadsheets became common, and doing the many trial-and-error calculations required to determine internal rate of return so daunting that most classes taught theory or shortcuts rather than practical applications. The advent of cheap computing has radically transformed the day-to-day work of financial analysis, making it possible to determine the NPV and IRR of even the most complicated sets of cash flows within a few minutes.

The most important, and most difficult, step is to set out all of the cash flows in an organized way. To do so, a timeline is used, conventionally running left to right, as in Table 12.1. The top row shows the periods (for this example, it can be assumed that they are years). The left-border column(s) are used for labels and formulas. The first column after that is year 0 or today. Year 1 is a year from now, and so on. The second row shows the present value of a dollar in that period. A dollar today has a present value of 1.000, a dollar in year 1 has a present value of 1.000 ÷ (1 + interest rate). The present value of a dollar in year 2 is (PV year 1) ÷ (1 + interest rate). Year 3 is (PV year 2) ÷ (1 + interest rate), and so on, for as many periods as are needed.

The easiest way to accomplish this calculation is to write the formula for PV year 1 and copy it across the row (remembering to use a fixed reference to the cell A1 with the interest rate). In the third row, put the net cash flow (CF). (If one wanted to be more detailed, one could use separate rows for cash in, cash out, and then net; or multiple rows for different types of revenues and expenses; but here we will keep it simple and just use one net cash flow

TABLE 12.1   Spreadsheet Timeline for NPV and IRR

6%	Year 0	Year 1	Year 2	Year 3	Year 4
PV of $1 @	1.000	0.943	0.890	0.840	0.792
Net CF	$ (1,000)	250	300	400	450
PV of CF	$(1,000.00)	$235.85	$267.00	$335.85	$356.44
NPV (sum)	$ 195.14				
Formulas	*(Copy cells across to the right for as many columns as needed to get to the end)*				
(Type in interest rate)	0	+ (cell to left) + 1		. . . + (cell to left) +1	
PV of $1	1.000	+ (cell to left)/(1 + A1)		. . . + (cell to left)/(1 + A1)	
Net CF	(Cash In − Cash Out)	(Net CF year 1)		. . . (Net CF year n)	
PV of CF in year	Multiply cell above by PV of $1	Multiply by PV $1 in year 1 . . . Multiply by PV of $1 in year n			
Net present value	= (sum across row above all the way to the last year)				

(Continued)

SPREADSHEET TIMELINE FOR NPV AND INTERNAL RATE OF RETURN (CONTINUED)

entry for each year). In this example, there is a net investment of ($1,000) today, and net operating cash flow (revenues minus expenses) of $250, $300, $400, and $450, respectively, in years 1 to 4. In the next row, multiply the present value of $1 times the net cash flow for the year to get the present value of cash flows in each year. Finally, sum across that row to obtain the NPV of $195.14.

That was a bit tiresome, but, when the spreadsheet timeline is set up for NPV once, it can be used over and over and over. To change the interest rate, simply type a new interest rate (in cell A1 if you used the indicated format) and immediately the new NPV is calculated. Want to find NPV for a different set of cash flows? Just type the new cash in and cash out into the appropriate cells. Want to find NPV for 10, 20, 250 years? Just copy the formulas across (it takes a single set of clicks—less than 10 seconds once you get the hang of it).

Oh yes, finding IRR—that is now a snap. If the NPV is positive, raise the interest rate until NPV is just zero (or near enough). If the NPV is negative, reduce the interest rate until NPV becomes positive. Usually you can get to within three or four decimal points in a few tries, and rarely more than a dozen (which, given the speed of most computers, takes less than a minute). Try it with the example above, and you should converge on 8.6 percent pretty quickly.

Internal rates of return provide a shorthand measure of how financially desirable a project is. If the rough measurement makes it seem worthwhile, then other elements such as taxes, working conditions, probability of getting laid off, and the prestige and satisfaction obtained with a higher degree can be factored in.

Human Capital: Medical Education as an Investment

We can use the **human capital** approach to evaluate whether going to medical school is a sacrifice, a sound investment, or both.[2] The returns on medical education are estimated from the increased annual earnings, relative to a person's opportunity cost, that flow from the decision to go to medical school. The costs are all the things that are given up, which include tuition, but mostly the forgone earnings and leisure from working 80 hours a week without pay in medical school or for below-market wages during residency. (Note that as with most education the implicit opportunity costs are greater than direct monetary costs). Real returns (after adjustment for inflation) on financial assets have historically been about 1 to 3 percent for savings accounts and treasury bonds and 3 to 6 percent for stocks, which are a bit riskier. Economic studies of the rates of return for high school and college education have typically shown substantially better returns, 8 to 10 percent or more.

Empirical studies of rate of return on education become complex in practice, because one must adjust for the superior earning power of above-average students, the costs of the excess hours worked by physicians, and so forth. Also important is the fact that the returns from a medical education are much less risky than from a bachelor of arts (BA), master of business administration (MBA), or doctor of law (JD) degree and thus should be adjusted accordingly (see the discussion of risk and expected returns below). In addition, becoming a medical doctor confers prestige and other valuable privileges. Empirical studies in labor economics have reached a consensus on some major conclusions, although many details are still subject to disagreement. The return on investment from a college education clearly exceeds the market rate of return on financial assets, and the premium for being a college graduate is rising. The return on investment from graduation from medical school, with real returns of

TABLE 12.2			Returns on Investment for a Professional Education		
Profession	Length of Training	Tuition ($)	Annual Income (age 40) ($)	Hours Worked (age 40)	Internal Rate of Return (%)
Business	2 years	34,452	$135,579	2,448	26%
Law	3 years	32,317	$139,616	1,959	23%
Dentistry	4 years	70,620	$133,050	1,781	22%
Primary medicine	4 years	74,504	$132,592	2,565	16%
Specialty medicine	4 years	74,504	$219,733	2,707	18%

Source: W.B. Weeks and A. E. Wallace, "The More Things Change: Revisiting a Comparison of Educational Costs and Incomes of Physicians and Other Professionals," *Academic Medicine* 77, no. 4 (2002): 312–319, 2002.

10 to 20 percent, is higher than that for graduation from college (see Table 12.2).[3] Returns on other graduate degrees, such as a doctor of philosophy (PhD) degree in biology or sociology, are much lower, and in some fields the returns are effectively zero. Returns on residency training follow incomes: They are high for surgical specialties (40 percent), intermediate for internal medicine (20 percent), and low for pediatrics (2 percent).

Risk

One of the benefits of medical education is the certainty that one will always have a job. Although the average income for lawyers might be similar to that of doctors, the variance is greater. Lawyers with salaries over $1 million are offset by other JDs who are barely getting by or have given up the practice of law entirely. Business incomes, particularly for entrepreneurs, are even more variable and extreme. Some are multimillionaires, and some are self-employed (and making less than minimum wage). Every investment carries risk to some degree or another. To calculate the internal rates of return using the spreadsheet timeline above, we first had to enter the cash flows for each future period, but we will never actually know what those cash flows are until after the fact. The precision of the calculations should not blind us to the reality that they are based on estimates, "best guesses" about what will (or might) happen in the future.

Some areas of medicine are relatively stable and provide low-risk earnings (physician, hospital administrator). Others, like biotechnology, have extremely high risks. Discovery of a new cure is worth hundreds of millions of dollars, but most biotechnology ventures end up disappointing their investors by producing little revenue and no profits. Rather than the stocks, bonds, and retained earnings used to finance large established companies, biotech firms get most of their funding from risk-taking specialists known as "venture capitalists" (VC) and the human capital of the doctors and scientists who believe enough in their own ideas to work very hard for very little money but many stock options. Biotech is too risky for bank loans, and investors must be quite knowledgeable and experienced in this specialized field to assess the likelihood that a real drug will ever get produced, or how much it could be worth. If a biotech start-up produces a potentially useful new drug within five years, the venture capitalists will "cash out" by selling the rights to a large pharmaceutical firm or to the public through an initial public offering (IPO). If the start-up has not found a product within five years, it will usually be shut down and the investment written off.

Suppose that a hypothetical VC obtains $95 million dollars from its backers (usually wealthy individuals or pension funds) and adds $5 million of its own funds to invest $100 million in exciting new projects. It chooses ten projects, investing $10 million in each one. At the end of five years one of the projects has a great drug that is sold to a pharmaceutical company for $140 million, another project seems promising and is sold for $60 million, two of the projects have some promise and are sold for $10 million each (i.e., breakeven), and six of the projects are terminated and thus valued at $0. At the end of five years, the $100 million invested has become $220 million. The internal rate of return is $220/$100 − 1.00 = 1.20 or 120 percent. Note that you must subtract 1.00 to account for the return of the original investment (i.e., if you invest $100 and get $103 back, that is a 3 percent IRR, not 103 percent). Note also that is a five-year return, so it is necessary to convert to an annualized rate of return by using the NPV timeline spreadsheet. There, you can see that turning $100 into $220 is an annualized rate of approximately 17 percent per year for five years.[4]

SPREADSHEET FOR EXPECTED NPV AND RISKY RETURNS

An NPV or IRR is certain only if one is certain of all future cash flows. Usually, the current (year 0) prices can be known with reasonable certainty. Future cash flows are almost always treated as risky unless they are interest payments on U.S. Treasury bonds or equivalents. The analyst must consider three things:

- What are the possible future outcomes (scenarios)?
- What are the cash flows for each outcome?
- What is the probability of each outcome?

An analyst considers several scenarios (*most likely, good, bad*) and determines the cash flows expected in each case. Then the analyst estimates the likelihood that each scenario will occur. After that, finding *expected* NPV and *expected* IRR is simply a matter of calculation.

In the example below, the most likely case is the same as in Table 12.1, whereas in the good scenario net operating cash flows are better ($300, $350, $450, and $500, respectively, in years 1 to 4) and in the bad scenario they are worse ($100 for each year; see Table 12.3). The analyst judges that the most likely scenario will happen 60 percent of the time, the good outcome 10 percent of the time, and the bad scenario the remaining 30 percent. The "expected cash flow" in year 0 is ($1,000) because regardless of the scenario, $1,000

TABLE 12.3 Spreadsheet Timeline for Expected NPV and Risky Rates of Return

6%	Probability	Year 0	Year 1	Year 2	Year 3	Year 4
PV of $1 @		1.000	0.943	0.890	0.840	0.792
Net CF (middle)	60%	(1,000)	250	300	400	450
Net CF (good)	10%	(1,000)	300	350	450	500
Net CF (bad)	30%	(1,000)	100	100	100	100
Expected CF	100%	(1,000)	210	245	315	350
PV of eCF		(1,000)	$198.11	$218.05	$264.48	$277.23
NPV (sum)		(42)				

Formulas	*(Copy cells across to the right for as many columns as needed to get to the end)*
(Type in interest rate)	
PV of $1	1.000 + (cell to left)/(1 + A1)...+ (cell to left)/(1 + A1)
Expected CF	Weighted average = (B3*C3) + (B4*C4) + (B5*C5)
PV of eCF in year	Multiply cell above by PV of $1 in year$_n$
Expected NPV	= (sum across row above all the way to the last year)

(Continued)

SPREADSHEET FOR EXPECTED NPV AND RISKY RETURNS (CONTINUED)

must be paid for the investment. In year 1, the expected cash flow is (60% × $250) + (10% × $300) + (30% × $100) = $210. This is a weighted average, with the weights being the likelihood for each scenario. Similarly for year 2, expected cash flow is (60% × $300) + (10% × $350) + (30% × $100) = $245, and so on for years 3 and 4. In setting up the spreadsheet, one needs to type in the formula for weighted average only once and copy it across (remembering to use fixed cell references for the probability weights).

This spreadsheet may seem like a bit much work to set up, but it only has to be done one time. With a single keystroke, the interest rate is changed. This makes it easy to determine expected IRR (here, since expected NPV is negative at 6%, the interest rate must be reduced to get NPV to zero, and that occurs at an interest rate of about 4.3%, which is thus determined to be the expected IRR). A few keystrokes and copying are all that is required to add on two or four or forty more years or to change the probabilities of each scenario or the cash flows that will occur in each scenario. More scenarios can be created by adding rows (remembering that probability must always sum to 100%) but in practice most analysts stay with less than a dozen. The venture capital example discussed previously has ten rows, but cash flows in only two columns, year 0 (initial investment) and year 5 (when projects are sold off).

It is worth noting how important the probability weights are: the expected NPV goes from positive to negative with a small shift in the likelihood of the good or bad scenario. This sensitivity is even more extreme when "bad" is something like a hurricane—or bankruptcy or a malpractice suit—as it often is in the real world. The job of the analyst is not so much to predict the future as to point out to management what the financial implications of different futures might be and how sensitive the financial strength of the organization is to both likely and extreme outcomes.

Valuing Assets

Finance is conceptually simple because **the only thing that ultimately matters is cash flow**. All other elements are considered only to help make estimates of cash flow better. The analyst only needs to know the cash flows in each period, and then makes the appropriate calculations to discount for when (*time*) and if (*risk*) the cash flows will occur. Although valuation is simple in theory, it is difficult and subject to large errors in practice, and it relies heavily on the judgment and expertise of the analyst.

What is an **asset**? Because cash flow is all that matters, from a financial point of view any item—a share of stock, a hospital building, a computer, or anything else—is an asset only to the extent that it provides future cash flow. The value of an MRI scanner is how much additional cash it can bring in before it is sold for scrap. Because the MS degree added to the future income of the therapist, is it an asset? Of course, but a medical education is just part of what makes a physician valuable. The most important assets of a physician's practice are intangible—not the building or the x-ray machine or the surgical instruments but the skill and reputation of the doctors practicing there. Patients will continue going to a practice where they feel the physicians are well qualified and caring. If patients stopped coming the stream of revenues would dry up, reducing the value of the practice to zero. Is reputation an asset? Just ask Tiger Woods how much his name is worth, or ask Kobe Bryant how much the value of his reputation has gone up and down over the years. Think how much a brand like "Coke" or "Tylenol" or "Nexium" or "Viagra" or "the Mayo Clinic" is worth.

Pharmaceutical R&D is placed on the books as an asset so long as the project is or could be viable. If it fails, then it is written off (valued at $0). Conversely, if it succeeds, then it is the patent that is the asset, which is recorded as having a value equal to the discounted profits from expected future sales. When a biotech firm is sold, the most valuable assets are the patents (or expected patents) to new drugs and the information about how they work and can be manufactured, not the actual chemicals or any equipment.

12.3 UNCORRELATED (INDEPENDENT) AND CORRELATED (SYSTEM) RISKS

Venture capitalists are a form of financial intermediary, pooling funds from a group of investors and using them to purchase a bundle of several projects, usually start-up firms. Putting ten biotech projects together averages out some of the risks: the expected value is the same, but the variance is reduced. In that way, VCs perform a function similar to insurance companies that pool the funds (premiums) of a large group of people to share risks so that no single person is bankrupted by catastrophic expense (see Chapter 4). Of course, insurance companies pool losses, whereas venture capitalists pool projects that have net gains (or at least, they hope they have gains). Financial intermediation is not cheap. A VC firm charges a management fee up front and then takes a big slice of the profits. (Note, however, that the VC is also usually investing a chunk of its own funds in the pool.) The projects chosen must be really good prospects in order to pay the VC so much off the top and still provide the 15 to 25 percent gains that investors in such risky pools expect. The VC is providing two functions: expert project selection and bundling funds together. A VC is like a mutual fund, which collects money from many individuals and invests in stocks chosen by the fund manager, except that the number of investors is much smaller (maybe 10 or 20 instead of thousands) and the VC invests in start-up companies rather than traded stocks.

Mutual funds help investors by diversifying risks. Rather than purchasing $10,000 worth of shares in one stock, an investor purchases $10,000 worth of shares in the "fund," which holds hundreds of stocks. Much financial theory is devoted to the analysis of such portfolio diversification. Rather than reviewing that extensive body of knowledge here, it is better to refer those who wish to know more to a finance textbook; for those who do not want to read finance theory, it is important to understand clearly why grandmother's admonition "not to put all your eggs in one basket" is sound financial advice. Portfolio diversification works to the extent that the risks of each stock are independent on one another. If Moleculetech happens to go up because a clinical trial was favorable, that does not affect the likelihood that Exxon or Biolyne will go up or down. Risks that are independent are also said to be uncorrelated. However, the CFO and the chief biologist for Moleculetech will both get rich, or not, depending upon the outcome of the same clinical trial—and thus their financial risks are highly (almost 100 percent) correlated. Perfect correlation exists between two shares of stock in the same company: if the price goes up, it goes up the same for both.

Some risks affect almost all stocks, so there is a high degree of correlation. If interest rates rise, the value of most stocks will decline because investors will start to sell stocks to buy the bonds that now pay more per year and also because the present value of future earnings is reduced when the discount rate is higher (see Section 12.2 and the NPV timeline spreadsheet above). Similarly, if the economy heads toward a recession, profits are likely to be lower for most companies, and the entire stock market will tend downward. Having bought a mutual fund with a thousand stocks rather than a single company stock does not help the investor minimize these systemic risks. Macroeconomic shifts affect all stocks, and hence this risk cannot be reduced by diversification.[5]

A risk may be correlated for a certain type of asset but not others. A hurricane might pose significant losses to all property insurance companies operating in Florida but not affect automobile insurers. A rise in the price of steel would affect automobile and appliance manufacturers but not movie companies or book publishers. The main macroeconomic risks (falling GDP or rising interest rates) actually have little effect on most health care stocks. People go to the hospital whether times are good or bad, and the future of Moleculetech is going to depend more on the results of a clinical trial than on the state of the economy. The major risks in health care often come from government action, as when Medicare Part D was enacted (affecting all drug companies) or cuts to Medicaid (affect all hospitals with high concentrations of poor patients) or changes in the RBRVS payment system (affected all physicians).

Which Is Riskier: Nursing Homes or Drug Companies?

The financial concepts of independent (uncorrelated) and systemic (correlated) risks can usefully be applied to the various kinds of health care organizations examined in previous chapters. Because it costs hundreds of millions of dollars to develop a new drug, and because most new drugs fail to even reach the marketplace, much less make any profits, it would seem that the pharmaceutical industry is very risky. The nursing home industry serves a growing number of elderly people with a product that does not require a lot of innovation or marketing to sell. Most nursing homes operate nearly full most of the time. Thus it would seem that the nursing home industry is quite stable and low risk.

First appearances can be deceiving, and the market evidence contradicts the propositions in the paragraph above. Pharmaceutical companies almost never go bankrupt and usually rank among the most consistently profitable industry groups in the S&P 500, whereas almost every publicly traded LTC company went bankrupt or became financially distressed during the 1990s. Why such discrepancy between first appearances and financial reality? Pharmaceutical companies are in fact diversified firms with many products: drugs for heart disease, drugs for cancer, drugs for skin conditions, and on and on. They are also geographically diversified, selling products not just across the United States but also in other countries. The portfolio of products means that in any given year at least some drugs are profitable and make up for the ones that fail. Overall the demand for drugs is stable and growing—higher interest rates or a looming recession might keep people from buying new cars or remodeling their homes but not from purchasing blood pressure medication, particularly now that most prescriptions are covered by insurance. An individual biotech company is a highly risky enterprise with a high likelihood of failure, but that failure is not correlated with the risk of biotech firm B or with the general stock market. It is specific to the particular drug the firm is investigating. However, the fact that most biotech firms are small start-up companies with few tangible assets does increase their relative risk. Big pharmaceutical firms are pretty resilient and only occasionally suffer setbacks.

Nursing homes, in contrast, all suffered together when the government cut Medicare and Medicaid reimbursements under the Balanced Budget Act of 1997. A single entry in the federal register caused Genesis, Manor Care, Beverly Enterprises, and the other major firms in this industry to suffer massive and unexpected losses. What had been a growth industry became a shambles of distressed assets almost overnight. The budget cuts pushed down revenues per bed everywhere, and expenses per bed could not be reduced fast enough to stave off disaster.

Assessing Business Risk

In the example above, a change in government policy hurt the nursing home industry by reducing revenues, which in turn reduced the value of the assets (value being the capitalized sum of future earnings an asset can generate). Financial analysts use a number of ways to assess the value and risks of a business. From an investor's point of view, the single most important issue is how much is earned for each dollar invested (called "return on equity" or ROE) and often analyzed using the "DuPont Equation."[6] This is appropriate for corporate finance based on the assumption that the most important objective (or even the only objective) is maximization of shareholder wealth. In health care, such an assumption is rarely justified. Even publicly traded for-profit health insurance companies, hospital chains, and pharmaceutical companies are often held to a higher standard (or other standards) than pure shareholder wealth maximization. Therefore a more conceptual and generalized approach to the assessment of business risk is more appropriate than a narrow focus on ROE. One conceptual structure used by managers in both for-profit and nonprofit enterprises is formulated as:

$$\text{Business Risk} = (\text{Revenue Risk}) \times (\text{Operating Expense Leverage}) \times (\text{Financial Leverage})$$

The overall financial risk to the organization is separated into components:

- How variable are revenues? Is there growth?
- Do expenses adjust a lot or only a little as revenue changes?
- Are the assets financed mostly with equity or debt? What kind of debt?

The first issue to face is how much revenue the organization will bring in. Is it stable, growing, or shrinking? Will revenue trend close to forecast, or will it be subject to lots of random fluctuations and variability? Is the generation of revenue under the control of management, perhaps because the organization can easily raise prices, serve more patients, or call upon donors? Having some handle on the range of risks in revenue, the organization must understand how readily it can adjust to unanticipated ups and downs. Will expenses automatically decline proportionately if there is a drop in revenue (as happens with variable costs when volume declines)? Can some expenses be easily cut or deferred for a while (R&D, maintenance, vanity projects, new product launch)? Operating leverage is often dominated by the fixed to variable cost ratio. Whereas a clinical laboratory or a physical therapy practice might find that many of its costs go up and down as patient volume rises or falls, nursing homes, hospitals, and pharmaceutical companies with large fixed costs tend to have inflexible expenses, so they make good profits when revenues surge and are sunk if revenues unexpectedly dip. To the extent that a hospital treats its labor force as permanent, it will have high operating leverage; management that is willing to quickly adjust nursing and other employment up and down to match patient flow is more flexible but may be perceived as ruthless cost-cutters rather than friendly patrons.

Revenues and expenses, the first two components, determine the cash flow from operations.[7] They establish the degree of risk in the business before any financial engineering to change the debt-to-equity structure takes place. Typically, businesses with a low degree of operational risk (utilities, real estate, nursing homes) take on more debt to increase leverage and raise the rate of return on equity, while businesses with a high degree of inherent risk (biotech, restaurants, moviemaking) must rely almost entirely on equity and thus have low leverage. Most corporate finance concentrates on the structuring of debt and equity. Although this issue has become increasingly important for hospitals, and was central to the problems of LTC companies with lots of highly leveraged debt-heavy real estate, it is relatively unimportant for physician practices (self-financed), pharmaceutical firms (equity financed with excess retained earnings), and insurance companies (more likely to be net creditors than debtors).

12.4   OWNERSHIP AND AGENCY

The original health care firm was the solo physician, taking care of patients and collecting fees. Even the author of the Hippocratic Oath was a businessperson.[8] Today's physicians, like Hippocrates, operate within an ethical context. The financial structure of ancient Greek medicine was fairly simple. There were no stocks and bonds. There were risks and rewards, and there was a form of debt and equity in the set of personal obligations that went with being part of an organized profession. The Oath talks about the physician's obligations (personal and financial) to the one who taught him (today, we might talk about medical school debts and junior partnerships), and the most valuable asset was the physician's reputation and that of the medical profession. Indeed, one of the goals of the Hippocratic Oath was to increase the value of this reputational equity. It is instructive to begin with this prototype, which is not so different from the single physician entering practice today, to see the elements that lead toward increasingly powerful financial structures and complex intermediaries.

Equity and Debt

A physician who starts a practice is an entrepreneur risking time and effort in the hope of doing well.[9] In common parlance, this is called "sweat equity." Some cash is required. In most cases, this comes from government-subsidized guaranteed student loans and from the parents who are proud of their daughter, the doctor. First come the tuition and living expenses during medical school, and then the expenses (rent, equipment, payroll) of furnishing a practice. The typical practice starts small and grows, paying for most of its expansion as more and more patients come in paying more and more fees (retained earnings).

In terms of finance, this physician practice is a 100 percent equity-financed sole proprietorship. Any profits go to the physician who started the practice and works there. Her employees might get paid better as the practice does better, but that is at her discretion. She, as **the owner, is the residual claimant to all of the money left after expenses are paid**. As the practice grows, she might want to add equipment or build a new office, and she approaches a bank for a loan. She is doing so because she expects the returns on the new computer system (increase in future cash flows) to be greater than the cost—perhaps a 15 percent return on funds borrowed at just 7 percent interest. Financial leverage is being used to increase the returns on equity (her hard work and MD degree). Of course if the computer system doesn't work, then she as the residual claimant is the one who suffers.

If the practice continues to grow, she will add other doctors. Initially, they will be on salary rather than sharing profit, both because (a) they do not want to take a risk, but want to be guaranteed they will earn enough to live if they move there to work, and (b) because she does not want to share the profits from her years of hard work and practice-building until the new doctors prove that they are worthwhile partners. As long as these additional doctors continue to work on salary, or even on some percentage of billings (if they were salespeople, we would call it a commission), the financial structure is still that of a sole proprietorship, even if she decides to buy the building and finances it with debt using a bank loan.

Once she finds a compatible doctor who wants to stick with the practice, the practice will undergo a legal change and become a **partnership**. Now there are multiple residual claimants to the profits, and this poses several challenges. The new doctor may be young and willing to work nights, while the founding doctor is close to retirement and wants more time off. She might feel that she is owed a bigger share since she built the practice up and bought all of the equipment. The potentials for conflicts are endless, but commonly people who want to work together find a way to do so. As there are more and more partners, it becomes increasingly necessary to use legal contracts and to regularize the role of partners: defining shares, relating pay to number of services each doctor bills for, making new doctors "buy in" over a period of years, and so on (see "Group Practice" in Section 7.4).

The clinic might decide to move aggressively into new technology by becoming a center for diagnostic imaging. The equipment is expensive and the task of running an operation with 40 exam rooms and many technicians is complex, so the medical group partnership decides to get help from an outside firm, DioTech. Also, the local bank has told the doctors they are not comfortable lending them more money because then the doctors would have too much debt relative to the value of their building and other liquid (i.e., easy to sell and convert into cash) assets, so any additional millions are a "maybe" and would carry a much higher interest rate. The imaging center will be set up separately from the medical group as an independent **corporation**. A corporation is a legal entity, like a person or a partnership, but with limited liability. Only the assets of the corporation can be taken if it goes bankrupt. The doctors and DioTech will both be residual claimants to the profits of the imaging center (according to some specified contract), but usually most of the financing is put up by the outside company.

DioTech might have been a project funded by some venture capitalists to build and operate imaging centers and is now ready for its IPO (initial public offering). Once DioTech decides to "**go public**" and have stock traded on NASDAQ, NYSE, or other exchange, all of its financial statements, including quarterly and annual reports, are made openly available on the Web at http://www.sec.gov/search/search.htm. Investors from around the world send in their money to buy shares and thus get fractional equity ownership. Some do not even know what business DioTech is in, only that it is supposed to be a hot stock. The better informed ones are hoping DioTech will get bought up by a large firm such as MegaMed and thus provide them with shares in a well-known established company or a quick profit by selling.

Who Owns the Business? Who Owns the Patient? Agency Issues

At this point it is appropriate to ask, who really owns this imaging center? The medical group, or at least the senior partners, usually have an active role in management and get a share of the profits, but profits also go the shareholders who have never been near the clinic. It should be apparent that "running the business," "making money off the business," and "owning the business" are no longer the same, as they were in the simple solo proprietorship with which Dr. Smith started. For a large publicly traded company like the hypothetical MegaMed (or a real company like Universal Healthcare or Johnson & Johnson), more than half of the "owners" are ordinary people whose money is in pension or mutual funds and do not even know that they are receiving the profits of this business.

The original equity was put up by the initial proprietor, Dr. Smith, and she had a triple role of working, managing, and investing. These roles become increasingly distinct as the organization grows. As the medical group gets larger, some differentiation of roles is likely to occur, with one or more senior physicians taking a leadership role, but each doctor is still doing some of each task. Even in the joint venture, the outside firm is putting in both management and operational expertise as well as money. A real bridge is crossed when a business goes public and the majority of investors are people who are not actually part of the company.

In financial theory, the **separation of ownership from control** is the subject of agency theory.[10] The managers of the business are supposed to make decisions on behalf of the shareholders, using their expertise and efforts to maximize shareholder wealth, but instead they might decide to take it easy, hire their friends, buy fancy corporate jets, or even engage in sweetheart deals that enrich the CEO and members of the board by draining money from the company. Agency theory was discussed in Chapter 6 with regard to physicians (agents) making decisions on behalf of patients (principals). In corporate finance, most of the attention is on managers making decisions on behalf of shareholders or other owners. For example, will the doctors do their best for DioTech? Will DioTech provide the physicians a fair share of the lucrative fees obtained from the hundreds of scans the center performs each day? What is "fair" in the distribution of a business profits?

In a legal sense, a "fair" distribution of profits is whatever the parties agree to. DioTech might feel that the medical group would never have made millions in the imaging business if it were not for their expertise and the $20 million in construction and equipment they provided. Smith Medical Group might feel that DioTech would not be making millions without their patients. Similar conflicts might have arisen when Dr. Smith first thought about taking on a partner.

Also, the answers change as business conditions change. For example, if there are five different publicly traded firms all offering to serve as joint venture partners in developing imaging centers (as there are now), then the medical group will have choices, get a competitive offer, and keep the bulk of the profits. Conversely, 20 years ago, DioTech might have been the pioneer taking all the risks and been the only game in town, leaving the medical group no choice but to accept a contract in which half the profits were permanently ceded to DioTech. More recently, Middletown HMO may be the payer for most of the patients coming to the clinic, and thus they can say "these patients are ours" and siphon off most of the profits by agreeing to let "their" patients be treated at the clinic only in return for reduced rates.

Current controversies over executive pay show that agency conflicts are quite serious. How much does the CEO deserve to get? Clearly, somebody has to run the company, and if he does a good job, he should benefit. Yet the CEO can award himself stock options and benefit just because the market goes up (carrying lazy MegaMed along with it). Even more egregious, the CEO can simply stack the board of directors with friends and ask them to vote him a bonus of $50 million or to provide an interest-free loan that he will never pay back. If the shareholders are not paying attention, then there are few consequences for such behavior. Even if the shareholders do think something is wrong, often the best they can do is simply sell their shares and hope the next company they invest in is better managed. This shows how difficult it is to determine who really "owns" a company.

Because the separation of ownership and control can create such problems, why is publicly traded stock used as equity? It is because the efficiencies gained more than outweigh the inefficiencies. How many single proprietors can come up with billions of dollars? And if they can, wouldn't they be wise to diversify, putting some of their money into other companies rather than letting their entire wealth ride just on their own company? The doctor with a great idea usually needs investors to make it a reality. Consider why patients allow the inefficiencies that come with having a doctor make decisions for them about which medicines to take, whether or not to have an operation, and whether an artificial knee is a better solution than ligament repair. Making decisions on one's own is too costly for most patients because they would have to spend many hours learning the relevant medical facts and because they would make more mistakes than a trained specialist. Most investors also need professional help to make good decisions.

The Role of Financial Intermediaries

Having a specialized entity act as an intermediary to deal with financing for many firms reduces the cost of doing business. Consider Dr. Smith's loan from the **bank**. The bank acts as an intermediary taking money from depositors and loaning to businesses. Why don't the depositors just lend their own money to Dr. Smith and get 8 percent instead of the 5 percent the bank pays them? By pooling the funds of many depositors, the bank is able to average out good and bad loans. The bank has expertise in credit assessment, choosing what businesses to loan to and which to avoid. The bank is also able to transfer funds from depositors to borrowers at much less cost than the parties could do on their own so that masses of legal and accounting transactions are done at low cost with standardized forms and computers.

Major **brokerage firms and stock markets** make it possible to raise large amounts of equity financing at low cost. They are far enough away from operations that they do not have to provide management expertise, just financial expertise. Modern business transactions go through hundreds of intermediaries, allowing each one to prosper by making all the other parties in the chain better off (another example of the fundamental theorem of exchange first discussed in Chapter 1). Money flows efficiently with rapid smoothness throughout the system at low cost—except occasionally, when a "kink" or stoppage suddenly occurs that makes each link in the chain worried about getting payment from the next link (insurance, credit card, hospital, bondholder, bank, **hedge fund**, **pension fund**, **mutual fund**, etc.), which can make the flow less "liquid" or even set off a chain reaction (as occurred in 2008–2009) in which the flow is so disrupted that everyone stops trading for no apparent reason, rather like a chance accident causing a traffic jam with massive tie-ups and multiple collisions as sometimes suddenly occurs on a busy freeway.

Health insurers, although discussed in Chapters 4 and 5 as "payers," are actually financial intermediaries, taking in cash (premiums) and then paying it out several months later (claims). Whereas the public thinks about insurance primarily in terms of the cost of covering claims, the earnings of an insurer often depend more on the investment returns from the money it holds and the efficiency of carrying out transactions. The residual left after medical costs and administrative expenses are paid is often less than 5 percent, and it may be near 0 percent. In a good year, the return on investments is much larger. That is one reason insurance companies are regulated as financial firms, with capital requirements related to liquidity (ability to pay) and investment risk, more than with regard to medical payments.

12.5   CAPITAL FINANCING: HOSPITALS

A frequent saying among hospital board members is "no margin, no mission," meaning that unless the hospital can keep expenses lower than revenues (margin), it will not be able to carry out its objectives (mission). Revenues must also be sufficiently above operating costs to compensate those who have invested capital. If a hospital borrows $10 million for construction, it must pay back the principal over time and pay interest on the loan each year. For a philanthropist making a donation, the returns on capital take the form of social services rather than interest or dividends. Having a nonprofit organization that is supposed to lose money each year, with the difference made up out of endowment or contributions, tends to blur the line between capital and operating funds. However, the conceptual requirement for a return on capital is clear. The philanthropist could always invest the money in financial assets and make a donation each year from the resulting interest if that were a more efficient way to achieve the charitable purpose than providing a lump-sum capital donation.

The start-up capital for most hospitals came from a combination of philanthropy and local government funds. Land and buildings were often donated. At the beginning of the 20th century, there were also a number of doctors' hospitals, usually started in a portion of the doctor's house or in a converted dwelling nearby. The capital financing for these small, private hospitals came from the doctor's own savings or from family members. Hospitals grew because they were successful in attracting funds or because they were successful in attracting paying patients and could build up reserves (which would be called "retained earnings" at a for-profit organization).

During World War II, millions of servicemen experienced the benefits of modern medical technology firsthand. The power of antibiotics and new surgical techniques to heal impressed many people, especially those from rural areas. This created a desire to spread hospitals across the land.[11] Yet only a few hospitals had been able to build up reserves during the Great Depression or World War II, and organizations that had conserved money wanted to expand their own operations, not help rural communities. The success of the New Deal and the victories of the military made it seem natural to mobilize government resources to meet this need. In 1946 the Hill–Burton Act was passed, making construction funds available to new hospitals in areas that had fewer than four beds per 1,000 people. As a form of repayment, hospitals receiving these funds were to give an equal or greater value in free care to indigent people. City and suburban hospitals were envious of the easy access rural areas had to capital and, because power tends to accrue to those who already have it (i.e., existing hospitals) and not necessarily to those who need it, subsequent changes were made to allow Hill–Burton funds to be used for expansion and renovation projects, as well as new construction.

Hill–Burton, retained earnings, and philanthropic fund drives provided most capital financing until the enactment of Medicare and Medicaid in 1965. Hospitals, which had chronically suffered operating losses, suddenly had steady revenue streams guaranteed by the government. They could meet the demand for new construction by borrowing against that promise, and they proceeded to do so. Borrowing increased from less than $100 million in 1960 to $200 million in 1970, $1,215 million in 1975, and $2.6 billion in 1977.[12] Three factors combined to make debt quickly become the dominant form of hospital capital:

- ■ Guaranteed revenues from Medicare and Medicaid that assured investor repayment
- ■ Tax exemption as municipal bonds made it cheap for nonprofit hospitals to borrow
- ■ Cost reimbursement for interest expenses

Medicare and Medicaid completely changed the financial picture of hospitals, from social organizations that had to beg for money each year, to solidly funded services backed by the government. For a time, it was virtually impossible for most hospitals to go bankrupt and hence for investors not to get repaid. States and localities created "health care financing authorities" that allowed nonprofit hospitals to qualify as municipal borrowers so that investors did not have to pay federal, state, and local taxes on the interest they received. This reduced the cost of borrowing by a third, making it possible for a hospital to issue bonds at 5 percent and invest at 7 percent while waiting to use the money for construction. Such arbitrage generated millions of dollars for astute hospital financial managers before being outlawed. The shift to cost reimbursement also favored borrowing. A hospital that used its own reserves to construct a new building could get reimbursed for depreciation, but the hospital that issued debt to do the same thing got reimbursed for interest expenses as well as depreciation.

In this environment with tax-exempt debt, willing investors, and cost reimbursement, it is not surprising that hospitals went on a borrowing spree, loading up with more than $10 billion in debt by 1980. However, any business that takes on lots of debt is more likely to come under financial pressure. Despite being organized as nonprofit organizations, hospitals were no exception. With millions of dollars of interest payments to make each year, hospital managers had to become more and more bottom-line oriented. As the threat of bankruptcy became more real, the social welfare and community benefit orientation that had prevailed since the turn of the century increasingly gave way to a business orientation.

Hospital borrowing rose so rapidly that it had to lose steam eventually. Too many new beds were added, and debt loads became insupportable. Also, pressures on the Medicare budget led to tighter and tighter reimbursement. In 1985, the first bond defaults began to occur. Investors quickly revised their expectations and treated hospital debt as risky, and hence they required a higher rate of interest. Municipalities were less and less pleased about the loss of property and income taxes, and calls were made to limit the use of tax-exempt revenue bonds such as those issued by hospital financing authorities. Access to capital became more difficult. Old and decrepit facilities could not tap the bond market and were acquired by for-profit hospital chains that could use the stock market to quickly raise equity, refurbish the physical plant, and make money. Many towns were willing to sell their hospitals for nothing, even provide special subsidies and tax breaks, rather than let them go bankrupt and disappear. The environment also had changed so that more hospitals felt it necessary to become part of a system covering all types of care over a broad geographic area. To do so, strong hospitals wanted to merge with or buy weaker ones and to buy nursing homes, home health agencies, physician practices, and medical office buildings. In most cases, it was not legal to use tax-exempt debt to do so, nor could the hospitals borrow the hundreds of millions of dollars necessary in the corporate (taxable) market.

THE ALLEGHENY BANKRUPTCY*

Allegheny General Hospital was one of the largest hospitals in the Pittsburgh, Pennsylvania, area.[13] It provided a broad range of services, had high occupancy, and generated large cash flows. In 1987, it merged with the cash-poor Medical College of Pennsylvania in Philadelphia to form Allegheny Health and Education Research Foundation (AHERF). The merger seemed to benefit both organizations: Allegheny General Hospital had the medical school affiliation it needed to enhance its image, and the Medical College of Pennsylvania had the cash it needed.

Medical schools have significant fixed costs. Shortly after the merger, AHERF began to look for more hospitals over which these fixed costs could be spread, and it went on a buying spree. It acquired a children's hospital, another Philadelphia medical college, and a number of community hospitals in the Philadelphia and Pittsburgh markets. All along the way, AHERF was leveraging the strong cash flows from its Allegheny General Hospital to buy up financially troubled hospitals. During the same period, many hospitals, fearful of the advent of managed care, had begun to purchase physician practices so as to lock in that physician's business and not lose admissions. AHERF was aggressive in doing so, trying to rapidly increase market share and thus driving up the prices paid for practices in the Philadelphia area. In the end, much money was spent, and few new admissions were gained as hospitals simply started paying extra for what they had received previously without payment: the inpatient business of doctors in the region.

AHERF also began competing aggressively for managed-care business during the 1990s, some of which were full-risk contracts under which the hospital contracts to take care of all HMO member health care needs for a percentage of that member's HMO policy premium. Competition with other hospital networks bid down the prices paid, and inexperience with full-risk management caused expenses to rise, resulting in substantial losses. Yet in the short run these contracts brought in additional cash (as HMO premiums were paid) that could be used for more acquisitions, and only in the long run, as services were paid for, did the losses appear on the balance sheet.

By 1996, AHERF was beginning to suffer on a number of fronts. Economies of scale from owning multiple facilities were not coming to fruition quickly enough because it takes time to consolidate operations. Bidding wars for physician practices resulted in lower returns. Bidding wars for HMO contracts resulted in lower reimbursement rates. To hide poor financial performance, AHERF executives transferred funds from one division to another trying to make each appear profitable at the time of the division's audit. Some transfers included restricted funds that were intended for use at one institution for a specific purpose; such transfers are illegal. Lack of diligence by AHERF's Board of Directors and their auditors left these transfers hidden. As with Enron, this financial shell game eventually unraveled. In 1997, AHERF became the largest not-for-profit bankruptcy in U.S. history, and its CEO, Sherif Abdelhak, was eventually sent to jail.

Hospital debt was subsequently viewed in the bond market as being much riskier, so all hospitals had to pay higher interest to compensate for the actions of this rogue entrepreneur.[14] Simple yet powerful economic forces put AHERF in jeopardy. AHERF leadership, through deliberate acts of top executives and passive acceptance by the Board of Directors, compounded the failure.

*This section was researched and prepared by Prof. Patrick M. Bernet, Florida Atlantic University.

The stand-alone community hospital was a good structure for creating a social contract.[15] Business leaders, citizens of the town, and the poor all participated in a visible symbol of community responsibility that was governed by a local board of directors. The move toward larger and more integrated health care systems has shown that this structure is inflexible and increasingly outmoded. People no longer identify primarily with a community or look to voluntary action to provide health care, and the solo hospital has no way to move capital from where the funds are (in wealthy suburbs) to where the needs are (in distressed urban and rural areas, in providing assistance to elderly people with disabilities). Creating a chain of hospitals is one way to regionalize and rationalize the allocation of capital. There has been a spurt of acquisitions and conversions of hospitals to for-profit status, although it is still unclear how far this trend will go and to what extent the government, as the primary payer for hospital care, will let it go. What has become clear is that private equity markets have far outstripped private philanthropy as a source of capital for meeting the demands for new health care services and new health care facility construction in the 21st century.

12.6 HMO OWNERSHIP AND CAPITAL MARKETS: SUCCESS AND FAILURE

Business Risks for an HMO

An HMO, especially a closed-panel group practice HMO, is a hybrid combining insurance (financial intermediary) with operations (hospitals, physicians, etc.). The major risks to the individual patient, random variation in illness, are diversified away. A group of 10,000 people has reasonably predictable health care costs, and a group of 100,000 has negligible variation in average costs due owing to the random variation among the individuals who make up the group. The more relevant risks to an HMO are related to marketing: selection and volume of patients. An HMO attracting a larger proportion of seriously ill people will suffer financially from adverse selection as much as any other insurer.[16] An even more serious marketing risk is the inability to attract a sufficient number of clients. To break even, a certain volume must be attained to cover fixed costs, and growth is a primary determinant of cash flow and profitability. In this regard, HMOs are similar to other insurance companies and most businesses. Indeed, the primary risks an investor must evaluate in considering HMO profitability are standard business risks: obtaining clients ("lives" or number of persons); pricing (capitation rate); expenses (e.g., wage rates, per diem hospital costs, cost of referrals); productivity (how much labor and capital it takes to run the HMO); and financial leverage (debt obligations relative to reserves).[17] The "core competency" of an HMO is the ability to keep the growth rate of medical costs below the rate of growth in premiums while maintaining or increasing patient satisfaction.

Kaiser Health Plan: The Evolution of an HMO

Kaiser Health Plan, with more than 9.8 million members, is the largest HMO in the United States and one of the largest medical delivery systems in the world. Its origins lie in the efforts of a young surgeon, Sydney R. Garfield, to find a place to practice when he completed residency at Los Angeles County Hospital in 1933.[18] The disastrous economy of the Depression made it impossible to open up a new solo fee-for-service practice in Los Angeles as he wished to do, so Dr. Garfield reluctantly began looking for a salaried job to tide him over until times improved. The Metropolitan Water District was building an aqueduct from the Colorado River to Los Angeles and was looking for a physician to staff a small clinic to treat construction workers in the desert. Garfield thought the salary they offered, $125 a month, was too little for someone as well trained as himself. With the support of a local doctor as partner, he decided to open his own hospital at Desert Center. The construction companies were very anxious to have a doctor for their workers and agreed to help Garfield and send all their industrial medicine cases, insured under the new workers' compensation plan, to his facility. Garfield opened a top-notch hospital, complete with modern operating facilities and air conditioning, an unheard of luxury for industrial workers at that time.

The injured workers and the construction companies loved the facility, but two financial problems quickly arose. The workers' compensation insurance companies thought Garfield treated the workers too well, and they argued over many of the bills submitted. Garfield also treated the men for nonindustrial illnesses, but few could afford to pay private practice fees for extended hospital stays or major surgery, even though Garfield felt obligated to treat them. Garfield threatened to close the hospital unless he could obtain a steady source of funding. The foundations of a major innovation in health care financing were laid when an executive of the major workers' compensation insurance companies suggested that they prepay Garfield by giving him one-eighth of the worker's compensation insurance premium, which amounted to $1.50 per month for each of the 5,000 construction workers on the project, and for workers to voluntarily prepay an additional $1.50 per month to cover all nonindustrial accidents and illnesses.[19] Garfield's experiment in prepaid HMO medicine was very successful. He added two more hospitals. At the end of five years, as construction slowed and the hospitals began to close, Garfield had made a net profit of more than $250,000 (equivalent to $4 million after adjustment for inflation to 2012).

Although Garfield intended to take his profits and set up a private practice in Los Angeles, he was lured north to open another prepaid workers' clinic by one of the aqueduct contractors, Henry J. Kaiser, who had just made a deal to complete the Grand Coulee Dam in Oregon. Kaiser was impressed by the efficiency and high quality of Garfield's operation in the desert and felt that establishing a similar facility would help him attract workers to another remote construction site. At Grand Coulee, SR Garfield & Associates provided 24-hour medical coverage to 15,000 workers and family members in a modernized and, once again, air-conditioned hospital with a group of five physicians and six nurses. Garfield himself, however, remained in Los Angeles, undergoing more medical training and looking after business interests, flying to Grand Coulee and working in the clinic only once every six weeks. It was as a manager that Garfield made the health plan successful, while his status as a physician gave him a special connection with the professionals who worked under his direction. He was, in the words of one of the physicians who worked for him, "a genius at keeping salaries and expenses down."

With Grand Coulee nearing completion and Garfield ordered up for service in the Army during World War II, it appeared that his days as an entrepreneur were over. However, Kaiser had just been given a new contract to construct 60 freighters at a hastily organized shipyard in Richmond, near San Francisco, and he wanted Garfield to provide the medical care for his wartime crew. Within a year, Garfield built a hospital and was caring for 90,000 workers. His commitment to staying at the forefront of medical practice is evidenced by the establishment of a research program and a new journal, the *Permanente* (Kaiser) *Foundation Medical Bulletin*, in 1943. By 1944, Garfield had a hundred doctors working for him to care for more than 200,000 workers and dependents. Although his first recruits were outstanding doctors from Stanford University, the University of Southern California, and other leading medical schools who wished to join a prepaid group practice, others were hired only because they were unfit for military service and needed a job. From them, Garfield learned an important management lesson, which he later stated as, "No matter how the principles of our plan are meant, if you don't have the physician group who have it in their hearts and who believe in prepaid practice, it won't work," emphasizing that it is the culture and the people even more than the financial contracts that define a successful HMO.[20]

As fast as the war had created a need for the Kaiser medical plan, the end of the war took it away. The only clinic not to suffer a major enrollment decline was the one at the new

Kaiser steel mill in Fontana, in the desert outside Los Angeles. The Alameda County and San Francisco medical societies, tolerant during the war emergency, grew openly hostile. Kaiser doctors were denied medical society membership, and hence could not join hospital medical staffs or participate in many forms of professional advancement. Yet Garfield, Kaiser, and many of their closest associates, including health economist Avram Yedidia, decided that the appropriate course of action was to regroup and expand their visionary health plan rather than shut it down. In the immediate postwar period, enrollment stabilized at fewer than 20,000. By 1948, it had rebounded to 60,000, with much of the growth coming from marketing to unions and firms whose employees would join as a group.

Yet the pressures of fluctuating enrollment, requirements for capital, and a need for clearer lines of authority made the entrepreneurial organization, with Sydney Garfield alone in charge of all the Kaiser health facilities, untenable. The new structure had three entities: a charitable corporation for the hospitals, a nonprofit foundation for the health plan, and a private for-profit partnership for the physician group. Garfield was paid $257,000 for his interest in the hospitals and subsequently gave up his interest in the partnership, so that by 1949 he was just an employee, albeit a very important one. By 1952, enrollment reached 250,000, but the organizational difficulties were not over, and financial disputes between the health plan and the physician groups had become serious. In 1955, Garfield resigned his post as executive director, and a new profit-sharing plan for the physician group was drafted.

The medical group was to be paid on a capitation basis, have a pension plan, and get half of all revenues in excess of the funds needed for expenses, capital replacement, and reserves for distribution as bonuses. This financial agreement between Kaiser Health Plan and the Permanente Medical Group has continued essentially unchanged for the past 50 years. In 1962, enrollment exceeded 1 million subscribers and dependents, 2.5 million in 1972, and 10 million in 2000. Kaiser health plans have maintained an enviable record of growth over 40 years, more than doubling in most decades. Although Kaiser remains strongest in its initial market areas around San Francisco, Los Angeles, and Portland, it has expanded to Hawaii, Colorado, Connecticut, North Carolina, and Washington, D.C.

Yet even as the forces of managed care began to revolutionize the U.S. health care system, Kaiser, the exemplar of prepaid organized medical practice, had begun to falter.[21] The Kaiser plan established in Hartford, Connecticut, was unable to grow past 30,000 members after ten years, below break-even size. To penetrate the competitive Washington, D.C., and North Carolina markets, Kaiser departed from its traditional closed-staff model and set up open IPA HMOs contracting with already-established local physicians. Despite—or because of—these changes, Kaiser in 1994 suffered its first enrollment decline in 50 years. A once-dominant and innovative organization had drifted, giving up its core competency as it imitated the newer IPA HMOs that could grow rapidly by just signing contracts. After losing hundreds of millions of dollars, Kaiser finally regrouped and recovered in 2000. When the federal HMO Act was passed in 1973, Kaiser accounted for more than 2 million of the 3 million total HMO enrollees in the United States, a market share of 70 percent. By 2002, although it was still the largest, Kaiser's 8 million enrollees represented less than a 15 percent market share.

The Kaiser Health Plan operated as a nonprofit foundation; thus, there were no stockholders or individual owners who stood to gain by expanding into new markets. To some extent, it might seem as though the physicians were shareholders, but in one important way they clearly were not owners. When each new region got started, it took capital from the existing Kaiser foundation. However, once the region was up and running, no "returns" were paid back. The physicians who had given up some current income to enable the new offshoot to grow gained nothing. Thus, it is not surprising that Kaiser plans grew robustly where they were already established (since that medical group stood to benefit) but had difficulty obtaining the resources to move into new areas. Garfield built Kaiser single-handedly, but after 1949, he held no legal ownership interest, and in 1955 he was forced out. Garfield was apparently willing to do it for the glory, but the fact is that someone of his talent and training would surely have ended up a wealthier man if he had stuck with his original plan to open a fee-for-service surgical practice in Los Angeles. The incomplete and complex ownership structure was not able to protect his interest, nor was it able to maximize the potential of the Kaiser Health Plan.

Group Health Association: A Consumer Co-op Gets Bought Out by a Franchise Chain

The history of another of the first HMOs makes a similar point regarding ownership. Group Health Association (GHA) of Washington, D.C., was founded in 1937 as a consumer's cooperative to provide physician services to its members, who were largely federal employees. The physicians were employees, not partners. The American Medical Association and the D.C. medical society sought to put GHA out of business, and GHA's victorious antitrust suit, which was affirmed by the U.S. Supreme Court in 1943, was considered crucial to the survival and growth of all HMOs, including Kaiser. Yet ten years later, GHA still had fewer than 20,000 members.

The cooperative structure legally made every subscriber an owner. Some existing members were ambivalent about letting large unions join, because it would change the dynamics of control. A basic management function, marketing, was the subject of great ideological debates rather than concerted action. GHA did become more solidly established after becoming an option in the Federal Employees Health Benefits Program, reaching 50,000 members in 1962 and 100,000 in 1975. An attempt by the physicians to set up a medical group partnership similar to that at Kaiser met with resistance from GHA members and their elected board. As a chronicle of GHA observes, the physicians "failed to comprehend GHA's special environment, in which the members instinctively reacted against the notion of a profit motive."[22]

Unable to form a corporate medical group, GHA's physicians formed a union in 1977 and went on strike in April 1978. GHA continued to suffer financial reversals and labor disagreements. The nurses and physical therapists went on strike in 1982, and the physicians struck again in 1986. GHA weathered the storm but continued to struggle. Enrollment reached 150,000 in 1986 and 200,000 in 1992. In 1994, unable to persevere in an increasingly competitive market, GHA was acquired by Humana. Thus, an organization that had begun as a consumer cooperative became part of a for-profit chain, one of whose founders had honed his business skills developing the Colonel Sanders Kentucky Fried Chicken franchise.

The rapid expansion of HMOs from 10 million enrollees in 1980 to 100 million in 2005 occurred mostly within the corporate for-profit structure. Many HMOs that started as nonprofits switched to for-profit to take better advantage of their market opportunities. Why have for-profit firms been more successful, and why didn't they emerge earlier? Sydney Garfield dreamed of "one organized integrality" that encompassed all of medicine as a business, including hospitals, laboratories, physicians, financing, and marketing under one roof. He was able to maintain unified control by force of personality during Kaiser's formative years, but he lost control when confronted by these vital questions: Who can borrow enough money to build a hospital? How are wages to be set once profits start rolling in? How can one physician single-handedly manage a group of doctors too large for all of them to be personal friends? The common answer to all of these questions lay in the "corporatization" of health care organizations.[23]

12.7   ENTREPRENEURSHIP AND PROFITS

In a corporation, control is more clearly defined. The board of directors has the power to appoint senior management, which, in turn, has the power to hire and fire employees, purchase assets, and borrow money. The stockholders have a clear right to the profits. However, being numerous and diffuse, these stockholders usually have little control over the management of operations. The corporate structure is able to delegate authority and establish accountability reasonably well. Opponents of for-profit health care might argue that nonprofit organizations can be very well managed. In fact, nonprofit and for-profit hospitals both have boards of directors and suites full of administrators who seem to look and act similarly in most ways. The difference is the nonprofit organization's lack of direct ownership. No one in a nonprofit organization has the incentive, or the power, to take a big risk in the hope of achieving a large capital gain. Furthermore, the lack of unified control makes it hard for any one person to make rapid and risky decisions on behalf of the whole organization in times of turbulent change and emerging opportunity.

A nonprofit structure with diffuse ownership might actually be an advantage when leadership requires achieving a consensus among a large number of stakeholder groups. Such a situation was characteristic for most community hospitals from 1950 to 1980. Yet when profits and survival depend on hard bargaining, innovation, and quick commitments to capture opportunities that expand and disappear in a moment, the diffuse voluntary structure is overwhelmed. It is simply harder for an entrepreneur to work in a nonprofit structure or to take the organization he or she has built and sell it for a large capital gain.

U.S. Healthcare: A Profitable Growth Company

U.S. Healthcare, founded by Leonard Abramson in 1975, is a good example of the new for-profit HMO firms that came to dominate the market. Abramson was from a South Philadelphia family of modest means and had driven a taxi to put himself through pharmacy school. After working as a detailer calling on physicians for a pharmaceutical firm (see Chapter 11), six years in retail pharmacy, and participation in equipment leasing and other health care businesses, Abramson was astounded by the freedom of doctors and hospitals to raise prices whenever they wanted. "It was a blank check," he said in a 1985 interview.[24] Abramson was much taken with the promise of HMOs to bring business methods to health care and knew a number of physicians who shared his enthusiasm. Taking advantage of the government loans made available by the HMO Act of 1973, the Health Maintenance Organization of Pennsylvania was incorporated as a nonprofit prepaid health plan in January 1975, obtained a state HMO license in 1976, and was designated a federally qualified HMO in 1977.[25] Operations started in April 1977 by taking over the assets of an existing prepaid health plan, Family Medical Care. HMO/PA began enrolling members and grew rapidly. In 1981, U.S. Healthcare left nonprofit status and went private using venture capital from Warburg, Pincus and Company to pay back a $2.5 million loan to the federal government. Its initial public offering of stock came in 1983, as did its expansion into New Jersey.

The Philadelphia market of the 1980s was old-style traditional medicine: lots of specialists, lots of hospital beds, and fee-for-service indemnity insurance. With changing medical trends and the advent of Medicare's prospective payment by DRG (see Chapter 8), it was becoming clear that there was a surplus of hospitals in the area and that even good specialists were having trouble attracting all the patients they wanted. There was room for an entrepreneur who could cut premiums by contracting in advance for surgery and beds at a discount. Abramson was a sharp negotiator. It often seemed that he came into a bargaining session knowing more about a hospital's operations and finances than its administrators did. Discounts of 20 percent, 30 percent, or more were often won. Abramson made information a weapon in the fight for market share and low prices, and he honed it to a fine edge in repeated competitive encounters.

Not everyone was enamored of U.S. Healthcare's tactics. Some hospitals were terrified that they would lose so much revenue that they might go out of business, and the Philadelphia Blue Cross plan was furious that an upstart was trying to invade its market by cutting prices.[26] The acrimony spilled over into name calling, then full-page attack advertisements in the newspapers, and finally a series of lawsuits charging libel and unfair trading on both sides (most of which were settled or won by U.S. Healthcare, although bad feelings between the two companies continued to run high). By 1985 U.S. Healthcare, with more than 500,000 enrollees, was the sixth-largest HMO in the nation, and probably the most profitable. Its medical loss ratio was only 75 percent, whereas the average was closer to 80 percent, and Kaiser was above 95 percent.[27] The formula of aggressive contracting, meticulous claims review, and conscientious client service made the company successful and financially sound, although with less than a 20 percent market share it was far from dominant and was not universally loved.

Abramson was not content to let the company rest on its laurels and pile up profits. He made a strategic decision to emphasize quality. Whereas most primary care physician incentive payments in the original HMO/PA reimbursement plan were cost controls dependent on reductions in the quantity of referrals and other services used, the Quality Care Compensation System (QCCS) for primary physicians, inaugurated in 1987, based 40 percent of practice bonuses on quality and consumer satisfaction measures. The 1992 QCCS revision raised the bar further, making 82 percent of incentives reliant on medical chart review, availability of evening hours, retention of existing patients, ability to attract new members, and ratings on questionnaires mailed to patients, with only 18 percent related to reductions in utilization.[28] For hospitals, the CapTainer payment system introduced in 1992 paid a quality- and diagnosis-adjusted per-diem rate. Quality incentive plans were introduced for obstetrician/gynecologists in 1994 and for other referral specialists in 1996.[29]

Central to the new strategy was the development of a corporate subsidiary in 1990, USQA, devoted solely to quality measurement. USQA created databanks based on millions of patient records, consumer surveys, pathology reports, and laboratory tests. The physician-information scientists working at USQA published significant studies on the cost-effectiveness of laparoscopic cholecystectomy, asthma treatment, influenza immunization, and autologous bone marrow transplantation for treatment of breast cancer. It used $2 million to fund a fellowship in Managed Care and Quality Assessment at Jefferson Medical College. In 1993, U.S. Healthcare was the first HMO to release the full 1992 Health Employer Data and Information Set (HEDIS) report and, in 1994, the first to provide members with a detailed report card on each participating physician.[30] U.S. Healthcare had clearly gone far beyond compliance and had established a leading presence in the quality assurance and health care information field.[31]

Growth continued to climb, reaching 1 million members in 1989 and 2 million members in 1995. In the face of such rising demand, Abramson's announcement that he would cut premiums in order to build market share came as quite a surprise.[32] Publicly traded HMO stocks fell by as much as 16 percent the following day. Yet the strategy of favoring long-term growth over short-term profitability was sound, and share prices soon recovered. U.S. Healthcare ended the year trading at $46\frac{1}{2}$, with a total market capitalization of $7.1 billion. In April 1996, Aetna Life & Casualty declared that it would acquire Abramson's company, paying more than $8 billion.[33] The information and quality-assurance systems of USQA would now be deployed to serve 14 million members, reaching roughly one out of every twelve people with health insurance in the United States.

Why did Abramson decide to sell if U.S. Healthcare was such a successful company? Although any analysis of internal motivations and assessments is largely speculative, some plausible reasons do appear upon reflection. Although U.S. Healthcare had created start-ups and/or joint ventures in Florida, Illinois, Delaware, and Maryland, as well as ten other states and even in Europe, by 1996 it was becoming more difficult to maintain the 10 to 20 percent annual growth it had enjoyed. Every major market now had an established HMO, often several, and the indemnity insurers such as Blue Cross, CIGNA, and New York Life had developed their own HMO plans; therefore, signing up each additional employer group was a struggle. Merger with Aetna meant that 11 million (mostly indemnity) members could be transferred over rather than fought for. Tremendous economies of scale in the use of USQA's software and statistical profiles could be immediately obtained. In 1992, heady with success, the management of U.S. Healthcare had envisioned that USQA would attract other HMOs as clients and be spun off as a separate company, perhaps growing larger than its parent. Later, it became clear why such a strategy was not viable. Monitoring quality and developing information systems is intimately intertwined with the core business of an HMO, so much so that most HMOs would never allow a competitor to participate in that task or to access such sensitive data. Hence, USQA technology could only be used in-house or sold in regions (such as England) where U.S. Healthcare would never be a competitive threat.

In the end, it may have been Abramson himself who was the most compelling reason for selling the company. U.S. Healthcare never developed a faceless corporate style; it was always Leonard Abramson's company, where he personally made most of the important decisions. Although he had groomed several of his children for leadership roles and brought in a number of senior executives, there was no clear successor in sight.[34] The genius and prime mover of the company was now 63. He sold the company—at the peak— for $8 billion.

Even though U.S. Healthcare was bought by Aetna, it was assumed that the smaller company, U.S. Healthcare, would colonize the larger old-line insurer from within, with those executives taking leading roles to spread managed-care quality measurement techniques and thereby transform the older and much larger indemnity insurer. How well did the deal work? It vaulted Abramson into the role of leading philanthropist and threw Aetna/U.S. Healthcare into a tailspin. Most of the U.S. Healthcare executives targeted as leaders drifted away or were let go. An Aetna insurance executive took the reins, tightened controls, cut payments, and drove the hospitals and physicians into revolt. The market had changed, and providers were no longer willing to make sacrifices for an HMO contract. Providers threatened to pull out, and Aetna had to pull back. Finally, a new CEO, a doctor from academia with almost no insurance experience, was brought in to restore confidence and rebuild relationships. Marginal lines of business were cut or sold. Aetna/U.S. Healthcare kept losing money, and after five years its total market capitalization had fallen below $6 billion—less than it had paid for U.S. Healthcare.

Aetna is no longer the largest health insurer in the United States. It reformed operations and turned the company around to become profitable. By 2005 its share price had increased 600 percent. However, the Aetna of today is not the ultimate managed-care company envisioned in the waning years of the last millennium but simply a strong, solid health insurance company servicing clients and earning a good return. Aetna suffered because it overpaid for U.S. Healthcare's assets. Those in control lacked business acumen, despite the expertise of their staff and financial consultants.

This chapter reviewed a number of financial concepts and techniques, serving as a mere introduction to the intricacies of legal structure, corporate finance, risk, and the time value of money. Yet perhaps even these simple lessons can be a caution to help someone avoid making big mistakes with billions of dollars.

12.8   HEALH CARE FOR PROFIT, OR NOT

There is no such thing as a free lunch, even for economic incentives. The promise of wealth can be a tremendous spur to entrepreneurship. Competition for profits forces firms to strive for efficiency with an intensity that rarely happens in a voluntary nonprofit organization run for community benefit, as the examination of the HMO history above illustrates. Yet money is not everything. Who wants the surgeon deciding whether to operate, or how much tissue to remove, thinking about the fees? Should an internist deciding which statin to prescribe be considering how large a rebate the manufacturer offers? Is the psychiatric facility where your friend is admitted for panic attacks and a drug overdose an oasis of caring and concern, or a factory maximizing occupancy and insurance reimbursement? There are things that money cannot buy, or whose value would be seriously eroded if they were purchased for cash.[35] Consider the following story reported by Bloomberg News in the *Washington Post:*

> Janet Stubbs was grateful when the nursing home recommended hospice care for her aunt Midge. Although Stubbs knew her aunt was not dying, the offer of free, Medicare-paid hospice visits from a nurse and chaplain, plus an extra weekly bath, was too good to pass up. Stubbs did not know that her aunt, Doris Midge Appling, was admitted to Hospice Care of Kansas during the company's "Summer Sizzle" promotion drive, which paid employees as much as $100 a head for referrals, according to the Department of Justice. Stubbs said she had no clue that the nursing home doctor who referred her aunt for hospice moonlighted as medical director for the hospice company. "It doesn't seem right," said Stubbs, who had Appling's power of attorney to make medical decisions. "What incentive did the doctor have to put my aunt on hospice? How much was she being paid?"
>
> —"Aided by Referral Bonuses, Hospice Industry Booms." Peter Waldman, Bloomberg News, published in the *Washington Post*, December 17, 2011.

Medical care is about "caring" as well as cure. Hospice especially so, because patients are transitioning to death and have renounced most intrusive treatments. "The Financial Reimbursement Cycle" (Chapter 10, Section 10) discussed how hospitals, nursing homes, home health, and now hospices were becoming more businesslike and for-profit. Palliative care of the dying, carried out by family members and volunteers for years with little recompense has, with the availability of generous Medicare reimbursement, become a billion-dollar growth industry. Hospices are now mostly for-profit, and many of the largest groups are divisions of public-traded corporations.

The purpose of a for-profit corporation is to maximize discounted cash flows for the owners. The social purpose of such companies is to allocate capital and generate profits, not help the community, cure disease, or care with kindness. As Adam Smith pointed out in *The Wealth of Nations*, benevolence is a side effect. The goal is wealth maximization. Voluntary (nonprofit) organizations are fundamentally different in that they are not allowed to distribute profits to the owners or managers; the residual claimant is society rather than an individual (the technical term for giving board members or managers a share of profits is "inurement," and it is illegal). Because the capital structure is different, the market discipline on nonprofits is weak; there are no stockholders clamoring for better earnings, cost-cutting layoffs, or sale of underperforming divisions, nor can the organization be bought out and sold to replace management and improve results unless the voluntary board should choose to do so or is forced to by bankruptcy.

Competitive pursuit of profits will crowd out human kindness and moral scruples unless regulated by social norms and legal restraints.[36] The use of incentive payments for surgical implants, drug prescribing, home health visits, and nursing home admissions has often been questioned. The $100 bonus for admitting the elderly aunt described above is not just distasteful, it violates regulations intended to stop providers from treating Medicare as OPM (other people's money), there for the taking. Each of these medical industries has seen one or more waves of indictments and convictions for pushing the boundaries too far, stepping over into fraud and abuse.

Voluntary nonprofits can also break the law, but historically they have been less likely to do so precisely because they do not face such powerful financial incentives. The goals of voluntary organizations are complex and are often more attuned to respect, moral satisfaction, community relations, or politics; they are not so focused on cash flow. A market environment that becomes more competitive and threatens the growth or survival of the institution will push voluntaries to act with more concern for the bottom line and hence behave more like their for-profit peers, but the pressure is not so intense.

Differences Between For-Profit and Nonprofit Behavior

Many studies have been done comparing for-profits with nonprofits. Some show large effects and others show small or negligible effects, yet almost all point in the same direction: Nonprofits tend to be somewhat less efficient, more willing to sacrifice profits to raise quality, and slower to respond to changing financial incentives. Typical is a recent MedPAC (Medicare Payment Advisory Committee) report finding that for-profit skilled nursing facilities (SNFs) had lower costs per day ($266 versus $280) and had lower quality as measured by the percentage of patients for whom rehospitalization was necessary (18.7 percent versus 14.8 percent), but they seemed to charge more per day as operating margins were significantly higher (20.7 percent versus 9.5 percent).[37] Analogous results have been shown in other studies in other contexts: For-profit hospices had longer lengths of stay but provided fewer visits, profitable surgical patients were differentially steered to private centers, doctors with ownership interest in laboratories or imaging centers ordered more tests, dialysis patients and prisoners receiving medical care from for-profit companies were more likely to die, patenting human genes to establish private ownership made sequencing go faster but reduced subsequent dissemination and use, and so on.[38]

For each study cited above one can find similar research showing no significant effect. A paper by Dafny and Ramanarayanan looking at the effects of converting a local Blue Cross plan to for-profit status helps to sort out the confusion.[39] In most regions they found little or no effect, but in areas where the converting plan had significant monopolistic market power, being for-profit led to higher premiums and less coverage. This accords with the conclusions from a comprehensive review of for-profit versus nonprofit hospitals carried out by Eggleston and colleagues, which states "the 'true' effect of ownership appears to depend upon institutional context, including differences across regions, markets and over time."[40]

Charity Care: For Real or for Show?

The social burden of caring for the poor is often used as an explanation for the special treatment given doctors and hospitals. Charity was obviously of great importance in financing medicine a hundred years ago, but it is much smaller today. A study of physician offices providing care to the uninsured showed that the higher prices (full charges) paid by those with no insurance more than made up for the higher likelihood that they would not pay. That is, these doctors made more per patient from those who were poor and had no insurance than from the better-off patients where insurance companies were competitively negotiating lower prices. This is rather like the credit card business, where banks charge poor people with bad scores enough extra fees to more than offset a higher rate of losses and hence keep subprime lending profitable.

Hospitals clearly do provide charity care, especially hospitals in the inner city. However, do they provide enough uncompensated care to the uninsured to make up for the tax breaks they receive? The IRS changed the rules on form 990 (the main financial report required of nonprofits) to make hospitals account for charity care. The results, first reported in December of 2011, were revealing and perhaps surprising: on average, charity accounted for just 1.5 percent of hospital gross revenues.[41] The vast majority of voluntary hospitals had operating margins greater than the amount of charity care provided. In the following year, as the economy continued to tank and unemployment reached 9 percent, hospitals had their best financial performance in thirty years, $53 billion in profits for a margin of 7.2 percent.

For-Profit or Not-for-Profit: Which is Better?

Health care is filled with dedicated doctors, nurses, and aides who strive to care for patients with compassion and science. Yet the practice of medicine is as compromised and competitive as any other human activity. Both for-profits and nonprofits have strengths and weaknesses.

Some health care organizations are innovative, with great management and outstanding performance (Intermountain Health, Geisinger, and the Cleveland and Mayo clinics are often mentioned), but most are ordinary, and quite a few are mediocre. There are bad actors on both sides. Some for-profits have enriched themselves by defrauding patients and occasionally had to pay the price (Healthsouth, ColumbiaHCA, Tenet, Stryker), as have some nonprofits (St. Barnabas, Cooper), although the more common abuse among nonprofits has been complacent boards that pampered friends while they allowed quality and efficiency to deteriorate.

The basic findings reported above will probably not change: For-profits tend to respond quicker, have lower costs, higher prices, and thus greater profits. They avoid patients who are sicker, uninsured, or poor; emphasize amenities to focus on the most profitable services (cream skimming); and are less likely to carry out undercompensated activities like teaching, research, or community outreach. Voluntary organizations often show higher costs, sicker patients, some lower fees, and thus lower operating margins, but they tend to practice medicine that is more caring, kinder, and gentler, even if a bit less efficient.

The relevant questions for economists are to determine why, and then what, if anything, can be done to improve the situation. As was pointed out in the discussion of the financial reimbursement cycle, the deficiencies of aggressive profit-seeking are usually ameliorated over time by regulation, social approbation, and the negative effects of a bad reputation. For example, the GAO found that for-profit nursing homes had more violations and deficiencies than not-for-profits, but that when acquired by new investors the staffing mix and facility quality tended to move up toward the mean (and also make these nursing homes more attractive to higher-paying residents).[42] The health care system needs both types of ownership. Over time, patients' expectations, social norms, and financial market pressures tend to force for-profits and nonprofits toward similar behavior, but never quite to converge. The best that we can do is to maintain a dynamic balance, recognizing the strengths and weaknesses of each form, and applying them differentially as conditions change.

Medical Care is Difficult: Risk, Information Asymmetry, Social Justice

The underlying reasons for the organizational and operational problems of medical care have been examined at length in previous chapters: the necessity of pooled third-party financing means that most transactions are carried out with other people's money, for which neither the patient nor the provided feels much concern. Information asymmetry and fear of illness and death leads to reliance on physicians as agents, making patients uninformed about the value or cost of the care their receive. Hospitals cover costs of teaching, research, and emergency care through extensive cost shifting, with reimbursement based on charges or administered prices (DRGS) that do not convey dynamically changing information the way most markets would. Pharmaceutical companies face cost-shifting requirements that are even more challenging as the billion-dollar expense of finding a new drug must be recouped from a pill costing a few cents to make and must be accomplished before the patent runs out. Long-term care further exposes the fallacy of a natural price, demonstrating that economic truism that providing more money to solve a problem will lead to more care—and to more aggressive profiteering that must be regulated.[43] These issues are inherent, part of the biology or DNA of medical care. Health is different, it will always be different (although certainly in different ways over time). Insurance and licensure cannot be wished or wiped away any more than bacteria, cancer, or dementia can. Hence the organizational struggles will follow the underlying problems: most difficult where informational asymmetry is greatest, where marginal and average costs are most divergent, where emotional distress is most painful, where considerations of fairness, charity, and social obligation are most contentious.

SUGGESTIONS FOR FURTHER READING

CFO Magazine, http://www.cfo.com

Fitch Ratings, Rating Process for Nonprofit Health Care Credits, http://www.fitchratings.com/

Louis C. Gapenski, *Healthcare Finance: An Introduction to Accounting and Financial Management* (Chicago: Health Administration Press, 2004).

Healthcare Financial Management Association, http://www.hfma.org

Moody's U.S. Municipal Bond Rating Scale, http://www.moodys.com/

Kristin R. Reiter, John R. C. Wheeler, and Dean G. Smith, "Liquidity Constraints on Hospital Investment When Credit Markets are Tight," *Journal of Health Care Finance* 35, no. 1 (2008): 24–33.

J. B. Silvers, "The Role of Capital Markets in Restructuring Health Care," *Journal of Health Politics, Policy and Law* 26, no. 5 (2001): 1019–1030.

Standard & Poors, Understanding Capital Markets, http://www2.standardandpoors.com

Burton Weisbrod, *The Nonprofit Economy* (Cambridge, Mass.: Harvard University Press, 1988); "Rewarding Performance That Is Hard to Measure: The Private Non-Profit Sector," *Science* 244, no. 4904 (1989): 541–546.

David Cutler, "Where Are The Health Care Entrepreneurs? The Failure of Organizational Innovation in Health Care," NBER working paper#16030, May 2010.

SUMMARY

1. Every organization must have cash inflows that exceed cumulative cash outflows (**no margin, no mission**). This means that start-up funds are required, that regular operations (plus fundraising and/or reserves) must generate a surplus, and that at the close of operations, some entity must be designated as residual claimant (owner) of remaining funds.

2. The value of an asset is the cash flow it generates. Anything that increases earnings, such as a medical degree, can be evaluated in terms of financial rate of return. Considering all present and future costs and benefits, **the internal rate of return (IRR) of a project is the interest rate at which the sum of the present value of all cash flows (NPV) is zero**.

3. Although medical school tuition is expensive, running as much as $50,000 per year, it is still a very good **investment in human capital**. The average medical student will graduate with a debt of about $85,000, but this is less than six months of the average physician's earnings. Overall, taking into account the tuition, years of training, extra hard work, and other factors, going to medical school provides an annual inflation-adjusted return of about 12 percent, three or four times what one could expect if one invested in financial assets rather than education, and about 1.5 to 2 times as much as one gains from most undergraduate and graduate education.

4. Assets with risks that are independent (uncorrelated) can be bundled together into **a diversified portfolio that reduces variability**. Insurance companies are financial intermediaries pooling individual risks, and pharmaceutical companies are diversified corporations with multiple projects and are thus able to maintain profitability in most years. However, if the risks are correlated, then bundling assets together can increase volatility and lead to a system-wide financial crisis.

5. If equity capital is replaced by borrowed funds, that **debt increases financial leverage**, raising returns on equity when outcomes are better than expected but reducing returns when outcomes are worse, and they can even bankrupt the company, leaving stockholders with nothing under adverse circumstances.

6. The largest sources of **risk in health care are changes in regulation and reimbursement** rather than the changes in interest rates or GDP that are the most important risks for most financial markets.

7. In a sole proprietorship, the owner is responsible for everything and can claim all the profits, but in larger organizations **agency problems arise where there is a separation of ownership from control**. Management can behave in ways that are not in the interest of the stockholders (publicly traded firms) or the community (nonprofits).

8. Although accounting for just 9 percent of operating costs, **access to capital** has been crucial in shaping the growth of hospitals. Philanthropy was first replaced by government construction grants through the **Hill–Burton Act** of 1946 and subsequently by **tax-exempt municipal revenue bonds** in the 1970s. **Equity** financing through the stock market is becoming increasingly important as hospitals try to acquire nursing homes, physician practices, and other hospitals to form integrated health care systems.

9. Most HMOs started as nonprofit organizations. Some were explicitly collectivist and anticapitalist in origin, but they have become increasingly businesslike. **Kaiser**, founded just after World War II, is **the largest HMO**, with more than 10 million members. However, the lack of a clearly defined ownership structure, limited access to capital, and resistance to capital mobility between regions have been major impediments to further growth. Over time, the more rapid **growth of for-profit firms** has led them to dominate the industry, and now even many nonprofit HMOs have for-profit subsidiaries.

10. Growth and/or downsizing through mergers and acquisitions are inherently more complex for nonprofits. With no market for corporate control there are no forced takeovers; **ownership changes and reorganization among nonprofits is limited mainly to distressed facilities** in financial trouble that need capital to survive.

PROBLEMS

1. {*financial definitions*} What is the value of an asset? What is its NPV? Its IRR?

2. {*annualized returns*} If the rate of return on human capital is 15 percent and the opportunity cost of time for a newly graduated physician is $60,000 per year, how large an incremental increase in annual earnings should the physician expect to obtain from a four-year postgraduate residency?

3. {*NPV, IRR*} If a project requires an initial investment of $25,000 and then is sold for $42,000 after five years, what is its NPV at an interest rate of 6 percent? What is its IRR?

4. {*NPV, IRR*} If Dr. Smith buys a machine for $5,000 and is able to improve the earnings of her practice by $2,000 a year for five years, and then can sell the machine for $600 as scrap, what is the NPV at 15 percent? What is the IRR?

5. {*NPV, IRR*} Dr. Smith opens a lab at a cost of $10,000 that provides revenues of $3,000 in the first year, with revenue growing by 15 percent a year after that. Expenses in each year are equal to 20 percent of revenues. In five years the lab is obsolete and worthless. What is the NPV of the lab at 8 percent? What is its IRR? What would the value be if you kept all the other assumptions the same, but sales in the first year were $2,000? What if instead of growing by 15 percent each year, revenues shrank by 15 percent each year?

6. {*ownership*} Are doctors usually employees, owners, or managers of hospitals?

7. {*ownership*} Who owns most hospitals? Who gets the profit when a nonprofit hospital makes money? Can nonprofit hospitals be bought and sold?

8. {*capital financing*} Are the ways hospitals obtain capital different from the ways doctors obtain capital? Why?

9. {*rate of return, incidence*} How does a philanthropist who donates funds to a hospital get "returns on capital"? Are these returns measured as a dollar amount, as an annualized percentage rate, or by some other method?

10. {*ownership, nonprofit, capital financing*} Hospitals received special treatment from the government and were able to borrow subsidized capital using tax-exempt municipal revenue bonds. During the 1970s and 1980s, billions of dollars of tax-free capital flowed into nonprofit hospitals. Did this make them more or less like for-profit firms?

11. {*financial reporting*} Which is more important in determining the type of financial reports a hospital must prepare: the type of ownership or the major sources of funding? If capital is attracted from different sources, are different types of financial reports required?

12. {*property rights*} What are the advantages and disadvantages of (a) nonprofit status and (b) publicly traded stock that provides incentives to physicians?

13. {*property rights*} Who owns Kaiser Permanente? Is there stock? Have ownership rights ever been sold?

14. {*property rights*} Why were HMOs formed in the 1930s often collectives attracting physicians with liberal or socialist leanings, whereas today HMOs are most often formed by entrepreneurs with capitalist ideals?

15. {*pricing*} How did Sidney Garfield set the monthly premiums for his first prepaid health plan? How are premiums set for Kaiser today?

16. {*regulation*} Did the HMO Act of 1973 affect competition and capital expenditure in a manner similar to the certificate of need (CON) acts passed during the same period?

ENDNOTES

1. Good general sources of information include *CFO* magazine at www.CFO.com and *HFM* magazine at www.hfma.org.
2. Gary S. Becker, *Human Capital* (Cambridge, Mass: Harvard University Press, 1975).
3. William B. Weeks and Amy E. Wallace, "The More Things Change: Revisiting a Comparison of Educational Costs and Incomes of Physicians and Other Professionals," *Academic Medicine* 77, no. 4 (2002): 312–319; see also Sean Nicholson, "Medical Career Choices and Rates of Return," in F. A. Sloan and H. Kasper, eds., *Incentives and Choice in Health Care* (Cambridge. Mass.: MIT Press, 2008), 195–225.
4. The calculation would be $(1.17) \times (1.17) \times (1.17) \times (1.17) \times (1.17) = 2.1924$, which is slightly less than 2.20, so a more precise answer would be 17.0805 percent; it just depends upon how exact you try to make your approximation.
5. Diversification that would help to reduce risk due to macroeconomic shifts in the U.S. economy would be foreign stocks (especially emerging markets), commodities, special purpose arbitrage funds, and other investments relatively uncorrelated with movements in the stock and bond markets. See also Joseph H. Golec and John A. Vernon, "Financial Risk in the Biotechnology Industry," NBER working paper #13604, November 2007.
6. The classic DuPont Equation for Return on Equity is:

$$ROE = \text{Net Income/Equity} = (\text{Net})/(\text{Sales}) \times (\text{Sales})/(\text{Assets}) \times (\text{Assets})/(\text{Equity})$$

7. Some beginning corporate finance texts refer to revenue risk and operating leverage together as "business risk" or "enterprise risk" and assume that one knows in advance all cash flows from operations. This allows them to focus solely on how financial leverage affects earnings without having to worry about revenues and expenses. In understanding the finances of health care organizations, that particular simplification is usually untenable. Most of the action is on the "revenue and expense" side, with pure financial engineering having limited relevance. It was important in the case of the nursing home industry because it is largely for-profit, publicly traded, and asset heavy with simple services and limited technology that doesn't change very rapidly—that is, compared to most of medicine.
8. There are several references to economics in the Oath. The classic translation is W. H. S. Jones, *Hippocrates*, The Loeb Classical Library (Cambridge, Mass.: Harvard University Press, 1923). A more recent translation is provided by Heinrich von Staden, "in a pure and holy way:" "Personal and Professional Conduct in the Hippocratic Oath," *Journal of the History of Medicine and Allied Sciences* 51, no. 4 (1996): 404–437.

9. "Entrepreneur" is taken from the French and means one who undertakes a venture, who grabs the chance, who organizes resources and brings an idea to business fruition.

10. Michael C. Jensen and William H. Meckling, "Theory of the Firm: Managerial Behavior, Agency Costs and Ownership Structure," *Journal of Financial Economics* 3, no. 4 (1976): 305–360.

11. Odin W. Anderson, *Health Services as a Growth Enterprise in the United States since 1875* (Ann Arbor: Health Administration Press, 1990).

12. Jonathan Betz Brown, *Health Capital Financing* (Ann Arbor: Health Administration Press, 1988), 14–18.

13. Patrick M. Bernet and Thomas E. Getzen, "The Company You Keep: Spreading Effects of Financial Fraud on Investor Trust," *Journal of Health Care Finance* 33, no. 3 (2007): 48–66; Cain Brothers, *Strategies in Capital Finance* 27 (Summer): 1–26, 1999; Lawton Burns and John Cacciamani, "The Fall of the House of AHERF: The Allegheny Bankruptcy," *Health Affairs* 19, no. 1 (2000): 7–42.

14. Mary Chris Jaklevic, "Pricier, Less Plentiful," *Modern Healthcare* 30, no. 21 (2000): 52–56.

15. Robert Sigmond, "From Charity Care to Community Benefit," *Hospitals & Health Services Administration* 39, no. 2 (Summer 1994): 141–142.

16. Charles Wrightson, "Selection Bias and Premium Rate Setting," in *HMO Rate Setting and Financial Strategy* (Ann Arbor: Health Administration Press, 1990), 245–292.

17. The term "risk" is used to mean many different things. The technical definition often used in finance is "random variation over which managers have no control" and is equated with the standard deviation of some statistical series. Most businesspeople use "risk" to mean something such as "all of the things that can happen." In health care, "taking on risk" means accepting capitation—and taking a fixed monthly payment would be seen by most businesses as getting rid of the risk from an uneven flow of FFS payments. A leading health care business consultant said, "What cannot be controlled should not be assumed as risk," (Joseph Coyne, *Healthcare Financial Management*, August 1994, p 33). This definition, relying on managerial control over clinical processes, is quite at odds with the definition of risk used by currency and bond traders, who strive to make money contracting strictly for things they cannot control.

18. Much of the information in this section comes from John G. Smillie, MD, *Can Physicians Manage the Quality and Costs of Health Care: The Story of the Permanente Medical Group* (New York: McGraw–Hill, 1991); and Paul de Kruif, *Kaiser Wakes the Doctors* (New York: Harcourt, Brace & Co., 1943).

19. Prepaid medical group practice had existed in America since at least 1790, when such a plan was used at the Boston Dispensary. The innovative prepayment contract between the City of Los Angeles Department of Water and Power and Drs. Ross and Loos to provide all medical services to 12,000 employees and 25,000 dependents for $2 per month (excluding hospitalization) was a more proximate example that probably influenced Garfield.

20. Quoted in John G. Smillie, MD, *Can Physicians Manage the Quality and Costs of Health Care: The Story of the Permanente Medical Group* (New York, McGraw–Hill, 1991), 55.

21. Louise Kertesz, "Kaiser Retools to Fight for Lost Ground," *Modern Healthcare*, 25, no. 29 (1995): 34–40.

22. Edward D. Berkowitz and Wendy Wolff, *Group Health Association: A Portrait of a Health Maintenance Organization* (Philadelphia: Temple University Press, 1988), 144.

23. Paul Starr, *The Social Transformation of American Medicine* (New York: Basic Books, 1982).

24. As quoted in Gilbert Gaul, "U.S. Healthcare's Abramson: Dedicated, Perhaps Ruthless," *Philadelphia Inquirer*, April 2, 1996: A5.

25. Much of the information in this case study comes from interviews with Sandra Harmon-Weiss, MD, Medical Director of U.S. Healthcare, and other executives, "A Brief Overview: U.S. Healthcare," by Hyman R. Kahn, M.D. (mimeo, November 28, 1994), and annual financial reports of U.S. Healthcare.

26. In the words of Pulitzer Prize–winning journalist Gilbert Gaul, "For years, some of the most prestigious hospitals in Philadelphia refused to sign contracts with U.S. Healthcare. Those that did often complained bitterly about the hard-line negotiating style of Abramson and his colleagues, which resulted in lower reimbursement rates for the hospitals." in "U.S. Healthcare's Abramson: Dedicated, Perhaps Ruthless," *Philadelphia Inquirer*, April 2, 1996: A5.

27. Accounting practices are significantly different in the nonprofit Kaiser plan, so the figures are not entirely comparable. It is, however, generally accepted that of the major HMOs, Kaiser probably has the highest percentage of premiums going to medical costs, whereas U.S. Healthcare had among the lowest.

28. Neil Schlackman, "Evolution of a Quality-Based Compensation Model: The Third Generation," *American Journal of Medical Quality* 8, no. 2 (1993): 103–110.

29. Nicholas Hanchak, Neil Schlackman, and Sandra Harmon-Weiss, *U.S. Healthcare's Quality-Based Compensation Model*, 32 pages (mimeo) (Blue Bell, Pa.: U.S. Healthcare, 1996).

30. Paul Kenkel, "U.S. Healthcare 'Report Cards' Expanded to Primary-Care Docs," *Modern Healthcare* April 11, 1994.

31. Eleanor H. Kerns, health care analyst for Alex Brown & Sons, a leading investment banking firm, has opined publicly that U.S. Healthcare's information systems were superior to those of competitors. See Marian Uhlman and Andrea Knox, "Aetna, U.S. Healthcare Plan Merger," *Philadelphia Inquirer* April 2, 1996: A1; A5.

32. George Anders and Ron Winslow, "HMO Stocks Skid on U.S. Healthcare Announcement," *Wall Street Journal*, April 20, 1995.

33. Leslie Scism and Steven Lipin, "Aetna Near $8 Billion Deal to Acquire U.S. Healthcare," *Wall Street Journal*, April 1, 1996: A3.

34. Gilbert Gaul, "U.S. Healthcare's Abramson: Dedicated, Perhaps Ruthless," *Philadelphia Inquirer*, April 2, 1996: A5.

35. E.g., love, a college degree, medal of honor, or sex.

36. However, see Markus Kitzmueller and Jay Shimshack, "Economic Perspectives on Corporate Social Responsibility," *Journal of Economic Literature* 50, no. 1 (2012):51–84.

37. Medicare Payment Advisory Commission, *Medicare Payment Policy: Report to Congress*, March 12, 2011. www.medpac.gov.

38. Y Zhang, DJ Cotter, M Thamer, "The Effect of Dialysis Chains on Mortality among Patients Receiving Hemodialysis," *Health Services Research* 46, no. 3 (2011): 747–767; M. W. Wachterman et al., "Association of Hospice Agency Profit Status With Patient Diagnosis, Location of Care, and Length of Stay," *Journal of the American Medical Association* 305, no. 5 (2011): 427–479, 2011; M. R. Plotzke and C. Courtemanche, "Does Procedure Profitability Impact Whether an Oupatient Surgery is Performed at an Ambulatory Surgery Center or Hospital?" *Health Economics* 20, no. 7 (2011): 817–830; Melanie Evans, "Juggling the Lineup: Seeking Better Financial Results, Providers Change Services," *Modern Healthcare*, 42, no. 3 (2012): 6-16, 2012; Sujoy Chakravarty, Martin Gaynor, Steven Klepper, and William B. Vogt, "Does the Profit Motive Make Jack Nimble? Ownership Form and the Evolution of the U.S. Hospital Industry," NBER working paper #11705, October 2005; Heidi Williams, "Intellectual Property Rights and Innovation: Evidence from the Human Genome," NBER working paper #16213, July 2010; David Dranove, "Is there Underinvestment in R&D about Prevention?" *Journal of Health Economics* 17, no. 1 (1998): 117–127; P. J. Devereaux et al., "Comparison of Mortality Between Private For-Profit and Private Not-For Profit Hemodialysis Centers," *Journal of the American Medical Association* 288, no. 19 (2002):2449–2457.

39. Leemore Dafny, "Does it Matter if Your Health Insurer is For-Profit? Effects of Ownership on Premiums, Medical Spending, and Insurance Coverage." Paper presented at the American Society of Health Economists and the American Economic Association/ASSA, December 2011.

40. Karen Eggleston et al., "Hospital Ownership and Quality of Care: What Explains the Different Results in the Literature," *Health Economics* 17, no. 12 (2008): 1345-1362; David M. Cutler, ed., *The Changing Hospital Industry: Comparing Not-for-Profit and For-Profit Institutions* (Chicago: University of Chicago Press, 2000).

41. Melanie Evans and Joe Carlson, "Out in the Open: Not-For-Profit Hospital's Charity Spending Revealed," *Modern Healthcare* 41, no. 51 (2011): 6–16; Ashok Selvan, "One for the Record Books: Hospital Profit Margins Hit Highest Level in Decades," *Modern Healthcare* 42, no. 2 (2012): 12; Jonathan Gruber and David Rodriguez, "How Much Uncompensated Care do Doctors Provide?" NBER working paper #13585, November 2007.

42. Government Accountability Office, *Nursing Homes: Private Investment Homes Sometimes Differed from Others in Deficiencies, Staffing and Financial Performance*, GAO-11-571 (Washington, DC: Government Accountability Office, 2011).

43. Maureen Farrell, "Medicare Passes on Big Profits to Insurers," CNN MoneyMarkets, December 22, 2011; John K. Iglehart, "A New Era of For-Profit Hospice Care—The Medicare Benefit," *New England Journal of Medicine* 360, no. 26 (2009): 2701–2703.

CHAPTER 13

MACROECONOMICS OF MEDICAL CARE

QUESTIONS

1. Does inflation affect health care spending? If so, does it affect health care spending permanently or temporarily?

2. How does a person decide what is the right amount to spend each year on health care?

3. How does a nation decide the right amount to spend on health care?

4. Is community health the same as individual health?

5. Why do general tax revenues pay for so much personal health care? Who will pay if the Medicare trust fund runs out of money?

6. Which is more important in determining how much to spend on medical care: how sick people are or how much money is available?

7. Do price controls work? If not, why might people think that they do?

8. Do professional licensure, third-party reimbursement, and nonprofit organizations make it easier or harder to adjust health care spending to changes in prices?

9. What determines wage levels in the health care industry?

10. Is it easier to adjust to growth or to a recession?

13.1 WHAT IS MACRO?

Macro means large. Macroeconomics deals with large-scale properties and institutions that characterize the system as a whole. Individuals become an economic system only when they start to trade with one another. In doing so, they create a whole that is larger than the sum of its parts, develop a government to set the rules under which trade will occur, and create a special medium, money, for conducting trade.[1] Macroeconomics evaluates gross domestic product (GDP) as a measure of national economic activity, whether growing (expansion) or falling (recession), and the dynamics of the process by which change occurs (investment, trade, unemployment, bankruptcy). Rather than investigating the income of a particular individual or firm, macroeconomics investigates growth and distribution of income. Macroeconomics seeks to determine how many people are rich, how many people are poor, whether the same people always make up the same groups over time, and whether the gap is widening or narrowing toward more economic equality.

Macroeconomic (system) properties

- Growth
- Dynamics
- Distribution

Macro (system) institutions

- Government
- Laws
- Money

The macroeconomics of health is concerned with a parallel set of large-scale system issues dealing with (a) spending, employment, and other aspects of medical care as a part of the economy and (b) the biological health status of the population as a whole and its relation to economic changes. Thus, it must address how GDP growth affects the number and income of physicians as well as how GDP growth affects the health (longevity, morbidity) of the population and, consequently, how an increase in longevity affects both spending on medical care and growth in overall GDP.

Health System Properties

Economic	*Biological*
Spending	Longevity
Employment	Fertility
Prices	Productivity

Health (System) Institutions

- Medical professions
- Hospitals and caring organizations
- Financing (insurance and reimbursement) structure

The central issues in the macroeconomics of medical care are growth and distribution: how much, for whom, by whom? Where is more money spent on medical care: Bangladesh or Boston? Why? Who gets the care? Who pays for it? Although these issues are clearly related, they can also usefully be distinguished.

Micro and Macro Perspectives on Spending

The main reason people in Boston spend more on medical care than people in Bangladesh is that they have more money. Medical expenditures depend upon the size of the available budget, as do most other types of spending (housing, food, transportation, entertainment). This simple budgetary dynamic also explains why more is spent on health care in 2010 than in 1910, and more will certainly be spent in 2050 than today (see Figure 13.1). From the graph, it is apparent that the amount spent per person on health care is aligned very closely to the amount of income per person. Income explains a lot of the growth in health spending over time; so much so that once an analyst takes account of income, there is not a lot of variation to be explained by other factors. However, if we ask how much is spent on this particular person in Boston compared to that person in Boston, the answer will be about illness and the need for medical care, not about budgets or per capita income. Even if we compare this person in 2010 with the same person in 2000, or 2020, most of the answers will be in terms of differences in health, not differences in income.

Why is there such a big difference in the answer when we ask about a particular person rather than the per-person national average? Note that the discussion made a subtle shift, from

FIGURE 13.1   U.S. Income per Capita and Health Expenditures per Capita, 1950–2005

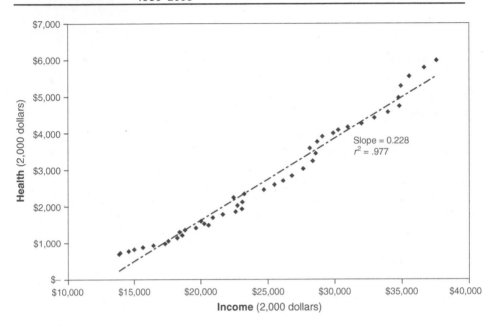

"how much this person spends" to "how much is spent on this person," and therein lies part of the answer. Most medical expenditures in Boston are paid by insurance rather than by the individual.[2] Budgets matter, for health as for other types of spending, but whose budget? The person? Their employer? The insurance company? The state of Massachusetts or the United States of America? All of these matter. For candy or cars, it is likely to be the personal budget (or maybe the family budget) that matters most, but for health care the most important budget is the national budget. For candy and cars, I have to spend my own money. For medical care, expenditures come from insurance, pooled funds from many people, and assistance from tax subsidies. The constraint that matters is not how much I earn; it is how much everybody else earns and contributes to "our" health insurance.

13.2 THE CONSUMPTION FUNCTION

The relationship between income and spending is known as the **consumption function**. Some people spend less than they earn so that they can save. Some people spend more than they earn, dissaving or going into debt. What is always true is that *consumption + savings = income*.[3] This is an accounting identity, a definition that cannot be changed by obfuscation or by wishing it were not so. A corresponding accounting identity holds across people and nations: for each person who borrows, there must be someone who saves and can lend the borrower money. Unless there are people with savings to lend, people (or nations) that want to spend more than they earn cannot do so. This accounting identity is most easily obfuscated when dealing in money rather than goods; therefore, it is better to think in terms of a specific item, such as food. If country A wants to consume 80 tons of lettuce but produces only 60, it has to borrow 20 tons from country B. Country B can do so only if it produces more lettuce than it consumes. Country A will usually pay off the debt with oil or wheat or money instead of lettuce, but the mechanics of transfer are clear: total consumption of all people globally = total production (plus amount saved for next year or minus amount taken from storage). For services and perishables that cannot be stored, the relationship simplifies to *total production = consumption + investment*.

INCOME ELASTICITY

The income elasticity of medical care is measured by the percentage increase in spending relative to each percentage increase in income. Suppose that the income elasticity of medical care were 1.6; that would mean that for a 10 percent increase in income, spending on medical care would increase 16 percent. If the income elasticity were 0.2, then a 10 percent rise in income would lead to only a 2 percent rise in spending.

$$Income\ Elasticity = \frac{percent\ change\ in\ expenditure}{percent\ change\ in\ income}$$

On average, items have an income elasticity of about 1.0. Such "unit elasticity" has a special constancy: Because a 10 percent rise in income leads to a 10 percent rise in expenditures, the share of the total budget spent on that item remains unchanged. If 0.133 of all spending was on an item that had unit income elasticity, then the share spent on that item would remain 0.133 if income rose 10 percent, rose 20 percent, or fell 10 percent. Items whose income elasticity is less than unitary (0.999 or less) will take a smaller and smaller share of total spending as income grows. Food was the largest budget item when the USA was founded in 1776, and for many decades afterward. As the nation grew richer the amount spent on food increased, but not by as much as income was increasing. Therefore the share of total spending accounted for by food fell from over 60 percent to less than 15 percent today. Items with income elasticity greater than 1.0 will take up a larger share of the total budget as income rises. By convention, items with income elasticity greater than 1.0 are termed *luxuries*, whereas items with income elasticity less than 1 are termed *necessities*.[4] This does not mean that one group is more or less important, only that the relative rates of expenditure increase as income rises are different. An item may be a necessity at some times or places and a luxury at others; spending on automobiles as a share of total spending, for example, goes up and down for different groups and for different income levels.

The total income elasticity of all things (consumption + savings) necessarily must equal 1.0. If your income goes from \$30,000 to \$55,000, then the additional \$25,000 is either spent or saved. Spending might go up more for some types of goods than others (travel and entertainment maybe rising more than food and electricity), but overall every additional dollar of income is spent on something or saved. Mathematically, if one takes the budget share of each item (weight) multiplied by the income elasticity of that item, such a weighted sum must exactly add up to 1.0. To account for all possible expenditures, one must of course include savings and debt (and taxes, or count income only after taxes).

A 10 percent increase in income must logically and necessarily result in a 10 percent increase in expenditures if all possible uses of income (including savings) are counted. Mathematically, the average income elasticity for all goods (with each good weighted by its share of the total budget) must equal 1.0, unit elasticity (see the box section on "Income Elasticity" or a standard economics text for a discussion of income elasticity). Economists are interested in why spending on one good, such as food, entertainment, or medical care, increases more or less than spending on another good, or more or less than proportionately as income increases. For many years, economists were perplexed by the following observation: rich individuals tended to save a larger percentage of their incomes than the poor, making the income elasticity of individual savings greater than 1.0 (thus "saving" was categorized as a superior or luxury good). In contrast, rich countries do not save a larger percentage of income than poor countries do; both save about the same fraction of national income. Furthermore, when gross domestic product (GDP) rises over time, there is no tendency for a larger percentage of national income to be saved. The disparity between individual and national income elasticities of consumption and savings posed a major puzzle, one that forced economists to scrutinize and reconsider the relationship between individual and national spending.

The Permanent Income Hypothesis

A major conceptual advance coming from the micro and macro economic analysis of consumption is that of **permanent income**: the hypothesis that the amount consumed is determined by expected average earnings over the long term rather than current earnings today. Thus, a medical student entering a surgical residency buys a new Lexus and a house for a growing family because she is confident that although her current earnings are near $0, they will jump to $40,000 next year and to several hundred thousand dollars per year as soon as her residency is completed. Conversely, a trial lawyer who has just earned $15 million from a case will not spend it all this year. He is aware that such big paydays are rare and that the next major settlement, if it occurs, could take 5, 10, or 20 years. Hence, although earnings and consumption are matched in the long run, they can deviate widely in any given period.

Nobel Laureate Milton Friedman began his economics career as an assistant in the construction of the first national income and product accounts used to measure GDP.[5] His task was to measure the incomes of doctors, lawyers, and engineers. Measuring the incomes of these people was problematic because their spending did not seem to match their incomes. Employees with steady wages seemed to consume about the same amount each year—but so did these professionals, whose incomes fluctuated widely from year to year. Friedman hypothesized that the spending of doctors, lawyers, fishermen, farmers, and other groups with highly variable earnings was based not on their actual income but on their expected long-run income.[6] Franco Modigliani examined how people's income and spending varied over their lifetimes, showing that they typically began with a period of borrowing at the start (to buy a home, automobile, furniture, and other goods), followed a period of saving in their 50s and 60s, and then dissaving in retirement.[7] Like Friedman, Modigliani found that spending is related to average long-run income rather than the size of the current paycheck. Together, the ideas of Friedman and Modigliani have become known as the *life-cycle permanent income hypothesis*.

The permanent income hypothesis resolved the empirical inconsistency between micro and macro studies of consumption and savings. It recognized that a disproportionate number of high-income individuals are people who only temporarily earn so much money (such as the malpractice lawyer who just received $15 million, or the 59-year-old house carpenter saving for retirement) and hence would naturally hold some for later periods, whereas a disproportionate number of low-income individuals (such as the surgical resident, the carpenter in winter, and most undergraduate economics and finance students) are only temporarily poor and hence rationally spend more than they currently earn. For countries, however, the budget constraint is binding. Total national consumption is limited by what the country produces each year (except for the limited flexibility allowed by international borrowing and investment) and thus automatically adjusts to match national income.

Shared Income

What is your income? If you are not working and your parents are sending you to school, the more relevant question is: What is your family's income? For the child of the young surgical resident, it is the parents' or grandparents' earnings, not the child's, that matter. The surgeon might also eventually have to support her aged parents. Families tend to share income. Thus it is usually the resources available to all family members on average, not the amount earned by an individual family member, that determines personal consumption. How extensive is such sharing? Who counts as a member of your family? Do you owe anything to your brother, who moved to Alaska 12 years ago and only contacts you once a year when he sends a Christmas card? Do you owe him more if he loses his leg and his job due to an accident and moves back home? Do you owe anything to a neighbor who lost his job, or a homeless person sleeping on the street? The surgeon might or might not feel that she owes a lot to a neighbor or a homeless person, but she pays taxes that are used to help both of them.

Just as the permanent income hypothesis suggests that long-run expected earnings rather than current measured earnings determine current spending, a similar **shared-income hypothesis** suggests that the average income of a group of people who share determines their consumption, rather than the earnings of each person individually. Most consumption is shared within the family, and some public goods are shared within the community (schools, roads, fire and police protection). Clothes, food, entertainment, and most other private goods are shared within a family, and perhaps within a circle of friends, but not within a larger community. What about medical care? Although care of an individual might seem like a private good, the infrastructure (hospitals, medical education, pharmaceutical companies), clinical standards, and funding of care are arranged collectively. Shared group spending is not just the 45 percent paid by taxes, or the 5 percent paid by charity and community programs. The 35 percent paid by private insurance is regulated by the Employee Retirement Income Security Act of 1974 (ERISA) and state insurance commissioners to meet public policy objectives. Even the remaining 15 percent paid out of pocket by individuals is subject to special treatment in the tax code and thus is affected by collective political decisions. A physician office practice and a for-profit hospital may be private enterprises, but both are subject to regulation and social expectations much greater than those faced by other firms. Thus it could reasonably be said that almost all health spending is subject to collective decisions made on the basis of partially shared perceptions and incomes.

Studies of individuals show that utilization of medical resources is only slightly related to income (elasticities of 0.0–0.4), but studies of nations show that rich nations spend more on health than poor nations (with income elasticities >1.1). The reason for this disparity is that individuals' ability to consume medical care is based not on their own personal income but on the average income level of all the people in their family, in their community, in their insurance plan, and in the nation as a whole.

Consider two people employed by a company that provides insurance benefits. Both employees, who are covered by the same insurance plan, a file clerk and the chief financial officer, have the same illness. They do not live in the same type of house, drive the same type of car, or take the same vacations, but they will receive similar hospital care. Even if the clerk does not make much money, most of the hospital bill is already taken care of. It would be foolish for him not to take advantage of his employee benefits when he is sick just to save a few dollars on copayments. Now consider the chief financial officer. There is little more medical care that she can buy, no matter how much she is willing to spend. If she wants to have the new gene therapy or positron scans she has read about, the decision is up to the medical staff, not her. Indeed, every effort is made to keep such medical decisions from being influenced by payment considerations. This is not to say that there are no differences in the treatment of the rich and the poor, but the differences are deliberately kept small by professional ethics within the system. Government provision of care for the poor and tax subsidies to pay for health insurance are parts of that system. The consequences, relatively similar sorts of care for all people with the same illness, are not an accident—they are one of the reasons that these policies receive wide public support. Insurance converts personal medical care into a public good, and as a society we have collectively decided that all citizens should have reasonable access to quality medical care.

For public goods, such as clean air, national defense, and control of communicable diseases, society's willingness to pay determines how much will be provided (see Chapter 14). Because everyone is able to consume the same amount of a public good, individual income is irrelevant except for its contribution to the total tax base. For a public good, or within a group insurance plan, the individual's income is not a binding budget constraint. It is possible to spend more curing one sick child than the child could earn in three lifetimes, and the amount of money spent to clean up the air in Los Angeles is hundreds of times greater than the money earned by a Hollywood movie star. It is the resources available to the group as a whole that determines the average level of spending.

The shared-income hypothesis implies that income becomes more important in determining health care spending as the unit of observation gets larger and becomes similar to the budgetary unit.[8] For individuals, income is relatively unimportant, and the income elasticities of medical expenditures are near 0. For small areas, such as a census tract, average per capita income is somewhat more important, with income elasticities rising to perhaps 0.4. For counties or states, their budgets are a constraint, but it is still possible for them to obtain money from the federal government. Per capita income is significantly more important as a determinant of health care spending than health status, and elasticities are about 0.9. For the nation as a whole, the budget constraint is binding. No other country is going to reimburse us for our medical bills. Every dollar paid to doctors, nurses, and drug companies must be collected in taxes, insurance premiums, or direct fees. Income thus becomes the dominant determinant of spending at the national level, with elasticities greater than 1, usually about 1.3 (see Figure 16.2).

Public and Private Decisions

Economics is a decision science. The implications of shared income are that an economist must consider who is making the decision, a person or a group, and even how that decision gets made and implemented (tradition, majority vote, popular will, law). Most individual and family decisions are private. Corporate employers are "private" in the sense of not being government entities, but insofar as they use rules and incentives to regulate and coordinate the behavior of many people, they are obviously public in nature. As soon as we begin to consider larger and/or less well defined groups of people, the simple utility maximization model is more difficult to implement and less plausible. What is "the" utility of the people living in Flagstaff, or Arizona, or the United States? Should we count immigrants, legal or illegal? How does a group such as "General Motors employees and their dependents" make up its mind about what medical benefits it wants and how much to pay for them? The role of government is discussed in Chapter 14, but the ramifications of public decision making go far beyond anything that can be presented in a single chapter, and indeed much is still beyond the grasp of economic analysis. Certain economic ideas have proved very helpful in understanding politics and public decisions. The concept of budget constraint is central to this discussion and to an understanding of the determinants of health spending for individuals, for larger groups, and for the nation as a whole.

Budget Constraints: Borders that Matter

The financing of a health care system is a macro system characteristic. For most countries, including the United States, funding is national in scope. Thus, we do not expect to see major differences in health care as we cross the border from Texas into Arizona, or in Mexico as we cross the border from Sonora into Chihuahua. Yet crossing the national border from Arizona into Sonora, or Texas into Chihuahua, reveals a vast disparity in the use of medical resources, costs, and prices.

Disparities in health care of this sort were once found within a single country. At the end of the 19th century, New Yorkers living on Park Avenue and those living in the tenements of lower Manhattan occupied different social and medical worlds. To some extent, disparities still exist within a country today—between the suburbs and the inner city, between the mainstream medicine provided to most Americans and the care available to residents of isolated Indian reservations in the United States or the remote Inuit villages in Canada. Studies in Australia have demonstrated that the health and health care of aboriginal populations is much worse than that of the majority white population.[9] Studies in South Africa showed large differences in health spending per capita for blacks and whites under apartheid, which has been greatly reduced but not entirely removed under the new political system. The crucial determinant of the health care available to a group of people is the amount of resources available to that group, often measured by average income per capita. The essential question then becomes: What is a group? Why are Mexican-Americans living in San Diego getting more medical care than their relatives and friends across the border in Tijuana? Why are some Indian tribes not sharing in the wealth of the average American? Defining who is and who is not part of the group determines who does and who does not have access to health care.

13.3 ADJUSTING TO CHANGE: DYNAMICS

If income falls, health care spending must also fall. Yet it is impossible to make this economic adjustment all at once. Usually the country goes into debt during the transitional period. Even for an individual, adjustments to changes in income are not instantaneous. If you were to lose your job today, you would not immediately move into a smaller apartment, drive an older car, or wear less fashionable clothes. In fact, if you lose your job today, you will probably go out and spend a little extra money to keep up your spirits. Next week you will cut back, but not too much, because you probably expect to find another job soon. If you are still out of work six months later, you will find that your clothes, house, and car start getting shabby, and you think about downsizing your lifestyle. Once you do get a new job, it will take years to build your savings back up.

When college students graduate and begin to earn good wages, they find it easy to live and save part of their salary because their lifestyles are still somewhat geared to being a student. Their consumption does not move upward as quickly as their incomes. During this "I can't figure out how to spend it all" period, savings accumulate. Later on, with a fancy lifestyle suitable for a young stockbroker or lawyer, they find it difficult to see how one could have lived on so little money as a student, or even on what they earned three years ago. Consumption is geared to expected income, whether $15,000 or $150,000. The amount of income saved depends not so much on how high the income is but on transitional (permanent income/life-cycle) factors and the extent to which a person is willing to give up current pleasures for retirement or future consumption.[10] If a young lawyer who has just bought a new Mercedes loses his job, he will discover one of the underlying asymmetric truths of human behavior: It is a lot easier and more fun to adjust spending upward rather than downward.

The dynamics of adjustment for individuals (micro) and for nations (macro) are similar, except that it usually takes longer for macro adjustment, because the system as a whole must change. People who still have their jobs must be convinced that it is necessary to cut back, to reduce the provision of public goods, or to change the tax code. Achieving a consensus to alter organizations and revise institutional structures is extremely time-consuming. The health care system, based on professional ethics, institutional obligations, and shared public values, reliant on a complex set of public and private financing mechanisms, is even more difficult to change than most other sectors of the economy. In the stock market, expectations of the future are traded every day, and prices change by the minute. Commodity sectors, such as farming and metals, are forced to respond quickly owing to market discipline. Although the number of houses cannot change rapidly, housing sales are sensitive to macroeconomic conditions. The decision to buy a house is based on an individual's assessment of job prospects. The effective price of a house, the monthly mortgage payment, depends on interest rates, which are both volatile and forward-looking. For these reasons, housing tends to be one of the sectors that leads the economy into or out of a recession. Health care is slow to change, and it lags behind other sectors in adjusting to macroeconomic conditions.

How long does it take for health care to adjust? It takes at least one to five years, and major structural changes may take even longer. Even if everyone in Congress decided today that we need more health care or less health care, this decision could not be carried out for months, and its full effects would take years to work their way through the system. If a medical school decides to accept more students, it takes at least a year to enroll them, and building new medical schools takes much longer. Medical students take four years to graduate, and another three or four years to complete a residency and enter practice. Thus, eight years after a decision to expand a medical school has been made, there are still no extra doctors in practice. Something might be done to reduce the rate of retirement, but effectively the quantity of doctors in practice who graduated in a particular year in the past was fixed once they left school. It took until 1985, 20 years after the Health Professions Educational Assistance Act of 1963, before the expansion in physician supply was a real force in the market—and by then Congress had changed its mind. It takes 40 years, until all graduating physicians have retired, before the full effects of such decisions work through the system (see Chapter 7).

Not everything in health care takes as long to adjust as physician supply. The supply of nurses is much more flexible, because typically there are many licensed nurses who are temporarily not working or are working part-time; therefore, an increase or decrease in demand quickly translates into a change in the numbers employed. Clerical, maintenance, and other less specialized labor adjusts even more smoothly and rapidly, because people can move between health services and other sectors of the economy in response to changing conditions. Although we do not have data to look at each segment of the health care sector separately, the National Health Expenditure (NHE) Accounts, the analogue to the National Income and Product Accounts established by the U.S. Department of Commerce to track GDP and the economy as a whole, do categorize health care spending by type (hospitals, physicians, dental care, drugs, nursing homes) and enable us to examine the patterns of adjustment separately for each component.

Hospitals, the largest component of health care expenditure, are quite rigidly institutionalized and dependent upon public or third-party financing. In a study of how rapidly health spending adjusts over time, hospitals took longer than the average 2.7 years.[11] Physician services are somewhat more flexible and adjust a bit more quickly, with a lag of 2.5 years. Spending on drugs, much of which depends on direct consumer decisions and is paid for out of pocket with current income, takes only 1.3 years. Long-term care, a mixture of flexible personal spending and rather inflexible Medicaid spending, adjusts in 2.5 years on average. The component that takes the longest to adjust is construction, at 3.5 years. Capital must be accumulated in advance to fund new construction, and the decision to build depends on long-run future economic considerations, not just revenues and expenses today.

The estimated average lag for adjustment of dental spending, 2.5 years, seems longer than one would expect since most dental bills are paid by individuals with limited third-party reimbursement, are a result of personal decisions, and occur in an office setting rather than within the large institutions. However, this estimate is the least reliable statistically, and it may just reflect how hard it is to pinpoint the timing of adjustment in a complex area with many segments and subsegments. Consider hospital expenditures again. Because of the way NHE accounts are kept, construction is listed as a separate component, making it possible to see that construction took longer to adjust than labor. However, some construction (clinics, equipment installation) probably takes less time than others (new buildings), but we cannot tell because they are categorized together. If supplies were listed separately, they would probably be seen to adjust more quickly than labor.

The "average lag" is just that: an average. Some parts are moving faster and some slower. It is also an average over time—in some periods the organization responds more quickly than in others. In particular, it appears that managers are quicker to step up purchasing when the economy expands than they are to cut back when the economy contracts. Everyone hopes that a slowdown is just temporary and delays firing people or closing clinics. The time required to adjust also depends on the magnitude of the change. The statistical techniques used here can only detect changes in the one- to ten-year range, but a truly massive revision of the system, such as that which occurred in 1965, may take several decades to complete. Some argue that one reason health spending is so high in the United States is because it is still stuck with a health care system constructed on the lines of the Great Society envisioned during the 1960s, when economic growth was steady and strong. This system is not appropriate to the more constrained conditions and budget deficits prevailing in 2012.

Permanent Income and Adjustment of Health Spending to GDP

Government is based on stable rules that change slowly and only with the consent of citizens. For example, any amendment to Medicare must be approved through the courts, the legislature, and public opinion. What are the consequences of slow adjustment in the health care sector? Importantly, it buffers the economy. During a downturn, Medicare and Medicaid spending usually continue; therefore, health care workers are less likely to lose their jobs than workers in the farming, housing, or financial services sectors (Figure 13.2).[12] Conversely, an increase in employment during an economic recovery is delayed.

The delay in adjustment can have adverse budgetary consequences. Because spending continues to rise in a recession even though government tax revenues fall, a deficit builds up.

FIGURE 13.2 Annual Percentage Change in Employment, United States, 2005–2012

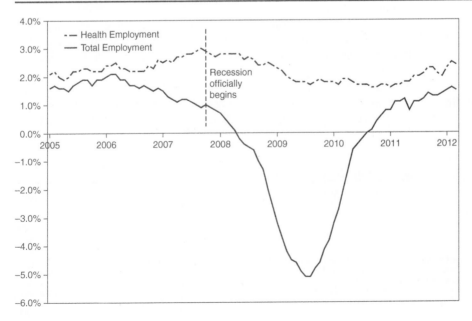

In theory, such periods of excess spending average out over time with underspending during periods of rapid growth. However, it is easier to obtain agreement to pour money into the health care sector and save jobs during a recession than it is to hold back and save money during good times. In a recession, people hope that normal growth will soon return, and they might bend their spending rules to temporarily soften the impact of macroeconomic disorder. An economic boom feels so good that people might not realize that such high growth rates are abnormal, that another recession is bound to come eventually. People might claim that this time around will be different and that we never have to worry about going hungry again, thus we do not need to save money for bad times or give up much to pay off old debts. As a consequence, it is much easier to accumulate deficits than build up surpluses.

Politicians want to get elected. They need results that will affect the economy and the voters in the near term. Extra government spending during a recession meets these needs; extra saving when the economy starts to grow again usually does not. The benefits of a balanced budget— low inflation, steady or falling interest rates, strengthening the dollar in foreign exchange, stability for businesses to invest in productivity improvements, and a modest but sustainable path of optimal growth—are long term. However, none of these benefits can be realized quickly enough to help the politician worried today about the next election. In a pinch, a politician (or a professor) will sacrifice the long-term good that helps others in favor of near-term benefits they can capture for themselves. It is difficult to get politicians to behave in a way that benefits the long-term public interest, because it is difficult to get voters to behave that way. One consequence of this is well known: a U.S. federal debt of $10 trillion. Eventually, just like the out-of-work lawyer running up his credit card balances, we will have to bring spending back into line and balance the budget. That is in the long term, though, and right now the elections keep coming up fast.

Adjustment to Inflation

Inflation is defined as a general rise in prices (or equivalently, a fall in the real value of the dollar). With 5 percent inflation, it will take 5 percent more dollars to purchase the same amount of real goods (pounds of butter, acres of land, hours of landscaping, gallons of gasoline, and everything else people buy) each year, and after 15 years of inflation at that rate, it will take more than $2 to buy what $1 used to buy.

The slow adjustment of the health care sector to inflation means that during a period of more rapidly rising prices, spending is less than expected.[13] To see why, we can trace the process of adjusting spending to changing price levels, as illustrated in Table 13.1. Suppose that a hospital spent $100,000 in 2000 and wanted to spend the same amount in real terms (e.g., full-time equivalents (FTEs) in labor, gallons of fuel, square feet of office space) in each succeeding year. If the expected rate of inflation is 5 percent, 105 percent of 2000 spending will be budgeted for 2001; that is, $105,000. If actual inflation equals the expected 5 percent, the

TABLE 13.1 Adjustment to Inflation			
	2000	**2001**	**2002**	**2003**
Nominal spending	$100	$105	$110	$123
Price index	100	105	117	123
Real spending	100	100	94	100

Note: Hypothetical example of adjustment to inflation. The hospital tries to spend exactly the same amount ($100 in year 2000 dollars) in each year. In the first year, inflation is 5 percent and spending increases 5 percent, so there is no change in real deflated expenditures. In the second year, spending increases by 5 percent again, but inflation is 12 percent, so the real spending power declines. In the third year, inflation is 5 percent, and the hospital catches up by increasing spending 12 percent (7 percent to catch up and 5 percent for current inflation).

same quantity of all inputs bought in 2000 can be bought with the 2001 budget. If inflation is again expected to be 5 percent in 2002, $110,250 is budgeted for that year. However, suppose that inflation actually turns out to be 12 percent in 2002. The budget does not buy $100,000 worth of goods in constant inflation-adjusted dollars, but only $110,250 ÷ (1.05 + .12) = $94,000. With a 12 percent rise in prices, the budgeted 5 percent wage increase leaves employees worse off, with less purchasing power. The budgeted 5 percent increase in the supply budget is not enough; thus, equipment purchases will have to be cut back. In 2003, inflation is expected to be, and actually is, 5 percent. However, the hospital has to make up for the lost purchasing power resulting from underestimating inflation the previous year. Therefore, the budget for 2003 will be up 12 percent to $123,480. Having caught up, spending will once again be $100,000 in real (year 2000) terms (see last line of Table 13.1).

ARE RECESSIONS GOOD FOR YOUR HEALTH?

Just as spending can respond differently to permanent and transitory income, it is possible that the effect of income on health may differ in the long run and the short run. The evidence reviewed in Chapters 16 and 17 makes it clear that long-term trends in health are strongly and positively related to growth in GDP per capita. Because that is well known to be the case, many economists assumed that disruptions in economic growth, recession, and the unemployment that accompanies it would temporarily cause health to worsen.

In a series of careful empirical articles Christopher Ruhm and other researchers have shown that exactly the opposite occurs.[14] For every 1 percent increase in unemployment, there was a 0.5 percent decrease in mortality rates. The primary reason that recessions appear to be good for health is that peoples' lifestyles improve; they exercise more, eat better, lose weight, and smoke less (however, they also appear to drink more). Motor vehicle fatalities show a large drop, in part because unemployment means less work and less money, so people drive less. Back injuries decline, perhaps because people no longer have to do so much heavy lifting. Diseases that are less affected by lifestyle, such as cancer, do not show much correlation.

Contrary to the general trend, suicides increase during recessions, as do some forms of mental illness. This is consistent with the common perception that the fact or threat of unemployment increases stress.

Related research shows that over the long run (20 years or more) job loss is strongly related to reduced life expectancy and increased mortality. What is fascinating about these studies is how clearly they illustrate the fallacy of composition. The short-run effects of macroeconomic fluctuations in this case are, for most conditions, exactly the opposite of the long-run effects.

National health care spending shows this type of lagging adjustment to unexpected changes in the price level for several reasons. First, government and nonprofit organizations such as hospitals usually set a budget at least a year in advance, which limits their flexibility. Second, most wage contracts run for at least one, and usually several, years. A set of inflation adjustments is already built into raises, and any difference between what negotiators expected to happen to prices and what actually happens falls on the workers. If inflation is less than expected, workers are lucky and can buy more. If inflation is worse, they have to tighten their belts. Estimates calculated from Bureau of Labor Statistics (BLS) data indicate that for any 1 percent change in the rate of inflation, only about 0.5 percent shows up in the wages of health workers in the first year, and another 0.3 percent in the following year. It takes three years for wages to fully adjust to a change in inflation. In the long run, all wages do adjust, making inflation neutral, neither raising nor lowering real health care spending. The government can only temporarily trick

TABLE 13.2		How Inflation Distorts Reported Health Expenditures			
Employment Canada	Inflation	Nurses Employed	Total Employment	Ratio	Health Share of GDP
1972	5.6%	152,005	8,447,000	.0180	7.3
1973	8.9%	159,274	8,860,000	.0180	7.0
1974	14.4%	168,530	9,220,000	.0183	6.9
1975	9.8%	177,182	9,364,000	.0189	7.4

Note: Inflation rates, nurses and total employment, and health spending as a share of GDP show how sudden price increases distort budgetary measurement of the relative size of the health sector.
Source: OECD 1990.

workers and firms into accepting a dollar that is only worth $0.90. Any government that tries to "save" money by printing lots of currency ends up with chronic inflation, as Argentina and Russia have had. Therefore, most governments aim for price stability and a sound currency. Yet the year-to-year fluctuations caused by temporary inflation adjustment problems may be larger than any real changes in health care spending due to GDP growth or changes in health care policy.

The distorting effects of a surge in inflation are shown in Table 13.2, which traces prices and employment in Canada during the oil price shock of 1973.[15] Inflation, which had previously been averaging 3 to 5 percent, suddenly leapt to 9 percent in 1973, peaked at 14 percent in 1974, and remained high at 10 percent in 1975. It looks as if spending, measured by the fraction of GDP devoted to health care, fell during 1973 and 1974. However, real resources, as measured by the number of nurses working in the Canadian health system, continued to rise throughout this period.[16] Indeed, employment for nursing rose not only in absolute numbers but also as a fraction of total employment. In terms of real labor, spending was rising. It only appeared to decline because the nurses were temporarily underpaid, getting raises smaller than the rate of inflation. Their wages had gone up somewhat during 1973 and 1974, but not as rapidly as the prices of the things they bought with those wages. Thus, the nurses' real purchasing power fell, which is why the health care fraction of GDP declined. This "decline" was entirely transitory, because the nurses were not willing to make less than everyone else and they were able to get their wages revised upward to take into account the increase in inflation during the next contract period. In the long run, whatever was taken away by a delay in adjustment had to be given back. When this was done, in 1975, there appeared to be a jump in the share of GDP spent on health care. Actually, this rapid rise is accounted for by the removal of the earlier distortion: Eventually the health care sector had to catch up with the rest of the economy.

Although expected inflation is built into contracts, a surge in overall prices is not immediately matched in the health care sector. Because wages are slow to adjust, workers bear the burden by being made worse off temporarily. Because budgets are slow to adjust, health care organizations must make do with fewer supplies, drugs, buildings, and so forth, or temporarily go into debt. However, in the long run, inflation has no effect on real health care spending. After about three years, health care wages and other contracts have fully taken account of earlier monetary shifts.[17]

Adjustment to GDP: Rates of Change and Time Series Analysis

It is evident from Figure 13.1 that there is a close relationship between per-capita income and health care spending per capita in the United States. A similar relationship will be seen across countries when an international comparison is made in Chapter 16 (see Figure 16.2). However, from the discussion regarding permanent income and the time required for adjustment of large systems, it should be apparent that one would not expect national health spending to respond

FIGURE 13.3   Annual Percentage Rates of Change

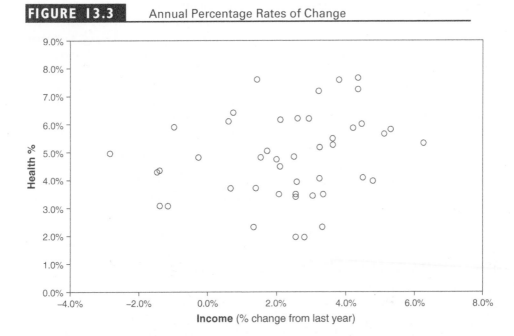

immediately to any rise or fall in GDP but rather to adjust over the long term. Looking at the current rate of growth in health expenditures from one year to the next compared to the growth in GDP makes it seem as if there is no relation at all (Figure 13.3). That is because the year-to-year change in GDP is a measure of current income, and the health system is responding to permanent income. Giving some time for adjustment to occur, and measuring not just the change in GDP over a single year but over three years, the relationship between health expenditures and per-capita income starts to become more visible (Figure 13.4). Adding a better measure of permanent income stretching over decades would increase the correlation.

FIGURE 13.4   Annual Percentage Rates of Change (Lagged Moving Average)

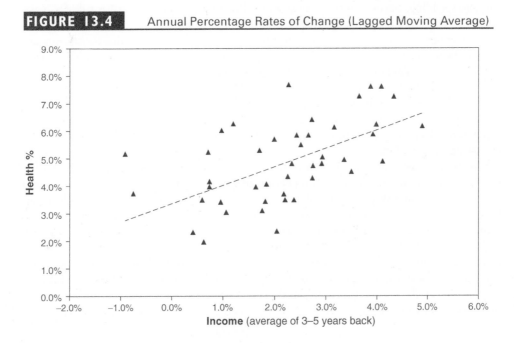

Reflection will indicate several reasons why there is so little connection between current income and current health spending. Government accounts for half of health expenditures, and government budgets must be proposed, debated, and passed well in advance of the current year. For the federal government, all money is committed at least 12 months in advance, if not more. A decision to build a hospital, create a medical school, or provide a new benefit involves a commitment to years and years of future spending. As shown in Tables 13.1 and 13.2, and as we will discuss in Section 13.6, wages of health care workers are slow to adjust to changing economic conditions, and thus it can be expected that spending in health care would lag a bit behind most sectors of the economy. The long-run trends in technology and organization are even more important. Decisions that affected spending in 2012 were made last year, the year before, and even decades ago. The enactment of Medicare in 1965, authorizing major increases in federal spending, was not unrelated to the surge of prosperity that the country was experiencing then. When times are bad, the public thinks more about cost controls than about providing new benefits.

13.4 FORECASTING FUTURE HEALTH EXPENDITURES

Using the permanent income hypothesis and lagging inflation adjustment allows economists to create a model to project future national health expenditures.[18] Analysis of the correlation among actual spending, fluctuations in prices, and per-capita income indicates that health expenditures are a function of the average percentage rate of growth in real per-capita GDP during each of the preceding five years (but not the current year) and over the preceding 25 years. This analysis also indicates that health care expenditures lag by 40 percent of the change in inflation for the current year and 20 percent of the change in inflation for the previous year. This model can be used to project future national health care spending quite well for the next three to five years, and it is fairly satisfactory for a 10-year or maybe even a 20-year projection.[19]

The fact that the health care system is slow to adjust is an advantage in forecasting. Next year will usually look a lot like last year, and the trend over the last few years is a pretty good guide to spending, wages, and prices next year. Also, for a one-year forecast it will not make much of a difference if the average growth in health expenditures exceeds the rate of inflation by 2 percent or 3 percent; factors specific to a particular person, group, or disease category are likely to be more important for decisions than general trends. However, that relatively minor difference between inflation plus 2 percent and inflation plus 3 percent would gain importance over time, and after 35 years it could amount to a 40 percent difference, more than enough to make up the shortfall in the Medicare trust fund (see Chapters 12 and 18).

A rule of thumb applied by forecasters is that for each year into the future, one needs comparable data going back three years in order to make a good forecast. In other words, to make a five-year forecast, the analyst would want at least 15 years of data. The trustees of the Medicare Trust fund are required to make not just a forecast for next year, or past the next election, but for a sufficiently long period to cover the life of current beneficiaries and taxpayers—70 years. With a "times three" rule of thumb for forecasting, that would mean looking at 210 years of historical data, all the way back to 1800. This emphasizes that long-run planning for the future of Medicare involves not only fluctuations in trend but also major shifts in the entire medical system (consider how different medicine and paying for care was 200 years ago). Most of today's college students will face their largest medical expenses in retirement, and they may be in a nursing home (or making use of a titanium hip replacement to hike the Appalachian Trail) 70 years from now. The possibility of major change in the health care system becomes a near certainty given that kind of time span.

13.5 COST CONTROLS: SPENDING GAPS AND THE PUSH TO REGULATE

Analysts have questioned why a cost-control policy that seems so successful in one instance, or so successful among individuals or physicians or hospitals alone, fails to reduce total costs. It is because the consequences of income for spending are established only at the level where the budget constraint is fixed. For some types of health care, this is the individual household. For other types of spending, it is the hospital, the region, or the insurance plan. However, for most medical care it is the national budget constraint that is most relevant.

The lagging response of the health care sector to macroeconomic changes creates spending inertia that makes it difficult to balance the budget. In a recession, expenditures continue to climb even as revenues fall. The budgetary gaps created by delays in the adjustment of spending to changing macroeconomic conditions might force governments to put cost controls on health care. Almost every inflationary spike or sharp recession is followed by a new attempt to regulate hospital rates, ration health care, establish price controls, cap revenues, or use another method to stem rising costs. The recession of 1970 pushed President Nixon to impose wage and price controls on the economy and to keep hospital prices under control for an extra period. Afterward it became clear that the U.S. experience from 1971 to 1975 served mostly to confirm the lessons learned from wage and price controls imposed by other governments around the world over the last two millennia. The underlying pressures created by excess monetary growth and the fiscal imprudence of waging a war without raising taxes could not be contained, controls were routinely evaded, and prices shot up as soon as controls ended in April 1974.[20]

After the expiration of the Nixon price controls, health care costs were freed from external economy-wide controls, although they continued to be regulated by cost reimbursement rules (see Chapters 5, 6, and 8). Then in April 1977 President Carter proposed a "voluntary effort" (VE) to constrain costs. Flyers and buttons were printed to promote voluntary efforts to have hospitals reduce prices and to lobby Congress. In November 1979 the Carter bill was soundly defeated by the legislature. This tale of voluntary regulation would normally have been forgotten and relegated to footnotes, yet the story lingered on because claims of effectiveness were uncritically accepted. Three reasons for the persistence of the impression that VE worked are that hospital price increases did moderate in 1978 and 1979, claims of VE's effectiveness were loudly voiced, and Congress cited these claims in debate before Carter's legislation was defeated. It is difficult to understand how flyers and buttons could accomplish what the force of law could not, but the claim appeared plausible until the data were examined more closely. Hospital costs had already begun falling in 1977 before VE. They declined further in 1978 and were below the target when the legislation failed. Even VE believers referred to the American Hospital Association's luck, because the VE coalition did not even convene a meeting until December 1977 and therefore had no time to directly affect hospital behavior.

Luck, however, was only one factor in the fortuitous "success" of VE. The main reason that nominal health care expenses were lower than expected was that hospital wages and supply prices, because they lag the CPI, had not yet caught up with the surge of inflation that began in 1977. There was no decline in hospitals' use of real inputs (labor FTEs, supply items), only a delay in price adjustment that made nurses and technicians temporarily cheap relative to the CPI (as in the Canadian example in Table 13.2).

In October 1983, Medicare radically changed its method of paying hospitals from cost reimbursement to a new prospective payment system (PPS) based on the expected cost of each admission, categorized into diagnosis-related groups (DRGs). This new cost control plan did work in some ways. There was a significant reduction in the rate of increase in Medicare Part A (inpatient) expenses and in hospital expenses generally. However, this was accomplished primarily by hospitals shifting services to outpatient and day surgery categories covered under

Medicare Part B. Total health care expenditures per capita continued to rise at historically high rates. In 1985, 16.9 percent of the $407.2 billion spent on health care was paid for by the federal government, and by 1990, the fraction actually increased to 17.7 percent of the $643.4 billion spent that year, even though reduction in the federal deficit was an explicit objective of the Medicare legislation. PPS clearly had a large effect on the health care system. Administrators and doctors panicked, employment was (temporarily) held below trends, and the average length of stay for patients fell sharply. However, there were no long-run reductions in the total cost of health care.[21]

The Balanced Budget Act of 1997 imposing significant cuts on Medicare payments was initially more successful in controlling costs. Yet by 2001 total spending was again rising in line with long-run trends (with the exception of home health, which had been specifically targeted for reform in this legislation; see Chapter 10, section 10).

The idea that ESP, VE, and PPS regulations were "effective" in reducing expenditures lingers because a superficial before-and-after comparison in each case showed a decline in spending that the public and legislators could understand and that was quickly reported in the newspapers. People did not recognize that these declines were delayed effects of the adverse macroeconomic conditions that had caused the regulations to be proposed in the first place. Also, the declines in spending in one reimbursement category (Part A) resulting from regulations look like effective cost controls, until it is realized that these costs were just shifted to another area (Part B). A more human reason for the persistence of this belief is that many analysts and politicians worked thousands of hours to draft and implement these regulations, becoming so personally committed that it was hard for them to accept that so much well intentioned effort had so little effect over the long run.[22]

Health care expenditures are never too high or too low in an absolute sense; rather, they are out of line with the spending that can be afforded under current economic conditions. A theory of health care cost regulation must start with the realization that shared costs, and governmental expenditures in particular, are always regulated even when no external regulatory agency is in operation. Furthermore, costs can be ratcheted up or down within the existing framework by making administrative procedures tighter or looser, even if no legislation is passed. Regulation is always an integral component of health care system management in a modern nation. It is part of the process, not an external shock. What an economist can evaluate is a *change* in the regulatory regime. To do so, one must first ask why the change took place at a particular time.

Legislatures don't get together to pass cost control measures for health care because the economy is doing well. Macroeconomic crises bring about a call for legislatures to do something, but these crises eventually push spending down, regardless of whether legislatures act. The ability of politicians to dictate spending independent of the rest of the economy is limited, particularly during the next one to four years, which are usually all that remain before the next election. The process of adjustment is shown in Figure 13.5. Incomplete adjustment to inflation and recession is apt to simultaneously exert pressure on legislatures to do something about excessive health care costs and force future spending downward, thus often creating a spurious correlation between the enactment of regulation and the temporary moderation in costs. This does not mean that cost controls have no effect but rather that much of the decline is due to the underlying process of macroeconomic adjustment rather than an explicit effect of regulation.

FIGURE 13.5   Macroeconomic Shock

Capacity Constraints and Budget Constraints

The slow adjustment of the health care sector is one reason that cost controls are ineffective. The number of doctors and hospitals is essentially fixed for the time span of most political action (one to four years). If twice as many people got sick next year, there would be no major increase in physician supply or the number of hospital beds. If the hospital is full, admitting another patient means discharging someone the doctors feel is less in need of care. Conversely, maintaining capacity means keeping nurses and technicians available even if there are fewer patients than expected, or treating more patients who are perhaps not quite so severely ill. Capacity in health care tends to be constrained rather than flexible. Although it is possible, even easy, to shift costs from one organization to another or to move a few billion dollars back and forth across budget years, real change in the capital and labor employed takes longer and is much harder to achieve. Only a small fraction of the total cost of hospital care (including drugs and supplies, food, nursing overtime) varies with the number of patients. Therefore any changes in the total expenditures show up as mostly short-run changes in employee wages and perhaps some temporary hiring or layoffs (although there is usually considerable reluctance on the part of administrators to adding permanent staff when there is a surge in demand, and an even stronger resistance from unions to cutting staff when demand falls).

13.6   WORKFORCE DYNAMICS: "SPENDING" IS MOSTLY LABOR

What does it mean to control costs? Because health services are mostly labor, costs are primarily a function of the number of people employed in the health care sector and the wages (or professional incomes) that they are paid. Cost control must be employment control. Yet it is easier for politicians to say that they will control costs than to say that they will have people laid off or cut wages, which is one reason that there is so much more rhetoric than action in health care cost control.

The most significant government interventions in the health care labor markets have been (1) cooperating with the medical profession in formulating effective licensure laws and making medical schools the restrictive gateway for entry into the profession during 1910 to 1930, (2) extending the medical licensure model to other health professions throughout the remainder of the 20th century, and (3) enacting the Health Professions Education Act of 1963 to expand health care labor (see Chapter 7).

Every occupation within the health services field has its supply and demand most strongly influenced by the particulars of licensure statutes and relations with the dominant medical profession. Yet what is true of each of the parts is not true of the whole. Most of the growth in health employment comes from adding new occupational categories rather than by expanding numbers within an existing occupation. Therefore, to study how health care labor is related to the economy as a whole, it is necessary to look at aggregate employment in the health sector rather than a single occupational category.

Employment

There are two separate sources of data on U.S. health care employment. The decennial census began recording information on the occupation of respondents in 1850 and thus can be used to create a long series of health-related occupations with 15 observations over the past 150 years (Table 13.3). The Bureau of Labor Statistics (BLS) records employment within industries by Standard Industrial Classification (SIC) codes and has identified health care services (SIC 808) as a category since 1958 (SIC 80806 is the subcategory "hospital employment"),

TABLE 13.3 U.S. Health Care Employment, 1850–2000

	1850	1860	1870	1880	1890	1900	1910	1920	1930	1940	1950	1960	1970	1980	1990	2000
Population	23,192	31,443	39,818	50,156	62,948	75,995	91,972	105,711	122,775	131,669	150,697	180,671	205,052	227,726	249,973	275,372
Employed Civilians	5,372		12,925	17,392	23,318	29,073	37,371	42,434	48,830	51,742	59,230	67,990	79,802	104,058	123,473	131,720
All Health Occupations	46	61	103	114	170	346	486	634	900	1,020	1,450	2,064	3,277	5,403	7,580	10,103
Fraction	0.8%	0.8%	0.8%	0.7%	0.7%	1.2%	1.3%	1.5%	1.8%	2.0%	2.4%	3.0%	4.1%	5.2%	6.1%	7.7%
H/pop	1.97	1.93	2.58	2.26	2.70	4.55	5.29	6.00	7.33	7.75	9.62	11.42	15.98	23.73	30.32	36.69
MD/pop	1.76	1.75	1.62	1.71	1.66	1.73	1.66	1.43	1.33	1.33	1.31	1.29	1.45	1.90	2.35	2.80
Aid/MD			0.2	0.2	0.5	1.0	1.4	2.1	3.2	3.7	5.1	6.7	8.7	10.1	10.6	10.9
Physicians	41	55	64	86	105	131	152	151	163	175	198	234	297	433	587	772
Dentists	3	6	8	12	17	30	40	56	71	71	76	83	95	125	156	168
Diagnosticians, NEC							8	22	38	40	53	68	40	54	132	94
Pharmacists	2		18	15		46	54	64	84	83	89	93	116	146	182	208
Nurse (practical)			13		47	120	166	212	236	200	224	276	267	435	429	679
RN-nurses				1	1	12	51	104	214	284	406	592	762	1,285	1,885	2,290
Att-Hosp/Nurse Aides, Orderlies									41	102	212	409	951	1,378	1,860	1,834
Att-Phy/Health Aid									14	35	42	73	134	292	249	490
Dent Asst							2	7					100	158	216	251
Dent Hygienist													17	46	72	148
Opticians, Lens Grinders						6	9	11	13	12	20	21	31	47	38	67
Therapists (licensed)							4	8	14	18	25	37	78	224	332	296
Psychologists											5	12	30	93	192	***
Dieticians											23	27	43	67	90	97
Med Technicians											78	141	260	508	927	1,057
Managers, Medicine & Health													58	111	234	***

U.S. Health Labor: Annual % Rates of Growth

	1850	1860	1870	1880	1890	1900	1910	1920	1930	1940	1950	1960	1970	1980	1990	2000
Population		3.1%	2.4%	2.3%	2.3%	1.9%	1.9%	1.4%	1.5%	0.7%	1.4%	1.8%	1.3%	1.1%	0.9%	1.0%
Employed Civilians		4%	4.5%	3.0%	3.0%	2.2%	2.5%	1.3%	1.4%	0.6%	1.4%	1.4%	1.6%	2.7%	1.7%	1.9%
All Health Occupations		2.9%	5.4%	1.0%	4.1%	7.4%	3.5%	2.7%	3.6%	1.3%	3.6%	3.6%	4.7%	5.1%	3.4%	2.6%
Physicians		3.1%	1.6%	2.9%	2.0%	2.3%	1.5%	-0.1%	0.7%	0.7%	1.3%	1.7%	2.4%	3.8%	3.1%	3.1%
Dentists		6.7%	3.6%	4.4%	3.6%	5.4%	3.0%	3.5%	2.4%	0.0%	0.6%	1.0%	1.4%	2.8%	2.2%	1.3%
Nurse (practical)						10.0%	3.3%	2.5%	1.1%	-1.6%	1.1%	2.1%	-0.3%	5.0%	-0.1%	
RN-nurses						28.0%	15.6%	7.5%	7.5%	2.9%	3.6%	3.9%	2.6%	5.4%	3.9%	2.7%
Att-Hosp/Nurse Aides, Orderlies										9.6%	7.6%	6.8%	8.8%	3.8%	3.0%	
Att-Phy/Health Aid										9.7%	1.7%	5.6%	6.3%	8.1%	-1.6%	
Therapists (licensed)								7.1%	5.5%	2.5%	3.3%	4.0%	7.7%	11.2%	4.0%	
Psychologists												9.4%	9.3%	12.1%	7.5%	
Dieticians												1.5%	4.9%	4.5%	3.0%	
Med Technicians												6.0%	6.3%	6.7%	6.2%	3.8%
Managers, Medicine & Health															7.8%	

Source: U.S. Census and Bureau of Labor Statistics, various publications.

TABLE 13.4	Trends in Employment in the Health Care Sector			
Year	Total U.S. (1000s)	Health Services	% of Total	Hospitals
1960	54,189	1,548	2.9%	1,030
1970	70,880	3,053	4.3%	1,863
1980	90,528	5,278	5.8%	2,750
1990	109,487	8,211	7.5%	3,513
1995	117,298	9,809	8.4%	3,734
2000	131,785	10,858	8.2%	3,954
2001	131,826	11,188	8.5%	4,051
2002	130,341	11,536	8.9%	4,160
2003	129,999	11,817	9.1%	4,245
2004	131,435	12,055	9.2%	4,285
2005	133,703	12,314	9.2%	4,345
2006	136,086	12,602	9.3%	4,423
2007	137,598	12,947	9.4%	4,515
2008	136,790	13,290	9.7%	4,627
2009	130,807	13,543	10.4%	4,667
2010	129,874	13,777	10.6%	4,679
2011	131,359	14,046	10.7%	4,731

Source: Bureau of Labor Statistics, *Employment and Earnings.*

providing annual and monthly observations (Table 13.4). The definition of the two series is quite different. The census data are based on *occupation of the individual* so that a secretary, chemist, or accountant employed at a hospital would not be counted as a health care employee. The BLS data are based on the *SIC code of the firm (employer)*; therefore, a nurse, medical technician, or doctor employed at a manufacturing firm would not be counted as a health care employee, but a hospital secretary would.

Employment in health care has grown more than twice as rapidly as total U.S. employment over the past hundred years, 3.4 percent versus 1.5 percent for the period 1900–2000. Consequently, the share of total employment accounted for by health care has increased from 1.2 percent at the turn of the century to 11 percent (1 out of every 9 workers) now. Yet the 0.6 percent of total employment accounted for by physicians in 2012 was up only slightly from 0.5 percent in 1900. The health care sector has enjoyed positive employment growth every year for the past three decades. The average annual growth rate of this sector between 1960 and 2011 was 4.4 percent, more than double the annual average growth of total U.S. employment. During this period, health care sector employment never contracted (see Figure 13.6), in

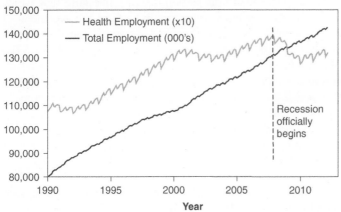

FIGURE 13.6   U.S. Employment 1990–2012

FIGURE 13.7   Health Employment Adjusts Slowly

Effect of a 1% Increase in Total U.S. Employment on
Health Sector Employment

contrast to total employment, which experienced four major contractionary episodes. Total U.S. employment contracted in the 1960s, after the oil price shocks of the 1970s, at the start of the 1980s and 1990s, and especially during the "great recession" starting in 2008 (from which employment is still struggling to recover.). Although health sector employment grew more slowly during the mid-1970s and early 1980s, annualized year-on-year growth never fell below 2 percent. Health care employment shows less fluctuation because it adjusts more slowly and gradually to macroeconomic shocks (see Figures 13.2 and 13.6). When total employment is shifted upward or downward 1 percent from trend, health care employment moves by only 0.2 percent after one year, 0.17 percent after two years, and so on (Figure 13.7).[23] The cumulative rise or fall in health care is proportionately larger, about 1.2 percent for each 1 percent shift in total employment, but spread out over the entire decade that follows, so that on average shifts in health employment lag by 2.6 years.

The slow rate of adjustment to government intervention is shown in Figure 13.8, which presents the estimated impact on health care employment resulting from the enactment of Medicare and Medicaid in 1965. Although this legislation created a fundamental change in reimbursement and flow of money into the system and was ultimately responsible for a rise of more than 10 percent in the number of health care jobs, it had no visible effect on health employment during 1965 or 1966. Not until 1967 did employment begin to soar, leaping 3.7 percent above trend in that year, 2.4 percent in 1968, 1.2 percent in 1969, 0.6 percent in 1970, and 0.4 percent in 1971 (see Figure 13.7). The average lag between the enactment of Medicare and the creation of an additional job was 3.5 years.

Wages

Health care wage data for the United States are available from the BLS for hospitals from 1968 on and for all health employment from 1972 on. There were rapid increases in real

FIGURE 13.8   Effect of Medicare on Health Employment in Subsequent Years

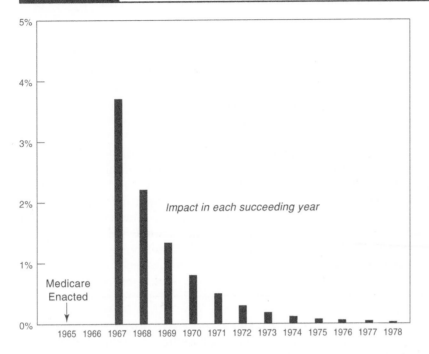

Impact in each succeeding year

Medicare
Enacted

inflation-adjusted wages of more than 5 percent per year in the late 1960s post-Medicare period. During the 1970s, health care wages were essentially flat, just keeping pace with wages in other industries and with inflation, and growing less than 0.5 percent per year. From 1980 to 2008, while real wages in the rest of the economy were essentially flat (rising by less than 3 percent), average health care wages rose by 27 percent, and the increases for hospital employees and self-employed physicians were even greater. There does not appear to be any consistent correlation between economic growth (GDP) and health care wages, but the 30 years of data available are not enough to be certain of this. Other than the apparent surge due to Medicare (which occurred before health care wage data were collected) no government policy appears to have significantly altered the health care wage trend. The adjustment of health care wages to changes in the rate of inflation is slow. More than 60 percent of the rise (or fall) in inflation from one year to the next was not incorporated in health care wages until the following year, and 11 percent was still missing after two years, indicating substantial contractual rigidity in health care wages.

THE IRON LAW: MEDICAL COSTS = MEDICAL INCOMES

One person's expenses are another person's income. This economic observation, seemingly obvious, is often overlooked. The circular flow of funds that makes trade possible (Chapter 1) and the structure of the National Income and Product Accounts used to measure GDP and other macroeconomic activity are based on the principle that when a dollar gets paid, it gets paid to someone.

every $100 income = $100 costs

The largest element in health care costs is labor, and it is reasonably clear that the $235 that gets paid for a visit is "expense" on the patient side and "revenue" on the provider

(Continued)

THE IRON LAW: MEDICAL COSTS = MEDICAL INCOMES (CONTINUED)

side. It is also evident that the salary of nurses, technicians, and administrators must come from patient revenues. What about the payments to suppliers or banks? They too have employees, and for them to pay the rent (and taxes) they must get paid from patient fees (or government subsidies or philanthropy or some other source of revenues). Isn't it possible to improve the efficiency of the health care system so that one can simultaneously reduce the cost of health care and maintain the incomes of doctors and nurses? Nope. The only way an organization can cut its labor bill is to either reduce wages or lay some people off, neither of which is very popular. Increased productivity could make it possible to employ fewer people in medicine, even at higher salary, and thus reduce the total wage bill (and hence reduce the total cost of care). Increased productivity could also mean providing more health care with the same costs (but not less). It is always worth remembering that any reductions in the cost of medical care only come through reductions in the incomes of providers, and that making medicine more productive, or getting people to lead healthier lives, only leads to a reduction in the cost of care and health insurance premiums or taxes if the number or salary of health care workers is decreased. Even after technology provided an answer to the Malthusian dilemma (see Chapter 16), economics is able to live up to its name as the "dismal science."

Real health expenditures per capita in the United States grew 5 percent a year from 1960 to 2012, outpacing the 2 percent rate of growth in per-capita incomes and thus consuming an ever-larger share of GDP. The labor portion of this 5 percent annual increase can be decomposed into a 4 percent increase in employment and a 1 percent annual increase in real wages; therefore, increased intensity of medical services, more nurses and perfusionists and occupational therapists per patient-day, is by far the more important cause of increased spending over this time span. With both wages and employment increasing faster than in other occupations, it may well be that health care professionals are getting more than a fair share of the nation's economic growth, a concern that health economist Uwe Reinhardt of Princeton University has humorously identified as "feasting on healthcare, or the allocation of lifestyles to providers."

Although the power of licensed health professions to control entry and wages is a major cause of delayed adjustment, it is not the only one. The dominance of nonprofit firms and third-party financing are also important factors in creating labor market rigidity. Health care in the United States is currently undergoing significant institutional changes. The pattern of slow and delayed adjustment over the last 40 years indicates that the ultimate outcome of these changes will not be revealed for a considerable period of time (see Chapters 17 and 18).

SUGGESTIONS FOR FURTHER READING

Centers for Medicare and Medicaid Services, NHE Projections 2007–2017, www.cms.hhs.gov/NationalHealthExpendData.

Cynthia Engel, "Health Services Industry: Still a Job Machine?" *Monthly Labor Review* (122, no. 3 (1999): 3–14 (www.bls.gov).

Milton Friedman, *A Theory of the Consumption Function* (Princeton: Princeton University Press, 1957) and with Simon Kuznets, *Income from Independent Professional Practice* (New York: National Bureau of Economic Research, 1945).

Thomas E. Getzen, "Aggregation and the Measurement of Health Care Costs," *Health Services Research* 41, no. 5 (2006):1938-1954; and "Health Care Is an Individual Necessity and a National Luxury: Applying Multilevel Decision Models to the Analysis of Health Care Expenditures," *Journal of Health Economics* 19, no. 2 (2000): 259–270.

Marian Osterweis et al., eds., *The U.S. Health Workforce: Power, Politics, and Policy* (Washington, D.C.: Association of Academic Health Centers, 1996).

SUMMARY

1. Consumption and savings decisions are not based on current income but on expected **permanent income** over the entire life cycle.

2. Shared financing through government and insurance makes health care into a **quasi-public good**, so that group or national income is the relevant budget constraint, not individual income.

3. The major determinants of total health spending are macroeconomic (inflation, population, and GDP).

4. Professional licensure, nonprofit organization, third-party reimbursement, and other institutional features **make the health care sector slow in adjusting to changes** in macroeconomic conditions.

5. These delays in response create **pressures for regulatory change**.

6. Many of the effects associated with the passage of health care cost control regulations are actually **delayed effects** of inflation and recession.

7. Real **increases in health care spending** are largely **increases in labor**. Much of the growth shows up in the form of new occupations, and some shows up as higher wages and professional incomes.

PROBLEMS

1. {*competition, welfare maximization*} Does the "invisible hand" work in health care markets? Give an example that clearly illustrates the welfare-maximizing effects of self-interested competition and one that calls self-interested competition into question. Is health care more, or less, nonprofit than other types of human productivity and exchange?

2. {*dynamics*} Explain the difference between the comparative statics and dynamics of a market, such as physician services or long-term care.

3. {*transaction costs*} Do all economic exchanges have a monetary price? How would a politician pay the price of changing insurance legislation to cover hospital-sponsored health maintenance organizations (HMOs)? To whom would the price be paid? Do laws regulating exchange make trade more expensive or less expensive?

4. {*dynamics, productivity*} How many nonphysicians are currently employed in the health care sector for each MD? Is this ratio more than or less than it was 50 years ago? Does the change in the ratio of physician to nonphysician labor imply that productivity has increased or decreased? Which adjusts more rapidly to changes in demand: ancillary employment or physician supply?

5. {*flow of funds*} Which factor has accounted for more of the increase in the cost of hospital care per patient: increases in the number of physicians, the number of days of care, physician incomes, wages of nonphysician employees, or number of nonphysician employees?

6. {*dynamics*} Do delays in adjustment cause deficits, surpluses, or both?

7. {*elasticity*} If the income elasticity of NHE spending is 1.4 and per-capita income increases from $12,000 to $15,000, how much will health care spending increase? How much will it increase if income elasticity is 0.9?

8. {*elasticity, aggregation*} Since the amount of income spent on health care for a group is just the sum of the amounts spent on each member, why would the income elasticity be

different if the economist measured one person, or groups of 10, or 100, or 1 million? Is individual income elasticity for health care spending larger or smaller than national income elasticity for health care spending? If so, why?

9. {*fallacy of composition*} What determines how much is spent on your health care: how sick you are or how much money you earn? What determines how much is spent on average in the United States: how sick people are or how much money they earn?

10. {*price controls*} Suppose that you read Sunday's newspaper and learn that price controls have been placed limiting the cost of health insurance to $2,500 per employee, significantly below the current average. What effects would you predict to occur?

11. {*inflation*}

    a. Assume that inflation is 4 percent for the years 2010 to 2014, jumps to 14 percent for the years 2015 and 2016, and then falls to 3 percent for 2017 to 2019. Calculate the price index using 2000 as the base year. What is the price in each year of a good whose price changes matched the overall level of inflation and cost $27.42 in 2012?

    b. Suppose that service L's price adjusts with a lag, causing a third of the change in the rate of inflation to show up in L's price in each succeeding year. Calculate the annual percentage rates of price increase for L.

    c. Suppose that good A anticipates future price increases, causing half the change in next year's inflation rate to show up in its price in advance. Calculate the annual rate of price increase for good A.

    d. Which prices in the health care system might show delayed adjustment, lagging behind changes in the general rate of inflation? Which prices might show anticipatory response, changing in advance of the general rate of inflation? (*Hint:* Who sets premiums in advance?) What problems would this pattern of delay/advance present to administrators trying to work within a budget?

12. {*inflation*} Will changes in the rate of inflation affect health care spending? In your answer, distinguish between real and nominal expenditures and between short- and long-run effects.

13. {*dynamics*} Are decisions regarding health care budgets and medical school enrollments based on the past or the future?

14. {*consumption*} What is the permanent income hypothesis? For which type of person would the permanent income hypothesis lead one to expect the greatest error from using tax returns to predict consumption?

    a. Assistant manager at Macy's
    b. Management intern at Macy's
    c. Chief executive officer at Macy's
    d. Retired vice president of Macy's
    e. College student
    f. Medical student
    g. High school teacher
    h. Retired college professor

15. {*dynamics*} Why might it take longer to adjust health care expenditures downward than upward? Frame your answer in terms of the economic incentives facing those who make the decisions.

16. {*equilibrium, segregation*} What determines the level of wages among health care occupations?

17. {*public good*} Why does insurance turn private medical care into a public good?

18. {*price controls, dynamics*} Did health care costs rise less rapidly after President Nixon introduced price controls in 1971? Why or why not?

19. {*dynamics, price controls*} Which forces cause the public to want price controls?

20. {*price controls*} What do you think was the effect of Medicare PPS, which paid a fixed price per DRG after 1983, on the length of hospital stay? What was the effect on the number of outpatient surgeries? On nursing home admissions? On total Medicare hospital expenditures? On total Medicare expenditures for all types of care?

21. {*voting*} If price controls and crazy tax proposals are the economic equivalent of voodoo, why do such proposals continue to gain support? For that matter, why has voodoo continued to be profitable?

22. {*dynamics*} How long is the "long run"? How much difference can the length of the period used for measurement make on the estimates of price and income elasticity?

23. {*productivity*} Is it be possible to raise both employment and wages while still controlling total costs through the development of new technology that increases the productivity of medical care? Why or why not?

ENDNOTES

1. This chapter borrows selectively from a number of authors, including James S. Coleman, *Foundations of Social Theory* (Cambridge, Mass.: Harvard University Press, 1990); Douglass North, *Structure and Change in Economic History* (New York: W. W. Norton, 1981); and Oliver Williamson, *Markets and Hierarchies* (New York: The Free Press, 1975).

2. Thomas E. Getzen, "Health Care is an Individual Necessity and a National Luxury: Applying Multilevel Decision Models to the Analysis of Health Care Expenditures," *Journal of Health Economics* 19, no. 2 (2000): 259–270.

3. The economic definitions of "necessity" or "inferior good" and of "superior" or "luxury goods" depend solely on consumer buying behavior, whether income elasticity is less than or greater than 1.0, and not on any judgments regarding the usefulness or importance of the items or how most people think of them. Thus bottled water, new cars, and organic baby food all qualify as luxuries, whereas hot dogs, cheap costume jewelry, and bus tickets are all termed necessities. This is an example of economists' occasional bad habit of taking a common term and giving it a very narrow meaning within the profession that is at odds with common usage. This twisted professional definition tends to confuse rather than communicate unless a reader has fully interiorized the profession's specific definition (e.g., "luxury" for income elastic, "marginal" for incremental, "rents" for payments for fixed resources).

4. Note that savings may temporarily be negative, as they are for many students who go into debt to support a lifestyle. Yet in the long run, savings aggregated across all people must be positive (or at least zero). It is not possible for everyone everywhere to have more by going into debt. Note also that economists consider savings very different from food, clothing, and other consumer goods because savings determine investment, interest rates, growth, the price level, and many other macroeconomic variables.

5. Milton Friedman and Simon Kuznets, *Income from Independent Professional Practice* (New York: National Bureau of Economic Research, 1945).

6. Milton Friedman, *A Theory of the Consumption Function* (Princeton, N.J.: Princeton University Press, 1957).

7. Franco Modigliani, *The Collected Papers of Franco Modigliani: Vol. 2: The Life-Cycle Hypothesis of Saving* (Cambridge, Mass.: MIT Press, 1980).

8. Thomas E. Getzen, "Aggregation and the Measurement of Health Care Costs," *Health Services Research* 41, no. 5 (2006): 1938–1954.

9. David Mayston, "Disadvantaged Populations, Equity, and the Determinants of Health: Lessons from Down Under," in Morris L. Barer, Thomas E. Getzen, and Greg L. Stoddart, eds., *Health, Health Care and Health Economics: Perspectives on Distribution* (Chichester, U.K.: John Wiley & Sons, 1998).

10. Take-home advice: if you want to become rich, get in the habit of saving now, while you are still in school.

11. Thomas E. Getzen, "Macro Forecasting of National Health Expenditures," *Advances in Health Economics and Health Services Research* 11(1990): 27–48.

12. William C. Goodman, "Employment in Services Industries Affected by Recessions and Expansions," *Monthly Labor Review* 124, no. 10 (2001): 1–15 (www.bls.gov).

13. Christopher J. Ruhm, "Are Recessions Good For Your Health?" *The Quarterly Journal of Economics* 115, no. 2 (2000): 617–650; "Good Times Make You Sick," *Journal of Health Economics* 22(4): 637–658, 2003; and "Healthy Living in Hard Times," *Journal of Health Economics* 24, no. 2 (2005): 341–363. Daniel Sullivan and Till von Wachter, "Mortality, Mass-Layoffs, and Career Outcomes: An Analysis Using Administrative Data," NBER working paper #13626, November 2007.

14. Angus Deaton, "Involuntary Savings Through Unanticipated Inflation," *American Economic Review* 67, no. 5 (1977): 899–910.

15. Although it would be nice to have a more recent example, economists are rather grateful that there has been no need to make rapid adjustments to surging inflation in the last 20 years. However, the increasing federal budget deficit and declining trade balance make the prospect that a future edition of this textbook will have a current example of necessary adjustment to rapid inflation within the U.S. somewhat more likely.

16. The changes in the numbers of RNs are used because the data for all health care workers are, unfortunately, not readily comparable across these years.

17. Sheila Smith et al., "The Next Ten Years of Health Spending: What Does the Future Hold?" *Health Affairs* 17, no. 5 (1998): 128–141.

18. Thomas E. Getzen, "Macro Forecasting of National Health Expenditures," *Advances in Health Economics and Health Services Research* 11(1990): 27–48; see the methodology paper and current projections at www.cms.hhs.gov/NationalHealthExpendData/projected/.

19. Thomas E. Getzen, "Forecasting Health Expenditures: Short, Medium and Long (Long) Term," *Journal of Health Care Finance* 26, no. 3 (2000): 56–72.

20. Paul Ginsburg, "Impact of the Hospital Stabilization Program on Hospitals," in M. Zubkoff, I. E. Raskin, and R. S. Hanft, eds., *Hospital Cost Containment: Selected Notes for Future Policy* (New York: PRODIST for Milbank Memorial Fund, 1978), pp. 293–323. See also the first and second editions of this textbook, which contained more extended analysis of these historical events.

21. Congressional Budget Office, *Rising Health Care Costs: Causes, Implications and Strategies* (Washington, D.C.: U.S. Government Printing Office, 1991).

22. David Dranove and Kenneth Cone, "Do State Rate Regulations Really Lower Hospital Expenses?" *Journal of Health Economics* 4, no. 2 (1985): 159–165; C. Eby and D. Cohodes, "What Do We Know about Rate Setting?" *Journal of Health Politics, Policy & Law* 10, no. 2 (1985): 299–327; Michael Morrisey, Douglas Conrad, Steven Shortell, and Karen Cook, "Hospital Rate Review: A Theory and Empirical Review," *Journal of Health Economics* 3, no. 1 (1984): 24–47. Karen Davis, Gerard Anderson, Diane Rowland, and Earl Steinberg, *Health Care Cost Containment* (Baltimore: Johns Hopkins University Press, 1990).

23. Michael Kendix and Thomas Getzen, "U.S. Health Services Employment: A Time Series Analysis," *Health Economics* 3, no. 3 (1994): 169–181.

CHAPTER 14

THE ROLE OF GOVERNMENT AND PUBLIC GOODS

"To do for the people what needs to be done, but which they cannot, by individual effort, do at all, or do so well, for themselves."

—Abraham Lincoln

"In the evolution of economic enterprise, the things which could be produced and sold for a price were taken over by private producers. Those that were not, but which were in the end no less urgent for that reason, remained with the state."

—John Kenneth Galbraith

QUESTIONS

1. Who paid for Pasteur to discover bacteria?
2. Are clean water or the theory of relativity public goods? Are they free or costly?
3. Should treatment of syphilis be part of the public health system or private medical care? What about psoriasis? Psychosis? Scoliosis?
4. Why not charge people full price for vaccinations?
5. Why are new surgical techniques developed with public funds whereas pharmaceutical research and development is conducted privately by for-profit firms?
6. Why pay for cost–benefit analysis to decide which public programs are worthwhile instead of using prices to let the market decide?
7. Should I pay taxes to care for the poor?
8. Is medical care for homeless and terminally ill AIDS patients a public good or a waste of money?
9. Do the preferences of smokers, patients who are mentally ill, or unborn children count when assessing the efficiency of the public health system?
10. Does the Food and Drug Administration, or any other agency that regulates health, operate in the interest of the public, in the interest of the people who work there, or for the special-interest lobbies?
11. Do people vote for what is good for society or what is good for themselves?

As people go about their daily activities, trying to stay happy and healthy and save a few dollars, they are usually not aware of government. Suppose that you get a headache and go to the drugstore for some aspirin. You are making that choice individually, as a private citizen, and buying from a private company. Yet this simple transaction could not take place unless a government had already done many things to prepare for the welfare of you and the company. To begin with, government provides a medium of exchange (money) and maintains its value. Without money you would have to engage in barter and search for someone who wanted you to cut their lawn, or care for their children, or whatever, in exchange for the aspirin. Not only is the value of money determined by the government, so are the measurements of what you buy. You don't ask for "some" or a scoop of aspirin, but for 100 325-milligram tablets. Furthermore, without government policing, you could not be sure whether the white pills were made of aspirin instead of sugar or flour or some noxious chemical. In fact, you depend on your government to keep your local store from selling you anything that could kill you when ingested. Without this form of consumer protection, you would have to spend a lot of time and money making sure that the drugs you bought were safe. All of the government activities that make exchange easy and inexpensive are going on almost without notice.[1]

To make any transaction, you must be able to say, "I own this, and I will give it to you in exchange for that." The most fundamental function of government is to maintain law and order. Unless we can define and enforce rights, including property rights, there is no way for people to cooperate and move beyond the law of the jungle—each person for himself or herself alone. Being killed because somebody wants your house or your cow or your mate is the most basic of threats to your health. Government arose in response to such threats. Families banded together into tribes to protect one another. To do so, they had to agree on how to work together: Who would farm and who would fight, who would lead, and when it was OK to disagree with the leader. Douglass North, the 1993 Nobel Laureate in economics, defines the state as "an organization with a comparative advantage in violence, extending over a geographic area whose boundaries are determined by its power to tax constituents."[2]

The state monopoly on violence makes it less costly for citizens to defend themselves and their property. Government is there to produce those goods and services that markets cannot provide, or cannot provide as efficiently as government can.

14.1 THE ROLES OF GOVERNMENT

The best way to run the economy is usually to let people work, play, and consume what they want without restriction. This interaction of supply and demand in the market leads to a point where marginal benefits equal marginal costs. The prices that arise direct people to work at the jobs in which their skills provide the most value to society, find the most efficient means of production, limit the consumption of goods that are most scarce, and save and invest for the future. If there were no special problems or difficulties, the entire economy could be coordinated without any central control or direction from the government.

Markets are Perfectly Efficient, but Only with Perfect Competition

The power of market prices to organize production and consumption to maximize welfare is expressed in the two fundamental theorems of welfare economics: Under "perfect" conditions, (1) competitive markets will always lead to an efficient allocation of resources for production and consumption and (2) any efficient allocation can be obtained through a market system without any central government control by adjusting initial distribution.[3] These theoretical results emerged from a continuing debate among economists and politicians of all persuasions, from monetarist to Marxist, conservative to liberal, during the early 20th century. They provide the prime intellectual underpinning for advocating the use of markets rather than government intervention to solve most economic problems. Although "perfectly competitive" conditions, like absolute zero or perfect vacuums, can never be obtained in the world of real human societies, markets are usually pretty useful—but they always need help, sometime lots of help, to get there.

Government in a Mixed Economy

Government has four primary tasks in all economies:

- Create laws and maintain order.
- Provide public goods.
- Deal with market failures.
- Build trust through fair and equitable distribution of goods and services.

To achieve these goals, a government may *produce* services, *finance* services that are provided by private contractors, or *regulate* the private market. In practice, programs usually serve several functions and use a combination of methods. The Medicare program, for example, deals with market failure due to adverse selection and redistributes services to the sick elderly, but it is implemented through contracts with private firms. Although functioning primarily as a financing mechanism, Medicare also uses regulation to enforce compliance and participation.

How Government Works

Government influence on various parts of the economy ranges from watchful oversight to total control (Table 14.1). Government is least intrusive when it confines its activities to creating a foundation of property rights and contract enforcement within which the market can operate freely. Government is most controlling when it takes over production and replaces private ownership completely. Through regulation and third-party financing, the health care sector has a high degree of government involvement. **Government production** is mostly limited to certain core public health functions, such as setting and monitoring standards, collecting statistics, controlling infectious disease, and conducting medical research.[4] Direct contracting with production tailored to government specifications, which occurs in military health insurance, federally qualified neighborhood health centers, immunization programs, and so on, offers extensive, yet not complete, public control because the workers are employed by private firms. With **subsidies**, government can exert influence but rarely control. For example, tax-exempt municipal bond financing can encourage construction of hospital facilities, but only rarely and indirectly does it affect the type of clinical services offered. **Entitlement financing**, such

TABLE 14.1	Varieties of Government Action
Type	**Examples**
Public production	*Centers for Disease Control and Prevention*
	Veterans Administration Hospitals
Public Financing	
• **Contract**	*Neighborhood health center*
• **Producer subsidy**	*Vaccine liability insurance*
• **Consumer subsidy**	*Employee health benefits*
• **Entitlement**	*Medicare*
Public Regulation	
• **For the market**	*Financial standards for insurance companies*
• **Superseding market**	*Price controls*
• **Private production**	*Self-paid visit to the therapist*

as Medicare, might leave behavior essentially unconstrained because it is designed to be the equivalent of privately purchased insurance.

A large part of **health regulation** is intended *to make markets more efficient* by providing standard definitions, quality assurance, uniform insurance contracts, and other measures that reduce transactions costs. Other regulations attempt to change the shape of the market *or to supersede the market entirely* and dictate prices and quantities. The regulatory apparatus can be tightened or loosened to allow government to exert more or less control, and it can be made compelling without resorting to legal action by combining regulation with financing. Medicare, initially a passive entitlement financing program that provided essentially private funding for the purchase of physician services, now sets prices within a narrow range and can virtually prohibit the use of some medical technology by refusing to pay for it. Direct regulatory control is exercised by government in only a few areas where the threat to public safety is compelling: water and air quality, production and prescribing of pharmaceuticals, and performance of surgery. For the most part, medical care is "regulated" through control over finances rather than laws.

The Voluntary Sector

The public good is sometimes best served neither by a government bureaucracy nor by a private firm but by independent **voluntary** organizations. Nonprofit status can free hospitals, social service agencies, professional societies, and other voluntary organizations from the dictates of profit maximization and make it easier for them to pursue the goal of maximizing health. Independence from government often makes voluntary organizations more flexible and creative than the public sector in meeting social needs.[5]

Government is Necessary, and Costly

Even when markets are suppressed, there is always competition. Physicians try to attract patients with their reputations for quality and with evening office hours. Hospitals try to attract physicians with subsidized office rentals, access to new equipment, and helpful staff. HMOs try to attract enrollees with special benefits, picnics, or free yoga classes. Conversely, even the most open market in health care is highly regulated, with oversight of safety, professional qualifications, and long-term side effects, even when prices are freely set. The issue is not "regulation" or "competition," but what combination and compromises to make.

Many problems are created by reliance on government intervention. First, regulation itself costs money: Agencies must be staffed, salaries must be paid, and information systems must be maintained. Many of these costs have to be paid for with taxes. Other costs, such as for the compilation of mandated reports and time spent in preparing for regulatory inspections, are imposed on private firms, which then pass them on to the public in the form of higher prices. When government takes over production from private firms, it has sometimes been inefficient and inept at customer service. Even if the market is superseded by direct government provision of services, some form of rationing must still take place. Because prices are not used to match demand and supply, the amount distributed often is too large or too small, and the people served might not be the ones who value the services most highly. Both discrepancies cause deadweight losses of consumer welfare. Government suppression of the price mechanism prevents desirable trades from occurring, and it also distorts related markets for inputs and substitute goods.

Government responds well, perhaps too well, to focused interest groups willing to lobby for their positions. Markets are better able to respond to diverse and diffuse consumer groups, and the prices people pay are a superior mechanism for publicly revealing the value of the services they use. Politicians are constrained by public scrutiny to "do no harm," and every dollar spent becomes a "federal case," therefore services that are valued by consumers and raise average health levels (e.g., mass immunizations, fluoridation, birth control) might not be available. Government is subject to so much criticism that agencies can become very risk averse. This exacerbates bureaucratic formalism. Government programs designed to deal with the public must impose universal standards and thus are less able to respond to the variation in individual preferences or to make individual exceptions. Legal constraints make bureaucracies rigid and may stifle innovation. A central failing of regulation is its reliance on precedent. There is no flexible equilibration of supply and demand through prices to create automatic adjustments as conditions change, and there is little scope for entrepreneurs who are willing to make mistakes and go out on a limb to create the next generation of technology.

Markets are Costly, Limited, and Always Regulated

Markets are also costly to operate, and they have flaws. Markets are *always* regulated. Just try to imagine the stock market without the SEC, or the Superbowl without referees. Regulations are necessary to create a market, to reduce some of the costs, and to make people trust the market enough to trade there. Every trade in the market requires salespeople, billing systems, and policing mechanisms. Entrepreneurs are apt to push the newest and most expensive technology because it is the most profitable rather than a more cost-effective substitute that would do more to improve health.[6] Markets reward those who provide what consumers want, not those who provide public goods such as medical research, infection control, and ethical standards of professional education. Furthermore, markets for health do not appear to be very price sensitive, perhaps because of information problems and the potential for death from even small errors; therefore, reliance on prices to motivate behavior seems ill placed. Even when people can use prices to make decisions about medical care, they seem to want to avoid doing so. For example, the elderly, although well insured with Medicare, overwhelmingly opt to obtain supplemental insurance that reduces the marginal price to zero.

Although advocates of competition emphasize the beneficial effect of creating incentives to win, what about the losers? Who will care for people with mental retardation, alert but alone and alienated 90-year-olds, people with genetic defects, or truly unlucky accident victims? Although markets can enable socially beneficial risk pooling through insurance, adverse selection may be so severe that insurance can become unstable or fail to cover many of those most in need unless government intervenes. Medical *care* is so grounded in a concern for the health of others that any competition sufficiently vicious to really cut costs and close all the unnecessary hospital beds could entail such a fundamental violation of human caring that it is socially unacceptable. One might also ask, "If the erosion of the marketplace due to licensure, insurance, and nonprofit organizations is so terrible, why are these anticompetitive features an integral part of every health care system in the civilized world?"

The approach to health care in the United States is among the most highly privatized and most responsive to individual needs. Yet even in the United States, government is the largest funding source, paying 50 percent of the bills directly, subsidizing much of the remainder through tax relief, and regulating virtually every dollar spent. It is the mixture of competition and market forces, the matching of programs to needs, that must be evaluated, not the pros and cons of one or the other alone.

14.2 GOVERNMENT HEALTH FINANCING

Federal, state, and local government funds are about half of all health spending in the United States. However, most "government" health care is actually third-party insurance payment to the highly regulated private health care industry composed of independent physicians, hospitals, nursing homes, insurance companies, and so on. More than 90 percent goes to such providers of personal health care services, and less than 10 percent goes to core government functions such as medical research, infectious disease control, collection of national health statistics, and public health. Government's share of the rapidly growing health care sector tripled from 14 percent in 1929 to 50 percent in 2012. If the tax subsidies for health insurance are included, the government share of total spending is 55 percent. In earlier years, state and local governments were larger sources of funding than the federal government. In 1965, the biggest single category of government spending was state and local hospitals, institutions providing care for both general medical conditions and chronic mental illness. Since then, Medicare and Medicaid have become much larger, and in 2012 they accounted for three-fourths of all government spending on health care.

The bulk of the $1,424,000,000,000 in 2012 government funds came from general tax revenues. Premiums paid by enrollees for supplemental Medicare insurance (set originally to pay a quarter of costs) brought in $37 billion, and the designated Medicare Hospital Insurance tax of 2.9 percent on the wages and self-employment income of all workers brought in another $186 billion. These funding schemes shift the incidence of the tax burden but do not change the total amount. Ultimately, all government spending must come at the expense of private consumption and investment.

Although the U.S. government provides the largest flow of funds into health care services, it has remained relatively passive. Both Medicare and Medicaid are **entitlement** programs, which are open-ended commitments for government to pay the bills incurred by any eligible patient (i.e., age 65 or over or indigent, respectively). Unlike budgeted programs, in which a fixed dollar amount is appropriated each year, there is no limit on the amount that can be spent on Medicaid and Medicare. Explosive growth in expenditures is a major cause of deficits in state and federal budgets and "crowds out" spending on vital infrastructure, including public health, research, and teaching activities. The future health and economic wellbeing of the United States is being compromised to pay for uncontrolled and excessive use of resources (see Figure 14.1 and Table 14.2).

FIGURE 14.1   Sources of Health Financing (% of GDP)

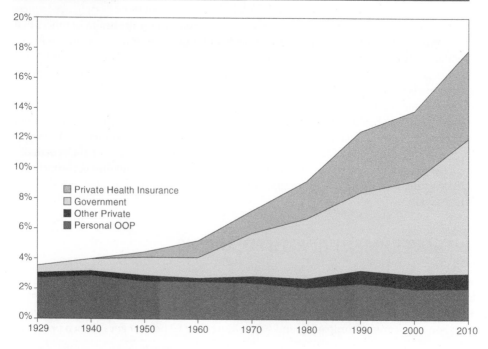

TABLE 14.2	Distribution of Government Funds	
	1965	**2012**
Total (millions)	$10,799	$1,424,000
Medicare	—	40%
Medicaid*	20%	32%
Veterans/DOD	18%	7%
Workers' compensation	8%	3%
State and local hospitals	22%	2%
Public health	8%	6%
Research	12%	4%
Construction	7%	4%
Other	5%	2%

*Medicaid category includes general assistance (welfare) payments for health care, and in 1965 it comprised a variety of medical care programs for the indigent, as Medicaid was not yet enacted.

Source: CMS National Health Accounts.

14.3 LAW AND ORDER

National defense and its complex domestic version—law and order—are the most fundamental tasks of governance. Without protection of life and property, society could not exist. A uniform interpretation of the law and a system of taxation must be enforced by the police and the courts. If the law applies to some and not to others, people are split into two different societies, even if they are nominally within the same nation. Coercive powers of taxation and law enforcement are freely given to the state by the citizens—we agree to have the government take our money and punish us if we break the law because we are better off that way. Each of us fighting our own battles is more expensive than all the taxes, parking fines, and so on that we love to complain about. Government is expensive, but anarchy, although it doesn't cost anything, is ruinous.

Getting people to agree that there should be law and order is much easier than reaching agreement on exactly what those laws should be, who pays how much tax, and so on. The philosopher John Rawls, in his book *A Theory of Justice,* suggests a useful way of looking at the problem of reaching a social consensus.[7] Rawls argues that much of the conflict over what is right and wrong is due not to differences in beliefs but to differences in the positions that people are coming from. Older people want government to provide subsidies for assisted living, and young families believe that better schools are more important. The rich want taxes to be kept low, and the poor (who hope to benefit from redistribution and government aid) want taxes to be higher. People with AIDS favor a national health insurance system that insures everyone, and healthy workers tend to favor higher take-home pay and insurance premiums based on expected costs. In each case, the supporters tend to be those who can expect to benefit, and the critics tend to be those who stand to lose (through higher taxation, less service, or loss of preference).

Consider the formation of policy on disability. It is expensive to provide home care, prostheses, therapy, and building modifications. Including students with disabilities in regular classrooms (mainstreaming) helps them become integrated into society, but it imposes costs on the other students in the diversion of teachers' attention, pacing of lectures, disruption, and so on. If everything that can possibly benefit the disabled students is done, it will cost too much. Yet providing only those benefits that reduce costs (e.g., a prostheses to help someone return to work) is not enough. Whether people focus primarily on the costs or emphasize the benefits depends mainly on whether they are disabled or care deeply about a child, parent, or friend who is. However, even people who are healthy recognize that there is some chance that they might become disabled in the future (e.g., after an automobile accident) and switch their focus. Rawls defines justice as a set of policies people would vote for "behind the veil of ignorance" (i.e., what people would consider an optimal balance of costs and benefits if they did not know whether they were disabled or healthy, farmers or lawyers, or young or old). Formally, Rawls's notion is a lot like insurance, where people willingly contribute enough to cover their expected losses to an insurance plan that spreads the risk. Most health care, disability, and pension financing systems in Europe and Asia are "social insurance" operating under principles of fairness and solidarity rather than private actuarial principles (such as rating and payment according to risk category) used in commercial insurance.

Justice is more than an abstract notion; it is necessary for the operation of society. Unless people believe that the system is fair and serves their needs, they will not trust the government, and it becomes prohibitively costly to force them to behave according to the rules. Pervasive cheating will cause the whole system to break down. If members of a group think they are not being treated fairly, the group will lose respect for the law. At the extreme, they will revolt and perhaps set up a separate government that conforms more closely to their ideal of a fair system.

14.4 PUBLIC GOODS AND EXTERNALITIES

A public good is something that everyone consumes collectively. National defense is a public good. So are clean air, the discovery of penicillin, and the publication of national health statistics. Public goods have two distinguishing properties. First, they are *inexhaustible*; therefore, once produced, there is no additional cost for having additional people use them (i.e., the marginal cost of additional users is $0). Second, they are *nonexclusive*; therefore, people cannot be stopped from using a public good once it is there. Private goods are exhaustible and get used up by consumption (a pill, an hour of a doctor's time), whereas public goods (the formula for the pill, the discovery that eating foods rich in vitamin C reduces certain diseases, clean air) do not. If one patient uses a doctor's time, another patient cannot. Yet if one patient uses a formula, clean air, or nutritional advice, the amount available for someone else is not reduced. Private goods are *exhaustible*; thus, if one person uses them, another person cannot. Usually it is easy to exclude those who do not pay, and thereby cover the costs of production.

Public goods tend to be nonexclusive and indivisible; thus, if anyone gets the benefits, everyone does. Since no one can be prevented from using a public good like clean air, no one has any incentive to pay for it. Selfishly, it makes sense for me to wait for someone else to clean up the air, discover a cure for AIDS, or build the Internet, because whether I contribute or not will make little difference. This is known as the free-rider problem. If no one is charged for public goods and no one voluntarily contributes, there is no way to conduct medical research, reduce pollution, or build highways. Therefore, governments are allowed to force everyone to "donate" taxes to pay for public goods.

Many goods are not purely private or purely public but somewhere in between, and the extent of "publicness" can change with market conditions. For people in an isolated rural area, building and staffing a hospital is mostly a public good. Without the hospital, they have no medical care, but once it is built, anyone who wants to can use the hospital without displacing or reducing anyone else's consumption because there is plenty of excess capacity (i.e., marginal cost of additional patients is near $0). However, if the population increases and the hospital becomes full, each additional patient displaces someone else who might have received care, and care becomes more like a private good (and marginal cost rises to approximately equal the average cost per unit). Highways, parks, and movie theaters show similar congestion effects, being almost pure public goods when they are mostly empty and more like private goods as they fill up.

Privatizing Public Goods

Prescription drugs and condominiums provide interesting cases of public goods being privatized. Once a discovery is made and validated through clinical trials, the actual costs of production are nearly zero. However, unlike a vaccine, which benefits the public by inhibiting communicable disease, most of the benefits from a prescription drug accrue to the user. Patent law gives the firm a monopoly on the drug for 17 years so that it can charge users for the sunk costs of discovery and testing.

Geographic enclosure privatizes condominiums. Thus all the residents of a resort community with a golf course pay privately for maintaining the cleanliness of a lake and have private agreements to limit noise and pollution. Members of a co-op in Manhattan pay fees to employ doormen, maintain public areas, and provide some utilities. Externalities arise primarily because the costs and benefits are borne by different people so that one or the other is external to the market transaction. Patent laws, enclosed communities, and membership clubs are examples of "internalizing" external effects so that owners rather than government pay for collective action.

Insurance Makes Any Good More Public

Whenever a service is financed through third-party insurance rather than directly by individual purchasers, the service becomes more of a public good. When individuals purchase a good, one person may choose high quality, another low or one may want the color to be blue while the other wants it to be green, and so on. Within a risk-pooling group, they are all the same. Whether the person being treated is a vice-president of marketing or an assistant janitor, the hospital gets paid the same amount. It is possible for insurance companies to provide extensive coverage for plastic surgery and 200 days of mental health coverage, but everyone in the benefit plan must get it. The differentiation between individuals by payment is eliminated. The quality of services covered by the insurance package is a public good. There is no gain to the janitor for seeking out a cheap hospital, because even if the company does obtain some savings, it won't make insurance any cheaper to the janitor personally. Once medical care is financed on a group basis, any change in quality or standards of service affects everyone and requires collective action.

Externalities

The production or consumption of a private good can have social consequences because it affects other people. A heavier car makes the driver safer but increases the risk of injury to other drivers.[8] A firm that produces cars might not pay for the exhaust they emit, an airport might not compensate residents in neighboring houses for the disruption caused by jets taking off at night, a student who cheats might not compensate classmates for the inconvenience caused by new test-taking rules, and a student who comes to class with a cold to take an exam might not compensate classmates for exposing them to illness. Externalities exist whenever a transaction affects an uncompensated party. The term *public good* focuses attention on the collective concerns that face all of us: a need for consensus, government control, and a universal tax system. The term *externalities* focuses attention on concerns in which the costs and benefits of actions are borne by different people, making private and social costs diverge. Whether considering public goods such as national defense and scientific research or externalities such as infection control and pollution, we end up with the same issue: how do we design appropriate institutions and governmental rules to align individual incentives with social welfare.

There are positive as well as negative externalities. Governments subsidize schools and colleges because they think that educated people will become better citizens (and able to pay more taxes). A person who fixes up an old house increases the value of all houses in the neighborhood, a cook who washes his hands reduces the risk of spreading infection, and a technological discovery that allows more efficient production by one firm creates external benefits for other firms that copy it. However, that same technology might create negative externalities for some corporations and people because it puts an obsolete factory out of business and causes workers to lose their jobs. In fact, whether an externality is positive or negative depends on the perspective from which it is viewed. The cook might have thought that he was doing his patrons a favor by washing his hands. The patrons might have thought that being clean is part of his job and that not washing his hands was an unwarranted burden to impose on them. This mirror-image aspect, that an action may be considered either a negative cost reduction or a positive benefit increase, leads to an important insight.

The Coase Theorem: Transaction Costs and Property Rights

If transacting were indeed costless, as is assumed under perfect competition, a factory would pay a fee for the smoke it emits, a cook with dirty hands would pay a fee to customers who became ill, and a student with the flu would not show up for an exam unless he or she was willing to pay each classmate $20 for exposing them to airborne viruses. These externalities would then be internalized by market transactions. If only one or two people are affected by an externality, individual transactions can be used to deal with it. For example, a person who dumps dirt in a neighbor's yard or who breaks a neighbor's window, or a doctor who negligently causes a leg fracture, will pay for it. If many people are affected by an externality, the cost of arranging thousands of individually negotiated transactions becomes prohibitive and **property rights** (who controls what, who must pay whom to use it) become unclear. No market develops to handle externalities at this scale. Therefore, government must act on behalf of many people by creating rules and regulations. It is cheaper to deal with a problem once and for all, despite some inefficiencies, than to make thousands of individual transactions with everyone who might be affected by the problem (e.g., pollution, infection, air traffic control).

Suppose that the socially optimal decision, in which marginal costs equal marginal benefits, is to force factories to reduce the pollution emitted from their smokestacks by 80 percent. The **Coase theorem** asserts that there would be *no difference* in outcome whether the factory has a right to pollute or the people have a right to clean air.[9] As long as all rights are well defined, there are no transacting costs and income distribution effects are ignored (two big "ifs"), the result will be the same. Thus when the neighbors have a right to clean air, the factory will pay each resident a fee to allow discharge of 20 percent of the smoke and will buy scrubbers to clean up the rest. If, instead, the factory has the right to pollute, the neighbors will pay the company a fee to install smokestack scrubbers until pollution has been reduced to 20 percent. Either way, the result will be the same: Air that is 80 percent cleaner. The ability to make mutually beneficial trades through the market guarantees that whoever values air quality more, whether positively or negatively, will "buy" it from the other party. The Coase theorem is important, not because outcomes would be the same under some hypothetically perfect conditions, but because it shows how transaction costs and the creation of winners and losers due to assignment of property rights will actually affect income distribution and efficiency in the real world.

14.5 MONOPOLY AND MARKET FAILURE

For public goods, the marginal cost of additional consumption is $0. The production of some private goods has such high fixed costs and low marginal costs that the average cost per unit continually falls as output increases. Such goods (telephone networks, power and water supply) are called **natural monopolies**. Declining average cost means that the largest firm can underbid all the others, and competition will lead to a single firm that dominates the whole market. However, to break even, that firm must charge a price above marginal cost (the high fixed cost overhead means that average cost per unit is always above marginal cost). Because there is no competition, the monopoly firm may push prices up to extract extra profits from consumers, stopping only when the profits are so great that another firm is tempted to enter the market, even at an inefficiently small scale. In a rural area, ambulance transport, hospital services, even a doctor's office, might all be natural monopolies. In addition to the technologically induced natural monopoly, there are monopolies created by political action. For example, a certificate-of-need law can give a hospital an effective monopoly in its local market by barring the construction of new competitors, licensure laws can give a profession monopoly control over supply, quality regulations can give a manufacturer monopoly control over a special medical device, and requirements to hold clinical trials demonstrating safety and efficacy can give a pharmaceutical firm monopoly control over a type of drug.

The desire to maximize profits and the lack of competition leads a monopolist, unlike a firm under perfectly competitive conditions, to charge prices above the average cost per unit, generating excess profits known as **monopoly rents**. Monopoly pricing causes the market to be inefficient. With prices above average cost, some consumers choose not to buy even though goods could have been produced and sold for an amount less than their willingness to pay. The amount of consumer welfare forgone is traditionally estimated by the "welfare triangle" (see Chapter 4, Section 5) which, under appropriate conditions, is approximately one-half the difference between the monopoly price and the average cost per unit ($P_{monopoly} - AC$) multiplied by the number of units not purchased owing to the excessive price ($Q_{optimum} - Q_{monopoly}$). The magnitude of inefficiency due to monopoly pricing is shown by the shaded welfare triangle in Figure 14.2. Monopoly rents (shown as the lightly shaded rectangle) resulting from high prices are a loss to consumers but are a gain to the seller and are regarded by most economists as a pure transfer that does not in itself create any loss of market efficiency. However, consumers tend to get upset about being charged extra just because a firm has a monopoly. Also, there is likely to be some fighting between firms for the right to become the monopolist that takes home the rents, and this fighting is a waste of resources that generates inefficiency.

FIGURE 14.2   Welfare Loss Due to Monopoly Pricing

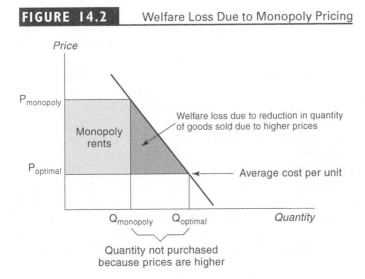

There are four ways for government to deal with the problems created by a natural monopoly:

- Take over the process and let government become the producer.
- Subsidize the fixed cost overhead and set a government-controlled price equal to the marginal cost per unit.
- Set a government-controlled price equal to the average cost, which causes some inefficiency but avoids using taxpayers' money to subsidize a monopoly firm.
- Do nothing and let the firm set a monopoly price.

Some economists claim that government production is so inefficient that the first option should always be avoided. The second and third options depend on the government's ability to accurately estimate marginal and average cost, which is always difficult and is inevitably made worse by firms' attempts to overstate costs and hide revenues to make extra profits. However, allowing firms to become monopolies often costs much more than the traditional welfare triangle loss, because firms waste millions of dollars making donations to politicians, hiring lawyers, and competing for (and competing away) the potential monopoly rents. Natural monopoly is a cornerstone of applied welfare economics, and of crucial importance in the analysis of pharmaceuticals (Chapter 11), yet many medical monopolies arise from government intervention (licensure, regulation, reimbursement rules, patents) designed to ameliorate market failures caused by risk and information difficulties (discussed in Chapter 6) rather than market failures caused by production conditions of declining average costs.

14.6   INFORMATION

Information is a quintessential public good: nonexclusive and inexhaustible. Once information is known (Pythagorean theorem, "Stairway to Heaven," Consumer Price Index, lemons cure scurvy) there is no way to stop people from using it, and there is no good reason to make them pay because the cost of additional users is zero. Statistics and scientific discoveries are almost pure public goods, yet they often serve important (and profitable) private functions as well. The discovery of bacteria by Louis Pasteur began a revolution in the treatment of disease. It also saved the wool industry from the plague of anthrax, which had been decimating sheep (Pasteur's original research project); the wine and beer industries, which were having trouble with fermentation irregularities; and the dairy industry, whose unpasteurized products caused diarrhea and many fatalities among infants.[10] Much of Pasteur's work was supported by government grants, just as medical research is today. No single person or firm could obtain enough benefits to justify spending the money required to fund such a large research and development project. It was a collective enterprise. However, there were still many free riders. Although the costs were paid mostly by France and, to a lesser extent, by industrial brewers and woolen manufacturers in Belgium and Germany, people in the United States, Africa, China, and the rest of the world benefited. To the extent that those who benefit do not contribute, there is underinvestment in the development of knowledge.

Research on new drugs, new surgical techniques, and new methods of diagnostic imaging have received billions of dollars in public funding. However, it is the collection of statistics over many years and from millions of patients that makes it possible to determine how medical discoveries work in practice. A landmark in the history of medicine and public health was the printing of *Observations on the Bills of Mortality*, by John Graunt, in 1662.[11] Graunt studied death records in the city of London and tabulated the number of people dying each year and their causes of death, thus creating the first modern work in the science of epidemiology. With the causes of death plainly laid out, the years of plague and the probable effects (or lack of effects) of government attempts to improve the health of citizens could be seen.

The National Institutes of Health (NIH) has overall responsibility for medical research in the United States, and the National Center for Health Statistics (NCHS) is responsible for data collection and distribution. NCHS's oldest and most important publication is its *Vital Statistics Reports* on births and deaths. NCHS also conducts surveys on health and nutrition status, insurance coverage, and the characteristics of patients treated in doctors' offices, and compiles statistics on patients discharged from hospitals using billing records. All this information is made available in "public use data tapes" and in free publications (which can be obtained online for your term paper) because it is a public good produced with public money. Those running the agency want to maximize the value of this "free" good so that they can argue for more funding from Congress—and, not incidentally, benefit all of us.

Measurement and statistics do not come into being just because it is a good thing to have them, they must serve an economic purpose. The census that recorded Mary and Joseph at the birth of Jesus of Nazareth was mandated to enable Caesar to collect taxes. Deaths historically have been recorded to establish inheritance, not to study the effects of medical treatment. The provision of universal public benefits, such as Social Security, made it possible for the United States to easily enforce the requirement that all deaths be recorded. The fact that collecting information is costly explains why there are more statistics on health care expenditures (which must be recorded on each transaction to pay employees, bill insurance companies, and so on) than on medical diagnosis or treatment effectiveness. The U.S. Centers for Medicare and Medicaid Services (CMS) (which has power because it controls the funds) is setting standards for a "uniform bill" that will be submitted electronically by all hospitals and doctors and thus provide an integrated database for comparing the costs and effects of all types of medical care. Potentially, this will not only reduce the administrative costs of running the system, it will also make it possible for researchers to tap into an online database with hundreds of millions of patient-years of experience and, therefore, rapidly determine which treatments, types of hospitals, drugs, and so on are most cost-effective.

Rational Consumer Ignorance

Why does the government have a better information base for making decisions than most citizens? Because the government paid for it. From safety standards for seatbelts to the efficacy of vitamin supplements, millions of dollars have been spent to determine the best possible answers. Massively wasteful duplication would result if each consumer collected such information individually. If consumers banded together to share the costs of gathering information, such banding would constitute a form of government. Consumers are rationally ignorant of many issues because it is more efficient to have the government collect information once than for each of us to do it separately. Rational consumer ignorance is sensible free riding. Even for a private good, such as a bottle of vitamins, it is cheaper to perform quality control once in a government laboratory than to do it over and over again in each individual's home. Consumers remain rationally ignorant by delegating their decision-making powers to the government because it is more efficient for them to do so—they are being smart by staying stupid! Thus, the Food and Drug Administration (FDA) tests the safety of food and drugs, the Environmental Protection Agency (EPA) conducts studies on the effects of pollution, and the Department of Transportation (DOT) monitors the safety of highways and motor vehicles.

Social Costs Depend on the Number of People

The extent of externalities depends on the magnitude of the costs and the number of people involved. Airplane accidents are scrutinized by government safety inspectors more carefully than automobile accidents, and nuclear power plant failures are even more closely scrutinized. The larger the number of people who could be hurt, the more thorough the investigation.

Garbage disposal is an example of how the treatment of public goods changes with the number of people involved.[12] In prehistoric times, people did whatever they pleased with their garbage and no one worried about a waste disposal system. The same is true today in isolated rural areas where people toss the garbage out in the woods or bury or burn it. Keeping one's own house tidy and the neighbors happy is sufficient incentive to maintain a social optimum, and no government rules are needed. As people move closer together, creating a town, the divergence between private and social costs widens. Dumping trash in fields or in the yards of strangers rapidly creates a problem. Therefore, rules are formulated designating when and where garbage may be dumped. As the town becomes larger, public spending becomes necessary to handle all the garbage produced. Land is purchased and set aside to serve as a dump. As the town becomes a city, it is not enough just to have a dump; the city must actively collect all the trash and carry it to the dump. Taxes are imposed and trucks come around to collect garbage at people's houses. In this way the private costs of conforming to the social optimum are minimized. Garbage collection is a public activity that requires collective financing through taxes, but the actual work can be done by a private firm and often is.

Milk or Bread: Which Is More Public?

Whether goods should fall in the public or private arena depends on the characteristics of the goods and the way they are produced and transacted. In general, if something is produced collectively so that one person's consumption cannot easily be separated from another's, more government intervention is called for. If the relevant characteristics are readily observable by consumers at the time of purchase, more reliance on private markets is appropriate. Consider two products that are consumed by almost everyone: milk and bread. Milk was subjected to government regulations more than a hundred years ago, and public milk-dispensing stations were set up in New York and other cities.[13] It is illegal in most states to sell milk that has not been inspected and processed according to government standards. Bread, although under routine surveillance as a food, is largely unregulated. Why this difference in treatment?

Bread may be mixed in batches, but each loaf is baked separately, and the baking process kills most germs. When bread gets old after sitting on the shelf too long, it becomes stale and hard, and green and white furry spots start growing on it. These signs of deterioration are readily visible to consumers. Milk from many dairies is mixed together when it is being processed for sale; so that contamination at any one dairy potentially threatens thousands of consumers. Contamination is most likely to occur during the milking process and can best be prevented by keeping the cows clean and the equipment sterilized and by removing manure from the barn. On-site inspection can be performed cheaply by government agents, but it would be prohibitively costly for consumers to visit all the dairies their milk comes from each week and check the floors. Bacteria are killed during the processing of milk, but how is a consumer to know that the "pasteurized" label on the carton is to be believed? When the crucial quality-control step can be monitored efficiently only during processing and compliance is not easily discernable at the point of sale, government oversight and labeling are called for. Most of the dangerous bacteria that people can get from milk, particularly salmonella, do not make milk curdle or smell bad and thus are hard to detect. Milk is an ideal culture medium for many bacteria, making milk distribution, in effect, a perfect way to spread disease. Contamination from one farm cannot be determined later because milk from all the farms is mixed together. The bacteria rapidly grow to infect all the milk and are delivered invisibly, with much of the product going to the most vulnerable segment of the population, children.

Many factors make milk more suitable for government regulation, but the crucial issue is information—what can consumers see or learn easily at the point of sale. Bad bread is visible to consumers; bad milk is not. The information necessary to protect the safety of the public is available at low cost if regulations are enforced *during production*, a process that would be prohibitively costly for consumers to carry out on their own. The asymmetry of information costs makes milk quality a public good, whereas the quality of bread is largely private.

Infectious Disease Externalities

Day care centers are a familiar and useful example of infection externalities. Parents with a child who is slightly sick, or who might be coming down with a cold, face a difficult choice. If they stay home with the child, they miss a day of work, but if they send the child to day care, other children will be exposed. The first cost is borne personally, but the costs of other children getting sick is a social cost borne by the other parents. Therefore, many busy parents faced with deadlines at work make a decision that is in their own best interests and drop the slightly sick child off at day care. Day care workers hate this and have developed a rule that if a child does get sick at day care, the parents must come immediately and take the child home or they will be fined and/or barred from the facility. The day care facility is forcing parents to "internalize" the risk of infecting others by deliberately increasing the penalty for bringing in a sick child.

Sexual transmission of diseases heightens the divergences between private and social costs of infection. The desire for privacy increases transaction costs. With the flu, everyone knows when you are sick. With syphilis or gonorrhea, the symptoms are usually unobservable, even by your sexual partner. Whereas coughing is a costless signal of flu infection, you must be told that you have been exposed to a sexually transmitted disease (STD). This is difficult for most people because it marks them as infected and involves the admission that they have been having sexual relations with others. Although it is beneficial to society as a whole that all your sexual partners be notified that you are infected, it is often costly to you personally. It could cost you some friends, a marriage, or a job. My first job was as an STD investigator for the city of New York. Why were tax dollars used to pay civil servants to find out who was infected, whom they had sex with, and to bring these people to the clinic for penicillin shots? Didn't people who were infected already have sufficient incentive to come in for treatment? No. Infection creates externalities. The one who is infected bears the personal costs of disease and treatment but does not bear the cost imposed on society by increasing other people's risk of infection. The divergence between private and social costs means that those currently infected are not sufficiently motivated to seek treatment. Whether someone gets treated this week or next might not make much difference to their own health, but it could significantly increase the risk imposed on others.

Stigmatization and embarrassment makes information harder to come by. The U.S. Public Health Service (PHS) developed a rule of anonymity to minimize the costs of acting in the interests of society. When sexual contacts are notified to come in for treatment, they are not told who has given their name. One client showed up with his wife and three girlfriends (yes, all at once, in the same room) and demanded to know who had been infected. Although it might have been in his interest to know, violating confidentiality would make it more difficult for the PHS to get people to divulge sensitive information. Anonymity made it easier for them to consider the well-being of society rather than just the personal risk to themselves.

Epidemics

Sudden upsurges in disease have had profound effects on the course of human civilization: Black Death in the Middle Ages, biblical plagues afflicted the people of Egypt under pharaohs, tuberculosis, syphilis, a pandemic (worldwide epidemic) flu outbreak in 1918 that killed hundreds of thousands of young people; and more recently, AIDS.[14] The externality imposed by contagion was recognized long before germs were identified as a cause of disease. Quarantine was among the earliest forms of public health action. In primitive societies, those who were visibly ill were sometimes banished from the tribe. As early as A.D. 1400, ships from ports where plague had been reported were kept out in the harbor for months to see whether any of the sailors would die. Only after sufficient time had passed for the authorities to convince themselves that the ship was not carrying disease was it allowed to unload. The public interest in disease reduction conflicted with the private interests of ship owners. Most of the costs of an epidemic (i.e., deaths) would fall on the population of the city, while the benefits of continuing to trade accrued to the merchants. *An Enemy of the People*, a famous play by Henrik Ibsen, centers on the disastrous consequences of a tannery ignoring the long-run risks of disease to pursue short-run profits.[15]

Leprosy may have been the first communicable disease brought under control by public health measures. Leprosy is a slow-growing bacterium that destroys the neural sheath and hence sensation. The infection itself is often less damaging than its side effects. People with leprosy cannot feel pain in the affected area, therefore they may scratch an itch until they gouge their flesh away, or get burned without even knowing it, and so on. The bacterium is hard to transmit from person to person thus infection usually requires intimate contact over an extended period of time. People with leprosy were isolated from the rest of the population to halt the spread of the disease. Although the United States still had leper colonies until 1953, effective treatment with antibiotics has now removed the threat of contagion.

In the 12th century, there were more than 200 hospitals for the confinement of lepers in France alone. Leprosy almost disappeared from medieval Europe, and permanent quarantine in hospitals appears to have played a significant role in reducing the incidence of disease. But consider the cost. Leprosy is a progressive disease. Without treatment, the person sent to a hospital was put away for life, without visitors. The church would hold a funeral for the leper, the family would mourn, and all the person's property would be passed on through inheritance, just as if that person had died. The signs and symptoms of leprosy (a scaly rash) are common to a variety of ordinary, nonserious disorders (psoriasis, scabies, skin allergy), making diagnosis difficult. Therefore many people without leprosy must also have been permanently confined in such hospitals (where presumably they caught leprosy after awhile anyway). The uncertainty of diagnosis and the severe consequences probably made people very reluctant to visit the doctor for a rash or to share information with neighbors. Claims of leprosy were more apt to be made against people who were not welcome within society (gypsies, Jews), and a disgruntled family member or impatient heir might assert that a wealthy grandfather had leprosy purely out of self-interest. Permanent quarantine probably did help protect the community, but at the cost of making a person with leprosy, or who was suspected of having leprosy, a nonperson. Only when epidemics caused high rates of mortality did the interests of the community (disease prevention) outweigh the interests of the individual (property, freedom). Similar discrimination and social turbulence arose when the AIDs epidemic arrived thirty years ago.

The Sanitary Revolution: A Moral Campaign for Public Health

The public health reforms that reduced the threat of cholera, diphtheria, typhoid, and other communicable diseases were part of the 19th-century social revolution that imposed Victorian middle-class values on society as a whole.[16] Posters that attacked working conditions in the coal mines did not stress that workers had to eat stooped over while standing in pools of water that collected human waste, but instead the fact that women working underground were stripped to the waist because of the heat. Mandating that children younger than 12 years work no more than 10 hours a day seemed an act of kindness, not an attempt to prevent premature disability. Above all else Victorians hated dirt. Social reformers wanted cleanliness and light, which happened to be effective in reducing the spread of infectious disease, although there was no way to know that given the science of the time. A belief in what was morally right, not scientific evidence, underlay the English sanitary revolution.

Not all attempts to remove dirt and immorality proved to be healthful. Sending women to maternity hospitals instead of having a midwife attend birth at home caused the spread of puerperal (childbirth) fever and a rapid increase in maternal mortality. The replacement of breastfeeding with sterile bottles deprived middle-class infants of maternal immunities. Diseases of poverty, such as pellagra, were so consistently blamed on lack of cleanliness and insects that the mounting evidence of dietary deficiency was ignored. The sanitary revolution did much to clean up the environmental mess created as industrial urbanization brought masses of people together in cities, but science was decidedly secondary to morality and ideology. The net result was beneficial overall, but it was quite unbalanced. These historical lessons are worth remembering as we attempt to evaluate the hazards of environmental carcinogens and other public health issues today.

Formation of the U.S. Public Health Service

The U.S. Public Health Service had it origins in the merchant seamen's hospital founded in 1798.[17] The rationale for government involvement was threefold. First, seamen were engaged in international trade and ships commonly carried diseases between countries, so the government had an interest in making sure that the seamen were willing to report any illnesses. Second, medical care was mostly provided at home by one's family, but sailors spent years abroad on ships and rarely had families to depend on. Ordinary laborers without kin who became sick or disabled were the responsibility of local communities, but sailors were travelers who might have been born in Boston or Chicago or Kankakee or anywhere, and thus they could not rely on any town to support them in their time of need. Third, international trade was vital to the economic growth of the nation. Unless the national government was willing to take care of people who became ill or disabled, few would have been willing to leave home and become sailors.

Public health activity was much more limited in the United States than in England during the 19th century. American cities were not as old or as crowded. There were fewer innovations in the United States, but European social programs and sanitary reforms were quickly adopted. Massachusetts set up the first state board of health following the Shattuck report in 1850. By 1900 the New York City health department had become an active center with special support programs for immigrants and free sterile milk distribution for mothers and children. The Pure Food and Drug Act was passed in 1906, and in 1920 the Shepard–Towner Act provided the first national government-sponsored medical care for mothers and dependent children. Other milestones in U.S. public health include the formation in 1952 of the National Institutes of Health, now by far the largest public health agency, to conduct medical research; the 1965 passage of amendments XVIII and XIX to the Social Security Act, which established Medicare and Medicaid; and the 1970 acts creating the Environmental Protection Agency (EPA) and the Occupational Safety and Health Administration (OSHA).

14.7 DRUGS, SEX, AND WAR: PUBLIC HEALTH IN ACTION

Market efficiency depends on consumers' ability to choose, to correctly balance their demands with prices and available income. Some types of consumers—notably children, the mentally ill, addicts—are considered incapable of making reasonable choices. There is a biological necessity for parents to care for and make decisions on behalf a child, forcing the child to learn by doing many things he or she does not initially want to do (hence the term *paternalism*). Market failure due to mental incapacity is dealt with by having a parent, legal guardian, social service agency, or government bureau make decisions on behalf of those individuals rather than allowing them to do so for themselves. To that extent, children and others judged deficient or dependent are wards of the state, not fully participating citizens.

Addiction

Addicts are prohibited by law from buying drugs they are willing to pay for. However, the legal distinctions regarding addiction are sometimes as much historical and political as they are biological. Heavy alcohol use is probably more likely to impair judgment and lead to injury than marijuana, and heroin taken regularly over years has fewer adverse physical effects than cigarettes. Yet heroin is such a powerful drug that addicts will do almost anything to get it, and illegality raises the price so high that it becomes necessary for many to steal to stay high. It is the externalities (stealing, dirty needles) rather than use that makes heroin so harmful to society. Cigarettes may be bad for your health, but they provide income to farmers, bring us sporting events, elect senators and representatives, and contribute mightily to the profits of large multinational firms. In trying to understand how morality is shaped by economics, it is useful to point out that the British Empire started a war with China to enforce its "right" to cross the border and sell opium to Chinese workers, a practice the Emperor wanted to prevent.

Sexual Behavior

Sexual behavior reveals some of the underlying value judgments that are at the heart of any paternalistic decision to override individual decision-making authority. For centuries, children's sexual behavior fell under the control of parents because inheritance was a major form of economic exchange. Thus, the rules regarding whom to have sex with for the aristocracy (who had inheritable land) were much different from the rules for the peasantry. Aristocrats, who were not allowed to have sex with the 17-year-old sons and daughters of neighboring lords, could have sex with their serfs because any children born from such a union had no property rights.

Sexual preferences are value laden, with active debates over homosexual marriage and the acceptability of gays and lesbians serving in the military and holding public office. The American Psychiatric Association until 1974 listed homosexuality as a disease and, although difficult to imagine today on a college campus with prominent gay organizations, young men and women then were treated for having the illness of "abnormal" desires. The labeling of behavior as illness is not limited to homosexuality. Activities such as eating pork, piercing lips and noses, circumcision, lying down to sleep with the dead, taking hallucinogenic drugs, speaking in tongues, and mortification of the flesh are viewed as normal or exemplary in some cultures and as clear signs of illness in others. The line between using power to make someone "do something for your own good" and dictatorial thought control is not always easily drawn, and it is rarely more contentious than when it touches on the continuation of society through procreation. In one society, it may be routine for a young person to be taken to a prostitute or religious center for sexual initiation, whereas in another such behavior would be seen as cruel or immoral.

Advocates for people with mental illness and mental retardation are willing to push for the fullest participation in "normal" activities, but they are often placed in a quandary regarding the desire of the mentally disabled to have children, especially when the disability is genetically related. Can that person understand the consequences? Is it fair to the unborn child? Even if the child has no genetic abnormalities, is it fair to the child to be raised by parents whose capacity is severely constrained, making it likely that the child will be raised in a foster home? Externalities forcefully raise the question: Who counts, and do some count more than others?

Who Counts as a Citizen? Abortion and Other Dilemmas

Nowhere is the conflict over whose views are to count more apparent than in decisions regarding abortion. American society has been unable to achieve a clear resolution, and we will not attempt to do so here. What we can do is see how abortion poses a dilemma that affects many other problems in public health, and thus we will use it to clarify the nature of a general issue: Who is to be counted as a citizen, and do everyone's views count equally?

Difficult questions are posed by pregnancy. The right of a mother, as the one most proximately involved, to make decisions regarding her pregnancy seems reasonable, but it does elevate her rights over those of others. Could this position, if accepted logically, be used to claim that someone else is even more proximate (a grandparent for example, especially if the mother is incapacitated by substance abuse or illness)? This position is also directly in conflict with what pro-life activists describe as the right to life of the unborn child—*if* such an entity can be said to be a citizen. In general, societies seem to accede that mothers have special rights over their infants, and this extends with even greater force to before their birth. Yet this interest is not absolute. Similarly, it is accepted that a fetus does not have the same standing as a child. Consider how differently a court would treat a pregnant woman who took heroin because she was anxious and upset and a mother who gave the drug to her baby to keep the baby quiet. There is no social resolution to these issues other than in crafting some new set of rules and in agreeing to live, however uneasily, within them. It is possible that for many years two or more sets of rules will be in effect for different groups of people who can only agree not to talk about the issue or to fight in the courts rather than in the streets.

Ultimately the question of who counts as a citizen, and how much, is a moral one, but it is heavily conditioned by economic considerations, and transaction costs in particular. Experience has shown that it is virtually impossible to stop women who desperately want an abortion from having one. Making the practice illegal leads to many unsafe operations that cause infertility, disability, and death. Furthermore, any woman who can afford an airplane ticket to a place where abortions are legal can choose that option, thus the practical effect may be to limit access for those who are young and poor and perhaps less able to care for a child. Indeed, the cost–benefit argument (that abortion is much cheaper than years of social services) may have sufficient appeal to some people that their moral positions are influenced by it. How strongly we support another person's right to self determination depends in part on our own self-interest.

In the marketplace of 3rd century Rome, there was a law stating that no citizen could be sold a fish that was more than three days old (which, given the lack of refrigeration, seems plenty). What happened to fish more than three days old? They were sold to noncitizens. Although this kind of blatantly discriminatory behavior seems inconceivable to us today, most countries follow similar policies. Pharmaceuticals that are not approved for use in the United States are routinely sold overseas, and for years many drugs whose shelf lives had expired were disposed of profitably this way. The most forceful statement regarding who is not a citizen, and what the country is willing to do to protect and enrich those who are its citizens, is war.

War and Public Health

A common wall poster during the 1960s read, "War is not healthy for children or other living things." Activity dedicated to killing seems obviously inimical to public health, and indeed, the American Public Health Association has passed several resolutions condemning war. Yet many advances in public health have been associated with war: Florence Nightingale's reform of field hospitals during the Crimean War led to modern nursing, malaria was eradicated during the Spanish–American War, and the campaign against venereal disease and the development of rapid psychotherapy occurred during World Wars I and II. The number of times that medical breakthroughs occurred during or because of a war raises the question: How (un)healthy is war?

As economic historian Douglass North points out, competition between states forces them to meet the needs of the people.[18] A government with no rivals does not need to develop new technologies. When kings or countries are vying for people's loyalty, it is in their interest to build hospitals, clean up the water supply, and perform all the other public health activities that are costly but also yield net benefits to society. North points out that we cannot understand the development of laws and political organization unless we recognize that rulers put their own interests first. War has a positive long-term effect on medical science because it heightens the interest of rulers in the health of the population. In other words, sick civilians make lousy soldiers.

In every war throughout history, at least until the 20th century, many more soldiers died from diseases than from wounds inflicted on the battlefield. Armies of 20,000 or more would gather and camp in open fields with no toilets or running water. Contamination of food and drink were a more likely cause of death than enemy attack. Even in battle it was often infection rather than bullets that killed, because lack of sanitation made minor wounds fatal. Conscripts were often drawn from isolated villages and so had never been exposed to common diseases. The result was uniform disaster. Armies that spent any long period together were decimated by disease.

War changes the calculus of individual costs and benefits. As the collective interest looms larger, massive investments in new knowledge and infrastructure are made. The attempt to place as many men as possible on the front lines leads to the rapid acquisition of knowledge on nutrition, surgery, psychology, and infectious disease. Without ignoring the shameful horror of death and destruction that wars impose on humankind, the fact that they have been a powerful force in advancing medicine and public health must be recognized.

14.8 POLITICS, REGULATION, AND COMPETITION

Politicians: Entrepreneurs Who Try to Get Votes

Markets operate through voluntary exchange whereas public goods can be provided only through political intervention. You cannot go to the store and buy more clean air, better schools, or safer highways. We depend on politicians to act as entrepreneurs, to propose a plan of action that appeals to us so that we will put them in positions of power. Like all entrepreneurs, politicians expect to be paid for their efforts, extracting "rents" in the form of influence, prestige, perquisites, and salary. To an extent, the political arena can be viewed as a market, with people "spending" votes or influence. However, the correspondence is very imperfect: People are not allowed to buy and sell votes, borrow votes by paying interest, or trade votes by setting up joint-stock corporations. The property rights to votes are much less well defined and enforceable, and thus the transaction costs are very high.

Because it is difficult to make a political bargain, a lot of the effort and money must be wasted. Millions of dollars are used to win support or to keep a wavering supporter in line. Formally, economists talk about the problems of "rent capture." If ordinary entrepreneurs have a good idea, they can trade the idea to a firm for money. For example, inventors, biochemists, and screenwriters avoid the hassles of marketing and production by licensing the rights to their ideas and obtaining royalty payments in return. These profits are called *rents* because once the entrepreneur has the idea, no more work needs to be done to get the money. It is similar to collecting rent on a piece of land. Also, like land, the rent depends entirely on the demand. A good idea (Mickey Mouse, penicillin, mobile phones) is valuable the way land in downtown Tokyo is valuable, but bad ideas are like acreage in the Gobi Desert.

Rents and rent seeking are major obstacles to providing an optimal level of investment in public health. Many good ideas (well-child care, genetic counseling for parents, dietary change) offer no simple way for innovators to capture the benefits, and thus there is little incentive to produce them. On the other hand, when large sums of money are available to put good ideas into practice, most of the money is not well spent. The new road primarily benefits a construction company owned by a senator's brother-in-law, the new antismoking campaign is highly visible and impresses voters but doesn't keep children from lighting up, and the new sex education program for teenagers is so dreary that they only use it to make jokes. Even if we know exactly how much to spend on public goods, it is doubtful that all the money will be well spent. Because no single individual has much of an interest, those who are able to capture a piece of the action will distort the program to benefit themselves, and the objective of meeting the needs of the public will be compromised.

Government as the Citizen's Agent

Government exists, to paraphrase the quote from Abraham Lincoln at the opening of this chapter, to do for the people things that they cannot do for themselves. However, what guarantee is there that a government agency will act as the agent of the people rather than of special interest groups or of the bureaucrats themselves? When information problems cause market failure and thus preclude private action, governments will also have a difficult time collecting information and voters will have a difficult time evaluating the performance of an agency to make sure that it is, in fact, operating in the public interest. Economists examine the performance of government agencies from four perspectives:

- Maximizing public welfare
- "Capturing" regulatory agencies by profit-maximizing firms
- Maximizing bureaucratic objectives
- Balancing political interest groups

Public Welfare Maximization   The starting point for the economic analysis is to assume that regulation does what it says it does—maximize public welfare. The British Empire, the state of Pennsylvania, and other governments argue as much when they define themselves as a *commonwealth*. However, to define *public welfare*, assumptions about whose preferences count, and how much, must be made. Is everyone equal? Do people who harm themselves through drug use or lack of exercise deserve the same services as people who try to stay healthy? Do people with genetic defects that shorten their lives deserve more, or less, than people without genetic defects? Does a desire for life-saving heart surgery count as much as a desire for face-saving cosmetic surgery? Even if all these issues are resolved, there still may be no way to reach a decision about which government policy is best, as demonstrated in the proof of the famous "Arrow impossibility theorem."[19]

The theoretical problems of welfare maximization pale beside the practical problems of public incentives. Unlike a firm, which has an owner, no one has an interest in maximizing the benefits of government. An individual or group seeks to maximize its own welfare. Acts and votes are usually directed by self-interest, even when the cost to others far outweighs the benefits to the individual. This causes structural difficulties because it is much easier to gain approval for a program with *concentrated benefits* and *diffuse costs* since the winners will be loud and vocal and the losers will hardly care. For example, lengthening patent restrictions will mean billions to pharmaceutical companies, but would raise the price of health care by just a few cents per prescription, thus adding millions of dollars to the profits of a few pharmaceutical firms but causing just a slight, almost unnoticeable, rise in the medical bills and insurance premiums of millions of consumers. Conversely, the diffuse benefits to consumers of slightly cleaner air or water could cost millions of dollars to one particular firm, which will be motivated to fight hard to block that action.

Regulatory Capture   The concentrated interest of the firms most affected by a regulation makes it worthwhile for them to lobby the government and try to "capture" the regulatory agency. For example, a hearing on the safety of cardiac pacemakers is sure to be attended by lawyers for the device's manufacturers, but few patients will travel to Washington to testify and will not be paid $400 an hour for doing so. Contributing to political campaigns is an obvious way of attempting to exercise control, but usually it is not the most effective way. It is common for firms in regulated industries to appeal directly to bureaucrats, not with money or gifts (which are illegal) but by hiring former regulators and holding informational seminars in Hawaii. It is natural for someone who has worked for years in regulating health to take a job with a company in the same field, but such a **revolving door** is likely to compromise regulatory objectivity. How can a junior analyst in an agency remain unbiased when asked to make a difficult judgment call if the person on the other side of the table is the well-respected former chairman? Even a bureaucrat who wants to do a good job performing daily tasks can be influenced by the asymmetry between concentrated producer interests and diffuse consumer interests. There are many more patients than producers, yet most complaints to regulators (or complaints to politicians about regulatory decisions) come from producers, because they stand to gain so much from any change in the rules.

Bureaucratic Objectives Bureaucrats, just like consumers, profit-maximizing owners, union workers, and all other individuals in the economy, prefer not to be harassed. Most people get paid to do jobs that are occasionally unpleasant in order to maximize long-term gains (e.g., impose discipline on second-graders, redo a botched repair job for free, fire an incompetent employee, hold the HMO doctors within budget). The difficulty of evaluating how well a government agency is performing can reduce the competitive pressure to take on unpleasant tasks. This can lead to an agency that is bloated and excessively risk averse. Unlike an owner or leveraged buyout specialist, who can gain large profits from taking on risk and improving efficiency, a bureaucrat will continue to be compensated on a civil service pay scale. Any effort to make changes or take risks could go wrong and cost them their jobs, so they tend to play it safe. If an owner believes that the additional revenues gained are less than the additional cost in wages, then an employee may be let go. A bureaucrat, on the other hand, has almost no incentive to reduce the number of workers. Instead, an increase in employment usually means a larger salary for the director (who now runs a bigger agency) and better working conditions (since the tasks are spread out among more employees, giving them more time to do the job). Unlike a profit-maximizing firm, there is no internal incentive to limit the size of a government agency, therefore control must be imposed from the outside.

Unfortunately, outsiders are, by definition, less familiar with the tasks, workload, and performance of the agency than the employees and managers inside or the industry experts who lobby them. This does not mean that most government agencies are too large, because the fear of "waste" can lead legislators to preemptively cut regulatory budgets. What it does mean is that the difficulty of evaluating performance, which is why this task was taken out of the market and given to government in the first place, also makes it much harder to tell whether the agency is too big or too small or to manage the agency so that the use of employees and other resources is optimized.

Political Interest Group Balance The actual behavior of government agencies is not determined by the public interest, self-interest of the industry, or self-interest of the bureaucrats, but by a complex and shifting balance of all interest groups. Transaction costs shape politics just as they shape markets, and they are lower when interests are concentrated or uniform across a large group of people (e.g., all of the elderly tend to favor increased Medicare budgets). However, political deals cannot be negotiated, specified, and enforced by precisely weighing conflicting interests the way the market can so precisely and quickly weigh dollars, making outcomes less predictable. Economists and political scientists devote considerable attention to studying how the process of making decisions affects the decisions made. For example, a majority rule implies that 50 to 49 wins while 49 to 50 loses, thus providing politicians with a great incentive to seek the median (50th percentile) voter rather than maximize the average level of support. Other political structures favor different parts of the voting spectrum. In union representation, for example, seniority is important, thus the desires of older workers for more health benefits and higher pensions tend to outweigh the desires of younger workers for fewer benefits and higher wages. Several critiques of the health care industry claim that it is dominated by an "iron triangle" of providers, insurance companies, and government agencies, all of whom benefit from higher health care spending rather than difficult, but potentially worthwhile, cost cutting.[20]

Public Goods Make Almost Everybody Better Off But Nobody Happy

Private goods are provided through individual decisions of buyers and sellers based on price. Public goods, in contrast, must be provided and paid for collectively, and there is no necessary reason that any single person be happy with the decision or agree on how much the service is worth. Skiers want open mountains while developers want to build condominiums. Young parents want better playgrounds and primary schools, while disabled grandparents want wheelchair-accessible sidewalks and drug benefits. Even among art or music lovers there is likely to be disagreement about which galleries or concerts deserve support. Worse, almost everyone underestimates the cost of their favorite program, overestimates how much they pay for things they do not like (typically, foreign aid) and net taxes (i.e., after accounting for all the government benefits received). For example, Alaska is noted for citizens who are proud of standing on their own in the wilds—while each citizen receives a check for oil revenues (instead of paying state taxes) and receives $1.87 in federal dollars for each dollar paid in federal taxes.[21] The goal is to balance all of the demands and resources. In the apocryphal words of a politician, "If neither side is happy, then I must be doing something right."

Winners and Losers

Although economists try to evaluate how a regulation changes the overall efficiency of the system, most hospital administrators, physicians, and patients are far more concerned with how it affects them personally. Even if a change in Medicare reimbursement is good for the country, a medical equipment vendor will fight it with everything he owns if that regulation would force his business into bankruptcy. Changes in the regulatory structure often have more to do with finding paths that have less resistance than the achievement of noble ends. Many issues have solutions that are nearly the same in terms of overall efficiency but are quite different in terms of who bears the costs or receives the benefits. For example, it might not make a great deal of difference in terms of economic efficiency whether an expanded Medicare drug benefit is paid for through increases in enrollee premiums or an income tax surcharge for the elderly, but the former falls more heavily on the poor while the latter falls mostly on the wealthy (who pay more taxes), with predictable consequences in the political support for these alternatives by different groups. Research suggests that when a necessary change in policy involves two mutually exclusive options, the wealthy, even if less numerous and initially less powerful than the poor, may be able to hold out longer and obtain a result more favorable to their interests.[22] A disproportionate share of benefits, from Medicare reimbursement to subsidized medical education, goes to those in the highest income groups, who have the power to make their demands on government effective. Yet, without government intervention, the poor would surely be much worse off.

14.9 TRUST, CARE, AND DISTRIBUTION

What people want from government first and foremost is that it make them *safe*, that law and order reign rather than the four horsemen of the apocalypse. From Bismarck in 1883 to the Chinese Communist Party in 2012, providing health care to the people has been a tool for quelling dissent, of swaying the public to support the government instead of trying to tear it down or replace it. Medicine plays a special role as part of the "safety net" that protects the community, convincing people that the government cares for them. "Caring" is clearly a matter of degree. A parent loves and cares for a child; a nurse cares for a patient; a general is expected to care for the soldiers he orders into battle. Family ties are perhaps the closest and most essential, but some form of caring bond must be there for the government to exercise authority without routinely resorting to violence. When the laws are freely respected as just and fair, then transactions costs are greatly reduced. Trust in the government, unlike GDP, is not readily measurable (although open revolt is a good indicator of a deficit). Yet the trust of its people is probably the most valuable asset that any nation can have.

The start of this chapter on government noted that under the assumptions of perfect competition and *ignoring income distribution*, market competition would achieve a perfectly efficient outcome (and the corollary: that any efficient allocation of resources could be reached by markets alone *with appropriate redistribution of income*). Subsequent sections discussed a number of market imperfections that might require government action: public goods, monopoly, externalities, transactions costs, information. Distribution has not been discussed as much, other than to note in passing that real people tend to care a lot more about what they pay and what they get rather than the efficiency of the economy as a whole. Thus we have not yet addressed a giant issue that often dominates political economy and that is more influential in getting votes than economic growth or efficiency. Sometimes just pointing out that some group of "others" (immigrants, addicts, disabled vets, or children) will get more tends to make many people feel like they must be losing and creates opposition to any new policy.

Only the government can redistribute income. The market will reward whoever wins according to the rules then in place. There is no such thing as "neutral." Of course, the current distribution of income will tend to persist if the laws are not changed, but those laws are a result of a series of decisions made in the past—often under different conditions (What is "copyright" in a Google world?) or with unanticipated effects (prohibition of alcohol). The rules not only make markets possible, they also determine who the winners and losers are. In a pure monarchy, everything technically belongs to the king (although the king has to spread some around to keep the peasants and dissident nobles from revolting). The king, or the king's favorite, always seems to win the tournaments and beauty contests because the only way to earn a lot more is to gain more favor from the king. In a modern economy with markets and democratic voting, talent and looks count—but not as much as the ability to make the rules. Billions of dollars hinge on obscure portions of the tax code or patent determinations. NBA basketball can make or break stars by moving the three-point line. The courts can decide if you are a businessman or a crook. Obviously it is not just by manipulating the rules that people get ahead. However, your potential for inheriting money can go a long way in determining your attitude toward estate taxes, just as your genetic endowment can convince you whether you want to compete in an economy dominated by sword and shield, sales ability, or computer programming.

Taking care of needs to keep everyone alive and caring for those who cannot care for themselves is one definition of "civilization." A family will take care of all its members, and we tend to judge government as a kind of very extended family, creating a level playing field and caring even for the losers. Every civilized society takes care of its poor. However, exactly who belongs to "society," and how much each deserves just for being a member, can be quite contentious. Historically "citizenship" belonged only to a privileged few. Most societies no longer exclude women, minorities, fieldworkers, renters or slaves, although the extent of participation in government decisions surely varies, and it is almost always true that wealthy people have more political clout. Provision of law and order is universal, but even murder trials tend to favor the rich. Provision of other public goods can vary widely. Some countries provide health services as a public good just as they provide water and sanitation. Education and information access

(Internet, telephone, mail) may be public or mixed but are mostly private and unregulated only in poorer countries.

Every country at least pretends to provide health care to "all." In a pluralistic system where individual income affects access to medical care, an explicit mechanism to protect those least able to pay is required. It is generally accepted that no one in the United States should die because he or she cannot afford a necessary operation or medications. However, the poor cannot afford to buy insurance or medical care generally available to most members of society. Not being able to buy is what being "poor" means. All health insurance is redistributive—taking from the healthy workers who pay premiums to provide services to the sick. It is explicitly redistributive when benefits are independent of premiums, as is the case with government provision (Medicare) or subsidies (employer-provided health plans). As is discussed at more length in Chapters 17 and 18, almost any proposal for changing health insurance in the United States will have winners and losers and could thereby significantly affect the distribution of income among families.

SUGGESTIONS FOR FURTHER READING

American Journal of Public Health and *Public Health Reports*, published monthly.

U.S. Centers for Disease Control and Prevention (http://www.cdc.gov/).

Institute of Medicine, *For the Public's Health* (Washington, D.C.: National Academies Press, 2012).

Ronald Coase, "The Problem of Social Cost," *Journal of Law & Economics* 3 (1960): 1–44.

Paul Feldstein, *The Politics of Health Legislation: An Economic Perspective* (Ann Arbor, Mich.: Health Administration Press, 2006).

Theodore Marmor, *The Politics of Medicare* (Chicago: Aldine, 2000).

Douglass North, *Structure and Change in Economic History* (New York: W.W. Norton, 1981).

George Rosen, *A History of Public Health* (New York: MD Publications, 1958).

Paul Samuelson, "A Diagrammatic Exposition of a Theory of Public Expenditure," *Review of Economics and Statistics* 37, no. 4 (1955): 350–356.

Joseph Stiglitz, *Economics of the Public Sector* (New York: W. W. Norton, 2000).

SUMMARY

1. **Government accounts for 50 percent of health care spending**. Most government spending pays for private medical services of special populations (the aged, the indigent, veterans). **Only three percent goes to core public health** activities such as infectious disease control, research, and monitoring of drugs, food, air, and water.

2. Under certain conditions, a purely **competitive market allocation** of goods and services, where marginal benefits equal marginal costs enforced by the price mechanism, is most efficient. Perfect competition is rare in the real world. There are **market failures** resulting from uncertainty and information problems, transaction costs, externalities, and the existence of **public goods**. Government or another paternalistic agency must step in when an individual is incapable of making appropriate market choices owing to immaturity, substance abuse, or severe mental illness. Civilized societies modify the **distribution** of goods and services to protect the poor and disabled.

3. A **pure public good** is something that is **consumed collectively** by all. It is indivisible so that **no one can be excluded** (zero charges), and one person's consumption has no effect on another's **(zero marginal costs)**. Examples are clean air, statistics, and the discovery of penicillin. Because most benefits of government are public goods available to all without restriction, many people would be **free riders** who avoid paying unless forced to do so through **compulsory taxation**.

4. **Externalities** are said to exist when the actions of one person affect another (e.g., smoking, disposing of garbage). Infectious disease externalities have shaped public health, from the foundation of the U.S. Public Health Service as the homeless seaman's hospital to

the pasteurization of milk. The increased risk of infecting others is a cost the individual does not bear, and government intervention is required to achieve (or get closer to) an optimum level of prevention.

5. Many goods are both public and private. The degree of **publicness** of a good increases with the **number of people**, the use of **insurance**, and the **transactions, information, and measurement costs**.

6. **For the most part, government works with the market**, regulating and financing private activities. Government supersedes the market when it exerts control over prices and quantities and when it prohibits certain kinds of trades. Some critical functions, such as law and order (police and courts) and national defense (military), are produced directly by government employees. The important question is not whether government or markets are "better," but how to **balance and blend regulation and competition** to optimize social welfare and meet necessary constraints. To do this, a consensus about what constitutes a **just society** is needed.

7. Government is formed to act as the agent of the citizens to **maximize public welfare**. However, the ability of special interests to exert undue influence can lead to **regulatory capture**, where government favors the industry rather than the public. Also, the employees of a government agency can pursue **bureaucratic self-interest**, avoiding risks and controversy and increasing budgets to obtain higher salaries and more employees to ease workloads. The most realistic model of government action combines all three of these perspectives and a consideration of **transaction costs** in achieving **political interest group balance**.

8. Although decisions about private goods can be made through the market, the **indivisibility** of public goods means that **governments must make these decisions through voting**, political compromises, or cost-benefit analysis. Invariably, this means that there is a **moral or social justice** dimension as well as an economic one. Although people say that they want to do what is best for everyone, **they tend to vote for what is good for themselves**.

9. **Distribution** issues regarding "who gets" and "who pays" are usually contentious. People's attitudes toward a particular public good are always affected by their **private interests**. Universal access to high-quality medical care and redistribution of goods and services may be important public goods. Whether you think so depends a lot on whether you are poor or identify with those who are. To improve public health, it is necessary to determine exactly **who the public is**, and whether some people or **some preferences count more than others**. Conflict over who is and is not worthwhile and able to make decisions lies at the heart of some of the most contentious public health issues: abortion, substance abuse, and care of people with mental illness.

PROBLEMS

1. {*flow of funds*} What fraction of total health expenditures in the United States is paid for by government? Which government programs are the largest? Were the same, or similar, programs at the top of the list for government funding in 1900?

2. {*public goods*} Explain which item in the following pairs is more "public" and why:
    a. AIDS or lung cancer
    b. Milk or bread
    c. Saturday morning cartoons or a Sunday night late show
    d. Stroke or lung cancer

3. {*property rights, public goods*} Why is most drug research paid for by companies, whereas most medical research is paid for by the government?

4. {*externalities*} Why not charge people full price for vaccinations?

5. {*exclusivity, marginal cost*} Some forms of health care are public because the marginal cost of serving additional people is zero. Other types of health care are public, even though marginal costs are positive, because it is impossible to exclude beneficiaries who do not pay. Some forms of care meet both criteria—zero marginal costs and a lack of exclusivity. Give examples of all three categories (recognizing that no real goods or services are perfectly public or fall entirely in one category or another).

6. {*public goods*} Which has more externalities: cigars or chewing tobacco? Guns or knives? Laptop computers or mobile telephones?

7. {*transaction costs*} What is the Coase theorem? What does it imply about the extent of immunization among herds of cattle? What does it imply about the levels of immunization among schoolchildren in a classroom?

8. {*public goods*} Does the demand for public health increase or decrease as the size of a city increases?

9. {*market failure*} Which aspects of the economic organization of U.S. medical care result from market failure?

10. {*incidence*} Why is more dental care paid for privately whereas more hospital care is paid for publicly?

11. {*externalities*} What are the externalities of heroin addiction?

12. {*welfare*} Which results in lower prices: competition or regulation?

13. {*regulatory capture*} Explain how the Food and Drug Administration might be subject to regulatory capture. Who would favor, and who would be opposed to, regulations that limited regulatory capture?

14. {*regulatory capture*} Name several medical professional or trade organizations that have made large donations to political campaigns. Did they get their money's worth?

15. {*welfare*} Which type of good is apt to have a larger consumers' surplus: a public good or a private good? Why?

16. {*property rights, scale*} Why have wars often given rise to improvements in medical technology?

17. {*distribution*} Many goods are desired by some people and not by others. Because diversity of tastes is universal, why does it create more problems for public goods than for private goods?

18. {*welfare*} Why pay economists to conduct a cost–benefit analysis for a new medical technology if the market will show its value to consumers?

19. {*distribution*} In several marches on Washington, demonstrators have carried signs saying, "No Justice, No Peace." Explain what this slogan means and how it relates to the level of funding for Medicaid.

20. {*distribution, politics*} Who counts for more in political calculus:

     a. The sick or the well?
     b. The old or the young?
     c. The rich or the poor?

21. {*distribution*} Medical savings accounts (discussed in Section 5.3) tend to favor which groups of people?

ENDNOTES

1. Oliver Williamson, *Markets and Hierarchies* (New York: Free Press, 1975).
2. Douglass C. North, *Structure and Change in Economic History* (New York: Norton, 1981), 21.
3. Joseph E. Stiglitz, *Economies of the Public Sector* (New York: W.W. Norton, 1986), 77.
4. A significant exception is the Department of Defense/Veterans Administration health care system. Although national defense is a pure public good, the fact that VA/DOD health is an adjunct to defense does not necessarily make it public, and indeed large parts of the VA/DOD health care are now being privatized through subcontracting.
5. Burton Weisbrod, *The Non-Profit Economy* (Cambridge, Mass.: Harvard University Press, 1988).
6. Eleena de Lisser, "Ready or Not, Firms Rush to Sell the Public on Laser Eye Surgery," *Wall Street Journal*, August 24, 1995: A1, A8.
7. John Rawls, *A Theory of Justice* (Cambridge, Mass.: Harvard University Press, 1971).
8. Michael Anderson and Maximilian Aufflhammer, "Pound that Kill: The External Costs of Vehicle Weight," NBER working paper #17170, 2011.
9. Ronald H. Coase, "The Problem of Social Cost," *Journal of Law & Economics* 3 (1960): 1–44.
10. Bruno Latour, *The Pasteurization of France* (Cambridge, Mass: Harvard University Press, 1988).
11. John Graunt, *Natural and Political Observations on the Bills of Mortality* (London: John Martyn, Printer to the Royal Society, 1662); see Charles Creighton, *A History of Epidemics in Britain*, 2nd ed. (New York: Barnes & Noble, 1965), 532.
12. Elizabeth Fee and Steven Corey, *Garbage: The History and Politics of Trash in New York* (New York: New York Public Library, 1994).
13. George Rosen, *A History of Public Health* (New York: MD Publications, 1958), 354–360.
14. David Rosner, ed., *Hives of Sickness: Public Health and Epidemics in New York City* (New Brunswick, N.J.: Rutgers University Press, 1995).
15. Henrik Ibsen, *An Enemy of the People* (1882) in Henrik Ibsen, *The Complete Major Prose Plays*, translated by Rolf Fjelde (New York: Farrar, Strauss, Giroux, 1978), 277–388.
16. George Rosen, *A History of Public Health* (New York: MD Publications, 1958).
17. Fitzhugh Mullan, *Plagues and Politics: The Story of the United States Public Health Service* (Basic Books: New York, 1989); Odin Anderson, *Health Services as a Growth Enterprise in the U.S. Since 1875* (Ann Arbor, Mich.: Health Administration Press, 1990).
18. Douglass North, *Structure and Change in Economic History* (New York: Norton, 1981).
19. Peter J. Hammond, "Social Choice: The Science of the Impossible," in George R. Feiwel, *Arrow and the Foundations of the Theory of Economic Policy* (New York: New York University Press, 1987), 116–134.
20. Lawrence R. Jacobs, "The Politics of America's Supply State: Health Reform and Technology," *Health Affairs* 14, no. 2 (1995): 143–157. See also Lawrence D. Brown, "Who Shall Pay? Politics, Money and Health Care Reform," *Health Affairs* 13, no. 2 (1994): 175–184; and "Commissions, Clubs and Consensus: Reform in Florida," *Health Affairs* 12, no. 2 (1993): 7–26.
21. Federal Tax Spending per dollar of taxes paid by state, 2005. www.taxfoundation.org.
22. Alberto Alesina and Allan Drazen, "Why Are Stabilizations Delayed?" *American Economic Review* 81, no. 5 (1991): 1170–1188.

CHAPTER 15

HISTORY, DEMOGRAPHY, AND THE GROWTH OF MODERN MEDICINE

QUESTIONS

1. Does economic growth cause population growth?
2. Is medical care the main reason life expectancy is increasing?
3. Must a society be wealthy to invest in medical care?
4. Do economic failures cause plagues and other mortality?
5. Was Malthus right? Will populations continue to expand until food supplies are exhausted?
6. Why do families have fewer children today?
7. Does medical technology create economic growth or does economic growth create new medical technology?

15.1 ECONOMIC GROWTH HAS DETERMINED THE SHAPE OF HEALTH CARE

For a modern health care system to develop and be supported economically, four conditions must exist:

- A sufficiently low risk of death such that improving health is worthwhile
- Ample wealth to pay for advanced medical treatment
- Effective medical technology
- Financial organization through insurance and government programs to pool funds from many people

Although medical care has been provided for as long as human society has existed, these four conditions have been met only within the past hundred years and only in developed countries. Most of Africa and parts of Asia and Latin America are still characterized by high mortality, subsistence farming, and a lack of social and financial organization so that the risks of dying are high and heavily influenced by the amount of income available.[1] Economic development creates the foundation for modern medicine. As large numbers of people live longer and have more wealth, they become more willing to pay for medical care. They pool funds to finance care through insurance (Chapters 4 and 5) and to support medical research so that collectively they can obtain the technological wonders that none of them could afford individually (Chapter 14).

Food was the primary limitation on the number of people in a population and their health until perhaps 200 years ago. Only after the Industrial Revolution did medical technology become important. Yet close study indicates that changes in economic organization, from simple tribes to complex multinational corporations and global markets, have done as much to increase human health and welfare as have advances in medical technology.[2]

15.2   BIRTH RATES, DEATH RATES, AND POPULATION GROWTH

Population growth is determined by the number of births minus the number of deaths (ignoring immigration, which just transfers people between different parts of the world). Stated in percentage terms:

Natural Rate of Population Increase = Birth Rate − Death Rate

If the birth rate is 4.2 percent and the death rate is 3.9 percent, the rate of increase is 4.2 percent − 3.9 percent = 0.3 percent per year. As a first order of approximation, the death rate is 1/(life expectancy); thus a life expectancy of 25 years implies that 1/25, or 4 percent, of the population will die each year.[3] Birth and death rates fluctuated wildly through most of history, but were forced quite close to each other on average because of the uneasy equilibrium between population and food supply. If the birth rate was high for a while, there would be too many mouths to feed in the winter and starvation became more likely. If food was scarce for many years, people delayed marriage, thus reducing the birth rate. On the other hand, years of bumper crops meant people were more likely to survive and reproduce.

It is important to recognize the numerical effects of **compounding**; small differences in rates turn into large differences in size over time. If births and deaths are both 4 percent per year, the population is stable, neither growing nor shrinking. If there is a slight increase in births to 4.1 percent a year, the natural rate of increase becomes 0.1 percent and the population will double in 700 years, as it did through much of the Agricultural Age. If the birth rate rises further to 4.2 percent (i.e., a 0.2 percent net increase), the population will be four times larger in 700 years. A growth rate of 1.0 percent a year means the population will double every 70 years, a total population growth of 106,000 percent in a 700-year time span.[4]

15.3   THE STONE AGE

Time span: 5 million to 10,000 B.C.	**Economy:** Subsistence hunter-gatherer
Total population: Beginning to 4 million	**Distribution of income:** Roughly equal
Growth rate (doubles): .0007% (100,000 years)	**Medical care:** Shaman/witch doctor
Life expectancy: 28 years	**Medical $:** Not applicable

The **Stone Age** began with the emergence of the first hominids in Africa about 5 million years ago. People lived in small bands as hunter-gatherers, with a simple family/tribal social structure and little physical or intellectual capital to improve productivity. Population was limited by the amount of food in the immediate area. Life expectancy was less than 30 years, and more than half the children did not live long enough to start families, although some elders lived into their forties or fifties.[5] For millennia upon millennia, the rate of population growth was so slow as to be almost unnoticeable. It took about 100,000 years for global population to double, an annual growth rate of 0.0007 percent. At the end of the prehistoric Stone Age around 10,000 B.C. there were about 4 million people in the world, mostly in Asia, Africa, and the Near East, with some in the Americas. For Stone Age hunter-gatherers, everyone lived pretty much equally at a subsistence level. Violent death and starvation in the winter were constant threats, but during the good times, life was relatively easy. Studies of remaining hunter-gatherer tribes that rely on Stone Age "technology" in the Amazon, Philippine jungles, and Africa indicate that only three to six hours per day is required to obtain food and repair simple shelters and tools, with much of the rest of the time taken up by other pursuits. Exchange between groups was rare, so there were no organized trading systems.

Population growth during the Stone Age occurred primarily by expansion into new territory. As a tribe got too large for the local area, some family groups split off and occupied new land. Evolution and new technology (i.e., bows and arrows, flint knives) meant better exploitation of the existing food supply, not increased productivity. *Homo sapiens* displaced *Homo erectus* because the former was more efficient at hunting and killing, gathering and storing food, and building shelter. This increased efficiency did not increase the productivity of the land, and in some cases it even reduced it as large game species (mammoths, sloths) were exterminated. Each additional person required more land, and the ultimate size of the population was limited by the area under settlement. By the end of the Stone Age, those limits had already been reached in some fully populated areas. The rising population pressure in long-settled lands overfilled with people might have contributed to the development of animal husbandry and plant cultivation to feed the excess population, initiating the Agricultural Age.

15.4   THE AGRICULTURAL AGE

Time span: 10,000 B.C. to 1800 A.D.	**Economy:** Farming and harvesting
Total population: 4 million to 400 million	**Distribution of income:** Top-heavy, unequal
Growth rate (doubles): .046% (1,500 years)	**Medical care:** Empirical
Life expectancy: 24 years	**Medical $:** Perhaps 1%

Population growth accelerated with the development of agriculture, but only slowly at first. Agriculture appears to have originated around 10,000 B.C. to 7000 B.C. in the river valleys of the Tigris, the Euphrates, and the Nile, and it subsequently developed independently in China and the Peruvian highlands. People began to settle permanently in one place. Irrigation canals were dug and roads were built. The same acreage could support more permanent farmers than roaming hunter-gatherers. The productivity increases that made agriculture a stable way of life depended on countless and often incremental innovations occurring at different times and places. Furthermore, the geographic diffusion of ideas was slow, only about one kilometer a year. As late as 4000 B.C., global population was still growing at a rate of only about 0.01 percent a year (doubling in 7,000 years). Agriculture meant greater reliance on just one or a few crops so there was less diversity in foodstuffs and nutrients, reducing health. Cultivation of a single food also exposed the population of a village to catastrophic declines as drought or infestation caused crop failure. Thus, although the population grew larger, life expectancy sometimes declined.

Investment and Trade

Farming takes investment. Seed must be saved, fields plowed, and animal pens erected. A hunter might have worked at making a sharper spear or better root gatherer, but the increase in output was small compared with the gains obtained from farm improvements (building an irrigation ditch, selecting superior seed, inventing the harrow or plow). In the **Agricultural Age**, many farm investments, such as building a road or a large corral, were collective, benefiting the entire village. The returns on investment became larger when more people were involved. There is a synergy (economy of scale) in bringing people together. Whereas each person could know something about farming, a hundred could compare experiences and draw on the best ideas. Each person could make tools, but collectively, in a village of a hundred, the few people who were best at it could spend more time making tools for others and get food in return. Specialization, trade, and division of labor arose. Towns and cities were built. Trade between regions became a regular part of economic activity.

For trade and investment to occur, societies must develop property rights. To have farms, people needed to be able to stay on their land and improve it from year to year. They had to own a portion of the extra grain that was stored for times of famine or traded for tools, salt, and other necessary items. Stored grain had to be defended against the marauding bandits who showed up at harvest time. Once an agricultural society formed an army, it quickly discovered that force was useful for things other than defense. Neighboring tribes were displaced from their more productive lands or conquered and made into slaves. Leaders who successfully rallied the troops in battle gained power and, through a hierarchy of princes and priests, effectively controlled most of the wealth of society. Yet the development of governance was more than a military necessity. To grow, agricultural societies needed rulers who could accumulate and manage the excess output necessary for collective investments in irrigation, laws, and war making.

Civilization, War, and Government

With the advent of the first great civilization—the Sumerians—population began to increase rapidly. Population growth rates increased to .07 percent per year (doubling in 1,000 years), about a hundred times the hunter-gatherer growth rate. Although the Sumerian empire soon fell, the Pharoic theocracy established along the banks of the Nile in Egypt endured for centuries. Between 1000 B.C. and A.D. 1, many other large and vigorous civilizations developed. The classical Greeks rose to unprecedented heights, and Alexander conquered the world before being displaced by the Romans. In China, the Han dynasty unified 50 million people, and in the Americas the great Inca and the Olmec, Maya, and Aztec civilizations began. By A.D. 1, empires spanned continents and trade routes stretched for thousands of miles. World population exceeded 200 million and was growing about 0.12 percent per year (doubling every 600 years).

As cities grew, the population split into two classes: peasants who worked the land and continued to live at subsistence level, and rulers who controlled all the wealth. Whereas hunter-gatherers were all at the same level, working three to six hours a day to obtain subsistence plus a little extra, farmers had to work much harder, eight to 12 hours a day, to obtain the same amount of food. Why, then, did anyone become a farmer? People became farmers probably out of necessity rather than choice. When a climatic change caused a succession of bad years, or a stronger band of tribes pushed people out of favored territory, they were forced to try to get more out of what was at hand: husbanding animals rather than just hunting them, planting roots and grain rather than just picking them wild, and so on.

Many peasants were "recruited" as they were captured and placed under the domination of a warlord. Once the shift from hunting to farming occurred, farming acquired a momentum of its own and the trend became irreversible. There were too many people in the valley to go back to the old ways, and the kings did not want to give up the wealth they obtained by ruling others. Even if doubling the population of the city did not make the average person better off, it made the king and the court twice as well off.

Prosperity depended on the willingness of people to support (or at least tacitly cooperate with) the existing system and to work toward improving it. Although the king might coerce peasants into paying taxes, he had to deliver order and a stable standard of living in return or face rebellion. The taxes collected had to be directed toward appropriate public works and services to maintain progress. The rapid growth in population could only be sustained by new forms of social organization, by creating the cultural, political, and economic institutions that make up civilization. Having enough wealth left over to indulge idle priests and philosophers as they researched mathematics, astronomy, chemistry, physics, and medicine also fostered the conditions for technological advance. This process of economic development was mutually reinforcing, because growth required more government and investment and made it possible to free up resources to support them.

The Decline of Civilizations Leads to Population Declines

The amazing growth of classical civilizations was followed by almost equally sensational declines when social order decayed. There were more people in ancient Greece at its apex in 340 B.C. than at any time during the next 2,000 years, and it was not until A.D. 1850 that the population again exceeded 3 million. As the Roman Empire shrank, the total population of Europe fell from 44 million in A.D. 200 to 22 million in A.D. 600. Four hundred years later the European population had only partly recovered, to 30 million. Similar though less severe declines occurred in China and Africa. A recent example is found in the traumatic transition of the Soviet Union as communism disintegrated in 1990. The sharp drop in economic output, widespread moral and social disorder, and precipitous decline in life expectancy was catastrophic.

IMPLOSION OF THE SOVIET ECONOMY CAUSES DRAMATIC DECLINES IN LIFE EXPECTANCY

Life expectancy in Russia in 1989 was 64.2 years for males and 74.4 years for females, slightly higher than it had been 30 years previously.[6] The reconstruction *(perestroika)* of the Union of Soviet Socialist Republics (USSR) under Mikhail Gorbachev brought hope, and then disaster. The Soviet economy crumbled, the USSR fragmented, and quality of life declined. For some people on fixed incomes, hyperinflation took food prices beyond their reach, causing malnutrition. More important, the loss of jobs and hope meant despair. In such a grim situation, deaths from alcohol poisoning and accidents soared. By 1994, life expectancy had fallen 6.6 years for males (to 57.6 years) and 3.3 years for females (to 71.1 years), a decline that is virtually unprecedented in modern industrial countries. Fertility dropped below replacement level and total population declined. In 1992, births exceeded deaths by 184,000. By 1993, there were 800,000 more deaths than births.[7] For every live birth, there were 2.2 abortions. Only later were the true dimensions of this contemporary social and demographic catastrophe realized.

The Plague

As European populations began to recover robustly toward the end of the Middle Ages (A.D. 500–1500), they were hit by a new and rampantly destructive illness, the plague. Bubonic plague, or black death, swept through Europe in 1347–1352 and repeatedly thereafter, wiping out a quarter of the population.[8] Half the citizens of Genoa and Naples died as a result of the plague of 1656.[9] Although bouts of plague continued to appear until 1700, changes in immunity, social structure, the plague bacillus itself, or a combination of these, reduced the impact over time, and population growth resumed. The peoples of the New World were not as fortunate.

After contact with the Spanish conquistadors, plagues of measles and smallpox spread rapidly, with devastating effects. The native population of Aztecs dropped from 17 million in 1532 to 2 million in 1580 and fell to just 1 million by 1608. It was not just disease but also the collapse of social order that caused the permanent decline in numbers. Much of the repopulation of the Americas after 1600 came from the growth of immigrant populations from Europe and Africa.

Food Supply Determines Population

From 1500 to 1750 the European and world populations grew at an average annual rate of 0.25 percent (doubling in 300 years). Food supply was the fundamental constraint on growth because the great majority of people lived at a subsistence level. A study of the Italian district of Siena for the period 1550–1715 shows that increases in prices for grain were associated with malnutrition and death.[10] Each time the cost of food rose, the meager salaries of the residents were stretched thinner and mortality climbed. The cycle is self-correcting and self-reinforcing. As people die, there are fewer mouths to feed; therefore, demand falls and prices fall. When food is abundant and prices are low, peasants are more able to marry and have children, the number of mouths to feed rises, demand increases, prices jump, and the cycle starts over again.

As the Agricultural Age drew to a close and the transition to an urbanized modern society began, scarcity of food continued to be a major issue. Salaried workers were little better off than peasants because it took 80 percent of their salaries to get enough to eat. France in 1790 was a highly developed country with perhaps the greatest cultural and political influence in the Western world, yet most of its citizens were impoverished and undernourished. The average 30-year-old Frenchman of 1790 had to live on 2,250 calories per day, was just 5 feet 3 inches tall, and weighed only 110 pounds.[11] The bottom 10 percent of society had so little to eat that they were usually ill, and most people below the 20th percentile did not get enough food to meet the caloric energy demands of regular work. Even relatively well-off people at the 80th percentile were sufficiently stunted and wasted (height and weight below current U.S. standards) that they were at substantially higher risk of chronic health conditions and premature mortality.

The Rise of Economics

The intellectual ferment of the Renaissance (A.D. 1350–1650) and Enlightenment (A.D. 1650–1800) brought advances in government, science, and commerce (although major changes in medicine did not occur until 1900). In 1662, John Graunt published his *Natural and Political Observations on the Bills of Mortality* in London, a work now recognized as the beginning of the science of epidemiology. In 1671, Sir William Petty made the first estimate of national wealth (gross domestic product [GDP]) in his essay *Political Arithmetik* (economic statistics). As people moved from rural estates, where they had been cared for (and/or owned) by a feudal lord, into cities where they worked at jobs for wages, the economic organization of society evolved from one based on tradition to one based on money. Only after exchange became standardized through the use of money could regularities be observed and statistical analysis be performed.

The development of accounting and statistics marked the emergence of a new "information technology" that revolutionized trade. Financial markets in London and other cities traded government bonds and shares in joint stock companies, shifting tons of gold with the stroke of a pen. Factories were built, and thousands of people changed occupations and even nationalities to better their standard of living. Capital investment and labor mobility of this magnitude had been impossible during the Middle Ages because the necessary economic structure was not available or was too rudimentary. Corporations, rental contracts, taxes, ownership, and other property rights had to be refined before trade between individuals, firms, and governments could be conducted on a large scale. *The Wealth of Nations*, Adam Smith's insightful analysis published in 1776, is recognized as the start of modern economics.[12] Yet Thomas Malthus's *Essay on the Principle of Population* (1798) often has been more influential, clearly presenting the consensus of thinkers at the end of the agricultural age and frequently linked to labeling economics "the dismal science."[13]

The Malthusian Hypothesis

Malthus's hypothesis was that any increase in productivity could provide only a temporary boost to the standard of living. Over time, increases in the number of people to be fed would use up all the productivity increase, therefore people on average would be no better off than before—still living at a subsistence level. The **Malthusian hypothesis** is based on two key assumptions: (1) *food supply* is a primary constraint on population growth and (2) any increase in the number of people would inevitably lead to more crowding or to farming of less desirable land, so that the *declining marginal productivity of labor* (and hence, wages) would bring down the standard of living.

ECONOMIC MODELING

Malthusian Hypothesis: An increase in productivity will not make most people better off in the long run.

1. The total population is held in check by the food supply.
2. An external change (new land or new technology) increases food production. As (Total Food / Total Population) rises, the average welfare increases.
3. More food per person allows people to have more children (or for more of the children born to get enough to eat to live to maturity).
4. Increasing population means more workers per acre of land.
5. More workers per acre of land means that the additional output per person (marginal product) will be lower *("the law of diminishing returns")*.
6. Adding in a declining marginal product per person will make the average fall.
7. The population stabilizes with a larger number of people living at the same average "subsistence" level of welfare (food per person) as before the new land or new technology was discovered.

The Malthusian hypothesis is presented here in step-by-step detail to provide an example of what economists mean by "modeling" a process. The crucial insight (economic concept) articulated for the first time by Malthus is step 5, what is now generally known as *the law of diminishing returns*. This insight is what makes Malthus famous as a founder of economic thought.

Ireland became a natural experiment for testing the Malthusian hypothesis. The importation of a new crop from the Americas, potatoes, led to a tremendous increase in yields per acre. Using the new crop, the acreage that could support only one family in 1700 could be split up and support three families by 1800. Potato farming was so much more efficient than other types of agriculture that the peasants ate little else, consuming up to 10 pounds per day. The population of this small and already fully settled island grew 50 percent in the half century before Malthus wrote, and by another 50 percent over the next 30 years. Farms were divided into smaller and smaller parcels, and the Irish people, with a diet consisting almost entirely of potatoes, lived no better than before—there were just more of them. Then came the fungus blight that damaged the potato harvest of 1845 and destroyed the crop of 1846 entirely: 1.5 million people died and another 1.5 million people emigrated, mostly to America. Those who were left tightened their belts and stopped having children (the women born before the blight who remained in Ireland were four times as likely to remain unmarried as those who emigrated to America).[14] Out of a population of 8 million in 1840, there were only 4.5 million left by 1900, and by 1960, only 2.8 million.

The assumptions in the Malthusian hypothesis had been valid through the thousands of years that spanned the Agricultural Age and continued to apply in countries that remained essentially rural, such as Ireland. The law of diminishing returns, as elaborated by Malthus, was a major intellectual contribution to economics. However, it applies only if the technology of production stays similar in essential ways (as agriculture had up until then). In England, Germany, France, and the United States, the intellectual revolution that stirred Malthus to write his treatise led others to create a technological and commercial revolution so profound that productivity increases were continuous, and output grew much more rapidly than any natural increase in the number of people.[15] A continuous excess of food and other goods became available for all to enjoy.

15.5 THE INDUSTRIAL AGE

Time span: 1800 to 1950 A.D.	**Economy**: Manufacturing
Total population: 0.4 billion to 1.6 billion	**Distribution of income**: Mixed
Growth rate (doubles): *.65% (108 years)*	**Medical care**: Empirical
Life expectancy: 35–65 years	**Medical $**: 2% to 4%

Life was difficult at the start of the Industrial Revolution and often got worse for those who moved into cities to work in factories. Crowded slums and harsh working conditions caused disease. Whereas diets on a farm could be supplemented by gardens and occasional hunting, in the cities food was monotonous and lacking in vitamins. As the countryside became enclosed (put under ownership of a lord rather than held in common) and people moved into cities, illness increased. Life expectancy in England, about 38 years in A.D. 1600, declined throughout the next hundred years and did not regain earlier levels until about 1850.[16] Yet as the Industrial Revolution took hold, productivity increases caused the average person's standard of living to improve. There was a sharp rise in the rate of population growth to 0.43 percent for 1750–1800, almost twice the rate of the preceding three centuries, rising to 0.53 percent for 1800–1900, 0.88 percent per year for 1900–1950, and surging to 1.8 percent after 1950. World population tripled between 1750 and 1950, from about 650 million to more than 2 billion in 1950, and overall life expectancy rose by more than it had in the previous 2,000 years, going from 27 to 40 years. The rise in longevity was even more remarkable in the most-developed countries, such as Sweden, where life expectancy rose from 37 to 71.3 years.

Why Malthus Was Wrong

There are two reasons Malthus's gloomy predictions went wrong. First, technological advance, rather than being a one-shot improvement, became a continuous process. Output expanded at an exponential rate as one invention led to another. In the Agricultural Age, the primary productive inputs were land and labor. The total supply of land is fixed, and any increase in the supply of labor meant more mouths to feed. In the **Industrial Age**, capital equipment, skilled labor, and knowledge became more important than land and unskilled agricultural labor. By 1950 a single farmer, sitting in an air-conditioned cab operating a combine harvesting genetically engineered wheat, could feed more people per 100 acres than a dozen farmers could in 1750. Although the rate of productivity increase during the Agricultural Age averaged about 1 percent a year, in the Industrial Age it rapidly tripled and sometimes exceeded 5 percent a year. A second reason that Malthus's immiserating population growth failed to occur was that as death rates declined, birth rates also declined. With fewer children dying, parents chose to have fewer babies, and they invested more in the education, medical care, and nutrition of each one. Cumulatively, these individual decisions brought about a social revolution. They also changed the character of labor (more education, more skills, fewer new entrants) and accelerated technological advance, leading to higher wages and a rising standard of living.

Why did Ireland suffer a Malthusian catastrophe and lose two thirds of its population while most other European nations experienced surging growth during the Industrial Revolution? Ireland was not a self-governing nation but a colony exploited by absentee landlords from England. Profits from Irish estates were not invested in Ireland but used to build factories in England or sent overseas through joint stock companies. Irish farmers did not own their land but were tenants working the fields for the benefit of the landlord. As crop yields went up, rents were raised, keeping workers in subsistence conditions typical of the Agricultural Age. With no claim on the profits, the tenant farmer had no incentive to raise crop yields and had little ability to save and improve the lot of the family in the next generation. The only way for Irish farmers to capture any of the economic surplus created by increased agricultural productivity was to have more children, and so they did. Irish citizens wishing to leave the farm and build a better life in the city had to leave their country and go to New York. The lack of property rights for citizens and restrictive colonial economic organization were significant factors in keeping Ireland from joining the ranks of industrialized countries during the 19th century.

Malthus's predictions were never as dismal or as wrong as his critics claimed. He hoped that by clearly laying out the logical conclusions of agricultural demographics, he would encourage people to delay marriage and have fewer children. Birthrates did, in fact, decline, but for other reasons. Women gained more opportunities and spent less time on child rearing. More children survived, so fewer births were needed to make sure that one or two children in a family lived to maturity. Dependence on children in old age was replaced by reliance on savings. Children went from being a form of supplemental income (as productive family farmworkers) to a form of consumption (bringing joy but costing money). All these changes either raised the price of or reduced the demand for children. Average total fertility per mature female in England fell from 5.3 births in 1750, to 4.6 in 1850, to 1.96 in 1900. This is below the replacement rate of 2.0 and therefore national population would have decreased over time if not for the addition of foreign immigration).

Demographic Transition

The process of economic development is linked to a dramatic change in national population known as "demographic transition." When societies are in the agricultural stage, many children die before reaching adulthood. High rates of mortality (4 to 5 percent) are matched by high rates of fertility (also 4 to 5 percent), so the total number of people is stable or just slowly increasing. This equilibrium between births and deaths changes radically during the process of economic development. With greater material well-being, mortality rates decline toward 1 to 2 percent. Because birth rates are still high, the rate of population growth (births − deaths) is very rapid, 2 to 4 percent a year, enough to double the population in each generation (every 20 to 40 years). Such explosive growth does not continue indefinitely. Although constantly increasing economic output should not necessarily cause birth rates to fall, it is observed that birth rates do in fact fall in virtually every developed country. As children cease to be productive farm assets and become a costly form of family consumption, families decide to concentrate more care and investment on fewer children.[17] This decline in fertility does not necessarily

FIGURE 15.1   Demographic Transition

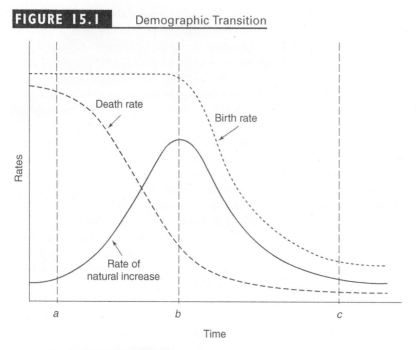

a = Beginning of the transition
b = Greatest difference between birth and death rates
c = End of the transition

require the use of modern birth control techniques. Delayed marriage, extended breastfeeding, infanticide, and other methods have been used to restrict population to desired levels in many countries without recourse to contraceptives. As economic development continues, low mortality (1–2 percent) is eventually matched by low fertility (1–2 percent) so that the total population is again stable or slowly growing, and the process of demographic transition is complete (see Figure 15.1).

Population growth spurts during the Agricultural Age occurred when settlement of new territories caused an increase in births, whereas population growth during demographic transition is caused by a decline in deaths. These two demographic patterns have different long-run consequences on the average level of individual wealth. When new territories are settled, the pioneers have much more land per person than in the country they came from and thus initially enjoy a much greater marginal productivity of labor and greater wealth. This advantage is eroded over time as more and more people are born in the new territories. Eventually, the new territories are just as crowded as the old country, the marginal productivity of labor is pushed back down to the subsistence level, and the total population, although larger, is not much better off. In contrast, the economic advances that mark demographic transition, rather than fading over time, are reinforced with each succeeding generation. Healthier adults can work longer and harder and thus accumulate more surplus for investment, while a smaller number of children means that each one receives more in the way of education, nutrition, and inheritance. These gains lead to even lower mortality, even fewer children, and so on. Each generation is better off and material advantage is concentrated among fewer offspring until the transition is complete. By then, the share of family income required to buy food has fallen from 80 percent to 20 percent. Getting enough to eat is no longer a significant factor in demographic change or labor productivity.

Demographic Change, Income Distribution, and the Rise of the Middle Classes

In a hunter-gatherer society, there are no wealthy people. The tribe as a whole is living at the subsistence level with only a little accumulated wealth in the form of weapons or religious objects. One or two bad years can spell disaster. An agricultural society, in contrast, is hierarchical and often has considerable wealth, almost all of it concentrated at the top. Most of the agricultural population consists of rural peasants. As agricultural civilizations develop, the number of traders, soldiers, craftspeople, merchants, and other members of the bourgeois who live as free "citizens" in (mostly small) cities increases, but they are always a minority. The king's authority is absolute, and almost all of the wealth stays under his control.

To industrialize, the bulk of the population has to move into cities. People who leave the land are no longer under the control of the lord, and they enter into wage-labor contracts with factories. As businesses and bureaucracies replace the feudal manor as a means of organizing production, the fruits of economic development are spread more widely. Although the wages of industrial workers are near the subsistence level at first, real earnings rise rapidly for two reasons. First, the decline in the number of births during demographic transition means fewer new workers entering the market; thus, the supply of labor grows less rapidly than demand, putting upward pressure on wages. Second, the labor market becomes specialized. Initially, the threat of starvation drove unskilled workers off the farm to take subsistence wages in the city. However, the later movement of skilled mechanics, clerks, and managers to the city was driven by the premium wages required to attract these workers. These well-paid workers and shopkeepers could afford some luxuries. They could also save for retirement, and in so doing, they could contribute to the pool of capital funds for investment and entrepreneurial ventures.

Although feudal blacksmiths took pride in their art, most of the benefits went to the lord. Master mechanics in the industrial era had a much greater incentive to improve their skills because they were paid directly and captured more value from increases in quality and productivity. They were apt to take the risk of innovating and start new businesses because they might become rich. Even when their ventures failed they could get other jobs and keep their families from starving.[18]

In the city-states and empires of the Agricultural Age, lords and kings exercised centralized bureaucratic power to raise taxes, build roads, and support armies. Building factories and inventing new technologies in the industrial era required decentralized entrepreneurs who acted as managers on their own behalf rather than on behalf of the king. Working independently or in small groups, entrepreneurs convinced investors to put up capital and attracted skilled labor with high wages. By the end of the Industrial Age, even people of modest means could go to school, start a business, and save for retirement. A startling change in the distribution of income and wealth had occurred as the bulk of the money was now held by the large and growing middle class of laborers, tradespeople, and small-business owners. In 1750 the market for art, education, travel, housing, and almost everything except food was concentrated in the upper 4 percent of families who were truly wealthy. By 1950, the market for such goods in the United States, England, Germany, and other developed countries was dominated by the middle class. The wealthy bought luxury in a few shops, while the millions shopped in department stores (see Figure 15.2).[19]

FIGURE 15.2	Distribution of Income at Different Stages of Development			
Upper classes		$$$$$	$$	$$$$$$$$
Middle class	$	$$	$$$$$$	$$$$$$$$$$
Lower classes	$$$$	$	$$$	$$$$$$$
	Hunter-Gatherer	Agricultural	Industrial	Informational

The hierarchies that dominated the Agricultural Age were broken up by tremendous increases in economic mobility and a general improvement in wages. The crowd at the bottom was replaced by a bulging middle class of people who actively participated in a monetary economy. This shift in social and economic structure, rather than the discovery of new technology *per se*, was the driving force that powered growth of the Industrial Revolution. Many countries today remain poor and rural, struggling to make the demographic and economic transition to development. It is not because they lack technology (which can be found in many textbooks, ordered from catalogs, or shared in commercial joint ventures) but because they lack the property rights, social order, and administrative structure to create a context in which technology can be applied productively.[20] The deficit that allows starvation to remain a threat to people's health is not a lack of knowledge, machinery, or money for investment, it is a lack of organization.

15.6   THE INFORMATION AGE

Time span: 1950 to future
Total population: 1.6 billion to 20 billion?
Growth rate (doubles): 1.88% (40 years)
   but slowing (perhaps toward 0%)
Life expectancy: 70+ years

Economy: Services
Distribution of income: Not yet clear
Medical care: Scientific

Medical $: 6% to 16%+

The advent of a postindustrial **Information Age** is marked by the ubiquitous appearance of the television and the computer. The economy is global, linked by communications networks where massive amounts of capital flow between countries with a few keystrokes. Labor is concentrated in services rather than agriculture or manufacturing. Information specialists, the dominant workers, spend their entire childhood and many years of adulthood in school investing in skills. Such training can be prevalent only in a population with long life expectancies and few children per family. In this era, most people are healthy and wealthy enough that personal income affects longevity and fertility primarily through lifestyle choices, rather than lack of food or shelter. What was rare throughout history, the ability to retire with independent means and sufficient fitness to travel the world after age 65, has become not just attainable but an ordinary reality for most people in postindustrial economies.

U.S. life expectancy was about 35 years in 1750 and 49 years in 1900, and it rose to 68 years by 1950 and 78 years in 2008. Although people will continue to live longer, incremental years of life expectancy are added at a slower rate as infectious diseases and childhood maladies are removed as major causes of death. More important from a demographic point of view is that almost all the gains in longevity after 1950 occurred for mature adults who had already completed their families. Each generation might live longer but will not have more babies. Additional increases in life expectancy will not increase the number of children and thus will have little effect on the long-run total size of the population.

During the demographic transition of the Industrial Age and its final phase, the 1950s baby boom, rapid population increase created expansive economic growth as more houses, roads, and factories were built. However, expansion due to demographic transition is a one-time occurrence. After transition, population returns to a steady state of slow or zero growth, typically a small natural decrease offset by immigration of people from less developed countries seeking higher wages. It is important to recognize that the "normal" conditions of industrializing countries from 1770 to 1970 were actually abnormal periods of spectacular but transitory growth. In comparison, the 1 to 2 percent growth rates of recent decades can seem inadequate, particularly because most of the added value comes in the less visible form of service improvement and information content (HD television, the Internet, cheap mobile phones, and travel), rather than in the number of countable goods (cars, houses, tons of corn) that are more readily measured in GDP accounts.

Much of the world is still undeveloped, caught somewhere between an agricultural society and the modern information era. A world map shaded to show which nations today still have economies dominated by agriculture is almost identical to a world map showing which nations have the most premature mortality under age 30 years.[21] Such nations have the potential for fantastic growth as they industrialize (e.g., Korea, Singapore, Indonesia) but also for tragic population explosions without economic advancement, leading to starvation and social ruin (e.g., Somalia, Rwanda). In a developing country, such as Indonesia, the average age of the population is about 17 years, longevity is less than 70 years, many people still work on farms, and a sizable fraction still live at the subsistence level. Such countries have a tremendous "population momentum." Even if every family immediately limited fertility to the replacement level of 2.2 births, the total population would still double in size because so many young women have already been born. In the United States, as in most developed countries, the natural population growth is already zero to negative; thus, the increase in population is due to immigration from less developed countries. If current trends continue, almost every country in the world will be developed within a hundred years and have a steady or shrinking population.[22] Total world population will stabilize somewhere between 10 to 20 billion, Mexico City will be much larger than Los Angeles, and food supply will be a trivial health problem compared to pollution and congestion (see Table 15.1).

15.7   INCOME AND HEALTH

The connection between poverty and poor health was noted long ago. The connection is described in ancient Greek and Chinese commentaries, and detailed empirical studies were conducted in London and Paris in the 19th century.[23] As economic historians carefully review the data, it becomes clear that although economic growth might have been the major contributor in lengthening life expectancy, its effects were neither uniform across groups nor steady over time. Average health appears to have declined significantly in the United States during the early decades of the 19th century despite rising per capita incomes; therefore, life expectancy was probably not much greater in 1900 than it was in 1800.[24]

Most commentators assume that extreme poverty has the most deleterious effects and that the relationship between income and health is nonlinear, with gains in life expectancy becoming smaller as one moves up the income scale (see Figure 16.4). However, the famous "Black Report" on civil service employees in the United Kingdom established that even among high-income people, mortality was lower for those at the very top. In addition, the report established that although the absolute effect got smaller over time as general life expectancy increased, the relative importance of rank did not disappear and perhaps even widened between 1930 and 1981 (Table 15.2).[25] This finding is often viewed as indicating that health insurance alone cannot remove the effects of poverty on health because this period includes the formation of the National Health Service in the United Kingdom, which provides essentially free medical care for all citizens. Studies of U.S. populations show a similar gradient, with smaller but still significant income effects even at very high income levels.[26]

The relationship between income and health is strong, but the nature of that relationship is far from clear. Getting sick makes people earn less, thus observing that "sicker people are poorer on average" does not establish whether the lack of income led to poor health, or bad health led to less income.[27] It seems as if income can affect health more than vice versa for young people, but not for older people, for whom bad health is more likely to be responsible for a loss of income. The Social Security "notch" (workers who happened to be born one day earlier in 1918 than the rest received higher retirement incomes) provided a natural experiment, indicating

TABLE 15.1   Timeline: Economic History, Population Growth, and Medical Care

	Stone Age		Agricultural Age				Industrial Age			Information Age	
	5 million–10,000 B.C.	4000 B.C.	1 A.D.	250	1200 A.D.	1800 A.D.	1900	1950	1975	2000	????
World population	Beginnings to 4 million	8	250		400 million	950	1.6 billion	2.5 billion	4 billion	6 billion	Stops @ 20 billion
Rate of growth	*.0007%*	*.01%*	*.09%*		*.04%*	*.14%*	*.52%*	*.88%*	*1.88%*	*.20%*	
(years to double)	*(100,000)*	*(7,000)*	*(800)*		*Varies*	*(500)*	*(130)*	*(80)*	*(40)*	*(Slowing)*	
Life expectancy	28 years		24 years				40 years			80 years	
Organization	Family/tribe		Fief/city/empire				National states			Global village?	
Information	Oral		Written				Statistics			Electronic	
Economy	Hunter-gatherer		Farming & harvesting				Manufacturing			Services	
Incomes	Subsistence		Rich rulers/subsistence serfs				Wages			Wages & entitlements	
Equivalent $ per capita	$200		$300				$300 rising to $5,000			$35,000 (developed countries)	
% Spent on food	All		Almost all—90%				80% falling to 30%			12%	
Income distribution	Roughly equal		Highly unequal				Mixed			Not yet clear	
Type of medicine	Witch doctor/shaman		Healer priest				Empiricist			Scientifically trained physicians	
Medical spending	—		? maybe 1%				2% rising to 4%		6%	10%	?

TABLE 15.2	Mortality Ratios by Social Class 1931–1981				
Class	**1931**	**1951**	**1961**	**1971**	**1981**
I Professionals	90	86	76	77	66
II Managerial	94	92	81	81	76
III Skilled manual	97	101	100	104	103
IV Semi-skilled	102	104	103	114	116
V Unskilled	111	118	143	137	166

Source: The Black Report (note 25). Standardized Mortality Ratios, Men 15–64, England and Wales, age-adjusted: 100 = average mortality rate for that year.

that just giving people bigger checks did not make them live longer.[28] It is not income per se that makes people healthy but all the things associated with higher income: more education, better nutrition, social connections, family stability, and so on. For children, it appears that the things that tend to go along with income (better environment, better education, better-educated mothers) may be more important than money per se.

15.8 REDUCING UNCERTAINTY: THE VALUE OF LIFE AND ECONOMIC SECURITY

Economic development not only meant that most people had more, it also meant that the risks of losing it all were vastly reduced. For the first time it was both possible and reasonable for ordinary people to plan for the future, to decide how many children to have, whether or not to go to school or start a business, and to save for retirement. The improvements in health and income brought about by economic development had a powerful and paradoxical effect: The more secure the future became, the more afraid workers became of losing that security.

The Value of Risk Reduction

Even if medical care is responsible for only a small incremental improvement in health, the value of that increment is increasing as workers become healthier and wealthier. Consider how the value of reducing the risk of dying in the next 10 years by 1 percent changes as workers gain greater life expectancy. If the average person has a 50–50 chance of dying in 10 years, it is not worth much to change the probability to 51–49. Yet if a healthy person has only a 1 percent chance of dying, eliminating this risk, or just cutting it in half, is worth a lot.[29]

The value of risk reduction also depends on the level of income. In a subsistence economy where workers get paid only enough to buy food and rudimentary housing, they cannot afford to give up much of what they earn to buy medical care, even if such care would help them avoid future illness and death. On the other hand, a skilled industrial worker earning $65,000 a year can probably afford to pay $300 a month for health insurance and another $100 for vitamin supplements and a health-club membership. A rock star or corporate CEO earning $5 million a year can afford to spend hundreds of thousands of dollars just to keep looking young.

By reviewing a number of studies conducted during the 20th century, Dora Costa and Matthew Kahn constructed estimates of the value of life (reducing mortality risk) for workers. Valuation increased by 30-fold, from $427,000 to $12,000,000 in inflation-adjusted dollars, during the last 100 years (Table 15.3).[30] The value of life tends to increase more than proportionately as income rises, because life itself is necessary to enjoy the benefits of having goods. Costa and Kahn estimated that the income elasticity of the value of life is about 1.6 (i.e., a 160 percent increase in value for every 100 percent increase in income), indicating that life itself is a "luxury good" in economists' terms (see Section 13.2).

TABLE 15.3	Changes in the Estimated Value of Life, 1900–2000

Year	Value of Life (2002 dollars)
1900	$427,000
1920	895,000
1940	1,377,000
1950	2,426,000
1960	2,884,000
1970	5,176,000
1980	7,393,000
2000	12,053,000

Source: Dora L. Costa and Matthew E. Kahn, "Changes in the Value of Life, 1940–1980," *Journal of Risk and Uncertainty* 29, no. 2 (2004): 149–180.

It is not just the increase in the length of life expectancy that is valuable; a reduction in the variance is also important. Most people would rather be faced with a life that might vary from 73 to 83 years in length than a life that is equally long on average but varied from 53 to 103. Knowing approximately when one will die could alleviate substantial existential anxiety and would be incredibly helpful for pension and estate planning. A study estimated that for the current U.S. population with a life expectancy of 78 (SD, 15) years, a reduction in that standard deviation by two years (i.e., to 13 years) is worth almost as much as a one-year increase in average life expectancy.[31]

Social Security and Health Insurance

Whereas the poor agricultural masses might have been happy to get a chance to stay alive and perhaps get ahead, the industrial middle class expected progress. If their lives did not constantly improve, or if something went wrong, they expected their employers or the government to do something to correct the problem. Originally, coal miners went underground to work to get higher wages. They began to demand safe working conditions, compensation for accidents and disability, and retirement plans. As early as 1700, a few English industrialists offered health insurance to their workers. Such employee benefits made the workers loyal to these firms and willing to work harder. The risks of disability and sickness were no longer borne by the workers individually, but by the firm. This sharing of risk reduced the uncertainty and variability of wages to workers (Chapters 4 and 5).

Industrialization and the change to wage labor shifted the distribution of political power. Workers' revolts spread across Europe during the 19th century, stretching from Paris in 1789 to Russia in 1917. Economic, legal, and health security were fundamental demands of what became known as "socialism." In 1883, to forestall further labor unrest, Chancellor Bismarck created the first national social security system in Germany, providing pensions to workers older than 65 years, sick leave, and health insurance.[32] In the United States, private insurance provided by employers became the dominant mode of health care financing in the 1950s. These plans have been supplemented by the government Medicaid program for the poor and Medicare for the elderly. Today 89 percent of all health care spending and 97 percent of hospital costs are paid for through third-party financing mechanisms. In 1850, medical care was still largely a personal transaction. Workers paid, or did not pay, for what they thought they could afford, the way they bought clothes, food, or heating oil. This continues to be the case in less-developed countries where most medicine is still individually purchased. However, all of the developed countries now use pooled financing through government and private insurance to pay for most medical expenditures. The shape of the health care system is determined by negotiations over benefit packages and government appropriations, not consumers' personal purchasing decisions.

15.9   THE RISE OF MODERN MEDICINE

Medicine is as old as humankind. One of the earliest-known written documents, the "Code of Hammurabi," contains references to medical price controls and malpractice in the laws of this Assyrian kingdom circa 2200 B.C. The Hippocratic Oath, written down around 400 B.C. and still quoted in medical writings today, put forth the principle that physicians should "first, do no harm." This was good advice, because for thousands of years physicians could do little to cure illness or reduce the risk of death. Despite the vast amount written about medicine, and the great store of practical knowledge transmitted orally in many cultures, this knowledge was largely unsystematic and did not create therapies that made a significant impact on the health of most people.[33] Medical theory, such as it was, usually consisted of a strange mixture of mysticism, and some sound advice about eating, sleeping, and getting fresh air, combined with serious looks and kind words. Each physician had a few favorite remedies, some of which might sometimes be useful. Hospitals were places where sick or disabled people were housed, and little was expected in the way of treatment. Physicians were counselors who could make someone feel better and preside over the deaths they prognosticated, but they could do little to change the course of illness. Many were also priests, and the distinction between morality and medicine was often unclear. Plagues were more likely to be blamed on infidelity or blasphemy than on unseen organisms in the blood.

Preconditions for Change

This chapter began with a list of four preconditions for the development of modern medical care: low risk of death, sufficient wealth, effective technology, and insurance financing. These factors are not independent of one another but mutually reinforcing. Increasing wealth meant more food, which reduced the risk of dying. Increased longevity also meant greater productivity and hence even more wealth. As trade developed, financial markets increased in complexity and insurance contracts were needed to better manage capital. Broad participation in pooled financing could only occur when most workers were relatively healthy and well-off. The development of medical technology was the result of an interactive process, requiring advances in biology, chemistry, physics, statistics, and data management. Gaining knowledge and reducing the uncertainty caused by illness takes both science and economics. It is now quite reasonable to say that the most commonly used medical instrument is the computer.

The Growth of Medical Science and Technology

The change from mysticism and fear to scientific investigation was the defining characteristic of the Enlightenment. Some milestones include the demonstration of proteins in urine by Paracelsus in 1500, the discovery of the microscope and "little worms" (bacteria and protozoans) by Athanasius Kircher in 1569, William Harvey's discovery of the circulation of blood in 1619, and Anton von Leewenhoek's microscopic description of red blood cells in 1668. The growing accumulation of knowledge presaged a form of medical practice that eventually would be able to provide effective treatment against disease. The crucial link, however, was organizational rather than technical—more a matter of changing the way knowledge was collected, used, and transmitted than any particular scientific breakthrough or discovery.

The formation of "clinics" in the great hospitals of Paris around 1750 is particularly noteworthy.[34] These clinics were organized by what would now be called specialties: one for the eye, another for the hand, another for mental illness, and so on. Instead of trying to create a holistic theory that covered all aspects of health, the clinics broke medical problems into component parts. A single doctor would become an expert in diseases of the hand, or the eye, and so on, and then train others. The clinic provided the working classes with access to trained physicians whom they otherwise could not afford. The physician was provided with a large group of compliant patients all suffering similar illness so that he could experiment with new therapies, teach students, and perfect his techniques. Practicing on the masses of poor workers allowed him to charge higher fees to wealthy patients and to collect tuition from students eager to learn the latest advances. The creation of clinics was a success because they provided a social exchange mechanism that yielded gains to both parties.

Organizational innovation was complemented by an intellectual innovation: statistics. Clinic doctors began to count how many people were treated and how many got well. Numerical comparisons of outcomes began to replace doctors' personal assessments. Instead of evaluating quality of care by the reputation and experience of the physicians who vouched for it, now clinical experiments and statistical observation were used. The impact of this new approach to medical science is well illustrated by Edward Jenner's discovery of vaccination for smallpox in 1798. The act of making a healthy person sick (inoculating them with cowpox) to prevent possible future illness is a form of therapy that can only be defended statistically. No single patient feels better or gets cured because of what the doctor does.

Scientific advances accumulated rapidly throughout the latter part of the 19th century; Pasteur, Semmelweiss, and Koch determined that bacteria cause anthrax, childbirth fever, tuber-culosis, and other infectious diseases; Eijkman discovered vitamins; and Roentgen discovered x-rays. Whereas France was preeminent in the 18th century, Germany was arguably the world leader in medical technology by the end of the 19th century when Chancellor Bismarck provided the landmark social insurance legislation. American physicians tried to improve the quality of practice in the United States with the Flexner Report of 1910, promoting the "Johns Hopkins model" (actually the German model, but Americans needed a local champion to make it more acceptable). By the end of the 1930s, a modern scientific education and a license were required to enter the practice of medicine, and most doctors treated their difficult cases in the hospital using a range of technical devices and nursing support (Chapter 7), and by 1950 America had clearly become the world's leader in advancing medical technology.

Information systems and access to capital gave hospitals economies of scale and made them necessary institutional structures for medical practice. As modern surgical techniques using anesthesia and antiseptics turned what were formerly warehouses for the sick into technolog-ically sophisticated treatment facilities, written medical records became the locus for storage and communication of test results, diagnostic information, and treatment documentation that linked all the trained medical practitioners together. Florence Nightingale, through her work in military hospitals during the Crimean War and subsequent books, is most often credited with developing the hospital as an organization. Her patients might have seen nurses as "angels of mercy," but she saw them as soldiers gathering intelligence and carrying out orders as part of a grand campaign against disease. As technology became more advanced and specialized, it cost more—too much for individual physicians to purchase on their own. In 1816, Laennec invented the stethoscope to investigate the body, and every doctor bought one. In 1885, Roentgen's x-ray machines peered inside the body, but the equipment was so large and so expensive that most doctors had to join the staff of a hospital to use one. The computed axial tomography (CAT) scan developed in 1973 costs millions of dollars, depends on software that few radiologists understand, and can transmit images through the Internet to be digitally enhanced and read by a specialist thousands of miles away in another country.

Although medicine has been actively practiced since ancient times, only fragmentary tech-nological advances were made until the end of the industrial era. In the 18th and 19th centuries, scientific discoveries came more and more rapidly, yet there was still little improvement in treatment outcomes. **Only after 1900 did effective medicine start** to become widely available, 150 years after the productive expansion that marked the beginning of the Industrial Age. Between 1900 and 1950, a virtual revolution took place, and medicine became one of society's most valued occupations.

Medical progress resulted more from planned effort and massive public investment than serendipitous discovery or any preordained march of ideas: Florence Nightingale's scientific hospital was supported by kings who wished to cut the cost of putting soldiers into battle, Pasteur's discovery of bacteria was made under contract to the French wine and beer industry, and Walter Reed worked to conquer yellow fever so that construction of the Panama Canal could be completed in tropical jungles. Rising incomes, falling mortality, and commercial organization were more than just contributing factors; they were the central forces driving the demand that created medical technology.

Although all four conditions needed for the development of modern medicine (low mortality, wealth, technology, organized financing) operate concurrently and reinforce one another, medical technology is more a result of the process than a cause. Society's accumulation of the necessary prerequisites for modern medicine began with the rise in wealth brought about by trade and technology, which quickly led to a decline in mortality and subsequently to a decline in the birth rate. The application of science and industrial technology to medicine not only took time, it also took money and an independent profession dedicated to continuous improvement. Both organized medicine, with its schools and professional associations, and organized financing, with insurance risk pooling and government funding, were necessary to carry out that research and pay for years of trial and error as treatments were perfected. The development of integrated health care systems and decentralized contracting will bring medicine to the final stages of the Industrial Revolution's productivity enhancements, and will evolve in new directions to meet the challenges of the Information Age.[35]

Did Better Medical Care Increase Life Expectancy?

It seems obvious that providing more and better medical care improves life expectancy, but it is actually quite difficult to show conclusively that this is the case. Given the strong relationship between mortality and income, questions have arisen regarding the relative importance of medical care by itself. After all, the catastrophic decline in Russian life expectancy in 1989–1994 was not caused by any loss of medical technology or reduction in the number of hospitals. More and better medical care is usually associated with higher incomes and better public health, making the independent effect of medicine harder to disentangle.

It is clear that life expectancy has risen steadily over the last 150 years. The causes are not so clear or so steady, making it likely that the truth is complex, with different factors being more or less important at different times and places. Nutrition, housing, and other income-related factors were probably most important during the 18th and early 19th centuries. With the subsequent advance of science and the Sanitary Revolution, public health became a major factor, and one study estimates that one half of the gains in life expectancy during this period can be attributed to improvements in water supply alone.[36]

Prior to 1910, it is unlikely that medical care had much effect on life expectancy because it was so ineffective. In a famous study, Samuel Preston showed that around the turn of the century the mortality rate for the children of doctors was no different from that for children of factory workers because both died in great numbers due to untreatable infections.[37] Medical care became increasingly efficacious during the 20th century as the extensive availability of inexpensive fresh food, clean water, and advanced waste treatment meant that the major gains from income (nutrition) and public health had already been made (i.e., the law of diminishing returns was setting in with regard to these factors).[38] Since 1960, much of the +8-year gain in life expectancy has been due to reduced cardiac mortality, with perhaps two thirds of that attributable to better medical care and one third attributable to lifestyle changes (primarily decreased smoking).[39]

The gains from medical *science* are much larger than the gains from *care* because advances in knowledge improve nutrition and public health as well as medical therapy. Indeed, these boundaries can become blurred when vitamin deficiency diseases are treated by dietary supplements, fluoride in the water reduces dental caries, and infectious diseases get made less threatening with vaccination. What was once advanced treatment can become routine (treating ulcers with Zantac bought at Walmart, taking an aspirin every day to reduce heart attacks and strokes). In the future, a healthy lifestyle might mean using genetically engineered personal foods to replace prescription medication. The importance of knowledge as the underlying driver of increased life expectancy is demonstrated by the mortality trends in Africa during the 1970s and 1980s. There, despite disastrous decades in which dysfunctional governments and economies led to declining per capita income and closed many medical clinics, life expectancy continued to rise. However, note also that the HIV/AIDS plague of the 1990s caused heavy losses in Africa that are only now being reversed.

SUGGESTIONS FOR FURTHER READING

David M. Cutler, *Your Money or Your Life* (Oxford, UK: Oxford University Press, 2004).

David Cutler, Angus Deaton, and Adriana Lleras-Muney, "The Determinants of Mortality," *Journal of Economic Perspectives* 20, no. 3 (2006): 97–120.

Angus Deaton, "Health, Inequality and Economic Development," *Journal of Economic Literature* 41, no. 1 (2003): 113–158.

Robert G. Evans, Morris Barer, and Theodore Marmor, *Why Are Some People Healthy and Others Not? The Determinants of Health of Populations* (New York: Aldine De Gruyter, 1994).

Robert W. Fogel, "Economic Growth, Population Theory and Physiology: The Bearing of Long-Term Processes on the Marking of Economic Policy," *American Economic Review* 84, no. 3 (1994): 369–395.

Robert W. Fogel, *The Escape From Hunger and Premature Death, 1700–2100* (Cambridge, UK: Cambridge University Press, 2004).

Massimo Livi-Bacci, *A Concise History of World Population* (Cambridge, Mass.: Wiley-Blackwell, 2012).

Angus Maddison, *The World Economy: A Millennial Perspective* (Paris and Washington, D.C.: Organization for Economic Cooperation and Development, 2001). See also www.ggdc.net/maddison/madidison-project/

Douglass C. North, *Structure and Change in Economic History* (New York: Norton, 1981).

Mancur Olson, Jr., "Big Bills Left on the Sidewalk: Why Some Nations are Rich, and Others Poor," *Journal of Economic Perspectives* 10, no. 2 (1996): 3–24.

Roy Porter, *The Greatest Benefit of Mankind* (New York: Harper-Collins, 1998).

James P. Smith, "Healthy Bodies and Thick Wallets: The Dual Relation Between Health and Economic Status," *Journal of Economic Perspectives* 13, no. 2 (1999): 145–166.

Rodrigo R. Soares, "Mortality Reductions, Educational Attainment and Fertility Choice," *American Economics Review* 95, no. 3 (2005): 580–602.

SUMMARY

1.   Four conditions must be met for modern medicine to develop:

    a.   The risk of dying must be low enough (i.e., **life expectancy** long enough) that spending money to improve health is worthwhile.

    b.   People must have **sufficient income** to pay for medical care.

    c.   There must be a way to pool funds and **organize financing** for large numbers of people through insurance or government programs.

    d.   **Medical technology** must be effective enough at improving health to be worth paying for.

2.   **Life expectancy** averaged about 28 years from 10,000 B.C. to A.D. 1, and populations grew slowly, taking 100,000 years to double. From A.D.1 to 1750, life expectancy averaged 22 to 28 years, and population doubled every 1,000 years. From 1750 to 1900, life expectancy averaged 30 to 45 years, and population doubled every 200 years. Today, life expectancy in the United States is more than 70 years, and the number of births is almost identical

to the number of deaths, making the total population stable. In some less-developed countries, life expectancy is still less than 50 years, and population growth is still very rapid, doubling every 30 years.

3. **Demographic transition** involves the movement of the population into cities, a rise in output per capita and a decline in mortality rates followed by a decline in birth rates, all of which leads to the stable and well-off populations characteristic of developed countries.

4. **Development** has always had adverse effects such as crowding and pollution that may cause temporary declines in living standards, although improvements in nutrition, security, and technology eventually make the overall effect of economic development strongly positive.

5. The dismal hypothesis of **Thomas Malthus** was that any increase in productivity would bring an uncontrolled increase in population, eventually making people no better off than before as the number of mouths to feed expanded to match the increased food supply. Although Malthus's analysis provided insight into forces that had previously governed population growth, he did not foresee the rapid and continuous rise in productivity due to the Industrial Revolution, nor did he understand how the newly emerging middle-class families would choose to have fewer children so that they could invest more in their care and education.

6. In the hunter-gatherer economy of the prehistoric Stone Age, no one had much more than basic necessities. In the Agricultural Age, most people lived at a subsistence level, but the rulers controlled vast wealth and made major investments. In the Industrial Age, workers' wages rose rapidly above the subsistence level, economic organization became more complex, and most income was held by a large **middle class**.

7. A 1 percent reduction in mortality is worth more to people with a 70-year life expectancy than to people with a life expectancy of only 25 years. With good salaries and savings, people can afford to pay more to protect their health than could their grandparents, who barely earned enough to eat.

8. The **reduction in uncertainty** brought about by lower mortality and better jobs made it possible for ordinary people to plan for the future. Having a taste of freedom from fear and loss, they wanted more. In time, the demand for insurance and social security became universal.

9. The development of **medical technology** came after the industrial revolution was already well advanced. Improvements in the productivity of medicine (the ability to actually heal and extend life expectancy) began about 150 years after technological change had begun to raise industrial productivity. Although scientific advances are to some extent accidental, **the rate of technological change in medicine is largely determined by the economic resources** devoted to making new discoveries and applying them in practice.

10. The **economic organization** of medical care is rapidly evolving. From prehistoric times until 1900, most care was given by doctors practicing alone as independent practitioners. By 1950, the hospital and an organized medical staff funded through third-party payment were common. By 2030, most care probably will be provided by integrated health care systems with thousands of employees. **The most important medical advances are being brought about by improvements in information technology**, not pills and scalpels.

11. The astounding improvements in health that have more than **doubled life expectancy** over the last 200 years are attributable first to **better nutrition due to rising GDP**, second to improvements in **public health**, particularly water supply and sanitation, and third to better **medical technology**, especially for reducing cardiac mortality, the leading cause of death, over the last 50 years.

PROBLEMS

1. {*life expectancy*} What is the current average life expectancy? What was life expectancy 100 years ago? One thousand years ago? Ten thousand years ago? Is life expectancy likely to increase more rapidly or less rapidly during the next 100 years?

2. {*population growth*} How rapidly is the population growing in the United States? Is population growing more rapidly or less rapidly elsewhere in the world? Was it growing more rapidly or less rapidly 100 years ago? One thousand years ago?

3. {*population growth, dynamics*} What were the causes of the baby boom? How long did it last? How long will it affect the U.S. economy? Which part of the health care system was (is, will be) most affected?

4. {*population growth*} If the birth rate is 5 percent and the death rate is 3.5 percent, what is the rate of population increase? That death rate is consistent with a life expectancy of approximately how many years? The birth rate is consistent with approximately what family size? (Hint: Family size = number of children per year times number of fertile female years.)

5. {*population growth*} How long will it take the population to double if it is growing 1 percent a year? If it is growing 0.1 percent a year?

6. {*distribution*} Is the distribution of income per capita more equal or less equal now than in the past? Is the distribution of life expectancy more equal or less equal now than in the past?

7. {*life expectancy*} Which has been more influential in raising life expectancy: economic growth or the development of medical technology? What evidence would support your answer? What evidence would contradict your answer? What evidence would support either answer?

8. {*population growth*} What is the Malthusian hypothesis? How did Malthus link population growth to declining marginal productivity?

9. {*population growth*} What are the most common reasons for population declines in the world today? Give examples.

10. {*family dynamics*} Will a family with higher income have more or fewer children? Which other economic factors affect choice of family size?

11. {*demographic transition*} Why do birth rates fall during demographic transition? How can population growth be accelerating if birth rates are declining?

12. {*demographic transition*} Why might death rates rise at the end of demographic transition? Can you give an example of a country where death rates might be rising now for this reason? Would such a situation imply more or less growth in per capita income? Why?

13. {*flow of funds*} Why is the development of a middle class a precondition for the development of medical insurance? Why is insurance necessary for the development of a modern, high-technology medical care system?

14. {*risk*} Does an increase in uncertainty, especially life-threatening uncertainties such as famine and plague, make medical care more or less valuable?

15. {*dynamics*} Did the productivity of medical technology start to increase before or after improvements in the productivity of industrial technology? Why? What determines the rate of technological change in medicine?

16. {*productivity*} Assume that you are writing a science-fiction book that takes place in the year 2050. Which would be more devastating to the health of the world: loss of the drugs that cure HIV/AIDS or loss of computers?

17. {*statistics, productivity*} In which field was the application of statistics necessary to improve productivity: industry, agriculture, or medical care?

18. {*productivity*} Which has grown more rapidly: the productivity of farmers or the productivity of doctors?

19. {*health production*} If the cities were the growing centers of economic opportunity, why did many of the people that moved to the city during the Industrial Revolution experience shorter average life spans than those who remained in the country?

20. {*industrial organization, dynamics*} Was it economic organization, social organization, political organization, medical organization, or technology that led to the creation of a national medical insurance plan in Germany in 1883?

21. {*distribution*} Does health insurance make income distribution more equal or less equal? Who is favored by such redistribution? Will the Affordable Care Act of 2010 affect distribution in the United States? Which groups are most likely to benefit from the Obama plan? Which groups of people would be most likely to gain or lose from the plan by Congressman Paul Ryan and the Republican Budget Committee to replace current Medicare with premium support (vouchers)?

22. {*distribution*} What is the difference between income and wealth? Which has grown more rapidly in the United States?

23. {*social insurance*} What is the difference between "social security" and "insurance"?

24. {*pricing, productivity, risk*} To whom will a drug that provides a 1 percent increase in 10-year survival be most valuable? List factors that might expand or reduce the impact of a 1 percent survival effect of on the market value of the drug.

ENDNOTES

1. *Mortality* is the death rate—the number of deaths per 100 (or 1,000 or 100,000) persons alive at the beginning of the period. *Morbidity* is the incidence of illness or ill health—the number of cases per 100 (or 1,000 or 100,000) persons. Although clearly related to mortality, morbidity should also be clearly distinguished from mortality rates. Although it is possible to obtain mortality rates from a variety of sources throughout history and so to create a reliable record, morbidity rates were available only under special circumstances (e.g., epidemics, aboard ships, or in school or prison populations) until the advent of routine health surveys in the 20th century, and they are still lacking in many low-income countries with less comprehensive government statistical capabilities.

2. Douglass C. North, *Structure and Change in Economic History* (New York: Norton, 1981).

3. Note that this relationship, death rate = 1/(life expectancy), is a stock/flow equation analogous to the relationship between interest rates and the value of an annuity, interest = coupon/(price of bond), presented in finance texts, and it is also rather similar to the stock/flow relationship between medical graduates and physician supply discussed in Section 7.3.

4. A rule of thumb for compounding is known as the "rule of 72." If you divide 72 by the interest rate, it gives the approximate length of time required to double your money. For very small rates of increase, such as those discussed here, a better approximation is to use 70 rather than 72. Thus $70 \div 2 = 35$ years to double at 2 percent per year, $70 \div 0.35 = 200$ years to double at 0.35 percent, and $70 \div 0.1 = 700$ years to double at a 0.1 percent rate of growth. This rule is quite accurate for rates less than 5 percent, and can be computed by hand or with a simple calculator until you have time to check the result with a spreadsheet.

5. For a large empirical study of conditions in the Americas, see Richard H. Steckel and Jerome C. Rose, eds., *The Backbone of History: Health and Nutrition in the Western Hemisphere* (Cambridge, UK: Cambridge University Press, 2002). An earlier assessment is found in Mark Nathan Cohen and George J. Amelagos, eds., *Paleopathology at the Origins of Agriculture* (New York: Academic Press, 1984), and a general overview in Mark Nathan Cohen, *Health and the Rise of Civilization* (New Haven: Yale University Press, 1989). It must be recognized that "life expectancy" varied widely (plus or minus 10 years or more, even for groups living within a few miles of one another during the same time period). Hence any comparisons of relative health are only rough indicators subject to many caveats and assumptions. The demographic data in this chapter are drawn largely from the books and articles by Deaton, Fogel, and Livi-Bacci listed among the Suggestions for Further Reading, as well as Wrigley and Schofield (note 16), McKeown (note 33), and McEvedy and Jones (note 9).

6. Theodore Tulchinsky and Elena Varavikova, "Addressing the Epidemiologic Transition in the Former Soviet Union," *American Journal of Public Health* 86, no. 3 (1996): 313–320; Vladimir Shkolnikov, Martina McKee, and David Leon, "Changes in Life Expectancy in Russia in the Mid-1990s," *The Lancet* 357, no. 9260 (2001): 917–921; Elizabeth Brainerd and David M. Cutler, "Autopsy of an Empire: Understanding Mortality in Russia and the Former Soviet Union," NBER working paper #10868, October 2004.

7. Barrie Cassileth, Vasily Vlassov, and Christopher Chapman, "Health Care, Medical Practice, and Medical Ethics in Russia Today," *Journal of the American Medical Association* 273, no. 20 (1995): 1569–1573.

8. Johannes Nohl, *The Black Death: A Chronicle of the Plague, Compiled from Contemporary Sources* (London: Unwin Books, 1971); Philip Ziegler, *The Black Death* (New York: John Day Company, 1969).

9. Massimo Livi-Bacci, *A Concise History of World Population* (Cambridge Mass.: Blackwell, 1992), 47, 106; Colin McEvedy and Richard Jones, *Atlas of World Population History* (Middlesex: Penguin, 1978), 25.

10. Massimo Livi-Bacci, *Population and Nutrition* (Cambridge: Cambridge University Press, 1991).

11. Robert Fogel, "Economic Growth, Population Theory and Physiology: The Bearing of Long-Term Processes on the Making of Economic Policy," *American Economic Review* 84, no. 3 (1994): 369–395.

12. Maurice Brown, *Adam Smith's Economics: Its Place in the Development of Economic Thought* (London: Croon Helm, 1988); E. G. West, *Adam Smith and Modern Economics: From Market Behavior to Social Choice* (Aldershot, England: Edward Elgar Publishing, 1990).

13. Thomas Robert Malthus, *An Essay on the Principle of Population*, 1803, new edition by Patricia James for the Royal Economic Society (Cambridge: Cambridge University Press, 1992). The term "dismal science" was coined by Thomas Carlyle and would not have been disputed by Malthus. However, the first use of the exact phrase was in Carlyle's argument for the reintroduction of slavery into the Caribbean, rather than population control. See Robert Dixon, "The Origin of the Term 'Dismal Science' to Describe Economics," University of Melbourne Department of Economics Working Paper #715, 1999.

14. Livi-Bacci (1992), 65.

15. Gary D. Hansen and Edward C. Prescott, "Malthus to Solow," *American Economic Review* 92, no. 4 (2002): 1205–1217.

16. E. A. Wrigley and R. S. Schofield, *The Population History of England, 1541–1871: A Reconstruction* (Cambridge, Mass.: Harvard University Press, 1981).

17. Gary Becker, *A Treatise on the Family* (Cambridge, Mass.: Harvard University Press, 1981).

18. A surprisingly large number of successful entrepreneurs and inventors go bankrupt several times before and after they strike it rich. Such risk taking is not feasible if two bad years in a row means starvation.

19. Note that the rise of the middle-class economy applies only within the small subset of developed countries. For most of the world's population, sharp divisions between rich and poor continued to be the rule. Francois Bourguignon and Christian Morrisson, "Inequality Among World Citizens: 1820–1992," *American Economic Review* 92, no. 4 (2002): 727–744.

20. Mancur Olson, Jr. "Big Bills Left on the Sidewalk: Why Some Nations are Rich, and Others Poor," *Journal of Economic Perspectives* 10, no. 2 (1996): 3–24.

21. The World Bank, *World Development Report 1993: Investing in Health* (Oxford, UK: Oxford University Press for the World Bank, 1993), 237.

22. United Nations, *World Population Prospects* (New York: United Nations, 1989); The World Bank, *World Development Report 1986* (Oxford, UK: Oxford University Press, 1986); Livi-Bacci, op. cit. (1992): 199–208.

23. Angus Deaton, "Policy Implications of the Health and Wealth Gradient," *Health Affairs* 21, no. 2 (2002): 13–30.

24. Clayne L. Pope, "The Changing View of the Standard-of-Living Question in the United States," *American Economic Review* 83, no. 2 (1993): 331–336.

25. "The Black Report," reprinted in Richard G. Wilkinson, *Class and Health* (London: Tavistock, 1986). See also G.D. Smith, Mel Bartley, and David Blane, "The Black Report on Socioeconomic Inequalities in Health 10 Years On," *British Medical Journal* 301, no. 6748 (1990): 373–377.

26. E. Rogot et al., *A Mortality Study of 1.3 Million Persons by Demographic, Social and Economic Factors: 1979–1985 Follow-Up* (Bethesda, Md.: National Institutes of Health, 1992); P. McDonough et al., "Income Dynamics and Adult Mortality in the United States, 1972 through 1989," *American Journal of Public Health* 87, no. 9 (1997): 1476–1483; Angus Deaton, "Health, Inequality and Economic Development," *Journal of Economic Literature* 41, no. 1 (2003): 113–158.

27. James P. Smith, "Healthy Bodies and Thick Wallets: The Dual Relation Between Health and Economic Status," *Journal of Economic Perspectives* 13, no. 2 (1999): 145–166.

28. Stephen E. Snyder and Wiliam N. Evans, "The Impact of Income on Mortality: Evidence from the Social Security Notch," *Review of Economics and Statistics* 88, no. 3 (2006): 482–495.

29. The value of risk reduction is also high at the other extreme, where a person faces near certain death. If you knew that otherwise you would die, you might well be willing to give up half of your money for just a 1 percent chance of continuing to live. See also Tomas Philipson, Gary Becker, Dana Goldman, Kevin Murphy, "Terminal Care and the Value of Life Near its End," NBER working paper #15649, January 2010.

30. Dora L. Costa and Matthew E. Kahn, "Changes in the Value of Life, 1940–1980," *Journal of Risk and Uncertainty* 29, no. 2 (2004): 149–180; and "The Rising Price of Non-Market Goods," paper presented at the American Economic Association Annual Meetings, Washington, D.C., January 4, 2003.

31. Ryan D. Edwards, "The Cost of Uncertain Life Span," NBER working paper #14093, June 2008. The risk of dying between ages 18 and 38 is currently about .02 (2%). Eliminating that risk of "unfortunate young death" would increase life expectancy by a bit over one year. If we were get rid of the risk of dying from 18 through 38 by accepting that we could live no older than 90 or by doubling the risk of dying between 75 and 80, such a trade-off would leave average life expectancy unchanged, but most of us would consider ourselves much better off.

32. Isidore S. Falk, *Security Against Sickness* (New York: Doubleday, 1936); Jesse George Crownheart, *Sickness Insurance in Europe* (Madison, Wisc: Democrat Printing Company, 1938).

33. Thomas McKeown, *The Modern Rise of Population* (London: Edward Arnold, 1976).

34. Michel Foucault, *The Birth of the Clinic* (New York: Pantheon Books, 1973).

35. Institute of Medicine, *Crossing the Quality Chasm* (Washington, D.C.: National Academies Press, 2001).

36. David M. Cutler and Grant Miller, "The Role of Public Health Improvements in Health Advances: The Twentieth-Century United States," *Demography* 42, no. 1 (2005): 1–22.

37. Samuel H. Preston, *Fatal Years: Child Mortality in Late 19th Century America* (Princeton: Princeton University Press, 1991).

38. David Cutler, Angus Deaton, and Adriana Lleras-Muney, "The Determinants of Mortality," *Journal of Economic Perspectives* 20, no. 3 (2006): 97–120.

39. David M. Cutler, *Your Money or Your Life* (Oxford, UK: Oxford University Press, 2004); Robert Hall and Charles Jones, "The Value of Life and the Rise in Health Care Spending," *Quarterly Journal of Economics* 122, no. 1 (2007): 39–72; David M. Cutler, Allison Rose, and Sandeep Vijan, "The Value of Medical Spending in the U.S. 1960–2000," *New England Journal of Medicine* 355, no. 9 (2006): 920–927.

CHAPTER 16

INTERNATIONAL COMPARISONS OF HEALTH AND HEALTH EXPENDITURES

QUESTIONS

1. Which country is the healthiest?
2. Which country has the best medical care system?
3. Which country has the largest health care market?
4. Is health care trade more or less international than other goods and services?
5. Is there more trade between countries in goods, services, people, or ideas?
6. What differences are greatest across countries: disparities in doctor supply, hospital technology, life expectancy, or per capita spending?
7. Is it high income or high medical expenditures that makes wealthy countries more healthy?
8. Does the distribution of income within a country determine the distribution of health?

16.1 WIDE DIFFERENCES AMONG NATIONS

There were more than 6 billion people in the world in 2010, distributed across some 200 countries. Health care expenditures for these 6 billion people totaled $5.8 trillion that year.[1] The 315 million people living in the United States represented 5 percent of the worldwide total, but U.S. health care expenditures, $2.3 trillion, accounted for almost 40 percent of total spending (see Table 16.1). Although China was the world's most populous country, with 1.4 billion people, it accounted for only $0.2 trillion in health care spending. Health expenditures per person in the United States were 9 times the worldwide average in 2010, twice as much as the $3,190 per person spent in Japan, and 50 times the per-person average of $146 in China (approximately $265 in international purchasing power parity (PPP) exchange rates) (Table 16.1).[2] The extra $2,100 billion purchased a lot more hospitals, physicians, drugs, and technologically sophisticated equipment for U.S. citizens. But how many additional years of life, how much reduction in morbidity and mortality, did this provide? Could the United States have done as well or become even more healthy while spending less? Many factors other

TABLE 16.1 Comparison of Health and Expenditures across Nations, 2006

Country	Pop. (millions)	Growth Rate (%)	Life Expectancy	% of pop. Age 60+	Mortality Rate <5 yr of age	Mortality Rate 15–59 yr of age	Income ($) (per/capital/PPP)	Health % of GNP	Expenditures per Capita PPP ($)	Expenditures per Capita US $	Government	Distribution of Payments (%) Prepaid Plans	Distribution of Payments (%) Out of Pocket
World	6,817	1.2	68	11	.060	.176	10,597	8.5	899	$ 854	61	16	19
Ghana	24	2.2	60	6	.069	.332	1,530	7.8	114	$ 55	50	3	39
Sudan	42	2.1	59	6	.108	.283	1,990	6.9	147	$ 97	10	1	64
Pakistan	181	2.2	63	6	.087	.208	2,680	2.6	62	$ 22	32	0	54
India	1,198	1.6	65	7	.066	.212	3,250	4.2	122	$ 45	32	2	50
China	1,353	0.7	74	12	.019	.116	6,890	4.3	265	$ 146	47	3	42
Turkey	75	1.3	75	9	.020	.104	13,710	6.1	845	$ 623	73	2	17
Mexico	110	1.1	76	9	.017	.122	14,100	5.9	837	$ 588	47	4	49
Poland	38	(0.1)	76	19	.006	.137	18,440	7.0	1,271	$ 971	67	1	22
U.K.	62	0.5	80	22	.005	.077	37,230	8.7	3,222	$3,771	83	1	11
Canada	34	1.0	81	20	.006	.070	37,410	8.8	3,867	$4,445	70	14	16
Japan	127	0.1	83	30	.003	.064	33,470	8.3	2,817	$3,190	81	2	15
Germany	82	0.0	80	26	.004	.076	36,780	10.5	3,922	$4,720	75	9	12
U.S.	315	1.0	79	18	.008	.106	45,640	15.2	7,164	$7,164	48	36	13

Source: World Health Statistics Report, 2008.

than hospitals and doctors are responsible for differences in health among China, the United States, and other countries, but an extra $2,100 billion is a significant amount to spend on health care.

Any assessment of health economy across the world must take into account the tremendous diversity in population, economic growth, and health status. Mozambique, Tanzania, and Ethiopia are among the world's poorest countries. These predominantly rural countries depend on subsistence agriculture and have limited government, little accumulation of savings or investment, per-capita incomes of less than $1,000, and rapidly expanding populations facing repeated threats from starvation. One out of 10 children die before age five years, and life expectancy is less than 60 years. At the other extreme are Sweden and Switzerland, whose urbane citizens enjoy incomes of more than $40,000, where most deaths occur after age 75 years, and where average life expectancy exceeds 80 years.

Development economists categorize countries as low, middle, or high income. More than half the world's population still lives in low-income, rural, agricultural countries. Most countries in Africa are toward the bottom of the distribution. The two undeveloped giants, China and India, have 1.353 and 1.198 billion people, respectively. China's recent rapid development could, if maintained, transform the economy within 20 years. Middle-income countries ($2,500 to $10,000 per-capita income), in which 1.5 billion people live, include many Latin American countries, most of the formerly socialist countries of the former Soviet Union and Eastern Europe, South Africa, Saudi Arabia (and other oil-rich states of the Middle East), and Asian countries with emerging economies (such as Korea). High-income countries ($10,000+ per-capita income), in which 850 million people live, include Western European countries and the United States, Canada, Japan, Australia, and New Zealand.

A nation's health resources generally increase with income, and the extent of illness and need for medical care are reduced. The high-income countries had 2.5 doctors and 8.3 hospital beds per 1,000 people in 2006.[3] The average life expectancy was 78 years, with more than half of all deaths occurring after that age. The perinatal mortality rate was 9 per 1,000 births, and the rate of tuberculosis (TB) infection was 0.2 per 1,000 population. In contrast, the low-income countries of sub-Saharan Africa could afford to spend only $12 per person on health care and had just 0.1 doctors and 1.4 hospital beds per 1,000 people. Life expectancy averaged 50 years, the perinatal mortality rate was 68 per 1,000 births, half of all deaths occurred in children younger than six years, and the TB infection rate was 2.20 per 1,000 population.

Size of the Market

From the perspective of the marketing department of a profit-maximizing health care firm, the importance of a country is determined not by the number of people, illnesses treated, or unmet needs but by the number of dollars spent there. In these terms, the United States is by far the largest market in the world, with a 40 percent share. In contrast, the world's most populous country, China, has only a 3 percent share, and the second most populous, India, has only a 1 percent share. In dollar terms, China's market is roughly the same size as the state of California's. All of the very-low-income countries together, 2.5 billion people, account for less than 3 percent of the world's health care spending (about as much as the state of Florida) (Figure 16.1).

The disparity in health resources is not as great as the disparity in health spending because wages are lower in low-income countries, therefore 75 percent less health care spending usually translates into a somewhat less severe reduction in the number of doctors or nurses.[4] Still, the gap between high-income and low-income countries is substantial (Table 16.1). Some goods, such as pharmaceuticals, are traded internationally, and their prices are somewhat consistent across countries so that a decline in spending causes an equivalent decline in use. Such internationally traded items take a much larger portion of health care budgets in low-income

FIGURE 16.1   International Comparisons of Market Sizes

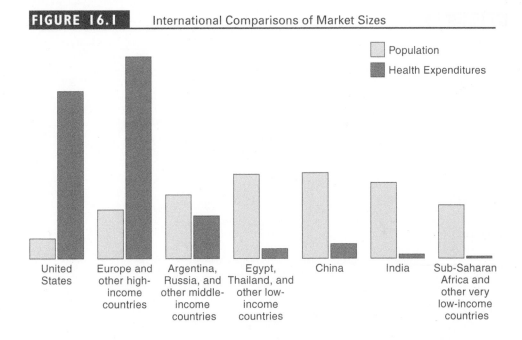

Population

Health Expenditures

United States | Europe and other high-income countries | Argentina, Russia, and other middle-income countries | Egypt, Thailand, and other low-income countries | China | India | Sub-Saharan Africa and other very low-income countries

countries (25 percent to 50 percent) than in high-income countries (5 percent to 15 percent). There are vast disparities between rich and poor. Haves and have-nots face such different choices that they almost seem like inhabitants of different planets or different centuries. What is common and readily accessible to most citizens of high-income countries are the favored privileges of a few government officials, industrialists, and celebrities in low-income countries. Medical care as practiced in the developed world is but a dream as distant as Hollywood for most of the world's population.

16.2 MICRO VERSUS MACRO ALLOCATION: HEALTH AS A NATIONAL LUXURY GOOD

Economists call entertainment, travel, and other expenditures "luxury goods," not as a judgment regarding the necessity or importance of such items but because they observe that the percentage of income spent on these goods increases as income increases. Items for which a 10 percent increase in income leads to a greater than 10 percent increase in spending (i.e., income elasticity >1.0) are labeled luxury goods, regardless of their use (see Section 13.2). Differences in relative wages between countries can complicate dollar comparisons, but a country that spends 12 percent of its gross domestic product (GDP) on health care is using more of its resources for medical care than a country spending 8 percent.[5]

Nations spend more money on health care because they have more money to spend, not because they have greater medical needs. This conclusion is not very surprising when considering whether Bangladesh (GDP $900 per capita) will spend more or less than Belgium (GDP $45,000 per capita) on health (Figure 16.2). Yet the finding that health care spending is unrelated or inverse to medical needs contradicts most personal experience: Individuals spend more on health care if they become sick. Decisions on how much will be spent by or for a particular individual (micro) are significantly different from, and based on different factors than, national decisions made collectively through the political process about how much of the budget or GDP should be spent on health (macro) (see Chapter 13).

FIGURE 16.2   Per-Capita Health Expenditures Related to Income

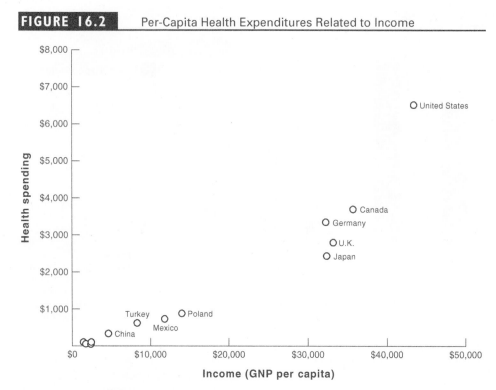

Source: World Health Statistics Report, 2008.

Health expenditures are made primarily with pooled funds raised through taxes and employee benefit plans. Decisions about how much to spend on each person from that pool will be based on individual medical needs. Insurance and government financing are ways to make sure that a person's ability to pay or family income does not limit the care they receive when they need it. Yet collectively the ability of everyone to pay, their aggregate prior contributions in taxes and insurance premiums, puts an absolute limit on how much can be spent in total on all the individuals treated. As the focus shifts from micro to macro allocation, the significant determinant of spending shifts from "medical need" to "available income" (Figure 16.3).

For example, most wealthy countries spend two to five times as much on elderly people as they do on young and middle-aged people. However, this does not mean that if a country's

FIGURE 16.3   Micro and Macro Determinants of Health Spending

Micro ◄━━━━━━━━━━━━━━━━━━━━━━━━━► Macro

Health status

Individual differences
in medical spending
are determined mostly
by differences in health
status, i.e., whether or
not the person is sick.

GDP per capita

National differences
in spending per person
are largely determined
by differences in income.

population is older it will spend more on health care (take it to the limit and suppose everyone were old and retired; who then would be working to pay for the extra nursing homes, hip replacements, and heart medications?).[6] As shown in Table 16.1, England has an older population than the United States and health statistics that are roughly equivalent on many measures (life expectancy 80 years versus 79 years, infant mortality 0.5 percent versus 0.8 percent), but England spends significantly less on health care on average ($3,771 versus $7,164), partly because per-capita income is lower ($43,570 versus $45,640).[7]

16.3 CAUSALITY: DOES MORE SPENDING IMPROVE HEALTH?

Wealthier countries are healthier, and they spend more on medical care. Can one then conclude that more spending buys better health? Not necessarily. Many factors associated with higher incomes, such as education, nutrition, and sanitation, are also known to improve health (see Chapter 15). Furthermore, life expectancy has increased greatly in many poor countries over the past 20 years, even when the availability of doctors and GDP per capita declined. A full assessment of all the influences on health status and relative contribution of each factor is not possible, but a rough appraisal of the relative importance of economic growth, advances in public health and medical research, and the use of medical care services can be made. However, it must be recognized that all these influences interact with and modify one another. With no knowledge of what to do, money is worthless, and medical knowledge alone is useless in the face of extreme poverty, which leads to death from starvation. Any specific estimate of how much each factor contributes to health is to some extent artificial and is also limited to what can readily be observed (i.e., differences noticeable within the range covered by statistics, such as those presented in Table 16.1).

Perusal of data from many countries indicates that only large differences, increases of two-fold or ten-fold, consistently affect health outcomes. Income differences on the order of 20 percent or 50 percent are not reliably associated with increases or decreases in life expectancy and appear to be within a range of indifference or minor variation or measurement error. Hence, they should either be treated with caution or ignored. It is the big picture that matters in this appraisal of relative importance.

Figure 16.4 illustrates that there is a relationship between per-capita income and average life expectancy, and that the relationship has changed over time. A plausible interpretation is that movements along the curve reflect the combined effects of more income and more medical care, while the shifting of the curve reflects the universal effect of increased knowledge, which is a public good. Between 1960 and 1990, life expectancy in Africa increased by about 10 years, from 43 to 52 years, despite the lack of improvement in living standards or incomes. Another piece of evidence for the effect of knowledge on health is provided by studies of childhood mortality in the United States around 1900.[8] In that era, children of well-to-do physicians were just as likely to die before age five years as children of poor laborers living in tenements, because both the wealthy and the poor used the same ineffectual health practices. As the importance of infection and nutrition were revealed, physicians' families were able to take advantage of their better education and resources so that child mortality declined much more rapidly in this group than among low-income laborers. In poor countries today, sanitation, basic nutrition supplements for infants, and control of preventable disease are still of primary importance. In these situations, studies have indicated that maternal education and literacy is often more important than income in preventing childhood disease and death.

Separate assessment of the effects of living standards and utilization of medical care is difficult because both generally rise or fall together. Japan, for example, has achieved a

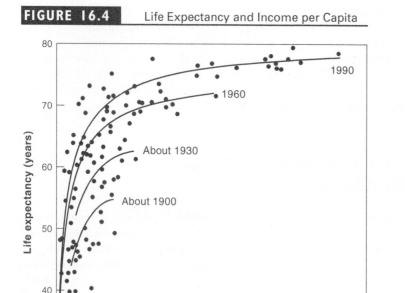

FIGURE 16.4   Life Expectancy and Income per Capita

phenomenal 25-year increase in life expectancy since World War II, but there is no easy way to determine how much is due to the rapid economic growth and how much is due to the deployment of modern medical care. The achievement of relatively high life expectancies in some low- or middle-income countries with relatively low use of sophisticated medical treatments (72 years in Malaysia, 75 years in the Czech Republic, 76 years in Costa Rica) suggests that the incremental effect of medical care alone is probably modest.

Analysis across many countries reveals that the absolute level of income might not be as important in some cases as **income distribution**.[9] It is not surprising that where there is greater equality of income, the average level of health is higher. The relationship between income and health is nonlinear. A 20 percent drop means much less at the middle or top of the distribution than it does toward the bottom. High rates of illness are a function not of poverty but of extreme deprivation. The greater the degree of inequality, the more likely it is that some families will be so lacking in food and amenities that deaths from infantile diarrhea, tuberculosis, and other preventable or treatable illnesses will occur.

16.4 LOW-INCOME COUNTRIES

Low-income countries face health care problems that are very different from those of wealthy industrialized countries. The populations of low-income countries are rural, with many children and a heavy burden of infectious disease and stunting (abnormally low height and/or small body size) due to occasional malnutrition. However, government officials living in the capital have incomes, tastes, and health care needs much more like those of developed countries. This can lead to a major misallocation of resources, such as building a modern research hospital in the capital providing excellent tertiary care, while much of the country lacks access to a doctor or a nurse and children remain unvaccinated so that preventable disease epidemics remain common. Occasionally half the entire health budget of a low-income country is spent in the capital city, with a large part going to equip and staff the leading hospital (in contrast, the Johns Hopkins University Hospital takes about 0.6 percent of the U.S. health care budget).

Convincing local medical leaders to change the allocation of resources to a more appropriate emphasis on low-technology primary care is difficult. They do not wish to give up their expensive research hospital that might bring the doctors and government officials prestige and international fame. The world may admire a European doctor trained at a leading university who spends years alone treating cases in an isolated river village, but a local physician who spends his days treating diarrhea and wound infections without any chance to practice in a modern surgical facility is simply considered to have minimal skills of little importance to outsiders. Incentives are not aligned with the health needs of the majority of citizens. Both ruling politicians and leaders of the medical profession naturally tend to favor maintaining a state-of-the-art facility with modern technology and capability for research, even when doing so drains funds from the village clinics and nursing care that can do more to reduce infant mortality and raise life expectancy. Even in very-low-income countries, medical schools train many specialists who want to perform technologically advanced procedures rather than primary care generalists able to treat most common illnesses.

Studies by the World Bank have found that the status of women is a major determinant of health in low-income countries. Access to knowledge is one factor. In countries where most women are illiterate and uneducated, there is no way for them to know about sterilization of water, proper nutrition, or care of childhood infections. Women are also more likely than men to make family health a priority. In subsistence economies where women have some control over spending (because of tradition or because they have a job with wages), a larger fraction of the household budget gets spent on food and less on alcohol and tobacco.

Starvation remains a problem in many of the lowest-income countries. In Nigeria, 43 percent of children aged two to six years are stunted (their height is low for their age), and the rate is 32 percent in Kenya, and 65 percent in India, compared with 22 percent in Mexico, 4 percent in Japan, and 2 percent in the United Kingdom and United States.[10] This situation occurs not because food supply is insufficient but because the supply is maldistributed. Organizational disarray, lack of transport, disruptions due to war and political upheaval, and poorly functioning markets mean that food does not get to where it is needed most. No simple solution presents itself, because the defects in economic organization that cause mismanagement of food are the same as those responsible for a lack of economic development in the first place. National governments that maintain order, handle their budgets and money supply prudently, and support market-oriented policies are able to grow out of the low-income category.

Health Care in Ghana*

Ghana has a population of 23.4 million (2008 figure) and an economy based on agriculture, services, and precious metals. Agriculture was the traditional backbone of the economy, constituting about 60 percent of GDP in the late 1970s, but its share has been steadily declining and now accounts for just a little more than 30 percent. However, smallholder agriculture still employs not less than half of the work force. The principal agricultural export is cocoa. Services account for the major share of GDP today, at more than 40 percent. Mineral extraction and exports, especially gold production, have also grown in importance. Manganese, bauxite,

---

*This section was prepared by Chris Atim, PhD, a Ghanaian senior health economist working in international public health and also the executive director of the African Health Economics and Policy Association. He can be contacted at chrisatim1@gmail.com.

and diamonds form the other major mineral exports. More recently, oil has been discovered; production began in 2011 and is expected to contribute around 7 percent to GDP.

In recent times, Ghana has moved from being a poor lower-income country, as measured by its GDP per capita, to being a lower-middle-income country (GDP estimated at US$1,600 in 2010 in current prices, from $670 in 2006, *Atlas method*). The official reclassification is the result of a rebasing of its national accounts, changing the base year of the calculation from 1993 to 2006. But the reclassification is also a reflection of considerable economic growth of the country since the mid-1980s following substantial reforms. For instance, between 1985 and 2008, Ghana's economy expanded by 170 percent, compared with the sub-Saharan Africa's average of 110 percent. At the same time, during the 1990s, national poverty dropped from 52 to 40 percent and extreme poverty from 37 to 27 percent. Life expectancy at 57 years is higher than sub-Saharan Africa's average of 52 years, and the population growth rate of 2.2 percent is lower than the regional average of 2.5 percent. Nearly half the population lives in urban areas and the literacy rate of adults (older than 15 years) is 65 percent. School enrollment rates have increased for primary and secondary schools. The net enrollment rate for primary school in Ghana is 78.6 percent, compared to the African average of 66.3 percent. Nearly 93 percent of those completing primary school in 2005–2006 continued to the next level.

The health system consists of public, private, and traditional sectors. The public sector provides nearly 60 percent of formal health care and is made up of the Ghana Health Service (GHS, which runs all primary to tertiary level institutions, mostly autonomously of the Ministry of Health), three Teaching Hospitals, and some quasi-Government and statutory bodies. GHS-run facilities include a large number of public health centers at the primary level, 110 secondary level district hospitals, and 10 tertiary level regional hospitals. Below the health centers are a network of community-based health planning and services (CHPS) compounds, each nominally staffed by a couple of nurses, midwives, and community volunteers for delivering preventive, promotive, and basic care to village communities. The private sector provides about 40 percent of health care and is dominated by primary and secondary level health facilities run by religious missions such as the Catholic Secretariat and Christian Health Association of Ghana, but there is also a vibrant and growing private for-profit sector in more urbanized areas of the country. Traditional healers operate in the informal sector but are officially recognized as a part of, although not integrated into, the country's health system. The World Health Organization estimates that such providers account for about 60 percent of the first line of treatment for children with malaria in Ghana and similar countries. Private pharmacies have proliferated all over the country including in rural areas although they are most visible and dominant in the urban areas (see Table 16.2).

After independence in 1957, Ghana's socialist-oriented CPP government followed a nominally free health care policy, but a new pro-liberal government in 1969 instituted some partial cost recovery in health and education. After a subsequent period of unstable governments and

TABLE 16.2	Health Economic Indicators for Ghana
Health Expenditures	**Percentage**
Out-of-pocket, % of total expenditure on health	43
Out-of-pocket, % of private expenditure on health	79
Per capita, current US$	45
Private, % of GDP	4
Public, % of total health expenditure	45
Public, % of government expenditure	9
Public, % of GDP	3
Total, % of GDP	7
External resources for health, % of total expenditure on health	17

steep economic decline, including partial reversal of the user fees policy, a populist military-led government with social democratic leanings emerged in 1981 that lasted until 1992 and which, untypically for such a regime, began to push through liberal market reforms. As a part of these reforms, user fees at health facilities were reintroduced in 1985. These fees aimed at recovering up to 20 percent of facilities' operational nonsalary costs from users. The user fees policy, popularly known as the "cash-and-carry" system, came to be felt as highly burdensome by many people.

In 1997, the government extended exemptions to its cash-and-carry policy in public health institutions beyond the so-called pauper category and with funding from debt relief. The new exemptions policy covered children up to five years, pregnant women, and the aged (older than 70 years). In practice, however, the system never really worked as intended, for two principal reasons that also serve to illustrate how incentives work in health care. The first reason is related to the incentives created for public providers whereby they were allowed to retain the revenue obtained from cash-and-carry and to use this retained revenue to pay for facility operational costs such as drugs and kerosene as well as to pay top-up allowances to staff. Because government transfers for operational costs and exemptions were less certain than user-fee income collected directly from patients, this fee-retention policy not only aligned the interests of provider staff neatly with those of the facilities (i.e., to maximize user fee revenue) but also meant in particular that providers had an incentive under the new system not to exempt whenever possible, because doing so meant a loss of their most secure form of revenue.[11] In fact, these incentives were so strong that a WHO survey in 2006 found a district health manager in Ghana admitting that districts were reluctant to report a local epidemic because it meant that they could no longer charge patients for the epidemic condition!

The second reason the system never worked as intended had to do with the fact that government budgetary transfers to facilities for exempted persons consistently fell far short of the costs of the scheme to providers, particularly for the increasing numbers of pregnant women making use of the exemption opportunities. This led to frequent and long delays in payment and sometimes even nonpayment for services rendered under the exemptions, a situation felt by both public and private providers alike. This was a further incentive not to exempt, and in the end many vulnerable persons entitled to free services continued to be denied needed care owing to lack of the means to pay for such care and the reluctance and refusal of facilities to exempt such persons as directed by the government. These problems were compounded by unclear guidelines and uneven implementation nationwide. Some regional directors of health made their own rules, setting the threshold age to benefit from the old-age exemption at 60 instead of 70 years, using the explanation that few people lived to 70 years and beyond in those regions. The lack of a clear definition of "old," "indigent," or "pauper" also gave rise to uneven interpretations of the rules and more comfort to those who did not want to exempt in any case.

At the end of 2000, a new government came to power on a promise to abolish cash-and-carry and a manifesto pledge to institute social health insurance. A law was finally passed in 2003 to set up the National Health Insurance Scheme (NHIS), a pioneering and bold effort at universal health coverage in a low-income context. The NHIS consists of decentralized district-level mutual health insurance schemes (DMHISs) that constitute the only avenue by which any Ghanaian can join and benefit from the publicly subsidized national health insurance system, as well as national-level institutions for, among other functions, the regulation, supervision, management, funding, and reinsurance of the district schemes. Those national institutions include the National Health Insurance Authority (NHIA) as the regulating and supervisory authority over the district schemes, the National Health Insurance Fund (NHIF), which receives tax and premium contributions for the funding and reinsurance of the schemes, and the National Health Insurance Council (NHIC) as the supervisory and oversight board of the NHIA.

Providers under the NHIS include all public health facilities of the GHS and accredited private facilities, including practically all mission-run facilities, accredited private for-profit providers, and numerous private pharmacies around the country. The benefit package is very generous, covering all outpatient and inpatient as well as diagnostic and specialist services for up to 95 percent of the medical conditions prevalent in the country.

The NHIS is mainly funded by a health insurance levy (a 2.5 percent earmarked addition to the VAT), 2.5 percent of workers' contributions to the Social Security and National Insurance Trust Fund (SSNIT Fund), considered the workers' premium contribution, and informal sector premium contributions of a minimum of around US$5 per annum per capita for adults in the informal sector. About 70 percent of NHIS income at the end of 2008 was derived from the VAT levy and about 23 percent from the social security contributions, making this scheme a largely tax-funded "insurance" system.

Reinforcing this character of a tax-funded insurance system is the extensive exemptions for key demographic and vulnerable groups, who are exempt from paying but are entitled to be covered by the NHIS for their health care. These are indigent persons, pregnant women, children younger than 18 years, pensioners, and elderly people older than 70 years.

Active NHIS membership rose from the scheme rollout around 2004 to just over 8 million at the end of 2010, or about 34 percent of the total population. This coverage represents a significant drop from previous figures based on faulty administrative records that put membership at about 65 percent of the population. A new methodology for assessing membership introduced in 2011 together with a cleanup of membership records enabled the new, more reliable, estimate. Not surprisingly, exempted categories dominate the NHIS membership, making up about two thirds of the total membership overall, with children younger than 18 years constituting nearly half of total scheme membership. Independent surveys and research have shown that the NHIS has brought about significant health sector benefits, including financial protection to the vulnerable and positive changes to health-seeking behavior. However there is also evidence and concern that scheme membership is skewed toward the better off so that the poorest are less well represented.

Sudan*

Sudan is a low-income, highly indebted poor country on the northeastern coast of sub-Saharan Africa. Sudan's population of 38 million people is spread out over 2.5 million square kilometers and is growing rapidly at a rate of 2.2 percent a year despite desperate poverty. Per-capita income is estimated at about $1,100 for 2006. As has been the case in most African countries, the public health system was the main provider of health care services, employing physicians, nurses, pharmacists, and paramedical and other support staff on a salary scale comparable to the public service salary scale. Physicians and facilities were overconcentrated in urban areas, although indicators point to the rural areas as being the most in need. Taxation was historically the primary source of funding, with all premises and equipment owned and maintained by the government.

Although historically services were offered free of charge at the time of use, economic retrenchments and severe natural and human-made disasters, including floods, droughts, and armed conflict in the southern part of the country, caused serious dislocations in the national health system. The promise of free health services for all citizens became increasingly hollow as inadequate budgets left buildings, equipment, and professional time of salaried health personnel seriously underutilized. Economic waste was further aggravated by purchases of capital equipment, building materials, and medical staff training using scarce foreign exchange. Spending on social services in general and on health in particular was low and declined during the 1980s and 1990s. In times of financial stringency, the obligations to pay salaries and rent and

*This section was contributed by Muneef Abdelbagi Babiker, Assistant Professor, Department of Economics, University of Khartoum.

to pay for maintenance and replenishment of assets commonly used by physicians (e.g., cars, stethoscopes) are given priority, making the impact of reduced spending on services even more severe than the financial figures alone indicate.

The adverse economic situation since the 1980s has had a great impact on health services, health status, and funding. The private sector in medical care witnessed a qualitative and quantitative expansion. Traditionally the private sector was restricted to after-hours consultations by government-employed doctors during their free time in the evening. However, more doctors have converted to full private practice, and private inpatient hospitals are being built. A World Health Organization (WHO) consultant estimated that the central government spent $2.50 per person on health care in 2002, about 0.65 percent of GDP.[12] Most total health spending, 62 percent, comes from fees paid by private households, 17 percent from the compulsory National Health Insurance Scheme, 19 percent from ministry of health and other central government ministries, and 2 percent from international organizations (mainly WHO and United Nations Children's Fund [UNICEF]). Other sources of financing for health services include small company-based health insurance schemes, humanitarian national and international nongovernmental organizations, and private expenditures on traditional healers.

According to a 2003 World Bank report, both in absolute and relative terms, government health spending in Sudan ranks among the lowest in the world at perhaps US$4 per capita and under or around 1 percent of GDP. This relatively low level of public health spending is supplemented by household out-of-pocket spending and health insurance spending. According to World Bank, "It is estimated that total out-of-pocket expenditures are as large [as] or larger than total government health spending (that is, 1 percent or more of GDP). In addition, the national health insurance scheme similarly spends around 1 percent of GDP, so that total health expenditures in Northern Sudan are likely in the range of 4 or 5 percent of GDP, or US$15 to 20 per capita. This level would be consistent with the lower range of total spending in countries in sub-Saharan Africa." Because most of the public and private health facilities and personnel are concentrated in urban areas, the actual coverage by health services is expected to be very low. By law the health insurance scheme is supposed to cover all employees of public and private enterprises that employ at least 10 people, but currently this plan covers only 6 percent of the population.

People who can afford to use the current fee-based health services system more tend to benefit most. Reliance on private funds has increased inequity. With less public funding, many individuals wait until their illness reaches a serious stage before contacting the health services system. There is less spending on routine care and prevention and more on catastrophic events. The trend toward privatization has even encroached on public health services. In Khartoum, the upkeep of a number of previously unattended, filthy, and deserted public lavatories attached to mosques, market areas, bus stops, and other public areas have been contracted to private individuals or institutions. The average annual rents for a lavatory unit are 615,000 Sudanese dinars (approximately $2,460). The contractors can charge a small fee ranging between 10 and 20 dinars (4–8 cents) for every episode of use. Although no formal study has been conducted to evaluate this privatization experiment, a limited survey revealed that contractors and users were satisfied. This, along with the fact that these arrangements have been functioning since 1995 and that more units are being constructed, indicates success.

16.5   MIDDLE-INCOME COUNTRIES

Turkey, Mexico, Thailand, and South Korea are examples of countries that are in the midst of development. Looming even larger are the emerging economies termed BRICs: Brazil, Russia, India, and China. Subsistence agriculture and poverty are still the norm in the remote rural regions, but the bulk of the population has moved into cities and works for wages. The shift from rural agricultural labor to urban wage labor presents a major organizational problem: How does a country develop a comprehensive health insurance system able to fund a higher level of health care? Rapid economic growth allows some countries to expand government services so that a predominantly public system is created. In other countries, such as Korea, a strong tradition of industrial paternalism leads to private insurance based on employment benefits. Some countries began with a public system and switched to reliance on the private sector, while others are moving in the opposite direction. In almost every middle-income developing country the health insurance system is in transition.

Even when coverage is universal by law, the reality is that access to medical care is very uneven. The urban ghettos and impoverished rural villages often lack sanitation. Restrictions and incompleteness in the health insurance system might prevent poor citizens from using medical facilities even when these facilities are accessible geographically. Thus, the disadvantaged populations are disproportionately represented in morbidity and mortality statistics. At the same time, expanding incomes have brought the lifestyle illnesses of the wealthy countries, such as heart disease and lung cancer, to prominence. The growth markets for cigarettes in the 21st century are China, India, and Asia, not Europe and North America. Finally, the middle-income countries are still likely to misallocate resources, emulating the advanced health care systems of high-income nations: large research hospitals in the cities matched by a lack of village clinics in the countryside and the training of too many specialists and not enough primary care physicians or public health experts.

China*

With a population of 1.3 billion, China is the largest developing country in the world. The country has experienced rapid economic and social development since its adoption of the "open the door" policy in 1978, which has laid a solid foundation for health system development. However, in a rapidly transitional context, the Chinese health care system has been confronted by many challenges brought by globalization, modernization, urbanization, and an aging population. Many rounds of health reforms were launched in the health sector to address these challenges. A new round of health reform was initiated in 2009, which has focused on people's welfare and health demands and aimed to provide universal health care.

With deepening of the health care reforms, the health status of the Chinese people has continuously improved, with remarkable development of key health indicators. The mortality rate of children younger than five years dropped from 61 per 1,000 births in 1991 to 17.2 in 2009. The maternal mortality ratio has dropped from 80 per 100,000 live births in 1991 to 31.9 in 2009. Life expectancy in 2005 was 73.0 years, and it is expected to reach 74.5 at the end of the 12th Five Year Plan period (2011–2015). The total expenditure on health (TEH) has seen a continuous increase (Figure 16.5). TEH in 2010 was $293.83 billion, 4.985 percent of the GDP.[13] Since 2003, the government has increased inputs to basic health insurance and the public health system so that the ratio of public inputs to the total health expenditure has seen constant increase (Figure 16.6). However, individual out-of-pocket health expenditure still accounts for a high percentage of health spending.

China has established a sound public health system and tiered health service network. Health facilities with public ownerships have occupied a dominant position (more than 90 percent). In urban areas, tertiary hospitals are leading in health technology and clinical skills, treating major or complicated illnesses, and secondary hospitals and community health centers provide care for common or minor illnesses. However, owing to lack of effective planning and steering mechanisms, health resources and patients all flow to big hospitals.

*This section was prepared by Zhengzhong Zang, Professor, China National Health Development Research Center, and Yue Xiao, Research Associate at CNHRDC.

FIGURE 16.5   Trends in Total Expenditure on Health in China, 1978–2010

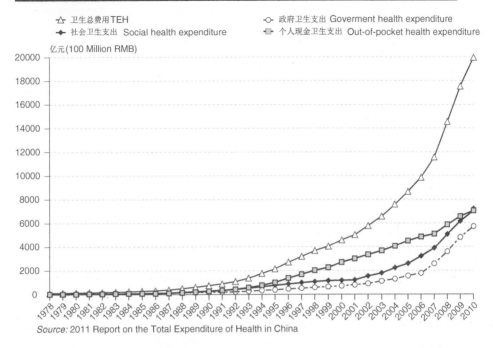

Source: 2011 Report on the Total Expenditure of Health in China

Three-tier rural health delivery relies heavily on township health centers and village clinics, but these facilities have poor capacity for providing quality public health and medical services owing to lack of professional capacity and equipment. Therefore, rural patients more often go to county hospitals for inpatient care.

FIGURE 16.6   Composition of Total Expenditure on Health in China, 1978–2010, Using International Calculation Methods

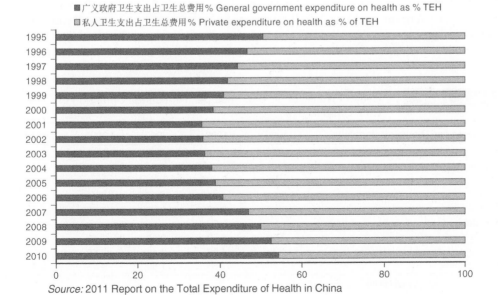

Source: 2011 Report on the Total Expenditure of Health in China

TABLE 16.3   Types and Numbers of Health Facilities in China, 2010

		Location		Economy Type	
Type	Number	Urban	Rural	Public	Nonpublic
Hospitals	20,918	11,297	9,621	13,850	7,068
Basic health facilities	901,709	115,636	786,073	460,927	440,782
Professional public health facilities	11,835	4,514	7,321	11,764	71
Total	936,927	132,465	804,462	488,932	447,995

Source: Yearbook of China Health Statistics in 2011

With development of health insurance schemes in recent years, health demands have rapidly increased. The total visits to health facilities reached 5.85 billion in 2010, with an increase of 350 million over the previous year (6.4 percent). The total number of inpatients amounted to more than 141.74 million, with an increase of 9.18 million over the previous year (6.9 percent).[14] Capacity of the health system has been greatly strengthened as well. Health professionals per thousand population was 2.85 in 1980 and 4.37 in 2010. Hospital beds per thousand population were 2.19 in 1980 and 3.56 in 2010. The total number of health facilities at all levels reached 937,000 at the end of 2010 (see Tables 16.3 and 16.4), and that of health staff amounted to about 8.21 million. Although there is a constant increase of health resources, there are still big disparities between urban and rural areas and different regions.

The national public health protection system in China can be summarized as "3 + 1": three basic national health protection schemes plus a medical financial assistance scheme covering more than 95 percent of the total population. The three health protection schemes are the Basic Health Insurance for urban employees (BMI), Social Medical Insurance for urban residents (SMI), and the New Rural Cooperative Medical Scheme (NRCMS). These have been financed mainly by public funds and supplemented by premiums and social funds, covering urban workers, the urban nonemployed population, and rural residents, respectively. The Medical Assistance for urban and rural residents (MA), publicly funded with society-wide contributions, has functioned as the bottom of the health safety net in the country.

The pattern of the 3+1 health protection system in China has been gradually formed along with implementation of several rounds of health reforms (see Figure 16.7). BMI, an employment-based insurance scheme established in 1998, has nearly 250 million enrollees. Employers are responsible for deducting insurance funds from individual employee's wages (about 6 percent of the total wage). SMI started its first pilot in 2007 and now 220 million unemployed people, university students, and school pupils in urban areas have enrolled in the program. NRCMS, launched in 2003 and scaled up nationwide in 2008, has provided basic

TABLE 16.4   Health Professionals and Beds per Thousand Population in China, 1980–2010

Resources per Thousand Population	1980	1990	2000	2005	2010
Health professionals	2.85	3.45	3.63	3.57	4.37
Physicians					
Total	1.17	1.56	1.68	1.60	1.79
Urban areas	3.22	2.95	2.31	2.46	2.97
Rural areas	0.76	0.98	1.17	1.26	1.32
Hospital beds					
Beds	2.19	2.53	2.47	2.63	3.56
Urban areas	4.70	4.18	3.49	3.59	5.33
Rural areas	1.48	1.55	1.50	1.43	2.44

Source: Yearbook of China Health Statistics in 2011

FIGURE 16.7 China's Major National Health Protection Schemes

Source: Yearbook of China health Statistics in 2009

health protection for more than 836 million rural residents. It started with a basic benefit package and now is exploring ways to upgrade protection for catastrophic illnesses. SMI and BMI, with prefectures and cities as basic units for fund pooling, are managed by human resource and social security agencies. NRCMS funds are pooled on a county basis and managed by health authorities. BMI enrollees enjoy the highest reimbursement and financing level, and NRCMS have enrollees the lowest.

Differences in financing level and management mechanisms led to inequality between beneficiaries of insurance schemes. MA pilots were initiated in 2003. After years of exploration, MA has integrated effectively with NRCMS and other insurance schemes, improved accessibility of health services to the poor, and reduced disease-induced poverty to a certain degree. One of the key components of the health reforms in 2009 was to establish and improve the basic health system. The main tasks included enhancing fund pooling and reimbursing capacity of NRCMS and SMI, exploring effective integration of various insurance schemes, and establishing a uniform health insurance scheme for all.

China's health system has undergone big changes since the launch of the reform in 2009 in terms of development of a public health system, medical delivery system, and drug supply system for urban and rural residents. Take the public health sector for instance. Nine public health programs have been fully launched nationwide, including programs on health records for all residents, health education, infant and child care, maternal care, planned immunization, reporting and management of communicable diseases, management of non-communicable diseases, and management of severe mental diseases. Public inputs on basic public health services have continuously increased. Per-capita funds for public health services increased from ¥15 (yuan) in 2009 ($2.20) to ¥25 in 2011 ($3.68), and will reach to ¥40 ($5.88) in 2015. Meanwhile, the public health service delivery system has been strengthened and more services have been provided. In two years, 190 million people have enjoyed services provided by the new public health programs.

Reforms of public hospitals are the most difficult part of the current health system reform in China. For a long period, public hospitals used drug markups to compensate medical revenue due to lack of public funds. The key to success of public hospital reforms is to reform compensation mechanisms while maintaining their basic features as public welfare hospitals. Meanwhile, payment reforms initiated by insurance agencies can propel changes of compensation mechanisms. Clinical pathways will contribute to streamlining internal management, regulating provider behavior, strengthening evidence-based clinical decision making, and containing unjustified increases in health expenditures while upgrading quality and efficiency. Currently, some secondary and tertiary hospitals have started reforms on case payment and clinical pathways. It is estimated that 100 percent of tertiary hospitals and 80 percent of secondary hospitals will implement case payment and clinical pathways by the end of 2015.

The Health Care System of Mexico

With a 2005 per capita GDP of $6,820, an average life expectancy of 73 years for males and 78 years for females, and a young population (30 percent younger than 15 years) of 106 million that is growing rapidly (1 percent per year), Mexico* is similar to many other countries with transitional economies. The bulk of the people have moved off the farms and into cities to find industrial and service jobs, but agriculture and export of raw commodities still make up a substantial part of the economy, and illiteracy is still a problem in rural areas. The government is politically stable, with a new party coming to power in 2000, shifting away from 80 years of single-party rule to a more open, multiparty democracy.

The government enacted a comprehensive social security system (IMSS, in 1943) relatively early for a transitional economy, but it only covered industrial workers and their dependents.[15] A nationwide network of IMSS health centers, polyclinics, and hospitals was built. The Ministry of Health and IMSS-Solidaridad provide services for around 40 million uninsured Mexicans, mainly the rural and urban poor. In 1960, a plan for government employees, ISSSTE, was established, and a modern and technologically sophisticated network of hospitals and clinics was built with generous funding to accommodate this favored group of employees. ISSSTE, IMSS, and the medical services for the armed forces and employees of the national oil company (PEMEX) provided the top tier of health insurance and covered about half the population (see Table 16.5).

The organization of services in Mexico is rigidly segregated, and quality is considerably heterogeneous. The Ministry of Health, IMSS, and ISSSTE provide primary, secondary, and tertiary services, with specialty services concentrated in the three largest cities: Mexico City, Guadalajara, and Monterrey. The private market provides services both at the bottom of the income distribution (where SSA is inadequate) and at the top (where wealthier people can buy state-of-the-art medical care); the middle is occupied by three separate tiers of public care. The private sector consists of providers working in hospitals, clinics, offices, and folk medicine units on a for-profit basis. In theory, this component should provide services for around 10 percent of the population. However, according to recent surveys, around 25 percent of the people enrolled in social security agencies report a private provider as their usual source of

TABLE 16.5   Health Insurance Coverage in Mexico

Insurance Plan	Population Covered (%)
Mexican Institute of Social Security (IMSS)	39%
Institute for Governmental Workers (ISSSTE)	8%
Other federal agency health plans	2%
Secretariat of Health and Welfare (SSA)	21%
Marginal families program	13%
Private medical care	5%
Unprotected population	12%

Source: Milton Roemer, *National Health Systems of the World* (New York: Oxford University Press, 1991).

*This section was revised by Julio Frenk, M.D., Ph.D., Minister of Health, and Octavio Gomez, M.D.

ambulatory care. In the same vein, around 40 percent of the uninsured population report a private practitioner as their usual source of primary care.

Most physicians in Mexico work in salaried positions for ISSSTE, IMSS, or SSA and also have a private practice. Yet even though Mexico has considerably fewer physicians per 100,000 population than the United States (about one-fourth as many), there is a large pool of unemployed or underemployed physicians (more than 30 percent of all physicians) who cannot find a government job or attract enough private patients to make a living from medicine.

The present administration promoted a major legislative reform establishing a system of social protection in health, which was approved by a large majority of the Mexican Congress in 2003. This system is reorganizing and increasing public funding by a full percentage point of GDP over seven years in order to provide universal health insurance and include the 50 million Mexicans, most of them poor, who had been excluded until now from formal social insurance plans because they are self-employed, are out of the labor market, or work in the informal sector of the economy. The increased funding is spearheading a major effort to realign incentives throughout the health system. Poor families can now enroll in a new scheme called Popular Health Insurance, which is the basis for allocating federal funds to states. The old model of bureaucratic budgeting, which subsidized providers without regard to performance, is being replaced by democratic budgeting, whereby money follows people through a demand-side subsidy. Capitated payments and freedom of choice ensure an optimal balance between quality and efficiency. To achieve this aim, the macro-level financial reform is being complemented by a micro-level management reform, which is strengthening delivery capacity through a series of specific interventions, such as long-term planning of new facilities, technology assessment, efficient schemes for drug supply, human resource development including managerial training, outcome-oriented information systems, facility accreditation, provider certification, quality assurance, and performance benchmarking at both the state and the provider levels.

Poland

Poland* has 38 million people, with an average per-capita income of $8,200 in 2005 and a life expectancy of 69 years for males and 78 years for females. There are about 22 doctors, 49 nurses, and 50 hospital beds per 10,000 people. Total expenses for health care in Poland were about $540 per capita (6.6 percent of GDP) in 2002.[16] The main sources of financing are public sickness funds (Kasy Chorych), but private resources have recently grown to contribute almost 40 percent. Since 1999, social insurance funds have accounted for 80 percent of public resources.

Insurance is mandatory for all workers. The amount of the premium (7.5 percent of wages) is established by Parliament as a part of personal income tax. Employers do not finance the premiums, but they withhold the amount from wages and submit it for collection by a nationwide public agency. The government pays premiums for about 35 percent of citizens (farmers, the unemployed, people collecting social security payments). Administrative information systems have many weak points; thus, these estimates must be used with caution. Payments between sickness funds are equalized to account for differences in participants' income and ages. The sickness funds practice cost control by establishing rates and limiting the number of services. However, administrative inefficiencies and the difficulty of enforcing agreements mean that budget limits are often exceeded.

Hospital services accounted for approximately 50 percent of the total expenditures of public funds in 2002. Cost shifting also takes place. Teaching hospitals receive financial resources for research from a special quasi-budget fund and from pharmaceutical company grants. Part of

*This section was contributed by Katarzyna Tymowska, Director of Postgraduate Study in Health Economics, Warsaw University.

these resources covers expenses for patients' treatment. Thanks to the extra funding, the quality of care rises, which attracts good physicians and more patients. Owing to the lack of standards, these specialized hospitals also admit patients with minor health problems.

Pharmaceuticals account for one-third of total health expenditures in Poland. The percentage is high not only because drug consumption is high but also because of the relatively low cost of medical staff. Half of households' private expenditures for health are for buying drugs. Among the causes for increasing pharmaceutical expenditures are the elimination of the state monopoly in the drug market, intensive marketing by pharmaceutical companies, and the strong belief of many Poles in the efficacy of expensive drugs produced by foreign companies. Hospital managers have responded to the squeeze caused by rising drug expenditures and limited budgets by introducing standardized pharmacologic procedures and prescription books and requiring approval by the head of a hospital unit to order expensive drugs.

In Poland, copayment for services is unimportant. Because patients incur few charges, services are overused (moral hazard). However, there exists a culturally conditioned custom of giving gifts to facilitate access to services or obtain greater kindness from hospital employees. Such informal gratuities constituted 36 percent of private out-of-pocket health spending in a recent study.

Private resources are of increasing importance in Poland. Earnings are going up, education levels are rising, and social expectations regarding easy access to health care (and to higher-quality care) are escalating. Medical services have become consumption goods, which has encouraged development of private medical companies. Unlike in the times of communist rule, one no longer needs administrative permits to establish a firm. These companies, often operating with foreign capital, react quickly to a growing demand for medical services. Some have signed contracts with public payers, and others are planning to take part in the competition offering medical services to the insured. Dissatisfaction with the low quality of public-sector medical services has been a major cause of increasing demand for the private companies. Large employers are able to buy services in advance, especially ambulatory care, using prepayments (called subscriptions). This is not the same as the workers' health plans, but it has similar benefits: tax advantages for employers and employees and "golden cuffs" to keep valued workers. Another factor favoring this development is the partial transfer of treatment costs so that the private sector does not bear full financial responsibility. High-risk patients are directed to specialized diagnostic centers and hospitals financed with public money. In Poland, private facilities act as a kind of gate through which patients can more easily get into a facility maintained by public resources.

The present system of contracts creates a special inducement for cost shifting through the use of capitation payments to primary care physicians. Primary physicians receive a fixed amount of funds to pay for their work, for the work of nurses and record-keepers, and for basic diagnostics (physicians are not allowed to own pharmacies but may own diagnostic centers). In some regions, capitation fees also cover specialized health care and diagnostic services. A primary care physician, especially one with an individual practice, prefers to send a patient to a specialist. The primary care physician keeps the capitation payment, the specialist takes over the patient's treatment, and public insurance pays a fee-for-service amount to the specialist.

Both primary and specialist physicians have reason to transfer diagnostic expenses to hospitals, especially when ambulatory diagnostics are underdeveloped or have a long waiting list. Patients, who eagerly accept hospital referrals, contribute to this situation. Despite attempts to limit the number of admissions, the number of hospitalized patients has increased greatly, as has the amount of hospital diagnostic testing. The contracts signed by ambulatory care physicians as well as those signed by hospitals create hidden incentives for cost shifting.

These comprehensive capitated payment plans, resembling managed care in the United States, have caused many conflicts between primary and specialist physicians. Primary care physicians created their own network of service providers, paying for the specialists' work and supervising them. This supervision, a type of utilization review, has brought many complaints from specialists. Very soon all capitation fees will cover primary medical care and an extended range of diagnostics. Some primary care physicians, having funds for a wide range of services, have been motivated to limit the number of referrals. These restrictions are seen as threats to the quality of care, particularly given the lack of standards and of treatment monitoring. Strong protests and lobbying by specialists have resulted in a number of changes, but it is unlikely that the problems of cost shifting and quality deterioration will go away soon.

16.6 HIGH-INCOME COUNTRIES

Among high-income countries, there is considerable variation in the use of medical care inputs (doctors per 1,000 population ranging from 1.4 to 4.3; hospital beds per 1,000 ranging from 3.9 to 16.1), organization of services, reliance on taxpayer financing, and total cost (from $450 to $4,500 per capita) but remarkably little variation in health outcomes. Life expectancy in the 22 high-income countries is between 76 and 81 years, and infant mortality is between four and eight per 1,000 births. Much greater variation in health statistics exists between regions within any one of these countries than across all 22 of them. Given the small differences in average health outcomes, it is difficult to say that one country's system is better or worse than another's. What is clear is that many health problems are concentrated in specific underserved populations, usually ethnic minorities or areas of extreme poverty.[17] Although tremendous resources are available for advanced experimental treatment, electronic scanning for diagnosis, and long-term rehabilitation, there is still a lack of primary care resources ensuring that every child is immunized, that all pregnant women receive adequate prenatal care, and that every person has a primary physician to contact when in need of advice or care. In many ways, high-income countries face the same problems of maldistribution and misallocation in the delivery of medical care as low-income countries, but at a different level (see Figure 16.8).

FIGURE 16.8   Health Expenditures and Life Expectancy across Countries

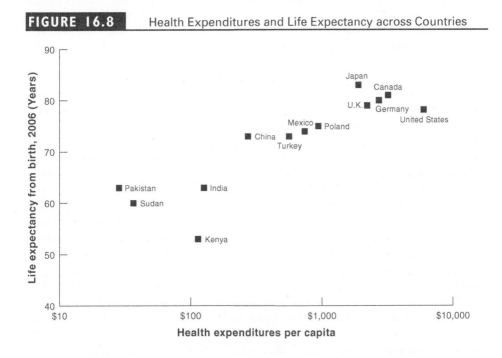

TABLE 16.6   Japan's Health Expenditures in 2010 by Type of System and by Fund

Source of Funding	Million Yen	Million Dollars	Contribution (%)
By Type of System			
Health care insurance	17,337	216.71	*48.1*
Advanced Elderly Medical Service System	11,031	137.88	*30.6*
Out of pocket	4,993	62.41	*13.9*
Public expense	2,406	30.08	*6.7*
Other	241	3.01	*0.7*
Total	36,007	450.09	*100.0*
By Source of Payment			
Insured person	10,182	127.28	*28.3*
National government	9,127	114.09	*25.3*
Employer	7,321	91.51	*20.3*
Patient sharing and other sources	5,011	62.63	*13.9*
Local government	4,366	54.58	*12.1*
Total	36,007	450.09	*100.0*

Health Care in Japan*

Japan's health care system provides comprehensive universal coverage, including free choice of health care providers by patients. Patients may choose a medical institution and visit a specialist without a referral from a primary care physician. Life expectancy in Japan is among the longest in the world, 78 years for men and 85 for women, making issues of aging of greater importance. In 2011, 23.1 percent of the population was 65 years or older and 11.4 percent was above 75. Despite this aging demography, Japanese health care expenditures as a percentage of GDP were 8.5 percent in 2008, lower than the OECD average of 8.8 percent, and much lower than the 16.8 percent in the United States.

Japan's Health Expenditures by Types and by Fund   Japanese health care expenditure in 2009 is estimated as ¥36,007 billion (yen) ($450.10 million converted at ¥80 per U.S. dollar, see Table 16.6), up 3.4 percent from the previous fiscal year.[18] The estimates of health care expenditure per capita were ¥282,400 ($3,530.00). In 2010, 48.1 percent of Japan's health expenditures came from health care insurance, followed by 30.6 percent from the Advanced Elderly Medical Service system. The medical fee paid by patients was 13.9 percent, and public expenses were a mere 6.7 percent. By funding, 28.3 percent of the expenditures came from the insured person, 20.3 percent from the employer, 13.9 percent from patient sharing, and national and local governments paid 25.3 percent and 12.1 percent, respectively.

There are six health insurance programs: two National Health Insurance programs (municipality controlled and country controlled), Japan Health Insurance Association, association- or union-administrated insurance, mutual aid associations, and the Advanced Elderly Medical Service system (see Table 16.7). The municipality controlled National Health Insurance, consisting of 1,723 insurers run by municipality, has the largest number of members (35.66 million members), and Japan Health Insurance Association, run by public companies, has the second largest number of members (29.95 million members). The premium rate of societies ranges from 3 percent to 10 percent of monthly wages (with a ceiling), shared equally by employees and employers. The Advanced Elderly Medical Service System has the highest average age of 81.9 years, and the municipality-controlled National Health Insurance has the second highest average age of 49.5 years old. The average age of the rest of insurers is below 40 years old. The age gaps between insurance programs have become a social issue that is discussed

*This section was prepared by Hirohisa Shimura, adjunct professor at Temple University, Japan.

TABLE 16.7	Characteristics of Health Insurance Plans in Japan					

		National Health Insurance				
	Municipality Controlled	Country Controlled	Japan Health Insurance Association	Association or Union	Mutual Aid Association	Advanced Elderly Medical Service System
Number of insurers	1,723	165	1	1,473	83	47
Number enrolled (millions)	35.7	3.4	35.0	30.0	9.0	14.0
Average age in FY2009	49.5	38.9	36.2	33.9	33.4	81.9
Average Income						
Per person (¥)	910,000	3,470,000	1,390,000	1,950,000	2,360,000	800,000
Per person ($)	11,375.00	43,375.00	17,375.00	24,375.00	29,500.00	10,000.00
Per household (¥)	1,580,000	7,430,000	2,450,000	3,700,000	4,790,000	N/A
Per household ($)	19,750.00	92,875.00	30,625.00	46,250.00	59,875.00	N/A
Average Premium						
Per person (¥)	83,000	124,000	86,000	133,000	135,000	63,000
Per household ($)	1,037.50	1,550.00	1,075.00	1,662.50	1,687.50	787.50
Including employers' contribution	N/A	N/A	152,000	N/A	N/A	N/A
Healthcare Expenses						
Per person (¥)	290,000	171,000	152,000	133,000	135,000	882,000
Per person ($)	3,625	2,138	1,900	1,663	1,688	11,025

later. Health care insurance premiums are based on income and ability to pay, but there is direct contribution from employers for municipality- and country-controlled national health insurance. The average premium per person varies from ¥63,000 ($787.50) per person to ¥124,000 ($1,550.00) per person, depending on program to which the person belongs. Regarding the health expenses per member, the Advanced Elderly Medical Service System has the highest expenditure of ¥882,000 ($11,025.00) per person, followed by the municipality-run National Health Insurance of ¥290,000 ($3,625) per person.

Copayment System Based on Age Group   In principle, medical services are provided to insured persons in the form of actual treatment rather than a cash reimbursement. The Japanese insurance system consists of 3,500 plans according to the person's place of residence and employment. There are uniform copayment rate systems except for elderly persons and children. There are four different copayment schedules based on age group. If a patient is yet to start compulsory education or is younger than 6 years, the copayment is 20 percent; and if a patient is between 6 and 69 years old, the copayment is 30 percent. In some prefectures, children up to 15 years of age or to the end of compulsory education pay nothing. If a patient is older than 70 years, the copayment is 10 percent for those with income below a specified limit, and 30 percent for those with income above the limit. (Before 2008 there were rates for persons aged 70 to 74 and those aged 75 or more, but now both groups of elderly are treated the same and subject to the income test). Subsidies for high-cost medical treatment are available to lessen the financial burden on the patient. Once the patient has paid the copayment, the government subsidizes the amount exceeding a fixed monthly limit, which is determined by income level. For example, if a patient between 15 and 64 years old and under the middle-income bracket spends the monthly medical expense of ¥1 million ($12,500), the patient pays 30 percent of the medical expense to the medical institution. The individual limit in this case is calculated as ¥87,430 (80,100 + (1,000,000 − 267,000) × 1%) or ($1,092.88), and the government pays ¥221,570 ($2,769.63) back to the patient.

Biannual Fee Schedule Review for Medical Treatment and Reimbursement Price

Once a patient is treated, the total medical service fees are calculated based on the Rules to Calculate Treatment Fees set by the Minister of Health, Labor, and Welfare (MHLW). These rules provide a point value assigned for each of the thousands of medical procedures, including medication and injection, and the list of reimbursement prices for drugs permitted under health insurance programs. The medical institution where the patient is treated applies for reimbursement of actual treatment fees after subtracting the amount paid directly by patients. The central government revises health services, drug prices, and a fee schedule every two years.

Many Challenges Ahead from Demographic Changes

Limited Generics Penetration.   A key challenge for sustaining the current universal coverage program in Japan is cost containment. An obvious policy is to promote generic drugs. Japan is the second largest pharmaceutical industry in the world and the use of generic medication is the lowest among Organization for Economic Cooperation and Development (OECD) member nations. According to data from the MHLW, sales share of generics was 7.6 percent and volume share of generics was 20.2 percent in September 2009. One factor that explains the low generic penetration was the existence of so-called long-term listed drugs. In Japan, Japanese pharmaceutical companies continue to sell their original products even after the patent expires, and sales of long-term listed drugs are often much greater than the generics. Sales shares of long-term listed drugs were 35.9 percent and volume share was 36.3 percent in September, 2009. The Japanese government has made several initiatives: two dispensing format changes in 2006 and 2008 and two incentive schemes to encourage pharmacists to change from patented original drugs to generics in 2008 and 2010. Because of these government efforts, the generic penetration rate in volume gradually increased from 15.4 percent in March 2006 to 22.7 percent in September 2011.

Financial Adjustment among Insurers and Introduction of the Public Long-Term Care Insurance Program.   The rapid aging of the Japanese population shifted the relative costs and subsidies of medical care across insurance plans. The introduction of the Long-Term Care Insurance Program and the Advanced Elderly Medical Service System was intended to correct these imbalances, along with other health system reforms and changes to the hospital reimbursement system.

All medical costs for the elderly were provided free of charge from 1973 to 1983. Because free medical care for the elderly resulted in a long-term deficit in the health insurance system, an imbalance in the contributions for medical costs of the elderly between the different health insurance programs due to differences in the proportion of elderly persons covered under each program became a big social issue. In 1982, the government introduced the Health Services for the Elderly Act to introduce a financial redistribution system by which medical costs for the elderly are shared fairly by public funding and contributions from individual insurance programs. This act alleviated the burden on the National Health Insurance, which had a high percentage of elderly insured.

Changes in family function and burden of home care on families due to the rapidly growing elderly population also became a social issue. In response to the increase in bedridden elderly and elderly people with dementia, the Long-Term Care Insurance Program was launched in April 2000 to provide care services on a community-wide basis. The system is managed by the city, with the premiums paid by residents who are 40 years old and older and public funds (taxes) used as revenue.

Introduction of the Advanced Elderly Medical Service System.   Even after the medical costs for the elderly were shared equally among insurers, contributions from insurers of employees have risen rapidly to cover the increase in the elderly population. The government introduced the Advanced Elderly Medical Service System in 2008. The system required the elderly aged 75 or older to pay a premium and a 10 percent copayment; 50 percent of the charge is covered by public expenditures and 40 percent by contributions from insurers of other insurance programs. The system is managed by wide-area cooperatives at the prefecture level, but the municipalities collect the premiums.

Cost Containment Implementation at Hospitals.   The average length of hospital stay is the highest among OECD nations (18.5 days, compared to 5.4 days in the United States). Two issues are related to this lengthy stay at hospitals: Elderly patients often stay at hospitals as an alternative to nursing care homes, and turnover of patients is low. To resolve the issue of social stays, the government introduced Long-Term Care Insurance in 2000.

To resolve the low turnover of patients, the Japanese government introduced the fixed fee basis system, called the Diagnosis Procedure Combination (DPC) system, which is similar to the Diagnosis Related Group/Prospective Payment System (DRG/PPS), beginning in April 2003. Under the DPC system, payment is on a fixed basis per day for each treatment, and if the actual length of stay exceeds the basic length of hospital stay, profitability could deteriorate.

The Health System in Germany*

The health care system in Germany has its roots in legislation initiated by Chancellor Bismarck in 1883 that made enrolment in pay-as-you-go sickness funds mandatory for certain groups of workers nationwide. This system of statutory social insurance financed by payroll taxes, has since been greatly expanded to include more and more groups of workers and now covers more than 90 percent of Germany's population. The remaining 9 percent have chosen private insurance. The objectives of the **social insurance system** are equality in access to medical care and a progressive distribution of the financial burden. Social insurance contributions are made through sickness funds (Krankenkassen) and set at a fixed percentage (15.5 percent) of gross wages, approximately half of which is deducted in the form of a payroll tax and half of which is paid by the insured to the sickness fund of his or her choice.

After the reunification of East Germany and West Germany in 1990, **the share of GDP** devoted to health rose to more than 10 percent, but it has been stable below or **around 11 percent since 1995.** As unemployment continued to rise until 2005, the government sought to limit the impact of health spending on nonwage labor costs by superimposing, in January 2009, a new national health fund (Gesundheitsfonds) that combines all revenue from the 15.5 percent payroll tax on the insured's gross wages with annual infusions from the government's budget and distributes the money among the 146 autonomous sickness funds that remain at the core of the statutory system. **Enrollees in the statutory system still make a personal choice for one of the sickness funds**, with family dependents without significant income of their own, such as homemaking spouses and underage children, covered free of extra charges.

Introduction of the health fund was part of a much broader reform effort that was implemented through the 2007 Gesetz zur Stärkung des Wettbewerbs in der gesetzlichen Krankenversicherung (GKV-WSG) and intended to foster competition within the health system and help to contain costs. Ninety-five percent of each sickness fund's expenditure must be covered by the flow of money from the health fund; in 2009, a flat monthly base payment of 185.64 per insured, and **an adjustment that depends on the insured's categorization into one of 152 risk groups**, including 40 age and sex categories, six earnings capacity categories, and 106 morbidity categories, which in turn are based on 80 well-defined chronic conditions, such as HIV/AIDS, diabetes, and schizophrenia, and in some cases differentiate the severity of the condition. For

---

*This section was contributed by Dr. Michael Stolpe, Kiel Institute for the World Economy and University of Kiel.

example, the adjustment for an insured man between the ages of 85 and 89 years is +€1.28, for dementia +€86.87, and for hypertension +€38.48, so that the total adjustment where all three conditions are met amounts to +€312.27. For younger people, the age adjustments are negative. In the case of a girl between the ages of 13 and 17 it is only −€117.45 as long as she does not suffer from a chronic condition. The Federal Insurance Office updates these adjustments as well as the base payments every year in line with changes in the underlying morbidity categories, although changes tend to be small. This morbidity-based risk adjustment scheme, nicknamed Morbi-RSA in German, is meant to eliminate the incentives for positive risk selection that Germany's sickness funds had under the previous rudimentary risk equalization system that was based only on the insured's age and sex. Under that plan, cream skimming, by providing inconvenient service for the chronically ill and by offering attractive extra services for the young and healthy, was a successful strategy. Free aerobics classes and health food cooking courses proved particularly popular.

Although sickness funds still use more than 90 percent of their budget for a long list of legally mandated medical services with little scope for product differentiation, the new law gives them much greater leeway to offer extra services, incentive plans for enrollees, and elements of managed care in relation to care providers. For example, all sickness funds are now required to offer at least two different elective contracts, one of which must offer reduced patient copayments in exchange for a binding agreement to see a registered primary physician, who acts as a gatekeeper, before consulting any specialist or a hospital (Hausarztmodell). In addition, sickness funds are allowed to offer contracts with retrospective bonus payments to the insured in exchange for pre-agreed deductibles. At the other end of the spectrum, sickness funds are allowed to offer supplementary insurance that may cover direct consultations with a specialist practitioner or expensive drugs not covered by the standard contract in exchange for a supplementary premium. Sickness funds can also design their own disease management programs for the chronically ill and make special deals with preferred providers, such as hospitals, rehabilitation clinics, pharmacies, and medical practitioner networks, that did not exist before.

All sickness funds whose expenditures exceed the income received from the health fund must charge a supplementary premium directly to their enrollees. However, the supplementary premium may not exceed one percent of the insured's income, or €8 per month in the absence of means testing. The insureds have the right to switch to another sickness fund in order to avoid paying the supplementary premium. Now sickness funds are allowed to go bankrupt, in which case the insureds are protected because they are seamlessly transferred to some other sickness fund of their choice.

The Morbi-RSA has been criticized for introducing incentives to manipulate the coding of medical diagnoses with the aim of obtaining more money from the central health fund. Some sickness funds reportedly pay doctors around €10 per case to provide "more detailed" diagnoses in the hope that more detail could justify claiming a chronic condition or a higher level of severity in one of the 80 predefined conditions that trigger the morbidity-based supplementary payments to the sickness fund. Diabetes mellitus, for example, triggers an annual supplementary payment per insured patient of €794 if it is diagnosed without any or with unspecified complications, but it triggers a payment of €1,825 if diagnosed with ophthalmologic manifestations, €2,022 with acute complications, €2,161 with neurologic or peripheral circulatory manifestations, and €2,887 with renal manifestations. Diagnoses follow the money, say the critics, raising the suspicion that sickness funds will want to reward expensive treatments and introduce innovative disease management programs that attract patients in financially attractive Morbi-RSA categories, at the expense of patients suffering diseases that are less profitable from the sickness funds' perspective. Doctors would have an incentive to collude, because treating more severe conditions is often more generously remunerated under the statutory system's new payment scheme for physicians' services. Hence, if the Morbi-RSA sets some of its morbidity adjustment payments too high, it could trigger the opposite of cream skimming: a hunt for the sickest.

Private health insurance is confined to the self-employed, civil servants, and the relatively small number of workers making more than approximately €50,000 per year who are allowed to opt out of the statutory system. Since 2009, the law requires every German to have full health insurance coverage, eliminating the approximately 200,000 who were previously uninsured in Germany. Anybody caught at a doctor's office or in a hospital without insurance may be fined and required to pay up to five years' worth of health insurance premiums. Private insurers assess premiums on the basis of the age, sex, and individual health risks of an applicant, who usually must answer a long health-related questionnaire and often undergo a medical examination.

After signing a contract, an insurer cannot unilaterally change its terms in response to changing health risks of the individual; the insurance promise is for the rest of the insured's life, and premiums are allowed to rise only by the same percentage as the general rise in medical care prices. In a similar vein, people opting for private insurance cannot revert to the statutory social insurance plan, but must remain with private insurance for the rest of their lives.

For those aged 55 years and older who can no longer bear the premiums for an existing health insurance contract, the new law requires all private insurers to offer a basic contract (Basistarif) that covers the same set of services covered in the statutory system. Because all people not in the statutory system must purchase private health insurance, the Basistarif is regulated to charge no more than the maximum wage-based premium in the statutory system, approximately €590 per month, regardless of individual health risks. Another regulated contract with similar conditions is offered for pensioners. These rules provide some protection against overestimating one's personal-earnings capacity at older ages or underestimating the rise in premiums that the generous care package of an insured's original private insurance contract might imply.

The government's aim of ruling out that any privately insured person ever moves back into the statutory system has not been fully achieved. Loopholes continue to exist for privately insured workers who become unemployed or accept (temporary) work remunerated below the ceiling of wage-income taxed in the statutory system.

The fee for medical services that private insurers reimburse can be three times higher than the official prices listed in the Federal Health Minister's list. Therefore doctors prefer to treat patients with private insurance. To lure them, waiting times in the physician's office tend to be shorter and treatment is sometimes more generous than for the socially insured. Many private health insurance plans provide strong financial incentives to refrain from seeing a doctor for small, self-limiting health problems. If an insured person makes no claims during a given year, many plans refund up to half of the annual premium payments. Because income is positively correlated with health status, the privately insured tend to be healthier and utilize medical services less frequently than the enrollees of statutory sickness funds. To foster consumer choice and competition, insurers are allowed to offer, in addition to regular full-coverage plans, a type of supplemental insurance, mainly used to upgrade the level of hospital amenities or dental care, to enrollees of any sickness fund.

There is still a relatively **strict separation of ambulatory care from hospital care in Germany**, but cooperation and competition between the two sectors is increasing. For example, hospitals are getting involved in outpatient care for chronically sick patients, such as cancer and AIDS patients, living at home. Moreover, the elderly have the right to rehabilitation services after an injury or disease that might otherwise prevent them from returning to their homes. Only one-third of doctors in the ambulatory sector are general practitioners, whereas two-thirds are specialists with their own private practices. Independent specialists often invest heavily in diagnostic and surgical technology, sometimes setting up their own clinics to rival the services offered by small hospitals. This high degree of medical specialization in ambulatory care has long been encouraged by Germany's system of **fee-for-service** payments. New technology creates more and more billable events, and patients are free to take themselves to any office-based physician but not to a hospital.

Remuneration for the individual physician treating statutory patients is a combination of fee-for-service and prospective health-status related payments. To prevent supplier-induced demand, the full price is paid only for services within predetermined volume limits (Regelleistungsvolumina) that are specific to each doctor or group practice and depend on the type of medical specialization, regional physician density, and morbidity of patients, approximated by age and sex. Additional selective contracting between individual doctors or groups of doctors and sickness funds is possible. However, many ambulatory care practitioners still rely on collective contracts, such as the Hausarztvertrag with individual sickness funds, which are negotiated by regional physician associations, called Kassenrztliche Vereinigungen, on their behalf. These associations also continue to allocate the funds to individual practitioners according to the official euro prices listed in the Federal Health Minister's list. Office-based physicians retain the opportunity to generate income from private patients.

The GKV-Versorgungsstrukturgesetz of 2011 tries to lure doctors into rural areas with low physician density by exempting them from volume limits. To counter physician oversupply in metropolitan agglomerations, the Kassenrztliche Vereinigungen have been given greater freedom to use financial incentives to induce elderly doctors to retire and to close down the offices of retiring doctors who do not have a qualified heir in their family.

German **hospitals** employ their own salaried physicians, and physicians in private practice do not have admitting privileges. However, chief physicians of German hospital departments have strong incentives to increase the amount and quality of care, because they are allowed to treat private patients and thereby supplement their personal income in proportion to the number of beds filled with patients with statutory insurance. Hospital reimbursement is generally according to a prospective payment (diagnostically related group, DRG) system that was implemented gradually between 2003 and 2005, accompanied by the obligation to publish regular quality audits. Most municipalities, especially in rural parts of Eastern Germany, have since seen their local public hospitals move into deficit. Also, because the municipalities find it difficult to make the investments that would move hospitals back into profit—for example, by improving quality and increasing specialization on a set of profitable hospital services—more and more hospitals have been put up for sale. This has created a profitable investment opportunity for the fast-growing private-sector hospital chains, especially those that can raise funds on the stock market. Private-sector hospital chains seem to be in a better position to make a profit under DRG because they can invest, restructure, and capture economies of scale from specialization and coordination among the different units in the chain. Some analysts predict that up to 40 percent of German hospital beds may be in private hands by 2015, compared to less than 15 percent in 2009. There is still a significant oversupply of hospital beds per capita, which has long encouraged the export of stationary care to foreign patients (mainly from Scandinavia and the United Kingdom, where rationing of hospital services has created long waiting lists for certain procedures).

In the **pharmaceutical sector** a *reference price* (set by the government) system limits drug spending. Sickness funds are required to reimburse retailers for part of the cost of any prescription drug that contains the chemical entity ordered by a medical practitioner for the insured; fixed reference prices are used for drugs with similar properties. The net effect on prices is unclear because drug competition almost collapsed as generic prices were brought into line with reference prices. Patient copayments are set at 10 percent of the price of the drug up to a maximum of €10 per refill. Some particularly low-priced drugs are dispensed without patient copayment. Sickness funds are free to negotiate volume and other rebates for branded prescription drugs directly with drug suppliers and to restrict reimbursement to one brand in each therapeutic category. This may be coupled with lower patient copayments or with a copayment waiver.

To further strengthen sickness funds' bargaining power vis-à-vis the pharmaceutical industry and prevent them from incurring steep cost increases for new drugs that might have only marginal improvements on the benefit side, comparative cost-effectiveness research has been given a much larger role than in the past. The mandate of the Cologne-based Institut für Qualität und Wirtschaftlichkeit im Gesundheitswesen (IQWiG), which since 2004 oversees and undertakes this type of research, has been extended so that it assesses not only the benefits of new drugs but also their costs. This enlarged mandate is likely to set an example for the handling of other issues in technology adoption of technologies and services in the future.

For new drugs, the Arzneimittelmarktneuordnungsgesetz (AMNOG), effective since January 2011, sets the rules for an interactive process of price setting on the basis of economic evaluations that is meant to be completed within six months upon market launch. Although initially free to set the price unilaterally, producers must submit a value dossier for each new drug to the G-BA, the key decision-making body within SHI made up of voting delegates from the Association of Statutory Sickness Funds, the Associations of Statutory Sickness Funds Physicians and Dentists, and the German Hospital Federation. The G-BA then asks IQWiG for an independent evaluation and organizes a hearing with the producer and outside experts before deciding whether the new drug provides sufficient incremental benefits, relative to existing therapies, to justify bilateral price negotiations between the producer and the G-BA taking these benefits into account. If no such incremental benefit is found, a nonnegotiable maximum reimbursement is determined by the reference price for existing drugs within the therapeutic class to which the new drug belongs. If no agreement is reached within six months, an arbitration panel, comprising the producer, the Association of Statutory Sickness Funds, and a neutral member, is given another three months to find a unanimous solution. Only if this also fails does the G-BA order IQWiG to perform a full cost-effectiveness analysis and decrees the drug's price on that basis. Producers may then challenge this price in court. In an extension of the original scope of AMNOG, Germany's private health insurers have persuaded the government to enforce the same rebates for private patients.

Although sickness funds' growing bargaining power vis-à-vis the pharmaceutical industry has resulted in substantial savings on generics over the past 20 years and might soon produce similar savings on new drugs, informed observers generally agree that many restrictions on sickness funds' ability to become efficient negotiators and buyers remain. Changing this would further undermine the corporatist cartel of ambulatory physicians and meet fierce resistance from this well organized and powerful political lobby. Should the government therefore choose to accommodate future hikes in per capita health expenditures by more generous infusions of general tax money, this would move the German system away from Bismarck's design of financially autonomous sickness funds.[19]

The Expensive Exception: The United States

In 1970, Denmark spent 7.9 percent of GDP on health care, and the United States spent just 7.0 percent. Since then, expenses have grown in every country, but they have soared far out of line in the United States. There has been a degree of convergence across the developed nations so that most spend between 8 percent and 12 percent of GDP on health care (Denmark spent $6,580 or 11.1 percent of GDP in 2010), with the notable exception of the United States, which rose to 18 percent in 2010. No other country spends as much on health care as the United States, yet the United States has still not been able to achieve the universal coverage that is standard in other developed countries, and life expectancy in the United States lags behind that of comparable countries.

Although the United States is considered to have the most "privatized" of major health systems, U.S. *government* spending on medical care exceeds that of every other country except

FIGURE 16.9   Female Life Expectancy at Age 50 Years: United States
Compared to 20 Countries 1980–2005

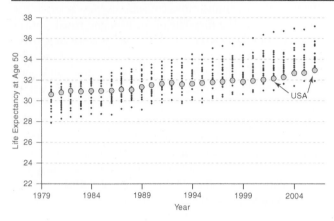

Luxembourg and Norway. The United States does not have more doctors or hospitals per capita than other developed countries. It ranks 22nd out of 23 countries in number of patient bed days per 1,000 population (only Greece is lower), ninth out of 14 in number of physician visits per person, and 12th out of 18 in number of prescriptions.[20] More important, the results of this very expensive care are hardly exceptional. Life expectancy at 78 years is lower than that of Canada (81), England (79), France (81), Germany (80), Sweden (81), Australia (82), or Japan (83) (see Figure 16.9).[21] American medicine does appear to be more dynamic and technology intensive, with more rapid introduction of new drugs, more tests, more complex surgical procedures, and more sophisticated diagnostic equipment. Health care in America also provides an extraordinarily wide range of insurance plans and contracts, whereas other countries might have only single national health insurance plan or a limited number of alternatives (although almost all countries offer free choice of physician). Although Americans express a desire for high-tech medicine with lots of choices and multiple insurance plans, they do not seem happy with what they get. Overall performance on a number of clinical and patient access measures is average or below average, and U.S. respondents' confidence and satisfaction with health care ranks in the bottom third in the Gallup World Poll.[22]

How were Canada, Japan and Europe able to keep health care costs so much lower than the United States while maintaining equal or better health outcomes and patient satisfaction? Many attempts to control costs in the United States have been motivated at the individual level, using deductibles and copayments to moderate demand, yet the use of pooled financing that protects patients from risks also insulates them from costs. Consumer choice does not lead to lower expenditures when consumers are spending someone else's money. European countries have operated largely on the supply side, constraining the provider system rather than individual demand. The number of health care workers and their wages has been limited and is often subject to nationwide bargaining and controls. Purchasing of expensive new diagnostic and therapeutic technology has been restricted.[23] Open-ended entitlements that reimburse patients for all bills have been avoided in favor of contracts for large groups of patients on a per-capita or fixed-budget basis. In analyzing the evolution of payment systems, it has been argued that the flaws of bureaucratic governmental control (lack of innovation and consumer responsiveness) and the flaws of insurance markets (lack of cost control and gaps in coverage) are leading toward a convergence of public and private in a blended contractual model, what is known in the United States as managed care (Chapter 5).[24] Government will be responsible for setting

TABLE 16.8	Procedure Prices Compared: Canada, Germany, United States				
			United States		
	Canada Average	Germany Average	Low (5th) Percentile)	Average	High (95th) Percentile)
Procedure					
CT scan, abdomen	$61	$374	$164	$536	$1,564
MRI	304	632	509	487	2,590
Cost per hospital day	340	554	1,595	3,612	14,306
Normal delivery	2,667	2,147	6,379	8,435	13,799
Appendectomy	3,810	3,286	7,758	13,123	25,344
Hip replacement	10,753	15,329	21,247	34,451	75,639
Coronary artery bypass graft	22,212	27,237	37,393	59,770	126,182
Physician Fees					
Routine office visit	$39	$15	$61	$86	$156
Cataract surgery*	502	560	632	954	2,210
Appendectomy*	356	271	647	959	2,072
Hip replacement*	815	679	2,008	2,834	5,280

*Included in procedure cost.
Source: International Federation of Health Plans, 2010 (2009 prices)

the rules and the overall limits on the amount to be spent and ensuring that everyone receives coverage, while market competition will be used to maintain the quality and amenity of services and provide local control. Four factors have been commonly cited as causes of higher spending in the United States[25]:

- Extensive use of the latest technological advances, even when benefits are marginal.
- Higher prices for medical procedures and for personnel (see Table 16.8).
- Administrative costs owing to multiple insurance plans and fragmented care.
- Lack of centralized cost control or expenditure regulation.

Whatever explains the lower cost and better statistics for health systems in other countries, it is clear that health care in the United States does not consistently provide more care or yield better results, and although it is very dynamic and high tech, it is also financially fragmented, managerially disorganized, and lacking in modern information technology. The public and patients express significant dissatisfaction with the current system, and expenditures are seriously out of line with what is spent in comparable systems in other countries.

16.7   INTERNATIONAL TRADE IN HEALTH CARE

Health care is among the world's largest industries, accounting for 10 percent of gross world product but only a tiny fraction of world trade. Products (drugs, equipment) are much more likely to be bought and sold across national boundaries than services. Although in principle there is no reason why an x-ray performed in Seoul cannot be read in San Francisco, licensure and other regulations currently make such international service flows difficult. Trade in services is usually limited to a small amount of border crossing—for example, when a Canadian citizen disgruntled with a long wait for elective surgery crosses into the United States or an uninsured Hispanic worker from Texas crosses to Mexico for cheaper hospital and physician care.[26] The part of the health care system most subject to international movement—trade in people and skills—does not appear in the world economic accounts.

People and Ideas

In stark contrast to the lack of international trade in medical services is the substantial movement of medical personnel and ideas across national boundaries. Most specialists in developing countries receive some of their training in Europe or the United States, bringing home skills of immense value. The extraordinary increase in life expectancy that has swept over the world is perhaps one of the greatest benefits of international trade. Information and scientific discoveries, as public goods, cannot be owned or charged for by a particular firm or country.

What is somewhat surprising is the extent of trade in the reverse direction—doctors and nurses who come to work in the United States from low-income countries. At its peak in 1978 more than half of all medical residents who were in training (and providing care) in urban U.S. teaching hospitals were foreign medical graduates. In the less remunerative and less attractive specialties, such as psychiatry, this is still the case today. More than 12 percent of all U.S. physicians are immigrant doctors. Similarly, a large number of licensed nurses were educated overseas. There are more Filipino nurses practicing in the United States and Canada than in the Philippines. This anomalous flow of highly trained labor from less-developed to more-developed countries has much to do with the economics of restrictions on labor supply and with the incentive structure created by the size of the market. Limits on the numbers of physicians and nurses imposed through the U.S. educational system mean that there is room for those who have received training overseas and are willing to work for less. Also, truly outstanding neurosurgeons are able to earn more in the United States than in Mexico, and they may be tempted to go where their skills command the highest reward, just as Latin baseball players and movie stars do. There is also a niche at the bottom of the market that attracts foreign labor. Caring for the elderly in nursing homes is so demanding and underpaid that it is difficult to find competent staff willing to work for the minimum wage. These positions are attractive to immigrants who are able to obtain steady employment and benefits in jobs that require a lot in the way of patience, endurance, and strength but not in language or education. The lack of dollar-denominated trade obscures the extent to which medicine and health became globalized in the 20th century.

Services

Health care is sharply demarcated at national boundaries. The U.S. Medicare program does not pay for operations in Mexico, nor will it cover Canadians who come to the United States. Therefore, the border-crossing trade in services that does occur is usually paid for privately. Private investment in the small fee-for-service or insured hospitals and clinics that exist alongside national health facilities in the United Kingdom, Sweden, and elsewhere is often international. The largest hospital in Singapore used to be owned by an American firm, National Medical Enterprises. Yet the true test of international trade in medical care looms in the proposals for full integration of service markets within the European Union. A Belgian patient might prefer heart surgery in one of the major Parisian hospitals, or a Swedish factory worker might decide to seek psychiatric care in Germany. Conversely, a German hospital would find it cheaper to obtain nurses or doctors from Greece and pay travel expenses rather than hire them locally. To date, every country has jealously guarded its health care system, and such freedom of choice is available only to a few employees of international companies.

Equipment

Medical equipment is less amenable to international trade because it cannot simply be packed in a box and shipped. Skilled technicians are required to maintain and use these sophisticated devices, and the ongoing labor costs are much larger than the manufacturing cost. Once a new technology is developed, it is usually produced and supported by a local firm or the local branch of a global firm within a few years.

Pharmaceuticals

The pharmaceutical trade is one of the world's truly global businesses (see Chapter 11). Drugs made in England or France cross pharmacy counters in the United States as readily as drugs made in Des Moines, and research is as likely to be conducted in Genoa or Geneva as it is in Georgia. Companies such as Rhone-Poulenc Rorer and AstraZeneca cross international boundaries and link major markets. Protectionist legislation still gives local firms an advantage, but it is common for more than 25 percent of a large pharmaceutical company's sales to occur outside the country where it is headquartered, and some, such as Ciba-Geigy, are mostly international. There are three major markets: Japan, the United States, and the European Union. The ability of Japanese doctors to profit from prescribing gave them the highest rate of prescription drug use in the world. Thus with only half as many consumers, the Japanese market was larger than the U.S. market in 1990 ($51 billion versus $48 billion). However, the decade-long recession in Japan has caused a relative decline even though the percentage of health expenditures spent on drugs there still exceeds that in the United States (16.8 percent versus 10.3 percent). The European Union accounted for about $40 billion, and all of the developing low- and middle-income countries accounted for $44 billion.[27]

Only the major market countries have the research infrastructure and a protected domestic market of sufficient size to cover the massive fixed costs of discovering and testing new drugs. Canada presents an interesting case. Because the nation lacked significant pharmaceutical development capacity, it decided to free-ride on the technology produced by the rest of the world. Canada refused to recognize the property rights created by patents and mandated that foreign companies license their drugs for manufacture or use in Canada in return for set royalty payments. This way the Canadians could obtain the benefits of research but not pay the cost. Vigorous protests eventually led to this system's being overturned, and now Canada recognizes international patent protection, as do other industrialized countries. However, free-riding is still the rule for many developing countries, either through mandatory licensing or simple failure to enforce patents, which allows local companies to make copycat versions of brand-name drugs. Clinical tests constitute a sizable portion of drug companies' costs and provide an interesting opportunity for international trade. By carrying out trials in a foreign country, a firm may be able to significantly reduce the cost per patient of developing a drug and might face lower liability from adverse reactions the experimental drug might produce.

One study showed how regulation of pharmaceutical prices in the European Union (one of the factors contributing to a lower cost of care) reduced profits of pharmaceutical companies in those countries, thus creating an incentive to move headquarters and R&D facilities into the United States.[28] EU citizens enjoyed lower pharmaceutical prices but lost some high-paying R&D jobs. The European share of pharmaceutical research dollars went from 24 percent above that of the United States ($4.8 billion versus $3.9 billion) in 1986 to 14 percent below ($26.8 billion versus $30.6 billion) in 2004. That is, the European pharmaceutical industry has continued to grow, but more expansive reimbursement overseas shifted a sizable part of that growth to the United States. The authors estimate that price regulation made European drugs 40 percent less expensive but shifted about 1,680 jobs from the European Union to the United States. The tradeoff between paying more for drugs and loss of jobs is inherently problematic. However, long-run growth in a dynamic global industry such as pharmaceuticals will inevitably tend to trail along the path of economic development in search of bigger markets and higher returns.

Although the future growth and evolution of the global pharmaceutical industry is inherently uncertain, past trends do allow some reasonable speculation. The United States has come to dominate the world pharmaceutical market to an increasing degree since 1950, but it is unlikely to continue to do so for the next 50 years. Previously the pharmaceutical industry had been centered in France, then Germany, and then England before moving to the United States. In each case, development of the pharmaceutical industry was preceded by growth in manufacturing, science, and industrial research. As global production moved toward America after World War II, so did the pharmaceutical companies, albeit with a lag. Europe and Japan retained strong pharmaceutical manufacturing centers long after their overall share of the global economy had begun to decline. Following the growth of the American economy and the extraordinarily generous reimbursements provided by an expensive open-ended health care system, a majority of the pharmaceutical industry had migrated to the United States by 2010. Just as the industry migrated from France and Germany as their economic power waned, it is likely to move on from the United States to the growing economic powerhouses of the 21st century: India and China.

SUGGESTIONS FOR FURTHER READING

OECD Health Data. www.oed.org

World Health Organization, *World Health Statistics 2011;* World Health Report 2010, 2012. www.who.int

Rupa Chandra, "Trade in Health Services," *Bulletin of the World Health Organization* 80, no. 2 (2002): 158–163.

David M. Cutler, "Equality, Efficiency and Market Fundamentals: The Dynamics of International Medical Care Reform," *Journal of Economic Literature* 40, no. 3 (2002): 881–906. "The Danish Health System through an American Lens," *Health Policy* 59, no. 2 (2002): 119–132.

Bruce J. Fried and Laura M. Gaydos, eds., *World Health Systems* (Chicago: AUPHA Press, 2002).

Alan Garber and Jonathan Skinner, "Is American Health Care Uniquely Inefficient?" *Journal of Economic Perspectives* 22, no. 4 (2008): 27–50.

Philip Musgrove, Riadh Zeramdini, and Guy Carrin, "Basic Patterns in National Health Expenditure," *Bulletin of the World Health Organization* 80, no. 2 (2002): 134–1146; www.who.org.

Wynand P. M. M. van de Ven and Frederik T. Schut, "Universal Mandatory Health Insurance in the Netherlands: A Model for the United States?" *Health Affairs* 27, no. 3 (2008): 771–781.

SUMMARY

1. There is a **tremendous disparity in health** between rich and poor nations. The poor countries of sub-Saharan Africa have very little health care and low life expectancies. Many people there die before the age of five years. The wealthier countries of Europe, North America, and Japan have more health resources to be applied to much less need. People in these countries have a longer life expectancy, with most deaths occurring after age 70 years.

2. Average **spending on health care is determined primarily by national income** per capita, not the health needs of individuals. Increased per capita income is also a major factor explaining increased life expectancy.

3. More health expenditures usually mean more health professionals and more use of technology, not more visits to physicians or days in the hospital. It is the **intensity of service, rather than quantity**, that increases as spending is increased.

4. **The United States is the world's largest health care market**, accounting for 40 percent of all health expenditures, even though it has only 5 percent of the world's population. U.S. health expenditures per person are 10 times the worldwide average and 100 times the average per person in India. With more than 15 percent of the world's population, India accounts for less than 1 percent of the global health care market.

5. Significantly **higher medical expenditures do not** appear to have made U.S. citizens significantly healthier. U.S. life expectancy ranks about in the middle of developed high-income countries.

6. The curve depicting the relationship between national income per capita and life expectancy has shifted upward over time. This illustrates the productive impact of **new knowledge** as well as the **transmission of that knowledge** across national boundaries.

7. The **distribution of income** across people and social groups, as well as the average, is important in explaining differences in health and life expectancy.

8. **Lack of organization, maldistribution, and political instability** are perhaps even more important than low income in causing poor health among many low-income countries. Even in middle- and high-income countries, many of the worst health problems result from the uneven distribution of health care and an inability to effectively target care to those most in need.

9. Most countries assert that their health care systems emphasize **primary care**, but their **funding favors specialty training and tertiary hospital care**.

10. **Cost control** in Europe, constraining supply and putting limits on the system as a whole, appears to have been more effective than in the United States. Japan's inexpensive health care system is much less technology-intensive than that of the United States, using only a third as much surgery but more drugs.

11. There is very little **international trade** in health care services. Global trade in health care is dominated by pharmaceuticals. However, the invisible trade in knowledge and health professionals has the largest effect on national health care systems.

PROBLEMS

1. {*flow of funds*} How many people are there in the world today? What fraction of them live in high-income developed economies? What fraction of total health expenditures is accounted for by high-income countries?

2. {*flow of funds*} How much is spent per person on health care in China? How much is spent per person on health care in the United States? In the United Kingdom? What are the primary factors accounting for these differences?

3. {*market size*} What is the largest global health care market?

4. {*correlation vs. causality*} Is more spending on health care associated with more health?

5. {*incidence*} As an officer of the World Health Organization with a budgetary allocation of $100 million, which programs would you fund if you wanted to make the greatest impact on health, measured as the increase in life expectancy multiplied by the number of people affected?

6. {*nominal vs. real*} Mexico spends less than a tenth as much per person on health care as the United States. Does it have more than or less than a tenth as many hospital beds? Physicians? Is the real amount of health care provided overestimated or underestimated by dollar comparisons? Why?

7. {*international trade*} Which types of health care labor are most likely to be traded between countries? Why?

8. {*international trade*} Which types of health care goods are most likely to be traded between countries? Are there more or fewer barriers to trade in health care than in other sectors?

9. {*trade*} Which aspects of medical care are most international? Which are the most parochial?

ENDNOTES

1. World Health Organization, World Health Report 2002, http://www.who.int/whr/2002/en.
2. In converting local expenditures and income into U.S. dollars, two methods are used. The value in local currency can be converted using the foreign exchange rate (the rate at which dollars are traded for local currency in the market) or it can be converted in terms of purchasing power parity (PPP), the amount required to purchase an equivalent amount of goods and services. In India, GNP per capita was $880 measured in terms of foreign exchange, but it was $2,460 in terms of the value of goods. This is largely because the cost of food, transportation, and so on is much lower than the price of such goods in the United States, converted at the currency market exchange rate. Whereas 100 rupees = $2.07, that amount cannot buy a good meal in the United States, but it would be sufficient to purchase more than three good meals in India.
3. The World Bank, *World Development Report 1993: Investing in Health* (New York: Oxford University Press for the World Bank, 1993). This report provides comparative data on a number of health issues not available elsewhere, and thus it is used here despite the age of the data (mostly from 1990). Making comparisons requires not only that the data exist but also that the data be made comparable in terms of definitions, time periods, etc., a tremendous task for 191 countries.
4. Victor Fuchs, "The Health Sector's Share of the Gross National Product," *Science* 247, no. 4942 (1990): 534–538.
5. Mark Pauly, "When Does Curbing Health Costs Really Help the Economy?" *Health Affairs* 14, no. 2 (1995): 68–82.
6. Thomas Getzen, "Population Aging and the Growth of Health Expenditures," *Journal of Gerontology* 47, no. 3 (1992): S98–S104.
7. Thomas E. Getzen, "An Income-Weighted International Average for Comparative Analysis of Health Expenditures," *International Journal of Health Planning and Management* 6, no. 1 (1991): 3–22.
8. Samuel H. Preston, *Fatal Years: Child Mortality in Late Nineteenth-Century America* (Princeton: Princeton University Press, 1991).
9. G. B. Rodgers, "Income and Inequality as Determinants of Mortality: An International Cross-Section Analysis," *Population Studies* 33, no. 2 (1979): 343–351; The World Bank, *Population Change and Economic Development* (New York: Oxford University Press, 1985).
10. The World Bank, *World Development Report 1993: Investing in Health* (New York: Oxford University Press for the World Bank, 1993).
11. Catriona Waddington, "Economics and Financial Management: What Do District Managers Need to Know?" WHO Series on Making Health Systems Work, working paper no. 6 (Geneva: World Health Organization, 2006).
12. Zineeldine Alidrissi, Summary Report of the Establishment of the Sudan Health Economics Unit, planning section, Sudan Federal Ministry of Health, November 7, 2002.
13. China National Health Development Research Center, *2010 Report on the Total Expenditure of Health in China* (Beijing: Peking University Health Science Center, 2011).
14. China Ministry of Health, *Statistics on China Health System Development in 2010* (Beijing: Center for Health Information and Statistics, 2011).
15. Milton Roemer, *National Health Systems of the World* (New York: Oxford University Press, 1991), 345–351.
16. Katarzyna Tymowska, "Health Care Under Transformation in Poland," *Health Policy* 56, no. 2 (2001): 85–98.
17. WHO Regional Office, European Health Report 2002, http://www.euro.who.int/europeanhealthreport.
18. Naoki Ikegami et al., "Japanese Universal Health Coverage: Evolution, Achievements, and Challenges," *The Lancet* 378, no. 9796 (2011): 1106–1115. Ministry of Health, Labor and Welfare, "Status of Insurance and Pensions," *Japanese Health and Welfare Statistics* 57, (2010): 46–47; *Basic Data about Health Insurance*, 52nd ed. (Tokyo: Ministry of Health, Labor and Welfare, 2007); Council for the Reform of Health System for Elders, *Cost Burden* (Tokyo: Ministry of Health, Labor and Welfare, 2010).
19. For an introduction to this debate, see Banafsheh Siadat and Michael Stolpe, "Reforming Health Care Finance: What Can Germany Learn from Other Countries?" Kiel Economic Policy Paper 5, Institut fr Weltwirtschaft an der Universitaet Kiel 2005, http://www.ifw-kiel.de/pub/kepp/2005/kepp05.pdf.
20. OECD Health Data (Paris: OECD, 2012). www.oecd.org.
21. Eileen M. Crimmins, Samuel H. Preston, Barney Cohen, eds, *Explaining Divergent Levels of Longevity in High-Income Countries*. (Washington, D.C., National Academies Press, 2011), 19 (Figure 1.8); Peter A Muenning and Sherry A Glied, "What Changes in Survival Rates Tell Us About US Health Care." *Health Affairs* 29, no. 11 (2010): 2105–2113.
22. Cathy Schoen et al., "Toward Higher Performance Health Systems: Adults' Health Care Experiences in Seven Countries, 2007," *Health Affairs* 26, no. 6 (2007): w717–w734; Angus Deaton, "Income, Aging, Health and Wellbeing Around the World: Evidence from the Gallup World Poll," NBER working paper #13317, August 2007.
23. Dale A. Rublee, "Medical Technology in Canada, Germany and the United States: An Update," *Health Affairs* 13, no. 4 (1994): 113–117.
24. Wynand P. Van De Ven and Frederik Schut, "Managed Competition in the Netherlands: Still Work-in-Progress," *Health Economics* 18, no. 3 (2009): 253–255; Jeremy Hurst, *The Reform of Health Care: A Comparative Analysis*

of Seven OECD Countries (Paris: OECD, 1992), 140–151. See also Alan Maynard and Karen Bloor' "Introducing a Market to the United Kingdom's National Health Service," *New England Journal of Medicine* 334, no. 9 (1996): 604–608, 1996. Anna Wilde Mathews, "The Future of U.S. Health Care." *Wall Street Journal* December 12, 2011: B1.

25. McKinsey Global Institute, *Why Americans Spend More,* December 2008; Alan Garber and Jonathan Skinner, "Is American Health Care Uniquely Inefficient?" *Journal of Economic Perspectives* 22, no. 4 (2008): 27–50; Jonathan Skinner and Douglas Staiger, "Technology Diffusion and Productivity Growth in Health Care," NBER working paper #14865, April 2009. Dante Morra et. al., "U.S. Physician Practices Versus Canadians: Spending Nearly Four Times As Much Money Interacting With Payers," *Health Affairs* 30, no. 8 (2011): 1443–1450; MJ Laugesen SA Glied, "Higher Fees Paid to US Physicians Drive Higher Spending," *Health Affairs* 30, no. 9 (2011): 1647–1656. Randall Cebul et. al., "Organizational Fragmentation and Care Quality in the U.S. Health Care System," NBER working paper #14212, 2008.

26. Theo Francis, "Medical Tourism Is Still Small," *Wall Street Journal,* May 6, 2008: D2.

27. The World Bank, *World Development Report 1993: Investing in Health* (New York: Oxford University Press for the World Bank, 1993), 145; Organisation for Economic Cooperation and Development: *OECD Health Data 2002* (Paris: OECD, 2002).

28. Joseph H. Golec and John A. Vernon, "European Pharmaceutical Price Regulation, Firm Profitability, and R&D Spending," NBER working paper #12676, November 2006; Eddy van Doorslaer et al., "Equity in the Delivery of Health Care in Europe and the U.S.," *Journal of Health Economics* 19, no. 5 (2000): 553–583.

CHAPTER 17

ECONOMIC EVALUATION OF HEALTH POLICY: THE PATIENT PROTECTION AND AFFORDABLE CARE ACT OF 2010

QUESTIONS

1. Which is a better model for national health reform, Massachusetts or Mississippi?
2. How much does it cost someone with a preexisting condition to buy health insurance?
3. Is the problem rising costs or the distribution of costs?
4. How long does it take to determine if a policy has met its objectives?
5. Did the changes in Obamacare prior to passage make it stronger or weaker?
6. Which companies stand to benefit from PPACA? Which companies are likely to lose?
7. Will insurance profits be increased, decreased, or stabilized under the act?
8. Does a rise in costs make the difference between mean and median household incomes more or less important?
9. "Defined contribution" plans define the risks for whom?

The "Patient Protection and Affordable Care Act of 2010" (Public Law 111-152, 111th Congress, also known as **"PPACA,"** the **"ACA,"** or "Obamacare") could be the most important health care legislation since the enactment of Medicare and Medicaid in 1965—or not. The intent of PPACA is to extend health insurance to almost all persons in the United States, make health insurance work better, control the cost of medical care, and incidentally avoid social, fiscal, and political catastrophe. That ambitious agenda is embedded in a long, complex, and dense document. If (a big if) PPACA marks a major turning point in the development of the U.S. health care system, only a few parts of the 974 pages of legalese in the law will prove to be of major importance, and the law will subsequently be found by courts or administrators to imply elements that are not discernable today, as was the case with Medicare, Medicaid, and most other major legislation.

This chapter is different from the others in this textbook. Instead of teaching you about incentives for moral hazard, hospital mergers, or pharmaceutical research, it illustrates some ways that economic concepts, models, and data might be used to construct a term paper on the assignment "evaluate PPACA." It is a bit more how-to and inevitably drifts into discussion of political and moral value judgments because this act is about health care, emergency care, medical bankruptcy, transplants, birth control, and the life-and-death choice of treatment, issues for which values and politics simply cannot be avoided as they are integral to making a decision. The big question left unanswered at the end of Chapter 5 was *"How much medicine can we afford and who will pay?"* Behind that were a series of unresolved issues: the uninsured, unfunded retiree plans, cost-shifting, price transparency, defined benefits or defined services, cancer drugs, organ transplants, disability, long-term care, and our willingness as citizens to pay for all these services through taxes or premiums.

The first task is to simply describe the major elements of PPACA. The historical background can then be used to frame the core problems the act is intended to address. This inevitably raises questions regarding the value of insurance and who should bear the risks.

17.1 PPACA 2010: DESCRIPTION OF MAIN ELEMENTS

The act is 974 pages long and contains many clauses, subclauses, exceptions, and transition rules. The first step is to obtain a copy (.pdf) of the act from one of the official U.S. government websites and some brief synopses or guides because the act is too long and complex to understand in less than 1,000 hours if you are starting from scratch.[1] Take care that the "guides" that you rely on are reasonably objective, and that you know the biases of the group putting out the guide.

This chapter relies heavily on official government guides and those of the independent Kaiser Family Foundation (kff.org). The U.S. government is quite divided by party affiliation, but because the official publications come from the executive branch they are likely to be at least guardedly supportive of the act. The Congressional Budget Office is respected for consistently providing objective, nonpartisan analysis for contentious legislation, and their projections of likely fiscal consequences are used here. Kff.org has become a go-to site for health care policy analysis by journalists and politicians of many different political persuasions, as has the publication *Health Affairs* and its blogs.

Once you are armed with a reasonable understanding of PPACA and its background and likely effects, it will be useful to sample a broader range of commentary (conservative, liberal, radical) to get an understanding of alternative perspectives and see what is potentially at stake. Please note that the description provided here is illustrative, not definitive. The description is a deliberately brief and incomplete guide meant to illustrate a complex and still-uncertain policy, skipping all the caveats, exceptions, transition periods, price changes, and other elements that are often critically important in implementing a new law. Readers requiring more precision should refer to the official copy of the law itself, as currently amended and legally interpreted.

Health insurance coverage as of 2012 and as projected by the CBO for 2021 is outlined in Table 17.1. (The percentages add to more than 100 percent owing to multiple coverages.) PPACA starts with the current insurance system and builds on that. It is evident that the main changes will have to come in the "remainder" category, the 18 million persons who must purchase individual insurance out-of-pocket or the 50 million uninsured. To stabilize and extend coverage among this group, the most vulnerable, PPACA proposes the creation of state insurance exchanges with federal subsidies for all individuals with incomes less than $44,000 {*$92,00 for families*} and a series of underwriting reforms.

TABLE 17.1	Health Insurance Coverage by Category, 2012 and 2021	
2012	**Coverage**	**2021**
52%	Employer	50%
16%	Medicare	18%
15%	Medicaid and other	19%
9%	Individual, exchange	14%
17%	Uninsured	8%

Source: Congressional Budget Office Projections.

Coverage Rules

PPACA requires that insurance companies meet a series of new rules or standards for coverage, requires people to obtain health insurance, and requires most companies to offer health insurance to their employees. As incentives, it provides a series of subsidies for obtaining health insurance and penalties for not doing so. Some of these vary substantially by type of coverage and so are listed separately below under individual and employer categories.

Nondiscrimination   Health insurance cannot be denied to anyone because of age, health status, preexisting conditions, genetic information, or disability. In particular, *all preexisting conditions are covered in full* and cannot be used to deny coverage or charge higher premiums.

Comprehensive Benefits   A health insurance plan must include all benefits described as essential in PPACA (inpatient, outpatient, emergency room, office visits, maternity, mental health, addiction, physical rehabilitation, pediatric vision and dental, laboratory and diagnostics, etc.), and cover at least 60 percent of the actuarial cost. Preventive services must be covered at no cost to the patient.

Limited Deductibles   Maximum deductible is related to income and must be no more than $2,000 for middle-income individuals and $4,000 for families.

No Dollar Limit on Benefits   The insurance plan must not include annual or lifetime maximum dollar limits on coverage.

Guaranteed Renewal   Once a plan provides coverage, the individual must have the option to continue coverage in force without regard to use of care, accidents, or other factors.

Dependents   Young adults remain covered under their parents' plan up to age 26.

Mandated Coverage (Penalty Tax)   Every U.S. citizen and legal resident must obtain health insurance or show that doing so would be unaffordable and create financial hardship. Those who fail to do so must pay a penalty ranging from $695 to $2,085 per year depending upon income.

Premium Rating Bands   Premiums must be independent of many factors typically used in underwriting (gender, blood pressure, family history, etc.). The act does allow premiums to increase with age (up to a limit of 3:1), tobacco use (1.5:1), and with family size or geographic area.

Medical Loss Ratios   All health plans must report how much is spent for medical services. The law requires rebates to consumers whenever spending is less than 80 percent of premiums (85 percent for large employer groups).

Uniform Benefit Descriptions   A brief (four pages or less), standardized, and comprehensible statement of plan benefits and costs are openly provided to all consumers.

Eligibility and Electronic Claims Submission   The law sets standards for rapid and transparent determinations of eligibility, electronic claims submission, patient smart cards, and automated fund transfers that can be easily verified by patients, hospitals, physicians, and insurers.

Other   The law includes other rules regarding cost-sharing, children, clinical trials, dentistry, underwriting, waiting periods, wellness plans, and more.

State Health Insurance Exchanges

The act provides funding support and requires that states establish "health benefit exchanges" as regulated markets where individuals and small groups can purchase health insurance plans. The plans must meet a number of conditions to become "qualified," and for many participants the premiums would be available at a reduced price that is subsidized by the employer or government. The state can have separate individual and small group exchanges, have a single combined exchange, join with other states to have a regional exchange, or create separate exchanges in different areas of the state. The act defines five tiers of coverage:

Plan Coverage Tiers

  Catastrophic is only available to individuals younger than 30 years or for demonstrable financial hardship.

  Bronze covers 60 percent of costs and limits out-pocket (OOP) payments to $5,950 {*$11,900 for families*}.

  Silver covers 70 percent of costs and has the same OOP limits.

  Gold covers 80 percent of costs and has the same OOP limits.

  Platinum covers 90 percent of costs and has the same OOP limits.

An illustrative example of the percentage of actuarial costs covered by differing combinations of copayments, coinsurance, deductibles, and OOP maximums is provided in Table 17.2. Each state exchange would have to offer at least one qualified silver and one gold plan. The Congressional Budget Office estimates that a silver plan would currently cost an individual $5,474 to $6,933 and would cost about twice that much for a family of four. A bronze plan would be 15 percent cheaper, a gold plan 15 percent more expensive. Exchanges are required to have multiple plans, and there are provisions for creating consumer cooperatives and other not-for-profit options. The percentage of actuarial costs covered can obviously be increased

TABLE 17.2   Examples of Differences in Estimated Percentage of Actuarial Cost Covered

	FEHBP, VA High	VA Medium	VA Low
Deductible	$ 0	$1,000	$ 5,000
Coinsurance	0%	0%	20%
Out-of-Pocket Max	$1,800	$1,000	$10,000
PCP Copay	$ 25	$ 25	$ 30
PCP Specialty Copay	$ 35	$ 50	$ 60
Estimated actuarial value	*84%*	*75%*	*55%*

Source: Institute of Medicine, *Essential Health Benefits, Balancing and Cost*, Figure 4-1 (2011), www.nap.edu.

or decreased by changing deductibles, copayments, or maximum on OOP costs, and plans are given some flexibility in shifting these parameters. The electronic data interchanges for determining eligibility, subsidies, and credits are created at the national level and then are coordinated and interfaced with all of the health plans, exchanges, and employers so that premiums, credits, and subsidies can all be automatically transferred and adjusted.

Individuals

The individual market will undergo a seismic change. Rather than submitting an application, receiving a medical examination, and then waiting to receive a premium quotation or denial of coverage for a policy that can have many pages of clauses, limits, and exclusions, a person buying from an exchange will purchase a qualified package at a fixed price (which varies only with age and smoking) with no waiting periods or exclusion of preexisting conditions and will probably receive better coverage at lower prices than are available today. Furthermore, if that person is earning less than $3,724 per month {*$7,684 for families*}, they will get a premium credit to reduce price even more, and a subsidy will reduce their maximum OOP payments. Assuming that the exchanges are successfully established, almost all of the individual market might migrate there because of lower prices, administrative simplification, ease of comparison, facilitated transactions, and generous federal subsidies. The schedule for income-related premium credits and cost-sharing subsidies is presented in Table 17.3. Note that the actual calculations will change over time and can be more complex.

CREDITS AND SUBSIDIES ON THE PPACA INSURANCE EXCHANGES

PPACA low-income credits are tied to the premium of the second-lowest silver plan. For example, if the plan premium is $500 per month, an individual earning $2,800 would be limited to a net 9.5% premium cost or $182. Thus the automatic premium credit would be $318 ($500 − $182) and the payment would be $182 for a plan that would cost $500 to someone making $100,000 a year. The implicit subsidy would also be increased by reducing the maximum OOP cost-sharing limit from $5,950 to $3,987. A person earning $1,400 a month would receive a larger credit of $446 ($500 − $56) and would pay $56. The maximum out-of-pocket limit for this person would be $2,975.

    The credit is fixed: If either person chose a better silver or gold plan costing $700, then he or she has to pay an extra $200. However, if either one chooses a bronze plan with a premium of $450, then he or she would pay $50 less.

Individuals with incomes less that than $14,856 {*families $30,56*} will generally be covered without annual premiums by Medicaid (see below), and states at their discretion may extend Medicaid or create a "State Basic Health Plan" for individuals with incomes between $14,856 − $22,340 {*families $30,567 − $46,100*}. Individuals with incomes greater than $46,800 {*families > $92,200*} no longer qualify for subsidies or credits, but are still eligible to buy health insurance through the exchanges, and thus will probably pay less than similar coverage would cost outside the exchange. People working at small firms will be able either to purchase insurance through the exchanges on their own or participate through the employer's plan (see the discussion of small business in the next section). People employed at firms that offer qualified health insurance benefits (i.e., with the employer contributing at 60 percent of cost) are generally not eligible to participate in the exchanges except through a specified premium credit or voucher program.

TABLE 17.3 PPACA Exchanges: Premiums (net of subsidy) and Maximums

Federal Poverty Level, 2012		Net Premium Contribution		Maximum OOP ($)	Actuarial Coverage (%)
		Percentage of Income	Amount ($)		
Individual	$11,170				
up to					
133%	$14,856	2.0%	$297	$1,983	94%
150%	$16,755	4.0%	$670	$1,983	94%
200%	$22,340	6.3%	$1,407	$2,975	87%
250%	$27,925	8.1%	$2,248	$2,975	73%
300%	$33,510	9.5%	$3,183	$3,967	70%
400%	$44,680	9.5%	$4,245	$3,967	70%
>400%*	≥ $44,681	N/A	N/A	$5,950	70%
Family of Four	$23,050				
up to					
133%	$30,657	2.0%	$613	$3,967	94%
150%	$34,575	4.0%	$1,383	$3,967	94%
200%	$46,100	6.3%	$2,904	$5,950	87%
250%	$57,625	8.1%	$4,639	$5,950	73%
300%	$69,150	9.5%	$6,569	$7,933	70%
400%	$92,200	9.5%	$8,759	$7,933	70%
>400%*	≥ $92,201	N/A	N/A	$11,900	70%

*Subsidies tied to Silver Plan, $ premium depends on other elements also.

Employers: Positive and Negative Incentives to Provide Benefits

Health insurance offered through an employer will undergo fewer changes under PPACA than the individual market will. Current health plans are grandfathered in (deemed acceptable) but eventually some firms will have to modify aspects of their current plans to meet PPACA standards for minimum essential benefits and affordability.

Large firms will be given incentives to offer health insurance, and those with more than 200 employees must automatically enroll the employee in a qualified plan. Although less than 2 percent of firms are this large, they employ more than 60 percent of the total workforce, and almost all (99 percent) already offer health insurance. Hence it is only at the margins that PPACA will make a difference. There is a significant fee (penalty tax) of $2,000 per employee for large firms that do **not** offer employees the opportunity to enroll in a plan meeting the minimum standards if even one employee used the state health insurance exchange and qualified for a premium credit, so the firms have a powerful incentive to offer health insurance.

If a firm offers health insurance but has at least one employee for whom those benefits are determined to be unqualified or **unaffordable** (generally, by requiring more than 9.5 percent of the employee's income as premium contribution) and therefore uses a premium credit on the exchange, the firm must pay a fee of $3,000 for each such employee, essentially compensating the government for the premium credits. Large firms may pay to provide "free choice vouchers" meeting certain criteria to avoid the fee. Either way, firms have an incentive to provide some contribution to employees who use subsidized care from the exchanges.

Small firms with 25 employees or fewer and average wages under $50,000 are eligible for subsides of up to 50 percent (35 percent for nonprofits) of the employer benefit contribution. This subsidy is phased out linearly between 10 and 25 employees and between $25,000 and $50,000 in average wages.

The choices of **medium-sized firms** remain somewhat open and uncertain. PPACA does not specify any subsidies or fees for firms with 26 to 49 employees. Every employer with 50 or more employees will be subject to the same fees as large firms. However, the exemption of the first 30 employees from the $2,000-per-employee fee could lead a firm with 70 or even 110 employees to decide to pay the government rather than provide benefits or vouchers. The firm will presumably have to make a choice as shown in the box below. How much employee loyalty is gained by providing benefits? How many of our employees would have low enough incomes to qualify, or to have our preferred plan deemed "unaffordable?" How do these trade-offs change as the firm gains or loses employees or as the relevant prices (silver premiums, fees) change?

WILL MEDIUM INC. CHOOSE TO PROVIDE HEALTH BENEFITS UNDER PPACA?

MEDium Inc. is a company with 45 employees. It distributes medical radium to hospitals and clinics throughout the Northwest, and its business is growing. The company has had a minimal health plan with very limited benefits, for which it contributed $1,800 for each employee (about one-third participate). Next year, MEDium expects to add nine employees for a total of 54, and it will come under PPACA rules. It estimates a conforming plan (i.e., equivalent to an exchange silver plan) will cost at least $4,500, and MEDium would have to contribute at least 60 percent, or $2,700. Should MEDium offer a conforming plan, stick with the old plan, or not offer employee health insurance? If MEDium chooses not to provide any benefits next year, and at least one employee chooses to take the state health insurance exchange subsidy (which someone is almost certain to do in this case), MEDium will pay a fine of $2,000 for every employee after 30, or $48,000. If MEDium offers better insurance to conform with PPACA standards, they expect the cost to them will be $2,700 for each of the 27 employees that participate, or $72,900. If MEDium stays with the current nonconforming plan, they will be contributing for 18 employees at $1,800 each or $32,400. However, because the plan is nonconforming, if even one employee chooses to receive state health insurance exchange subsidies, MEDium is again liable for the fine of $2,000 for every employee after 30, or $48,000.

Plan	Employer Premiums	Fines	Total
No insurance	$0	24 × $2,000	$48,000
Better insurance	27 × $2,700	$0	$72,900
Old insurance	18 × $1,800	24 × $2,000	$80,400

It is clear that MEDium will not stick with the previous cheap nonconforming policy, because that will end up costing them more than providing better benefits to a larger number of employees under the new conforming plan. MEDium already thought the $32,400 they were paying each year for the inferior plan was worthwhile in terms of attracting employees and building loyalty, so they would almost certainly step up to the new plan, because the marginal cost of doing so is only $24,900. The potential of a $3,000 fine for each employee choosing a state exchange subsidy for employers offering conforming plans appears to be not very relevant in most cases, because the employer insurance would usually be more attractive, and anyway, each employee opting to go that route is saving MEDium their $2,700 employer contribution. As MEDium continues to grow and adds more employees, then not offering insurance becomes less and less attractive. However, MEDium might decide to outsource some work to contractors to stay below the 50-employee cut-off for compliance with PPACA rules.

Medicare: ACOs, IPAB, Bundled Payments, and the Donut Hole

As with employer insurance, much of Medicare stays the same. There are a series of payment reductions for Medicare Advantage Plans, hospital annual updates, disproportionate share (DSH), excess admissions, and so on that are used to offset other PPACA costs and will make finances tighter for providers and insurance companies, but they will be little noticed by most patients. What many patients will quickly perceive is that the infamous "donut hole" in Medicare D forcing many patients to pay 100 percent of drug costs between $2,700 and $6,154 has been closed and that their Medicare premiums have changed. Over time the various reporting standards, payment reforms, and voluntary organizational innovations promulgated in PPACA might prove to be of greater importance.

Accountable care organizations (ACOs) are patient-centered teams that deliver comprehensive medical care (hospital, physician, diagnostic, etc.) to more than 5,000 assigned beneficiaries and agree to be accountable for overall quality and cost, and they thus become eligible for a share of any cost savings. There has been considerable excitement about the promise of ACOs to deliver better medicine, better patient satisfaction, and greater efficiency, but until the concept has been fully worked out and tested for a number of years it is difficult to tell if this will be a major breakthrough or just one more idea that comes and then goes.[2] Even more speculative is the **Center for Medicare and Medicaid Innovation**, a kind of internal think tank.

The **Independent Payment Advisory Board (IPAB)** represents an ambitious proposal to provide a technical solution to a political problem.[3] A panel of experts is to determine ways to reduce the rate of growth in Medicare expenditures over a 10-year span. If the Office of the Actuary projects per-capita Medicare cost to growth in excess of a specified target (GDP growth rate plus 1 percent), then the IPAB will deliver a set of proposals to Congress. According to PPACA, Congress must then either accept the recommendations or find a new set that provides an equivalent amount of cost savings. PPACA specifies that if Congress does not succeed in doing so within six months, the IPAB proposals will automatically be put into effect. However, given that Congress has repeatedly overridden limitations on Medical cost growth built into previous laws, the likelihood that the IPAB recommendations will effectively be able to limit costs should be questioned.

Medicaid: Major Expansions with Federal Funding

PPACA provides generous federal funding to expand the Medicaid program. Provisions ensuring coverage for all persons up to 133 percent of the poverty level ($14,856 for single adults), state "basic health plans," enrollment simplifications, enhancement of the Children's Health Insurance Program, and other elements could extend Medicaid to cover as many as 20 million additional persons by 2022. The Medicaid expansions are substantial, potentially second in scale only to the changes in the individual market. PPACA contains a number of specifications applied to various aspects of the Medicaid program. That complexity, and the fact that Medicaid varies so much from state to state, make it hard to generalize further or to add much detail to the brief summary provided here. (Note: the Supreme Court decision in June 2012 allows states to opt out of the Medicaid expansions, adding more uncertainty.)

Prevention and Other Provisions of PPACA

PPACA makes an investment in prevention and the promotion of population health as pathways to lower costs and increase quality by requiring that insurance fully cover preventive care and creating a National Prevention and Public Health Fund. There is also support for workplace wellness programs and of the network of community health centers providing primary care. ACA also makes some small attempts to improve and expand the education and placement of doctors, nurses, and other health care workers.

One portion of PPACA, the CLASS Act, was intended create a voluntary insurance program for employed adults to purchase assistance for long-term care at home and in the community during retirement, thus reducing reliance on Medicaid and pensions. Mounting political opposition and a recognition that the subsidies required would probably end up being much greater than anticipated brought repeal of the CLASS Act in February 2012.

Still Uninsured: The Undocumented and Some Other Outsiders

Even with a large set of incentives and regulations, PPACA will not insure everyone in the United States. In part, that is because it is designed as a voluntary program, leaving people free to make choices even if they are not in their own best interest or the interest of the country as a whole. A very small group, probably less than 1 percent, will have a job but no insurance and will choose to pay the specified penalty rather than purchase coverage. A somewhat larger group, perhaps 2 percent or more, chooses to live off the grid. These are marginal persons, many of whom do not have a regular job or pay income taxes. Whether surfing in Hawaii or suffering from mental illness, this group is hard to engage in regular administrative procedures. They do, however, show up in emergency departments needing care. This group of uninsured might be considered more of a problem if it were not for the fact that they would in any case contribute so few resources to the risk pool that the net financial status of the system is not much affected. Whatever premiums one might collect are smaller than the costs of doing so. The one group explicitly excluded from PPACA is immigrants who are undocumented or working illegally in the United States.

17.2   STATEMENT OF THE PROBLEM: AFFORDABILITY

The goal of this legislation, to make health insurance and medical care "affordable," is clearly stated in the title of the act. Economic evaluation might address affordability for the person or the nation. For people (or households), affordability could be assessed as an amount that does not threaten the family with bankruptcy either for obtaining health insurance or, if sick, for making whatever additional payments are required. Quantitatively, analysis could be framed in terms of the mean and variance relative to income and applied for both the average family and for households at the upper and lower ends of the distribution. A macro analysis must take account of these micro elements, but it is more concerned with the system as a whole, health insurance as financial intermediation and the trend in national health expenditures relative to inflation and GDP.

The definition and standards for affordability have been discussed and debated at great length. A definition that can be culled from the text of the PPACA is the limit on the employee contribution required to purchase basic coverage, 9.5 percent of income. This is reasonably close to amounts most often discussed in the press and research literature.[4] Because current national health expenditures are almost twice that percentage (18 percent of GDP), significant redistribution and cost-shifting is implied in order to make the financing system work (see Figure 17.1).

Rising Costs Slowly Create a Crisis

In 1960, the average income per person in the United States was $2,827, and the amount spent on health care averaged $147 per year. Even without insurance, such expenses were manageable. For those whose incomes were below average or who perhaps had a bad year so that their expenses were three times as much, or even ten times that much, it was still possible to find a way to cover the costs by relying on friends or family. Today the copays and coinsurance required even with a good employer-provided health plan take more than 5 percent of income—which is what workers had to pay out for everything back then. It is not reasonable to expect that someone making minimum wage pay $5,000 or $15,000 or $25,000 or more just for medical care and insurance. By 2012, income per capita rose to $49,917 but the cost of medical care had risen even more rapidly, to $8,936. Paying one or two weeks of salary for doctor bills and health insurance in 1960 did not seem unfair. Trying to put aside two months of paychecks today just for the insurance would make it hard to cover rent, food, and taxes. A serious illness requiring hospitalization could easily cost more than $100,000 and leave one bankrupt.[5]

Distributional problems are made more severe by the skewness of incomes. The "average" of $50,000 per person per year is pulled upward by a few very high incomes: lawyers, professional athletes, CEOs, investment bankers, and so on. The median, the middle of distribution at the 50th percentile that many would consider a more "typical" income, is less than the mean (mathematical average). The average household income in 2010 was $67,523, but the median household income was $49,445. The distribution of financial wealth, savings needed for unexpected emergencies, and long-term care in retirement, is even more skewed.[6]

Health insurance is expensive, $5,429 for a regular plan with single coverage and $15,073 for family coverage (see Table 5.2). Families fortunate enough to have someone working at a good job with employer health insurance pays only about one quarter of that ($3,750). Most other families were in trouble and very likely to fall into the pinched camp of those who were employed but uninsured, for whom any significant illness could mean financial catastrophe.

The Middle Class Gets Stretched: A Leveraged Gap in Coverage

In 1960 the median U.S. household income was $4,970, more than sufficient to cover the average national health expenditure of $147 several times over with little strain. Any household with at least one person working at minimum wage could afford health care (defining "affordability" as average health expenditures being less than 9.5 percent of income). Figure 17.1 shows the dashed "affordable" line crossing above income and opening a small gap after 1980. By 1981, medical costs had risen to $1,275 and only 65 percent of households could afford coverage on their own. Another 17 percent of households earned less than the minimum wage and presumably had Medicaid or other safety net coverage, leaving a "gap" of 18 percent—the working poor who could not really afford health insurance but would probably not qualify for assistance. The cost of medical care in 2010 was $8,402, and only one quarter of households earned enough income ($88,442) to meet the 9.5 percent definition of affordability. The percentage of households earning minimum wage or less was approximately 13 percent, meaning that the affordability gap had widened to 62 percent of all households in the United States, swallowing most of the middle class.

FIGURE 17.1   Affordability of Medical Care, 1960 to 2012

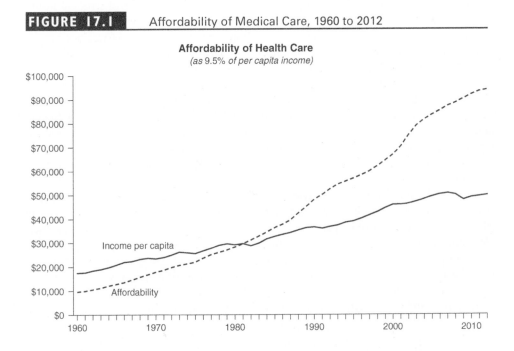

TABLE 17.4	A Widening Gap Between Medical Costs and Household Income		
	1960	**1981**	**2010**
Cost of Medical Care	$ 147	$ 1,275	$ 8,936
Median Household Income	$4,970	$19,074	$49,445
Below Minimum Wage (%)	22%	17%	13%
Household can Afford	85%	65%	25%
(less than 9.5% of Income)			
GAP	**_**	**18%**	**62%**

When health care costs were a problem only for the near-poor without decent jobs and a small segment of the lower middle class, they could be ignored by most people. Today, when affordable health care is a problem for one-half or three-quarters of all working families, the public and the politicians are forced to take notice. Some unions and a few firms adjust the employee contribution up or down with salary levels, but most are more like the Federal Employees Health Benefits (FEHB) plan, with a defined employer contribution. With a fixed defined contribution, workers with low salaries end up paying out a higher percentage of their already low income for medical care, even before they get sick. Global consulting firm McKinsey & Company estimated that the fraction of wages taken from workers in the lower income category was 10 times as much as from those with higher incomes and that this gap had widened substantially over the past decade.[7] Some economists estimate that almost all of the wage gains for middle-income working families since the turn of the 21st century have been wiped out by the increase in health insurance contributions. Well before 2012, affordable health care had become a problem, not for a few, but for most Americans.

Macro Affordability: The Growth Gap

For the federal government, the gap between the growth rate in national health expenditures (spending) and the growth rate in GDP (ability to pay) is the problem, even more pressing than some of the distributional issues it exacerbates. When Medicare and Medicaid were enacted in 1965, there was a consensus to increase national spending on medical care and to push the wages of nurses and doctors higher. From 1960 to 1990 the growth rate of national health expenditures exceeded GDP by +3%, taking one out of every eight dollars of national product and putting the federal budget in deficit. The Clinton health plan of 1993 was not passed, but the pressure for reform and the power of rule making and administrative procedures were sufficient to control cost until 2000 (growth less than GDP +1%). Cost pressures then exploded and expenditures rose quickly, helping to create a new budget deficit and the financial crisis of 2008. Deep recession meant negative GDP growth until 2010. Since then, health care costs have risen only slightly faster than GDP, but the lagged effect of income and inflation changes and the fact that health care employment has continued to increase more rapidly than regular job growth indicates that excess spending continues and will still be out of control in coming years unless additional tightening occurs. (See Chapter 13, especially section 13.3 on dynamics and Figure 13.2).

This trend cannot continue. Analyses by the Congressional Budget Office, U.S. Treasury, university researchers, and industry consultants all conclude that the expected increases in health expenditures, and most particularly in Medicare and Medicaid, are unsustainable.[8] Unless limited to the rate of increase in ability to pay (GDP growth), they will eventually bankrupt the federal government, the states, and large employers (such as the auto industry) with obligations to provide care for beneficiaries. Financing is ultimately a systemic problem. It must be solved at the system level, but will involve adjustments and sacrifice at every level, including state and city governments, businesses, individuals, and households.

17.3 USING EXISTING PLANS AS MODELS

To make projections, the CBO or any other analyst must start from somewhere, finding a program or situation that is analogous. With PPACA there were several examples, such as HMOs, the FEHB, and the Massachusetts health care law of 2006, that were obvious choices since they were models that had been used in designing and promoting the law.

States

Studies of the Massachusetts law are in agreement on a number of points.[9] Coverage has increased, and the premiums for individual coverage have dropped dramatically. Employers have adjusted with little problem or complaint. Use of doctors and hospitals has risen, as has reported health status, but there are no dramatic changes in mortality or morbidity, and disparities in care for the disadvantaged remain. The mandated fee or penalty for coverage has worked, and while the plan is well accepted by most of the public, it is not liked, and is even detested, by those who feel they are compelled to pay for something they do not want. This is a somewhat predictable result because the idea behind the mandate was to force healthy working people who previously chose not to participate to join in a covered group so as to better spread the risk (and hence subsidize the old, the sick, and the disabled).

Although Massachusetts was the primary state health program example, Hawaii and Oregon also created programs that were relevant to analysis of PPACA.[10] A long-standing mandate for employer coverage in Hawaii has kept employer group health insurance coverage from declining, but it has also, as theory would predict, forced adjustment along other margins: shifting employees from full-time to part-time work so the employer can escape the cost of mandated coverage, especially for small firms and low-wage workers. The Oregon experiment randomized expansion of Medicaid and showed a sizable increase in utilization and reported health among people previously uninsured, but changes in life expectancy, mortality, or morbidity were not discernible in such a short time span.

A major problem with the use of analogies is that *generalization* of results from one state to project results for the United States as a whole might not be accurate or even appropriate. Massachusetts is a high-income state that started health reform with 92 percent of population already covered. Conversely, Mississippi is a low-income state with more than a quarter of their much more needy population uninsured. Hawaii is an island, with a labor and employment market severely constrained because they are separated from other opportunities by thousands of miles of open ocean. Analysts understand such limitations and recognize the increased uncertainty caused by generalization, yet they also understand that a model and some data are better than nothing and that an educated estimate usually (but not always) beats an uniformed guess.

The Federal Employees Health Benefits Plan

The state health insurance exchanges in PPACA are modeled on the **FEHB** plan, a system that has operated successfully for more than 40 years with an unusual structure that provides for consumer choice and price competition among plans. Within each area many companies make bids (i.e., advertise a premium per month) to provide standard coverage plus additional optional benefits. Although employees can choose among any of the qualified plans, the FEHB pays only up to the cost of the lowest bid. The employee must personally pay the extra amount (if any) by which the chosen plan exceeds the premium for the low-cost plan. In this way the individual bears the full marginal cost of extra benefits, amenities, and inefficiencies.

Based on the experience of FEHB, economist Alain Enthoven published a provocative proposal for a consumer-choice health plan in the *New England Journal of Medicine* in 1978, envisioning a future in which managed care was the norm and fee for service was the secondary alternative.[11] His proposal was based on a recognition that consumers were confronted with thousands of possible illnesses, millions of possible prices, and indemnity coverage that was difficult to understand and comprehensive enough to make the effort of comparing costs not worthwhile. Because of this situation, most consumers actually made decisions based on reasons that were very remote from the market and the actuarial realities considered by employers and insurers. Consumers looked for plans with low copayments, or coverage of eyeglasses and orthodontics, or benefit maximums set at reassuringly astronomical amounts, factors that had nothing to do with the average total cost of most medical care or the rising premiums that employers had to pay each year.

In contrast, consumer choice as presented by Enthoven was based on making a choice between two or three competing plans, each with a price that was known in advance and for which the consumer would have to pay the full difference between the low-cost plan and the high-cost plan. Consumers who preferred to obtain greater choice, more coverage, or higher quality would have to pay extra. It is this concept of consumer choice that stands behind the accountable-care organization proposed in PPACA. However, the people in the FEHB plan, federal employees, might have attitudes toward work and risk, stability and level of income, or other characteristics that differ from attitudes of the uninsured, hence the issue of generalizability must again be considered.

17.4   UNRESOLVED ISSUES

PPACA as enacted by Congress represents a compromise, an incomplete and partial step toward reform of the U.S. health care system. Many of the core conflicts and issues mentioned at the end of Chapter 5 are still open. Perhaps the most important aspect of major new legislation, such as PPACA, is the indication that the problems of health care are actually going to be faced, closing the door on the various easy answers that offer deceptive false hope. The nation cannot simply turn the clock back to 1910 and do without a health care financing system. There is no secret answer. Other people's money, cost-shifting, more debt, government, investors, an AIDS vaccine, better food, more exercise, or miraculous technological advances will not remove the burden of paying more for medical care by 2020. Health care reform must begin with the bitter taste of reality; changes do have to be made, they will not be easy, and almost everyone will have to make some sacrifices. Furthermore, if the United States as a nation cannot agree upon a path, then indecision and delay will tend to make reform harder and more painful.

Equity

The technical aspects of insurance can never be fully separated from the emotional issues of medical care and health or from the normative and political values of the people involved. Opinions are very divided on the extent to which health care should be a public good or a private one, an entitlement or a purchase. This cannot be separated from risk bearing or other issues. If the patient bears the financial risks, then poorer patients will buy less care and will not be able to afford some advanced modern medicine. If the financial risks are borne publicly, then patients will not care about prices. The balance can be moved up or down. For example, the PPACA exchange subsidy tied to the cost of a silver health insurance package says that citizens are entitled to that much, but if they want any more, they have to pay for it. How high or low "that much" is depends greatly upon the definition of the minimum essential benefit package.

Within most companies, all employees get different wages but the same health insurance plan, whether they are custodians or comptrollers. This is common, and it indicates that most people want more equity in health insurance than in wages. How much more? At any given time, opinion polls show about one-quarter of Americans wanting all citizens to have the same access to care through universal coverage and willing to pay for public funding and one-quarter strongly opposed to being forced to pay anything to cover anyone but themselves. The majority appear to be undecided.

The two extremes are not compatible. Moving the balance up or down might allow us to arrive at a compromise with majority support, but it does not resolve the dilemma. An economic evaluation of PPACA or other health policy should always include an analysis of equity and distributional consequences. An economic evaluation could reasonably begin by identifying the winners and losers and then build from that to construct an analysis of implementation, efficiency, outcomes, externalities, and political reality.

Defining Essential Benefits

The first PPACA proposals envisioned replacing the vague "medically necessary" specification found in current health insurance contracts with a uniform national definition, or rather, with a dynamic process for doing so because the practice of medicine is constantly changing. Broadening or narrowing the scope of benefits can vastly change what the "minimum" is, and how much financial burden is left to the individual. Through inclusion or exclusion, it will also inevitably touch certain political trigger points. Every proposal quickly became controversial, tagged with powerful rhetoric ("death panels") and provoked contention rather than consensus.[12] Although PPACA retains a list of 10 minimum essential benefit categories that all qualified health insurance plans are required to cover, the task has been delegated to the states, with each allowed to come up with their own definition.

The OPM Legacy: Third-Party Payment and Cost Shifting

Over the years, a variety of mechanisms have been used to transfer funds and shift costs so that vital public goods such as medical education, research, community outreach, heroic (and expensive) trauma care, disaster preparedness, and so on could at least be partially paid for, even if not adequately funded. Almost any reform tends to take the cover off and reveal such flows. Currently, the public is unaware of how much such public goods cost, and they are unprepared to provide the hundreds of billions of dollars required to maintain adequate funding. Each group will try to have some other group pay (i.e., use **OPM**, "other people's money") or at least will complain when such previously hidden cost shifts are removed, forcing them to pay more. We will have to decide which legacy items built into the system deserve to remain funded as overhead or else identify charges or taxes to create a visible revenue stream.

Price Transparency: A Conspiracy of Silence

Most of the "price" of medical care is overhead. Every patient admitted to the hospital contributes something to covering the emergency department, and most of the nurses who work in the hospital have to be paid whether it is empty or full. Pharmaceutical costs are mostly research, administration, and marketing, not pill manufacture. In principle, patients could pay only for the direct costs of the care they receive, but that would leave most of the system costs (i.e., the other 80 percent) unfunded. The most valuable, immediate, and costly form of care—the undivided attention of a trained physician willing to listen, explain what the problem is, explore treatment options, and tolerantly help the patient and family find the best solution—is universally underpaid. Patients who willingly pay thousands of dollars for pills, transplants, and procedures usually balk when asked to spend a few hundred dollars to obtain thoughtful consideration and consultation.

Providers, patients, and insurance companies all benefit from the conspiracy of silence around the cost of medical care. Otherwise it would not be so pervasive or persistent. Hospitals cannot provide a bill that is comprehensible, and probably should not be asked to. Whether sick, dying, or emotionally disturbed, most patients do not want to start their care by bargaining over the price, nor do they have the tools to do so. Commercial Medigap and Medicare Advantage policies, among the most lucrative lines of health insurance, make much of those profits by positive selection and shifting costs to the government Medicare program rather than by cost efficiency. If granted, the request for price transparency would require a level of brutal honesty that is alien to the delivery of care and make everyone uncomfortable. Making prices transparent would reduce the ability of providers to shift costs, and the ability of patients to ignore costs. The question then becomes, who is going to pay?

The Uninsured: Still There, Still Have to be Paid For

PPACA will go a long way toward resolving the problem of the uninsured, but it will still leave millions of people who do not have coverage and who show up in hospitals and clinics needing care. Reforms will make it harder to shift costs or obscure the use of funds for unapproved purposes (i.e., those who choose to do without insurance, illegal immigrants, self-destructive addicts, or sick children with mentally disturbed parents).

UPDATE: AFTER THE SCOTUS DECISION

On June 30, 2012 the United States Supreme Court ruled that PPACA was constitutional and should remain the law of the land, but that states could choose whether to accept additional federal funding and expand their Medicaid programs as directed (covering up to 133 percent of poverty level) or not take more federal funds and maintain their old Medicaid programs. Since the Medicaid expansion is now voluntary, albeit heavily subsidized, it is likely that five to ten states will not expand, and hence about 6 million more American citizens will remain without medical insurance.

Although most sections of PPACA do not come into full effect until 2014, there have been some early results and indicators for provisions already in force. For example, the requirement that children can retain dependent coverage until age 26 has apparently provided several million young adults with coverage, and the requirement that 80 percent of premiums be used to provide benefits will result in $1.1 billion in rebate checks being sent back to individuals and companies that purchased health insurance in 2011.[13] Perhaps of broader importance in the long run is that the state of Massachusetts, whose health plan was a model for PPACA, has now passed a law limiting the rate of future growth in health spending to the rate of growth in state GDP, thus indicating one path federal cost controls may take in the future.

Unfunded Health and Retirement Benefits

In addition to the uninsured, there are the legacy costs of millions of retirees who have been promised extensive health care benefits. Revealing such previously hidden liabilities has already caused a number of major airlines, auto companies, steel mills, and other corporations to go through Chapter 11 bankruptcy reorganizations. The U.S. Army, Marine Corps, postal service, and state governments do not have that convenient option. And then there is Medicare, 42 million strong. Health reform must not only provide a viable financing mechanism for the future, it must also deal with the leftover costs from the past by imposing a hefty surcharge on future beneficiaries.

Defined Benefits, Defined Services, or Defined Contribution

Most companies have dealt with the problem of unfunded retiree benefits by dropping retiree health benefits and pensions in favor of 401k or similar plans. The uncertain liabilities created by "defined benefit" pensions that promised employees a specified monthly amount or percentage of salary were replaced by a "defined contribution." A contractual promise stretching years into the future was replaced by a flexible policy with smaller payments that could be reduced or eliminated at any time at the discretion of the firm. Instead of massive and uncertain future liabilities, the company no longer owed retirees anything at all. Of course, this did mean that the employees had to save, do retirement planning, and bear all risks for future lifespan and investment returns on their own.

Who Bears the Risk?

No one wants risks. People do not want to put their health or retirement at risk. Companies do not want to put their profits at risks. Governments do not want to put their leadership or budgets at risk. What can be done is to try to determine who can best bear the risk and "sell" it to them through insurance. When all else fails (war, flood, hurricanes, banking collapses, insurance insolvencies), the government is expected to take the risks and spread the burden publically to all of us.

The shift of pensions to defined-contribution plans means that the risk is removed from the employer and placed on the individual. This has pros and cons, many of which have been more sharply revealed over the last ten years. Pensions were popular with most large companies and their employees until companies were required to explicitly show them as liabilities in their financial statements. On paper, explicit recognition of future costs decreased stated profits by millions of dollars. Once the magnitude and risk of expected payments became clear, most companies moved to terminate defined-benefit pension plans, shifting investment and longevity risks to their employees. The personal risk of relying on investment returns only became clear to most employees as the financial markets collapsed in 2008. Retirees from companies whose pension plans went bankrupt at least had the benefit of a partial bailout by the federal government's Pension Benefit Guarantee Corporation. Those invested in the market made good or bad choices and took their chances. The actual risks of longevity and disability are still unknown to most current employees.

What has been learned during the great risk shift of the first decade of the 21st century is that most people, and especially poor and uneducated people, do not save enough, are not equipped to price or compare insurance policies, and are often overwhelmed by the administrative tasks and complexity of retirement, (which is much simpler than health insurance).[14] In trying to avoid risk, most financially uninformed people actually lose money and increase risk. They buy high and sell low, hold cash while inflation erodes the value of their money, and take on debt when they can least afford it. Insurance is overpurchased for events that are frightening (cancer, airplane crashes) or for benefits that "I am sure I will use" (eyeglasses, trip cancellation), and underpurchased where risks are complex and hard to understand.

PPACA is, above all, a plan for health insurance. The obvious problem is affordability. The more subtle problems are pooling, pricing, and risk bearing. Employers moved quickly to remove pension risks from their balance sheets and income statements. Patients and families always bear the risk of illness. How much of the financial risks they should bear remains a question still to be answered.

SUGGESTIONS FOR FURTHER READING

U.S. House of Representatives, *Patient Protection and Affordable Care Act of 2010*, www.healthcare.gov (accessed June 16, 2012).

Kaiser Family foundation, *Health Reform Source,* http://healthreform.kff.org (accessed June 16, 2012).

U.S. Congressional Budget Office, *CBO's Analysis of the Major Health Care Legislation Enacted in March 2010,* www.cbo.gov/publication/22077 (accessed June 16, 2012).

C Ullmer et. al. *Essential Health Benefits: Balancing Coverage and Cost* (Washington, D.C.: National Academy of Science, Institute of Medicine, 2011).

Austin Frakt, "What is the Economic Rationale for the Health Care Law's Individual Mandate?" *JAMA Forum,* March 26, 2012. http://newsatjama.jama.com/2012/03/26/jama-forum-what-is-the-economic-rationale-for-the-health-care-laws-individual-mandate/ (accessed June 16, 2012).

SUMMARY

1. The Patient Protection and Affordable Care Act of 2010, also known as **PPACA**, the **ACA** or "Obamacare," is a **complex** piece of legislation and represents a **compromise** among a number of health reform proposals. It creates subsidies to help buy health insurance for individuals that gradually phases out between incomes of $11,170 to $46,800 {*$23,050 to $92,200 for a family of four*}. However, anyone who could afford health insurance but did not get it would have to pay a **mandated penalty** of $695 for choosing not to buy any.

2. State **health insurance exchanges** would be created, making health insurance available **without regard to gender, pre-existing conditions, disability, or health status**. An essential set of benefits would be provided with guaranteed renewal, a $5,950 maximum limit on out-of-pocket cost-sharing, and no annual or lifetime dollar benefit limits.

3. **Large employers** would be required to offer health insurance to employees, but **small firms would receive subsidies for providing health insurance**. Medium-sized firms with more than 200 employees would face a variety of positive and negative incentives.

4. PPACA establishes an expert panel called the Independent Payment Advisory Board (**IPAB**) that would recommend changes to Congress subject only to a quick up-or-down vote if the growth in **Medicare** expenditures exceeded specified limits. Accountable care organizations (**ACOs**), patient-centered teams providing comprehensive hospital and physician benefits to groups of Medicare patients, are made eligible to share cost savings with the government.

5. **Medicaid** would be substantially expanded to **cover all persons up to 133 percent of the poverty** limit, $14,856 for individuals {*$30,656 for a family of four*}, with most of the funding coming from the federal government.

6. **Preventive services** will largely be available at **no charge to patients** under PPACA.

7. Rising costs have made the **affordability** of health insurance a problem for more and more people. In 1960 only one-quarter of households were unable to afford health insurance, and most of them had safety-net coverage through Medicaid or other programs. In 2010 three-quarters of the working households in America have problems affording insurance, and less than 15 percent are covered by Medicaid.

8. Even if PPACA is fully and successfully implemented, there will still be a number of unresolved issues: complex transactions with a lack of price transparency, unfunded retiree health benefits, some 10 million undocumented persons still uninsured, and controversies over cost shifting, who should pay, and who should bear the risk.

PROBLEMS

1. {*uninsured, subsidies*} What existing insurance plan will expand the most under PPACA?

2. {*affordability, cost-shifting*} How can people working at minimum-wage jobs get better health insurance and yet be paying less for premiums?

3. {*profitability*} Find a section (or subsection or clause) in PPACA. Explain how it helps a specific company to increase profits. Find another section and explain how it hurts the profits of a different company.

4. {*uninsured*} If PPACA is supposed to cover everyone, how could it still leave 10 million people uninsured?

5. {*marginal cost*} How was the structure of the Federal Employees Health Benefits plan incorporated into PPACA?

6. {*distribution*} Why did more families have trouble affording health insurance in 2010 than in 1995?

7. {*measurement, scope*} How can the definition of essential benefits change the cost of PPACA?

8. {*sustainability*} What is the "excess growth rate" and why does it worry the CBO so much?

9. {*competition*} Will PPACA make health care pricing more or less transparent?

10. {*distribution*} Which is more representative of the average family income: the median or the mean? Does random variation make a skewed distribution of costs more or less problematic with regard to affordability?

11. {*policy, incentives*} What policy questions is economics good at answering? What policy questions is economics bad at answering?

12. {*objective function*} What objectives of PPACA will be easiest to measure? Hardest?

13. {*distribution, risk*} A defined contribution plan makes risk more well defined for whom?

14. {*distribution, equity*} What is equity? What do winners and losers have to do with it?

ENDNOTES

1. U.S. House of Representatives, *Patient Protection and Affordable Care Act of 2010*. www.healthcare.gov; Kaiser Family Foundation, *Health Reform Source*, http://healthreform.kff.org; U.S. Congressional Budget Office, *CBO's Analysis of the Major Health Care Legislation Enacted in March 2010,* March 30, 2011, www.cbo.gov/publication/22077.

2. US Department of Health and Human Services, Centers for Medicare & Medicaid Services, "What Providers Need to Know: Accountable Care Organizations," *Medicare Fact Sheet,* March 31, 2011. Aparna Higgins et al, "Early Lessons from Accountable Care Models in the Private Sector," *Health Affairs* 30, no. 9 (2011): 1718–1727. S. M. Lieberman and J. M. Bertko, "Building Regulatory and Operational Flexibility into Accountable Care Organizations and 'Shared Savings,'" *Health Affairs* 30, no. 1 (2011): 23–31.

3. Kaiser Health News, "The IPAB: The Center of A Political Clash Over How to Change Medicare," www.kaiserhealthnews.org, March 22, 2012.

4. R. V. Burkhauser, S. Lyons, and K. Simon, "The Importance and Measurement of 'Affordable' in the Affordable Care Act," NBER working paper #17279. Daniel Polsky and David Grande, "The Burden of Health Care Costs for Working Families—Implications for Reform," *New England Journal of Medicine* 361, no. 5 (2009): 437–439; Didem M. Bernard, Jessica S. Banthin, and William Encinosa, "Wealth, Income and the Affordability for Health Insurance Coverage," *Health Affairs* 28, no. 3 (May 2009): 887–896. P Ketsche et al, "Lower Income Families Pay a Higher Share of Income," *Health Affairs* 30, no. 9 (2011): 1637–1646.

5. D. U. Himmelstein et al, "Medical Bankruptcy in the United States, 2007: Results of a National Study," *American Journal of Medicine* 122, no. 8 (2009): 741–746.

6. Brian K. Bucks, Arthur B. Kennickell, Traci L. Mach, and Kevin B. Moore, "Changes in U.S. Family Finances from 2004 to 2007: Evidence from the Survey of Consumer Finances," *Federal Reserve Bulletin* (2008), A8–38, http://www.federalreserve.gov/pubs/bulletin/.

7. B. G. Auguste, M. Laboissiere, and L. T. Mendonca, "How Health Care Costs Contribute to Income Disparity in the United States," *McKinsey Quarterly* April 2009, https://www.mckinseyquarterly.com/Economic_Studies/Country_Reports/How_health_care_costs_contribute_to_income_disparity_in_the_United_States_2328. David Auerbach and Arthur Kellerman, "A Decade of Health Care Cost Growth has Wiped Out Real Income Gains for an Average US Family," *Health Affairs* 30, no. 9 (2011): 1630–1636.

8. Congress Budget Office, CBO's 2011 Long Term Budget Outlook. www.cbo.gov.

9. J Gruber, "The Impacts of the Affordable Care Act: How Reasonable are the Projections?" NBER working paper #17168, June 2011. C. J. Courtemanche, D. Zapata, "Does Universal Coverage Improve Health? The Massachusetts Experience," NBER working paper #17893, 2012. S. K. Long, K. Stockley, H. Dahlen, "Massachusetts Health Reforms: Uninsurance Remains Low, Self-Reported health Status Improves as State Prepares to Tackle Costs," *Health Affairs* 31, no. 2 (2012): 444–451.

10. T. C. Buchmueller, J. DiNardo, R. G. Valletta, "The Effect of an Employer Health Insurance Mandate on Health Insurance Coverage and the Demand for Labor: Evidence from Hawaii," *American Economic Journal: Economic Policy* 3, no. 4 (2011): 25–51. Amy Finklestein et al, "The Oregon Health Insurance Experiment: Evidence from the First Year," NBER working paper #17190, July 2011.

11. Alain Enthoven, *Theory and Practice of Managed Competition in Health Care Finance* (Amsterdam: North-Holland, 1988).

12. C. Ullmer et. al. *Essential Health Benefits: Balancing Coverage and Cost* (Washington, D.C.: National Academy of Science, 2011).

13. Cantor J, AC Monheit, D. DeLia and K Lloyd, "The Role of Federal and State Dependent Coverage Eligibility Policies on the Health Insurance Status of Young Adults," NBER wp#18254, July 2012. Abby Goodnough, "Insurance Rebates Seen as Selling Point for Health Law," *The New York Times*, July 30, 2012.

14. J. Liebman and R. Zeckhauser, "Simple Humans, Complex Insurance, Subtle Subsidies," NBER working paper #14330, 2008. J. M. McWilliams et al, "Complex Medicare Advantage Choices may Overwhelm Seniors," *Health Affairs* 30, no. 9 (2011): 1786–1794.

CHAPTER 18

VALUE FOR MONEY IN THE FUTURE OF HEALTH CARE

QUESTIONS

1. What, how, and for whom is medical care provided?
2. Is Medicare likely to go broke or continue to grow?
3. Will investors put more money into biotechnology or nursing homes?
4. How will economists affect the allocation of health care? Of health care incomes?
5. Are people willing to spend more and get less health?
6. Why is it so hard to reach a consensus if everyone knows what the problem is?

18.1 FORCING THE QUESTION: WHO GETS HEALTHY AND WHO GETS PAID?

The most important contribution economists can make to the operation of the health care system is to be relentless in pointing out that every choice involves a trade-off: that difficult questions regarding who gets what, and who must give up what, are inevitable and must be faced even when politicians, the public, and patients would rather avoid them. In the words of Paul Samuelson, "Every economy must answer a triad of questions: *what*, *how*, and for *whom*."[1] In the case of cancer, for example, one could ask what symptoms or diagnoses are to be treated, should this treatment be inpatient or outpatient, by generalists or specialists, and who is to receive first priority for treatment (those who are most ill, those most likely to recover, those with the best insurance, or those who plan ahead and show up first). Although these questions can be asked independently, the answer to one influences all the others: "For whom" affects "what" and "how," and vice versa. Any answer also determines who pays, who gets paid, and how much. That is, it determines the distribution of income as well as the distribution of health care.

It is the job of economists to give advice, not patient care. They estimate, evaluate, and elucidate the decisions to be made, but do not make the decisions or carry them out. The analysis of decision making can be divided into three levels:

WHAT ARE THE QUESTIONS?

WHO IS GOING TO DECIDE?

WHAT ARE THE ANSWERS?

For most economists, it is necessary to work backward, starting with the data collection required to make comparisons among different treatments (i.e., cost–benefit analysis), then consider how different systems for making medical care decisions can affect efficiency (e.g., physician practices versus hospital IT systems, patients, or regulatory authorities), and only then approach the top level—framing the questions (What is fair? Public or private financing? Are new discoveries more important than caring for the elderly?). Tracing the flow of money over the last 17 chapters reveals that although data can be used for clarification, the questions are fundamentally *economic*: They are about choices and thus have to do with values as well as numbers. Are some lives worth more than others? How much should a surgeon be paid for a one-hour operation if it saves a life? If it fails to save a life? Which product of the health care system is more important: social justice or cancer mortality?

The pragmatic and detailed collection of data for comparing the costs and outcomes of different drugs, different surgical procedures, and different treatment settings has grown rapidly over the last decade. Doing such work requires a tremendous amount of clinical knowledge

---

BEHAVIORAL ECONOMICS: RATIONAL CHOICE WITH A NUDGE

Modern ("neoclassical") economics has been based on the logical structure of rational choice theory, which assumes that each person acts in a way that maximizes her or his own well-being (utility). It was always recognized that some behavior did not meet this standard of perfection, yet most economists assumed that deviations were random, resulting from a lack of experience or foresight, or were eventually brought into alignment with utility maximization over time. Two psychologists, Daniel Kahneman and Amos Tversky, demonstrated clearly that there were common and quite predictable deviations, "consistently irrational" choices.[2] The new "behavioral" economics has provided several interdisciplinary findings of great importance to health economics. Having more choices, which economists used to assume always makes consumers better off, frequently makes people less satisfied and more likely to make poor choices or none ("I just couldn't pick one—there were too many to choose from"). The Medicare supplemental market actually became more competitive and more satisfactory to many elderly participants once the options were limited to 10 well-defined choices. Paying people to attend smoking cessation or exercise classes gets much more participation than providing "equivalent" rewards in the form of tax breaks. Although economists used to assume that people would always make a deal, any deal, that made them better off, a series of experiments have shown that people often do not participate if they think the deal is unfair (e.g., two people split a reward, with one getting $2 and the other $998), and they sometimes use their own money to "punish" unfairness even though such acts of conscience do not benefit them directly. Although cost–benefit analyses often assume that "having" something and not losing it is worth the same as "getting" it, this turns out rarely to be the case. A person might only be willing to pay $2,000 to partially reverse a hearing loss caused by a birth defect but might want to sue for $500,000 if an accident causes the same loss.

These insights provide a more nuanced understanding of how incentives affect behavior and are beginning to be used in a number of practical ways to improve health policy: for example, automatically enrolling new employees in health insurance and then giving them options, rather than making them sign up and choose a plan, or paying a cash bonus of $500 to new mothers who get all of their baby's shots on time instead of a deduction on income taxes. Behavioral economics does not so much contradict the traditional rational choice model as supplement it, and it provides methods to improve efficiency in the real world.

and an understanding of basic economic principles: equilibrium at the margin, production functions, comparative advantage, opportunity cost, and so on. Increasingly, such work is being carried out by clinicians who have training in economic concepts, while economists concentrate on developing theory and new measurement techniques.

Upon this mass of detailed data collection and analysis rests the second layer of issues regarding how to design a better health care system. At this level, the question is not whether radiation is better than chemotherapy but whether capitation or fee for service leads to better decisions, or whether group practice is more efficient than solo practice. The focus shifts from the particular decision being made to the issue of who is making the decision: physicians, patients, or payers (see the box "Behavioral Economics").

As economists trace how the flow of money follows the path of decision making, the assumptions embedded in the current medical care system become more evident. Analysis at the third level becomes reflective. What does "better" mean? According to which value system? Better for whom? Is it fair? Analysis transcends the current system as it is by asking: "What are the questions?" Reaching beyond the veil of money and grasping the concept that every dollar spent on health care is a dollar earned by a health care provider helps clarify how the distribution of income and health are connected and suggests fruitful directions for assessing the health implications of changes in economic organization.

18.2 SPENDING MONEY OR PRODUCING HEALTH?

The distribution of health is unequal. This has a profound impact on economic well-being. Some people work productively for years and die contentedly with wealth and happiness in old age, while others struggle for a few months or decades in agony as they are relentlessly drawn down into premature mortality. The question is not whether the distribution of health is fair, or whether it determines or is determined by income, but whether and how it can be changed. More narrowly, one might ask how, and how much, change can be brought about by spending more on medical care? What is that change worth? The marginal productivity of medical care spending tends to decline as more is spent. Increasing spending from $7,000 to $8,000 per person increases average life expectancy, but not by as much as increasing spending from $2,000 to $3,000, and even that does not have as large an effect as going from $0 to $1,000.

Reaching a consensus on how much to spend becomes more complicated when there are two or more types of people who are to receive care. Suppose that one group is relatively healthy and would maintain a high level of health even if no money were spent on them, while another group begins at a disadvantage and even with maximal effort would still remain less healthy. If the same amount is spent per person on each group, the total and marginal impact of medical care will be very low in the healthy group, which seems wasteful, while the sicker group would still be forced to do without a lot of potentially beneficial care. To jointly maximize the average healthiness of all people for a given health care budget, it would be necessary to equalize the marginal productivity of medical care (increase in health per additional dollar spent) across both groups, spending much more per person on the sicker people. Such an allocation of medical care resources might seem both fair and efficient, but it also might not. Suppose that the healthy group consisted of employed people who paid insurance premiums, whereas the sicker group were heroin and cocaine users living on the streets. Most voters would not be willing to cut funding for those who take care of themselves and go to work every day in order to provide more funding to people who stick needles in their arms. Further complications are posed by groups such as infants born with genetic defects or severely wounded policemen who are likely to die even with the best medical care. Should they be denied treatment on the grounds that it would not do them much good anyway? Questions such as these evoke strong emotional reactions because they touch on deeply held beliefs and assumptions about humanity and the allocation of health.

The distinction between "medical decisions" and the "determinants of health" is important. Stating that the goal of medical care is to *maximize health* might appear both accurate and appropriate. However, some reflection and reading the last 17 chapters shows how inaccurate and irrelevant such a measure often is. If taken literally, maximizing health would mean that most hospitals in the United States would close so that more food, clothes, books, and medicine could be provided to Afghanistan, Indonesia, Mozambique, and other less-developed countries. It would also force most surgeons to give up their operating rooms in favor of sewage treatment plants and force psychiatrists to give up providing therapy and prescribing psychoactive drugs in favor of immunization campaigns and early childhood education. To assert that the goal of medical care is to maximize health for all is not only inaccurate but also profoundly misleading. It confuses a measure of social welfare with the incentives of the groups that make up society to maximize their own welfare. Doctors, nurses, hospital supply company executives, National Basketball Association players, healthy industrial workers, college students, and other definable groups have multiple objectives, including the health of their families and their own incomes, many of which are more important to them than the advancement of global health averages.

It is relatively easy to understand why most Americans do not want all of their hospitals to close and why most of the doctors who work in them are not eager to practice in Mozambique, even if they are certain that the number of additional life-years produced would be higher. It is less obvious why Americans keep spending so much more on medical care. Baseline life expectancy is much higher now than it was a century ago, making every extra year of life expectancy added more difficult and more expensive to obtain, implying that marginal productivity (gain in life expectancy per additional dollar spent) to be much lower today than it was 50 or 100 years ago. If society were actually optimizing by choosing the point at which the value of health matched the price of health, and the value of health were the same as before, then less money would be spent as technology improved (owing to diminishing marginal productivity).[3] Instead, we now spend more per person, implying that the incremental increase in health per additional dollar is even smaller. Extrapolating from the comparisons with Japan, Germany, and England in Chapter 16, it appears that it would be possible to cut spending by a third or more with only a minor impact on health, leaving average life expectancy in the United States almost unchanged at 79 years.[4]

The declining marginal productivity of health care dollars is offset by two demand effects. Technological advance and process improvements make existing medical treatments less costly over time, raising the quantity demanded as price per unit falls. Probably even more important is that rising aggregate wealth raises the dollar value of each additional year of health gained (see Table 15.3) and reduces the relative value of other goods.[5] There is also some augmentation of medical buying power among specific groups that are likely to be high users of care (the elderly, children with disabilities). Yet even considering all these factors, the vastness and rapidity of the increase in medical expenditure cannot easily be explained purely in terms of productivity and relative prices.

18.3   DYNAMIC EFFICIENCY

A major difficulty for health economics is that the question of "how to improve efficiency" is usually less relevant to reform than the question of "how to make a deal." Deals are tough to make because any significant change in the allocation of resources is going to hurt somebody and thus generate resistance. Groups that will be harmed are not sure that their concerns are adequately weighed or the harm done to them is balanced fairly by benefits gained from other programs and policies. Assurances of fair treatment are harder to believe the more distant in time and uncertain the compensating benefits are. A group of elderly people might be willing to accept less technologically advanced treatment for a reduction in their premiums and out-of-pocket costs, but they might not be willing to make such a sacrifice to fund research that will only bring results 20 or 30 years from now. Such reluctance may be short-sighted, but it is perfectly reasonable.

THE VALUE OF MEDICAL PROGRESS

Is the development of new medical technology worth the cost? Should we have spent so much money trying to improve health? William Nordhaus concluded that the growth in longevity in the United States during the 20th century was worth almost as much as all of the growth in GDP (market goods and services) in the economy.[6] However, a substantial portion of that increase in longevity was due to better housing, nutrition, heating, transportation, and other nonmedical factors. David Cutler and Mark McClellan examined technological advances in five conditions: heart attack, low birth weight, breast cancer, depression, and cataracts. Table 18.1 summarizes their findings. For heart attacks, the cost of treatment increased from $12,083 in 1984 to $21,714 in 1998 (inflation adjusted), a real increase of $9,631 per case.[7] Life expectancy increased from just under five years to a bit over six, a gain of more than a year. If society values an extra year of life at $10,000 or more, it appears that the gains in health are worth more than the cost. (Usual assumptions for the value of a year of life are in the range of $75,000 to $375,000 per additional year.) Conversely, treatment of breast and many other cancers has become substantially more expensive but has not reduced mortality rates or provided sizable increases in life expectancy. Overall assessment depends on the mix of treatments and individuals considered. On balance, averaged across all types of people and all kinds of treatments (the good, the mediocre, and the truly awful), investment in medical technology appears to have provided substantial net benefits to society, although it is also evident that some kinds of treatment still in use are not worth the costs.

TABLE 18.1   Costs and Gains of Medical Technology

Condition	Period	Incremental Cost	Gains from Treatment
Heart attack	1984 to 1998	$9,631	One more year of life
Low birth weight	1950 to 1990	$40,000	Twelve years of life
Depression	1991 to 1996	(decreased)	Better quality of life
Cataracts	1969 to 1998	($0 or decrease)	Better quality of life
Breast cancer	1985 to 1996	$20,000	Two months of life

Source: Cutler and McClellan (2001).

The problems of allocation are often formalized by economists in terms of technical productivity (maximizing the output from any given set of resource inputs), cost minimization (choosing the least expensive set of inputs), and current economic efficiency (balancing marginal costs and marginal benefits) (see "Efficiency" in Section 2.8 and "The Value of Medical Progress," above). More sophisticated analyses may also consider how systems are structured to deal with transaction costs and public goods. In medicine, the most important allocation may be that between current consumption and future productivity. The difference between adequate and outstanding current practice is far smaller than the gap between what was possible twenty years ago and what is expected within the next decade (e.g., gene therapy, real-time imaging, robotic laser surgery, in vitro diagnoses). The challenge is to structure a health care system for *dynamic efficiency*, creating technological and organizational change to improve health and productivity. Some current allocative efficiency must be sacrificed for scientists to spend time tinkering to make new discoveries and to give managers the slack to come up with ideas for new products and service delivery systems. A purely cost-minimizing organization is not creative enough to be economically efficient in the long run.

18.4   DISTRIBUTION, DISTRIBUTION, DISTRIBUTION

When asked which three factors are most important in determining value, real estate appraisers reply, "location, location, and location." In a similar vein, health economists asked to determine the value of the money spent on health care might say "allocation, allocation, and allocation," focusing repeatedly on distributional issues: the distribution of resources, the distribution of health, the distribution of medical care, and the distribution of provider incomes. Although a high value is often placed on the quality of nursing care, the skill of the physician, or the use of new medical technology, none of these matters much if the care is provided to the wrong person or at the wrong time. Health economists are asked to assess economic efficiency—how well the health care system has used the resources available to achieve its stated (and unstated) goals. The following short list contains a few of the questions that must be answered in this regard:

- Which diseases should be treated?
- Should we aim for more research or more primary care?
- Which people should be treated?
- How much care should be given?
- Who will pay?
- If the money is to come from taxes, who should be taxed most—those who benefit most or those who can most afford to pay?
- Should more money be spent on prevention or cure?
- How much should healers be paid?
- Should treatment be given by specialists or primary care providers?
- How should the power to make decisions be allocated?

Allocation is the subject of economics. Why then haven't economists been more successful in reforming health care? First, it must be recognized that the study of health economics has indeed improved efficiency to some degree. It has made the system better, although it is still far from perfect. Cost–benefit analysis has led to a reduction in the overinvestment in hospitals, to the support and improvement of immunization programs, and to the more rapid and objective evaluation of new drugs. Assessment of incentives and risk bearing has led to the creation of new types of insurance and to the refinement of managed care contracting. The application of microeconomics to decisions regarding individual allocation has only limited potential, however, because the most crucial issues in health are likely to involve personal values, public goods, macroallocation, contentious questions of how the costs and benefits are to be distributed between different groups of producers and consumers, and the political dynamics of change.

18.5   PATH DEPENDENCE AND THE POSSIBILITIES FOR REFORM

Path dependence is the term social scientists use to describe the fact that the current system is not only a function of current conditions but also a function of the path taken to get here. Whereas the external demographic, economic, and technological forces matter, so do the organizations, institutions, and culture that have developed over the years, as well as the habits and rules they have accumulated. What path dependence means for health care is that any reforms likely to actually take place will grow out of the existing system—perhaps removing some flaws and adding some innovative elements, but not creating anew from scratch.[8] The "new" will be a pragmatic extension of the old. Rather than a pure and idealized structure, a reformed U.S. health care system will make compromises with history and the give-and-take of American politics.

How Did We Get Here?

Two signature institutional characteristics of the U.S. health care system, professional licensure and voluntary community hospitals, gelled and formalized during the 1920s and 1930s. Medical care was just becoming scientific and therapeutically relevant (although most of our science was still borrowed from Europe). Costs were low at $30 per person per year (about $400 in 2012 dollars), and amounted to less than 4 percent of GDP. From 1935 to 1955 the prestige of medicine grew tremendously, although costs remained modest. Advances such as antibiotics and artificial kidneys were announced with awe as "medical miracles," and medical care got much of the credit for increases in life expectancy that were as much due to better nutrition, sanitation, and other public health measures as to therapeutic improvements (see Section 15.9). The major institutions of insurance and technology-driven academic medicine coalesced in the 1950s and 1960s (Medicare, Medicaid, NIH, Health Professions Educational Assistance). Flooding the system with money after 1965 created a new technocracy, with medical specialties growing as if on steroids. The fusty gentlemen's club of the 1920s with its quaint rules and traditions that largely excluded minorities and women from the profession was pushed aside in favor of selection by merit and scientific knowledge. Medical care grew rapidly, but GDP was also growing rapidly. With the help of employer-based health plans, most Americans could afford to pay for all of the new medical care available with little problem, since it still added up to less than 6 percent of GDP.

The story of American medicine in the 20th century would seem to be one of triumphant success if we were to stop there, but tensions inherent in the system created in 1965 began to appear soon afterward and have worsened over time. Too many specialists meant not enough individual attention from a family doctor. Costs kept rising even as some of the medical "miracles" began to lose their shine. Hospital bills became a major cause of personal bankruptcy. Health insurance from an employer became harder to obtain and kept requiring more copays and more paperwork, while the inability to cover 50 million uninsured persons nagged at the nation's conscience. Faith in technical progress and trust in the profession sagged. By 2008 it was common to see newspaper articles labeling the health care system "broken," and the Congressional Budget Office had already fingered rising health care costs as "unsustainable" and the major cause of future budget deficits.[9]

The United States still has the path-dependent remnants of a medical profession based on the reality of the 1920s, an insurance system based on the employee benefits of the 1950s and 1960s, and academic medical centers built on the expansive funding of the 1970s. The organizations built on those foundations were great back then but are now in need of a makeover. Yet change in the health care system is slow and inertial, with a delayed and drawn-out response to changes in the economic, social, scientific, and political environment.

What Did Medicine Miss?

Most of the economy has gone through substantial change since 1970, becoming leaner and more flexible to deal with inflation, foreign competition, and aggressive investors that moved capital and labor around to achieve greater efficiency. Not medicine. IBM was a giant of the 1960s that has been supplanted by a succession of firms over the decades: Intel, Microsoft, Google. Sears and A&P dominated retailing, and no one had heard of Wal-Mart, much less Amazon. In retrospect, it can be difficult to appreciate how painful and harsh this process is. Termed "creative destruction" by Joseph Schumpeter in his classic 1942 economic text *Capitalism, Socialism and Democracy*, technological and organizational change forces workers to lose jobs and find new careers. It is not fun to compete in the economy, just necessary. Losing hurts, and people do not always get to start over again from the same place and are often worse off for years.

In medicine, entrenched practices, revered traditions, and a rising flow of funds kept the profession from undergoing many of the changes in management, financing, workflow, and information processing that gradually revolutionized most of the rest of the economy. Long after bar codes and online ordering had become common elsewhere, medical professionals still shuffled paper records.[10] Medicare "Part A" and "Part B" enshrines a distinction between inpatient and ambulatory care from the 1960s that has become increasingly irrelevant and whose continuation makes it difficult to bundle prices meaningfully. Whatever else the emerging medical system accomplishes, it must bring **teamwork** and modern **information technology** to the practice of medicine. Inadequate management structure and IT means that administrative costs are higher, and the ability to track results lower, in the U.S. health system than in those of most other developed countries.[11]

What Went Wrong? Notable Failures and Unresolved Dilemmas

The United States was recognized throughout the 20th century as the technological leader in medicine, with more Nobel laureates than any other country. But it is also recognized as having developed a health care system that is overly expensive, does not deliver particularly good health (mortality and morbidity are average or below that for other developed countries), and leaves many citizens without insurance or lacking access to quality care. It has become increasingly apparent that the most critical problem is a continual increase in costs without commensurate improvement in health outcomes. Paying a lot might be worthwhile if people felt they were getting a lot out of the system, but they do not. Surveys show dissatisfaction with medical care as a whole and a pervasive sense that professional and business relationships have deteriorated.[12] For many Americans, it seems that health insurance premiums are becoming unaffordable, that hospitals and doctors do not "care" as personally for patients as they used to, that medical advances are increasingly of a "me-too" variety that provide only incremental gains—in short, that health care is not as good as it used to be.

Given the broad agreement that rising costs and falling satisfaction are the main problems in health care, it is a bit surprising that there is no consensus regarding what to do. Instead, health policy is faced with a series of contentious questions and enduring conflicts. Should funding be public or private? Do hospitals and doctors need more regulation or more competition? Are new drugs priced too high, or too low? How can we cover the uninsured? These conflicts can be traced to fundamental *unresolved dilemmas of dynamics and distribution*. Path dependence means following an American path, as determined by American culture and history: the frontier society that embraced liberty and innovation to become the capitalist leader of the free world and dominant economy of the year 2000. Sometimes this means aggressive free-market competition so that entrepreneurs can advance the process of creative destruction by which new technologies and new companies wipe out the old. However, path dependence also means that entrenched interests (professional monopolies, pharmaceutical firms, political parties) will fight to maintain profits by deflecting or stifling competition. Everyone admires competition and growth in theory, yet no one wants their job to be the one that is replaced by computerization or low-cost foreign labor. The conflict between open entrepreneurialism and closed protection of existing organizations creates sharp tensions.

Failures in health policy are best illustrated by looking at the extremes: an unregulated market of "consumer-driven health care" with purely private ownership at one end, and totally regulated "universal health care" organized and financed collectively by the government at the other. Plans emphasizing personal responsibility for medical costs (health savings accounts [HSAs], medical savings accounts [MSAs], and other consumer-directed health plans described in Section 5.3) were crafted during the 1990s in imitation of the "defined contribution" 401k, individually owned retirement plans that were increasingly being used to replace company-provided defined-benefit retirement plans. MSAs shifted risk and responsibility onto the individual, rather than relying on broad government or employer financing pools that covered thousands or millions of people. Originally a niche within the self-employed individual health insurance market, high-deductible MSAs were held by advocates of an "ownership society" to be a superior alternative to existing employer-provided health insurance because they would give patients "more skin in the game" (i.e., a larger financial stake in each episode of care) and hence be able to use consumer choice to control health care costs (and incidentally relieve employers and government from doing so, just as the 401k had shifted responsibility for retirement from the employer to the individual). Employees, however, did not embrace consumer-directed plans with much enthusiasm. The niche expanded but remained a niche rather than becoming the mainstream alternative.

As 401k plans got clobbered in 2008 and 2009 people had less enthusiasm for picking up another such financial vehicle in an MSA or HSA. The idea that the individual employee should take personal risk for retirement and health care rather than relying on large-scale risk pooling through employers or government became less appealing. Advocates still push to replace most existing health insurance with MSA-type plans, but the limited ability to attract more than a narrow segment of the market and a fear of financial crisis make it doubtful that any broad move to privatize most risks will become politically acceptable within the next few years. Even before the political reversals brought about by the 2008 election, legislation to privatize Social Security was unable to pass Congress. Privatizing Medicare is a nonstarter. Other factors that make regulation seem more appealing than purely market-driven for-profit solutions are the series of convictions and fines levied against private hospital chains (AMI, HealthSouth, National Medical Enterprises, Columbia-HCA, Tenet) and health insurance companies (Oxford Health Plans, United Health, Ingenix) for market abuse violations, as well as the accumulating evidence that private Medicare Advantage plans, rather than saving money, actually cost more than regular Medicare.[15]

The other extreme is represented by "universal health care," financed by government and uniformly available to everyone without charge. Many doctors feel that medical care should be allocated to those who need it most, not those who can afford to pay the most. They point to wasteful advertising of expensive new drugs (which have high profit margins) and elaborate surgical interventions yielding only slight improvements, while proven low-cost remedies (aspirin, vaccinations) are not promoted among the populations most at risk. Yet universal health care for the United States, despite persistent legislative efforts by advocates, has consistently failed to gather majority support at any time since it was first proposed in 1918. A minority has always been strongly in favor, but the majority of the public has refused to accept a purely public health care system. This political failure has been influenced by doctors, especially entrepreneurs in solo (or small group) practice fiercely protective of their independence and autonomy, and also by the public's generally negative perceptions of the post office, public housing, drivers' licensing bureaus, and other government-run enterprises.

The American electorate tends to value independence and personal liberties more, and trust government less, than do most Europeans, Asians, or citizens in the rest of the world. Rarely do people in the United States willingly allow government control over their daily lives or make it illegal to spend money on some service because it is not worthwhile.[16] "Managed care" generated a huge backlash in part because it crimped doctors' incomes but more because it was perceived as an interference with "freedom of practice," restricting what patients could obtain from their private doctors. Distributional issues create tensions and tradeoffs between the sick and the well, the old versus the new, urban versus rural, and the rich versus the poor. Even when it is agreed that everyone should have health care, it is hard to reach consensus on who is going to pay for it and how much each person should get.

18.6 THE PATH FORWARD: STEP BY STEP

Every country that has extended health insurance to the entire population and achieved some degree of success in controlling costs has built upon existing blocks of partial financing, filling in the cracks over time. The first national health insurance program in Germany in 1883 covered only miners and industrial workers (Chapter 4). Australia, France, Canada, and Japan similarly started with partial coverage of a limited group of workers. Later new plans (or expansions of existing ones) extended coverage to dependents, farmers, the elderly, the self-employed, and so on. The English National Health Service is perhaps a bit different in that virtually all of the hospitals had already been taken over by the government during the war, and most doctors and nurses had been in the military, so the step to a government-run system with doctors and nurses as public employees was just a small shuffle that rationalized an existing situation when the NHS began operations in 1948. Those who favor a government-run national health service for the United States must face the facts that the situation in 2012 is far different from that in postwar England and that legislation sponsoring universal health coverage has been repeatedly rejected by the U.S. Congress.

Private employer-based health insurance, along with voluntary hospital and insurance plans (Blue Cross and Blue Shield), became entrenched as pillars of health financing in the United States during the 20th century. The social insurance program that was tried and accepted in the United States is Medicare, which has become immensely popular and has strong political support. These forms of health financing may be supplemented or modified but are unlikely to suddenly disappear. Medicare was originally crafted in imitation of existing private medical insurance plans with UCR and indemnity reimbursement based on charges. As Medicare moved from a secondary role to become the biggest player in the health insurance market, it went from being guided by the private market to creating its own system of terminology and administered prices (DRGs, RBRVS, etc.) that are now guidelines leading the rest of the market.

Although each polar extreme is loved by its partisan advocates, neither government-provided health care (NHS) nor pure private ownership (HSAs) with vouchers is probable in the United States right now. New regulations and legislation are inevitable. The important long-run issue is, will they be used? In principle, Medicare officials could go ahead now and regulate payment so that only effective therapies are reimbursed using existing rule-making powers and technical advisory panels. So far, Medicare officials have usually backed away from such direct regulation. It is not the legislation that creates change but the change in organizations and institutions that creates a new "path."

As long as Americans believe that access to the latest medical technology is more important than the financial insecurity of escalating uncontrolled costs, as long as it is accepted that

American health care is obviously superior to that practiced in other countries where greater life expectancy and patient satisfaction are provided at less cost, then little will change. Until doctors and other medical professionals are willing to shift from autonomous cottage practices to modern management and information technology, very little systematic change can occur.

18.7   THE SHAPE OF HEALTH CARE SPENDING TO COME

It is never possible to predict the future with certainty, but a review of historical trends (Chapter 15) and the simple fact that spending is eventually constrained by the availability of funds make it likely that the long-run trend of health care spending will take on the S-shape that characterizes most growth curves. After a long period of unsteady growth with little cumulative increase, a tipping point or sudden acceleration pushes growth exponentially upward. Ever more steeply inclined growth meets inherent constraints that begin to bend the curve back (inflexion point) toward moderation and eventual stability. For medical expenditures, the long period of vacillating slow growth extends back before the founding of the United States. Health care accounted for perhaps 1 to 3 percent of total consumption for hundreds of years. During the period 1929 to 1955, U.S. spending grew at an annual rate of less than GDP +0.9 percent, and it amounted to less than a 5 percent share of total consumption. From 1955 through 1993, the average rate of growth exceeded GDP +3 percent, and health care accounted for more than 13 percent of total GDP. Since then, the rate of growth has slowed and averaged about GDP +1.5 percent. Exactly when or at what level health expenditures will finally stabilize is far from clear. Excessive growth is likely to continue at least for a decade, and perhaps beyond 2025. However, it is likely that the average rate of long-run growth will begin to level out in the range of GDP +0 to 1 percent sometime before 2050 (see Figure 18.1).

FIGURE 18.1   Growth Curve: Health Share of GDP 1850–2099?

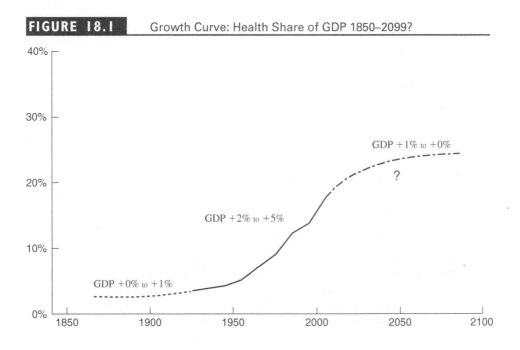

18.8   THE LONG RUN: 2050 AND BEYOND

What can be said about the future of health and medical care over the next 50 years? The box "Future Trends" lists some expected trends. It is relatively certain that there will be continued increases in longevity, greater technological capability to treat disease, and continuous increases in expenditure. Although there will be more spending overall, the sources and uses of funding will change rather markedly, and it is probable that at some point the annual rate of increase will moderate. An older and healthier population implies more long-term care, with greater emphasis on caring and rehabilitation. Thus, the fraction of medical spending accounted for by acute illnesses of the employed tax-paying population will fall. The tension between public and private financing is likely to remain unresolved, with payers operating under a mixture of market incentives and regulatory structures to provide a middle ground. Treatment and production will become less and less important relative to the provision of care and information management. Organization and teamwork will be more important as solo practice continues to fade. Quality control will rely on outcomes more than the initial qualifications and resource use by specialists and clinical technicians, with integrated assessment of processes in real time rather than examination of each part or profession separately. Some of these changes will be the disruptive consequences of medical and organizational entrepreneurship, but most will be slow, inertial, and incremental. The net effect of all these changes will on balance be beneficial, yet most are apt to be painful and resisted by some constituency.

FUTURE TRENDS

- Greater longevity, better health
- More long-term and chronic care, less acute illness
- More spending overall, but a smaller fraction spent on the working population
- Less ability to shift costs by overcharging for treatment
- A middle ground between public and private control
- More assessment of cost and outcomes
- Declining trust in organized professions
- Physicians leading teams within organizations and having less autonomy and independence
- Successful organizations based on information (e.g., biotechnology) and caring (e.g., hospice)
- Special characteristics previously found mostly in medical care becoming more typical of many service organizations in a post-industrial economy

---

The best prototypes for studying health economics in the 21st century are probably bio-technology and hospice. Physicians will become technical team leaders operating within a corporate organization, rather than independent medical practitioners. Cost shifting in the form of marked-up prices and open-ended reimbursement will continue to wither and be replaced by new forms, such as mandated benefits pools. The use of economic information and cost accounting for comparative decision making will continue to increase. Greater knowledge about actual costs and the actual effectiveness of clinical practice will provide greater clarity in the questions raised about the tradeoff between dollars and health. Some fields (dietary modification, parts of mental health and disability care) are being spun off and are less likely to be counted as an integral part of medicine. Others, such as information systems and genetic engineering, are becoming more integrated and will blur the traditional boundaries between what is medicine and what is information or environmental modification.

The special institutional features that set medicine and health apart from the rest of the economy might become less distinctively special over the coming years. In part, this is because medicine is becoming more organized and more corporate, more subject to a bottom-line assessment of costs and benefits. Yet the extent to which medicine is becoming like the rest of the economy may be of less importance than the extent to which the rest of the economy is becoming like medicine, where information, service, and public goods matter more than manufactured commodities. Previously, health economists have taken models from the study of industrial production and applied them to health and medical care. Ideas might increasingly flow in the other direction as the issues of special interest to health economists—uncertainty, agency, trust, service delivery, and quality—become central to the economy as a whole in a postindustrial era. Models developed for the study of medical care might in the future be applied to banking, entertainment, automation, fashion, and other industries, leading to applications and discoveries as spectacular as genomic sequencing and heart transplants.

SUGGESTIONS FOR FURTHER READING

David M. Cutler and Mark McClellan, "Is Technological Change in Medicine Worth It?" *Health Affairs* 20, no. 5 (September 2001): 11–29.

Victor Fuchs, "Economics, Values and Health Care Reform," *American Economic Review* 86, no. 1 (1996): 1–24.

Atul Gawande, "Getting There from Here: How Should Obama Reform Health Care?" *The New Yorker* (January 26, 2009), 26–33.

Institute of Medicine, *Crossing the Quality Chasm*, July 2001, http://www.newton.nap.edu/catalog/1027.html

Ian Morrison, *Health Care in the New Millennium* (San Francisco: Jossey-Bass, 2000).

Jonathan Skinner and Douglas Staiger, "Technology Diffusion and Productivity Growth in Health Care," NBER working paper 14865, April 2009.

SUMMARY

1. A primary role of health economists is to **force the public and politicians to consider the tradeoffs** implicit in every health and medical care decision. Who gets helped? Who gets hurt? Who makes money?

2. Health economics can be viewed as answering questions in levels of ascending generality. At the base are the questions, **Which treatments are better?** and **How much do they cost?** At an intermediate level, **Who is going to have the power to make decisions?** Finally, **Which questions should be asked** to shape and judge the health care system?

3. The purpose of the health care system is to **satisfy the interests of the groups that participate** in it. Maximizing health is but one of many objectives. The average health of the population often matters much less than who, in particular, gets healthy.

4. The increase in health and life expectancy that can be obtained from any given set of medical resources depends largely on the **allocation** of treatment to those most likely to benefit. Often, this is not the group that is most able or willing to pay.

5. Major **difficulties in economic appraisal** of health care policies arise because the most important issues often involve **public goods** and the **distribution of benefits and incomes** to different groups, as well as technical issues regarding productive efficiency.

6. Differences in the quality of care at a particular point in time are usually dwarfed by changes in the effectiveness of care over time. Hence, a health care system must

provide resources and slack to make room for experiments, fostering the technological and organizational changes that bring about **dynamic efficiency**.

7. The health care system is **path dependent**, with institutions and organizations embedded in a cultural and financial matrix. This makes progress **slow and inertial, with delayed responses** to changes in the political, economic, and scientific environment.

8. Medical care has not yet experienced the **information technology** revolution or **financial restructuring** that forced many organizations to become more efficient over the last 40 years. In the future, **teamwork** and linked information systems will matter more to medical professions than solo practices and piece-by-piece quality assurance.

9. **Values** ultimately mean more in health economics than the efficacy of medical technology or the estimation of costs. Analysis will increasingly focus on **the economics of caring and information**, not on production.

PROBLEMS

1. {*allocation*} Will health care be more efficient or less efficient in 2020? Will people spend more money or less money on health care?

2. {*budget* } Will Medicare go broke by 2030 as some analysts predict? Why or why not? What historical evidence could you give to support your answer?

3. {*distribution*} Which matters more: how healthy we are on average or who gets healthy?

4. {*distribution*} Why redistribute health insurance costs and not automobile insurance costs?

5. {*values*} Economists debate the future of Medicare by arguing about which set of numbers best represents reality. Do these numbers represent objective or subjective values?

6. {*economic organization, distribution*} Who will make the decisions regarding medical care in the year 2020? Which of these groups will have more or less power over those decisions in 2020?

    a. Physicians
    b. Nurses
    c. Pharmaceutical companies
    d. Biotechnology investors
    e. U.S. Senators
    f. AARP (formerly the American Association of Retired Persons)
    g. Disability advocates
    h. Children
    i. Economists

7. {*productivity*} As medical technology continues to develop, will the marginal productivity of each additional dollar spent on it increase or decrease? What about the average productivity per dollar spent on medical care?

8. {*economic organization, distribution*} Are health care funds spent to maximize health or to maximize the welfare of those who make the decisions?

9. {*allocation, budget*} Given the ever-increasing age of the population and advance of medical technology, why would anyone expect the growth of medical costs to slow down in the future?

ENDNOTES

1. Paul Samuelson and William Nordhaus, *Economics,* 14th ed. (New York: McGraw-Hill, 1992), 19.
2. Daniel Kahneman, Paul Slovic, and Amos Tversky, *Judgment Under Uncertainty: Heuristics and Biases* (New York: Cambridge University Press, 1982); this is the classic in the field. See also: Richard H. Thaler and Cass R. Sunstein, *Nudge: Improving Decisions About Health, Wealth and Happiness* (New Haven: Yale University Press, 2008); Richard Frank, "Behavioral Economics and Health Economics," NBER working paper 10881, November 2004; Jeffrey Liebman and Richard Zeckhauser, "Simple Humans, Complex Insurance, Subtle Subsidies," NBER working paper 14330, September 2008; Richard Frank and Karine Lamiraud, "Choice, Price Competition and Complexity in Markets for Health Insurance," NBER working paper 13817, February 2008; Jason Abaluck and Jonathan Gruber, "Choice Inconsistencies Among the Elderly: Evidence from Plan Choice in the Medicare Part D Program," NBER working paper 14759, February 2009; Emmanuel Saez, "Details Matter: The Impact of Presentation and Information on the Take-up of Financial Incentives for Retirement Saving," *American Economic Journal: Economic Policy* 1, no. 1 (2009): 204–228.
3. It is possible to construct a production function that moves up and yet is steeper, with greater average productivity and yet lower marginal productivity for a given set of inputs, but it requires some contortion to do so, and such quirks are unlikely to explain the large and persistent rise in health care spending that has accompanied the 20th century advance of health care technology. Some other explanation must be found if the attempt is to remain plausible.
4. Alan Garber and Jonathan Skinner, "Is American Health Care Uniquely Inefficient?" NBER working paper 14257, August 2008; Jonathan Skinner and Douglas Staiger, "Technology Diffusion and Productivity Growth in Health Care," NBER working paper 14865, April 2009.
5. Hall, Robert E., and Charles I Jones, "The Value of Life and the Rise in Health Spending," *The Quarterly Journal of Economics* 122, no. 1 (2007): 39–72; Kevin Murphy and Robert Topel, "The Value of Health and Longevity," *Journal of Political Economy,* 114, no. 5 (2006): 871–904.
6. William D. Nordhaus, "The Health of Nations: The Contribution of Improved Health to Living Standards," NBER working paper 8818, January 2002.
7. David M. Cutler and Mark McClellan, "Is Technological Change in Medicine Worth It?" *Health Affairs* 20, no. 5 (September 2001): 11–29.
8. Atul Gawande, "Getting There from Here: How Should Obama Reform Health Care?" *The New Yorker,* 26 January 2009: 26–33.
9. Congressional Budget Office, *The Budget and Economic Outlook: An Update,* September 2008: XII; Peter Orzag, "The Long-Term Budget Outlook and Options for Slowing the Growth of Health Care Costs: Testimony for the Senate Finance Committee," Congressional Budget Office, June 17, 2008.
10. The Economist, "Medicine Goes Digital: A Special Report on Health Care and Technology," *The Economist,* 18 pages, April 18, 2009.
11. Randall D. Cebul et al., "Organizational Fragmentation and Care Quality in the U.S. Health Care System," NBER working paper 14212, August 2008.
12. George D. Lundberg, *Severed Trust: Why American Medicine Hasn't Been Fixed* (New York: Basic Books, 2000); R. J. Blendon et al., "Satisfaction with Health Care Systems in Ten Nations," *Health Affairs* 9, no. 2 (Summer 1990): 185–192; R. J. Blendon et al., "Understanding the American Public's Health Priorities: A 2006 Perspective," *Health Affairs* 25, no. 6 (October 2006): w508–w515.

ACA Affordable Care Act of 2010: see **PPACA**.

Activities of Daily Living (ADLs) A checklist measure of the extent of disability and functional status.

Actuarially Fair Premium A premium equal to the expected value of the loss, although in practice all premiums must be set higher in order to cover overhead costs.

Actuary Accredited insurance mathematician who calculates premium rates and company reserve requirements using statistical studies.

Administered Prices Prices that are specified by an administrative agency, rather than being set in the market.

Administered Service Only (ASO) A self-insured health plan in which the employer bears all the risk of losses but hires an administrator to process claims.

Administratively Necessary Days (ANDs) Payment for days when a patient's medical status is such that they should have been discharged from the hospital but were not because no nursing home beds were available.

Adverse Selection A disproportionate share of bad risks. When given a choice, the people who choose to purchase insurance are likely to be a group with higher than average losses.

Agency The process of having one party (the agent) make decisions on behalf of another (the principal).

Aggregation The process of clumping together; the creation of summary measures for a population as a whole; study at the system or group level.

Allocative Efficiency Allowing those who value a good more to consume more. Total consumption value is maximized by allowing the process to continue toward an equilibrium where for each individual, marginal benefit = marginal cost. Also, targeting medical care to those most in need so as to maximize average life expectancy.

American Medical Association (AMA) The professional organization that represents the interest of MD physicians in the United States and lobbies government agencies on their behalf.

Antitrust Legal restrictions relating to collusion between firms and market domination.

Arbitrage The process by which the prices of a good selling to different persons or in different markets are brought together by trade. Also, the act of buying and selling in anticipation of price movements, which makes the price adjust more rapidly to information.

Assignment An agreement by a physician to take payment directly from Medicare and to accept the amount as payment in full (i.e., with no balance billing).

Average Cost The total cost divided by the number of units.

Balance Billing Making the patient pay for the balance of any charges in excess of the amount allowed by the insurance company.

Balanced Budget Act of 1997 An act passed by the U.S. Congress in 1997 that significantly reduced provider payments and expanded the role of managed care in the Medicare program.

Branded Drugs Drugs whose production and sale are protected by a patent. Also, the brand-name drug produced by the initial firm even after its patent expires and other firms begin to sell competing generic versions.

Cap A limit on the amount that an insurance company will pay. The cap may be an overall maximum, such as a lifetime maximum of $250,000, or it may apply to specific services, such as a $500-per-year cap on outpatient mental health counseling.

Capitation Paying a fixed amount per enrolled person per month for a defined set of services; the amount does not vary with utilization.

Case-Mix Reimbursement Adjustment of reimbursement to account for differences in patient diagnoses, and sometimes for the severity of illness as well.

Certificate of Need (CON) A legal requirement that approval from a state agency to certify need

(CON) must be obtained before a health care facility is built or remodeled.

Ceteris Paribus All other factors being held constant.

Charges The amount appearing on the patient's bill.

Chiropractic An alternative form of medical practice that emphasizes spinal manipulation in the treatment of disease, often to the exclusion of drugs and surgery. Although chiropractors are found in most communities, they are often not accepted by the organized medical profession.

Circular Flow of Funds The circulation of money facilitates exchange; it is not used up or consumed. Each dollar spent by a consumer goes to a producer, who in turn gives it to an owner, worker, or supplier, who as consumers send those dollars on to another producer, and so on in an unending circular flow.

Clinical Pathways A protocol, or defined standard set of tests and procedures to be used in diagnosing or treating a particular symptom or disease.

Clinical Trials Testing of new drugs or medical technology on humans.

Coase Theorem The hypothesis that the type of economic organization (for-profit or nonprofit, one firm or many, capitalist or socialist) and which party holds ownership rights (e.g., chemical firms or fishermen, homeowners or airport operators) would not matter if there were no transaction costs.

Coinsurance The amount of the bill not paid by insurance but paid by the patient. A plan with 15 percent coinsurance means that the insurance company pays 85 percent and the person pays 15 percent.

Community Rating Setting the same premium rate for every person in the community regardless of age, sex, or previous illness.

Comparative Statics The study of a system by comparing how the state of equilibrium differs when some set of parameters (incomes, prices, fertility) differs; in contrast to dynamics, in which the process of change is the focus of study.

Compounding Adding to; the accumulation of growth over time; how a small percentage increase eventually leads, with interest on the interest, to doubling, quadrupling, and many-fold increasing.

Concurrent Review Daily checks by an HMO on the status of a patient to monitor, and if necessary, modify or terminate, the provision of services.

Consumer Price Index (CPI) A measure of the average change in price over time in a fixed "market basket" of goods and service purchased either by urban wage earners and clerical workers or by all urban consumers.

Consumer Surplus The difference between what consumers are willing to pay for a product and the market clearing price. As such, consumer surplus is represented by the area under the demand curve but above market price.

Consumption Function The relationship between consumption and income as income changes; the fraction of total income saved as the level or composition of aggregate income changes.

Continuing Care Retirement Communities (CCRCs) Living quarters for elderly persons with provisions for meals, transportation, therapy, and other assistance, usually constructed with an adjacent nursing home. Financial risks to the individual are often reduced through prepayment. Also known as life-care communities.

Copayment A specified amount that the patient must pay with each service received, such as the $2 for each prescription that many drug plans make the pharmacist collect, $10 for each day in the hospital under Medicare, $5 for each visit to the doctor under some HMO plans, etc. One of the purposes of copayments is to discourage overutilization. Thus while deductibles and coinsurance are sometimes covered under a spouse's plan or other insurance, the insured must usually pay the copayment out of pocket.

Cost Reimbursement Retrospective payment for services based upon audited cost reports, often including complex limits and rules for allocation.

Cost Shifting The process of using excess revenues from one set of services or patients to subsidize other services or patient groups.

Cost–Benefit Analysis (CBA) A set of techniques for assisting in the making of decisions, which translates all relevant concerns into market (dollar) terms.

Cost-Effectiveness Analysis (CEA) Comparison of the costs of different ways of achieving an objective (cases prevented, years of life saved). Similar to CBA, except that CEA does not require benefits to be expressed in dollar terms.

Cream Skimming Choosing to provide only the most profitable services or to insure only the healthiest patients to avoid subsidizing public goods (education, research, indigent care) and to obtain extra profits.

Cross-Sectional Analysis   Statistics constructed using observations across different individuals or groups at one point in time, as opposed to longitudinal or time-series analysis.

Deductible   An amount that must be paid by the individual before the insurance company begins to pay. For example, many policies have a $100-per-year deductible. This means that if total insured medical bills were $730, the insurance would apply only after the person had paid the first $100, that is, to $630.

Demand   A schedule of the amount that will be consumed in the market at varying prices.

Demographic Transition   The period of rapidly increasing population that usually occurs during economic development as a poor society with high mortality and high birth rates transitions to a wealthy society with low mortality and low birth rates.

Demographics   Age, sex, and other characteristics of populations.

Derived Demand   The demand for an input due to the demand for output; demand for a good due to its use, rather than in itself (e.g., the demand for x-ray film is derived from the demand for medical diagnoses, which in turn are derived from a consumer's demand for health).

Detailing   Marketing of pharmaceuticals to physicians by drug company representatives (detailers); offers of free samples and advice in order to increase the number of times a drug is prescribed.

Diagnostically Related Grouping (DRG)   A system of reimbursement which compensates by the case (rather than per day or per charged item) based on the diagnosis of the patient.

Diminishing Marginal Returns   As additional amounts of a variable input are put into the production process, holding constant all other variables, the incremental amount added to total output becomes smaller and smaller.

Discounted FFS   Contracts with providers to pay a specified percentage of usual charges.

Discounting   Adjustment of valuation for the passage of time, reflecting the fact that the present value of a future good is smaller. Also, adjustments to reflect risk, reductions in the quality of life, and other factors.

Diseconomies of Scale   The average cost per unit rises as the quantity produced increases.

Distribution   How evenly things are shared, divided, or spread out. The amount or frequency in the top 10 percent, second 10 percent, and so

on. In statistics, the shape of the graph when the number or probability of observations is arranged in order of magnitude (e.g., normal distribution, skewed distribution).

Dynamic Efficiency   Use of inputs so as to maximize long-run value over time, taking account of the need for tinkering to bring about technological and organizational advances.

Dynamic Shortage   A temporary deficit in supply caused by a sudden increase in demand or a sudden drop in supply.

Dynamics   The process of change; the study of how change occurs over time, including the order, timing, and strength of interacting forces.

Economies of Scale   The average cost per unit decreases as output increases.

Efficacy   The ability to actually cure a disease; how well a treatment works in practice.

Elasticity   The percentage change in one variable when another variable changes by one percent.

Enrollee   A person covered by a health benefits plan.

Entitlements   Social insurance payments to which beneficiaries are entitled by law with little regard to actual contributions or premiums or income qualifications (i.e., Medicare, Social Security).

Entrepreneur   The person who undertakes the effort to create an organization and the network of contracts necessary for its success.

Equity   In health services research, equity is the extent of equality in health, income, or other resources. In finance, equity refers to the net worth of the organization (assets — liabilities); the capital belonging to the owners. (See **Leverage**.)

ERISA   The Employee Retirement and Income Security Act of 1974 and subsequent amendments, which govern most health insurance contracts and, in particular, exempt self-insured plans from most state regulation.

Expected Value   The value of an outcome multiplied by its probability of occurring. Also, the probability-weighted average of all possible outcomes.

Experience Rating   Setting a group premium based on the actual losses experienced by that group during the prior year or years.

Externalities   The effects of a transaction between parties on outsiders; the uncompensated effects of an action (e.g., pollution); side effects.

Fallacy of Composition   The logical error of assuming that what holds true for the individuals within a group must also hold true for the group collectively, or vice versa.

Fee Schedule A list of approved fees for each service promulgated by an insurance company, government agency, or professional society.

Fee for Service (FFS) Payment for health care based on the charges for each service or item used.

FEHBP The Federal Employees Health Benefits Plan (FEHBP) is the system through which all federal employees, including congresspeople and senators, obtain health insurance. In each area, several plans that meet or exceed the specified qualifications are offered, and the government pays an amount equal to the lowest-priced plan premium. The employee must pay the amount by which the plan chosen exceeds that of the lowest-cost plan.

Firm An organization that is responsible for coordinating the transformation of inputs, such as land, labor, capital, and entrepreneurship, into some final output or outputs.

Flexible Budget A budget that is adjusted for changes in the volume of service.

Flexner Report The critique written in 1910 that led to the reform of medical education and established the MD degree as a qualification for licensure.

Flow The amount over a period of time (i.e., income ($ per month), mortality rate (deaths per year)).

Food and Drug Administration (FDA) The federal agency with jurisdiction over labeling, manufacture, and sale of food and drugs for human consumption.

Formulary A list of approved drugs for reimbursement, with all nonapproved drugs paid at a lesser rate or not at all.

Free Rider A person who allows others to produce a public good, and then uses it without paying. For example, most poor country prevention programs are free-riders, dependent upon the research of rich countries to do the research and produce the vaccines needed to control infectious diseases.

Full-Time Equivalents (FTE) A measure of the quantity of labor used.

Fundamental Theorem of Exchange Any voluntary exchange between persons must make both of them better off since they willingly agreed to trade.

Gatekeeper A primary physician who manages and approves all services for the patient who enrolls in his practice.

Generic Drugs Drugs that are identical in chemical composition to a brand-name pharmaceutical preparation but produced by competitors after the firm's patent expires.

Global Budget A fixed total budget for all health services.

Grandfathering Approving those who are already in practice to continue even if they do not meet the new standards.

Gross Domestic Product (GDP) The total market value of all production in a nation.

Group Insurance Contract for insurance made with an employer or other entity, called the policyholder, that covers a group of persons as a single unit.

Health Maintenance Organization (HMO) An organization that contracts to provide comprehensive medical services (not reimbursement) for a specified fee each month. The term *health maintenance organization* arose because doctors under this arrangement have a financial incentive to keep their patients healthy because they are not paid extra for providing more services.

Health Insurance Portability and Accountability Act of 1996 (HIPAA) A legislated set of rules to increase efficiency by standardizing billing and making health care transactions paperless. HIPAA also specifies rules governing access to records, privacy, confidentiality; combating fraud; developing medical savings accounts; and other matters.

Homeopathy An alternative form of health practice emphasizing natural remedies used in extremely dilute solutions.

Hospital Privileges The rights of those doctors who have been approved for acceptance on the hospital's medical staff to admit patients and perform surgery.

Human Capital Analysis of investments of time, effort, and money in education or health that improve a person's productivity as analogous to investments of financial capital.

Income Distribution The fraction of all income earned by the top 10 percent of the population, the second 10 percent, and so on; the degree of disparity in incomes between the rich and the poor.

Income Elasticity The percentage change in expenditures due to a one percent change in income. Income elasticities below 1.0 mean that although spending on a good rises with income, it rises less than proportionately so that the fraction of total income spent on that good is reduced. With income elasticities greater than 1.0 (luxury goods), spending rises more than proportionately so that the share of total income spent on the good increases as income increases.

Indemnity Benefit A specified dollar amount reimbursed for a particular injury or type of care, such as $15 for each x-ray or $475 for gallbladder removal, is an indemnity benefit. Life insurance, which provides a specified dollar amount in case of death, has an indemnity benefit.

Independent Practice Association (IPA-HMO) An HMO formed by nonexclusive contracts with many providers who operate independently, as opposed to closed group staff HMO where physicians work exclusively for the HMO and are often on salary.

Inflation A measure of the reduction in the real purchasing power of currency over time.

Information Asymmetry The disparity in information between a buyer and a seller in a transaction.

Inpatient Services or goods provided within a hospital or nursing home.

Intensity (of Services) The amount of inputs used to provide each unit of service. For example, an urban university hospital typically provides complex services of high intensity, and a primary care doctor on an emergency call in an isolated rural area uses far fewer resources to treat the same injury.

Investigational New Drug (IND) A designation of FDA approval to begin the testing of a drug.

Kickbacks Surreptitious payments made in order to obtain business.

Leverage The ratio of debt to equity, or the amount of assets per dollar of net capital.

Licensure The establishment of legal restrictions specifying which individuals or firms have the rights to provide services or goods.

Life-Cycle Hypothesis Assertion that individual spending at any point in time is based on long-run expected income over the life cycle rather than just current income at that point in time; a common form of the **permanent income** hypothesis.

Loading Factor (or Load) The percentage of total premiums used for administrative costs, profits, and all items other than medical benefits.

Long-Term Care (LTC) Nursing homes, visiting nurses, home IV, and other services provided to chronically ill or disabled persons.

Longitudinal Analysis Study of a set of individuals or groups tracking how they change over time.

Macroeconomics (from the Greek *macro*, meaning "large") The branch of economics that studies how the economy as a whole operates, covering such topics as total output, employment, and price levels. See also **Microeconomics**.

Major Medical In order to compete with the Blue Cross service benefits, commercial insurance companies came up with plans with deductibles and coinsurance that could be sold for much less. Today major medical is sometimes used as a supplement, some basic services, such as hospital and doctor visits, are covered in full.

Malpractice The legal framework specifying failure to meet professional standards.

Malthusian Hypothesis The expectation that any increase in food supply would eventually lead to a matching increase in the number of people living at a subsistence level, so that on average, living conditions would be no better than before.

Managed Behavioral Health Mental health and substance abuse services managed by an MCO.

Managed Care The use of a manager to control utilization of medical services and control costs. Often associated with HMOs, other forms of managed care include peer-review panels, preapproval procedures for surgery, case management for the chronically ill, formularies limiting pharmacy reimbursement to an approved list, and other contractual provisions.

Managed-Care Organization (MCO) An HMO, PPO, or other organization that accepts financial risk and manages care.

Managed Competition A policy of increased reliance on competing HMOs and a fixed limit to tax subsidies so that employees would bear the full marginal cost of their health benefit plans.

Mandated Benefits Specific services (e.g., pregnancy, alcoholism detoxification) for which a state requires all health plans to provide coverage.

Marginal Incremental; a one-unit increase.

Marginal Propensity to Consume The fraction of an additional dollar that would be spent on consumption, and thus not invested as savings.

Marginal Productivity The incremental output obtained with one more unit of input.

Marginal Cost The increase in total costs caused by the production of one more unit of output.

Market Failure The inability of the market to arrive at a reasonably efficient equilibrium under certain conditions, notably the existence of public goods and externalities, lack of clear property rights, inability of some consumers to act in their own best interest, natural monopoly due to constantly declining average costs of production, and excessive transaction costs or information asymmetry.

Means Testing Setting a standard of low income in order to qualify for a government benefit, e.g., Medicaid.

Medicaid Combined state and federal program to insure people whose incomes are insufficient to pay for health care; primarily those on welfare or older people in nursing homes.

Medical Savings Account (MSA) A proposal to replace regular health insurance and HMOs by allowing people to place money in a tax-free savings account to be used for medical expenses, in conjunction with the purchase of a catastrophic stop-loss health insurance plan covering expenses in excess of a specified amount such as $3,000.

Medicare A Federal government insurance program that provides hospital benefits (part A), medical benefits (part B), and drug benefits (part D) to persons older than 65 years and some qualified widows and disabled persons.

Medigap A policy designed to pay coinsurance, deductibles, drugs, and other expenses not fully covered by Medicare.

Microeconomics (from the Greek *micro*, meaning "small") A field of economics that uses economic theory to study how individual consumers and firms make economic decisions.

Monopoly A market in which there is a single provider (seller).

Monopoly Rents Profits in excess of competitive market returns due to a monopolist's ability to unilaterally increase prices.

Monopsony A market characterized by a single buyer that has the ability to influence market price.

Moral Hazard Any behavioral change that results from having insurance and that increases expected losses, such as the higher utilization of covered medical services by employees or the acceptance of more risky loans by insured banks.

Morbidity Illness or disability, especially when expressed as a rate (e.g., sick days per year per 1,000 employees).

Mortality Death, usually expressed as a rate per 100, per 1,000, or per 100,000.

Need A professional determination of the quantity that should be supplied (as distinct from market demand).

NICE The National Institute for Clinical Effectiveness (NICE), an independent council operating in the United Kingdom to provide independent advice on the costs and benefits of new drugs and therapies and to make recommendations for the National Health Service regarding their use and reimbursement.

Normative Shortage When too little is supplied according to professional opinion, although not necessarily according to market behavior (e.g., a shortage of raw vegetables in the diet of teenagers).

Occupancy Rate The percentage of a hospital's beds filled at a specific time.

Off-Label The use of a prescription drug for diseases other than those for which it has been approved by the FDA.

Opportunity Cost What must be given up in order to do or obtain something; the highest-valued alternative that must be foregone; for example, the opportunity cost of taking the final exam may be missing out on a trip to Bermuda.

Option Demand Willingness to pay for access to a good that may or may not be used, e.g., emergency department, spare tire.

Osteopathy An alternative form of medical practice that emphasizes spinal adjustment as well as surgery and drugs in the treatment of disease. Originally quite distinct from mainstream allopathic medicine, osteopathy is now almost identical so that MDs and DOs usually practice together, although DOs are more likely to be generalists focusing on primary care.

Out of Pocket Payments made by individuals or their family, rather than an insurance company, HMO, government, or other third party, for medical care.

Outpatient Services provided in a physicians' office, clinic, or other ambulatory setting.

Over the Counter A drug that consumers can purchase without a prescription from a physician.

Patent A legal monopoly for a specified period of years given to a firm that makes a discovery.

Path Dependence The idea that the current situation develops out of the past and cannot be fully understood without considering the steps that led up to it. Also, an observation by social scientists that change in most systems tends to be slow and inertial, depending on people and organizations that are embedded in specific cultures and institutions facing durable legal and financial constraints. In geometry, it is the fact that the area under a curve depends not only on the starting and ending points but also on the path between these two points.

Per Diem Per-day payment for services.

Per Member per Month (PMPM) The standard form of HMO payment, also known as **capitation**.

Permanent Income Expected long-run average income, as opposed to the transitory income that a person (or group) might have during the current month or year.

Pharmacoeconomics Cost–benefit analysis of drugs; assessment of the market for a drug.

Point-of-Service Plan (POS) An HMO that offers partial reimbursement for services a patient chooses to obtain outside of the HMO network.

Population Medicine Analysis and assessment of health care on the basis of the community or group rather than the individual; design of a system with services targeted to those of greatest need; making trade-offs to optimize average health, rather than doing the best possible for one specific individual under treatment.

PPACA The *Patient Protection and Affordable Care Act of 2010*, also known as "Obamacare."

Practice Variation Differences in the number of medical services provided to a group of patients not explainable by any differences in the population served. Also known as small area variation.

Preauthorization A requirement that the doctor or the patient obtain approval from the HMO before the service is provided.

Preexisting Condition An insurance contract may specify that it will not pay for medical problems already diagnosed or under treatment before the policy is purchased, known as preexisting conditions. A person with AIDS who bought a policy with such a clause would find that it paid for his broken leg, and maybe even to have his tooth drilled, but not for anything related to AIDS. Often the preexisting condition exclusion only applies to the first 6 months or year of coverage. This, and other exclusionary clauses, are a major way of reducing adverse selection when medical insurance is marketed to individuals.

Preferred Provider Organization (PPO) A health insurance plan that offers enrollees a discount for using hospitals and physicians within an approved network of contracted providers.

Premiums Payments made in advance to provide medical services or reimbursement in the future.

Price Discrimination Charging different people different prices for the same good.

Price Index A measure of the purchasing power of money, usually set arbitrarily equal to 100 at one specific point in time (or space). The average change in prices weighted by the expenditure on each item.

Primary Care The basic medical attention provided by a physician to a patient seeking care, as distinct from referral services obtained from specialists, or tertiary care provided in technologically sophisticated hospitals.

Progressive A progressive policy is one that redistributes costs and benefits in favor of those toward the bottom. A progressive tax, such as the U.S. income tax, is one that takes a larger percentage from high-income persons or groups. (See **Regressive**.)

Property Rights The right to use, sell, or to derive income from a good.

Prospective Payment Payments set in advance, especially in contrast to retrospective **cost reimbursement**.

Provider Network The set of physicians, hospitals, and others with which an MCO has signed a contract to provide care for enrollees.

Public Goods Goods that are consumed or financed collectively (e.g., clean air, national defense, discovery of penicillin) either because it is impossible to include or exclude any consumer who does not pay (see **free rider**), or because once produced, there is no additional cost for additional consumers.

QALYs (Quality Adjusted Life-Years) A way of measuring the value of a medical intervention by the increase in life expectancy, adjusted for differences in disability and timing.

Rationality The notion that consumers (a) will never purposely make themselves worse off and (b) have the ability to rank preferences and allocate income in a fashion that derives the maximum level of utility.

RBRVS The *resource-based relative-value system* developed for Medicare to reimburse ambulatory services based on the estimated time, effort, skill, equipment, and other resources needed to provide each service.

RCCAC The *ratio of costs-to-charges applied to charges* methodology used to apportion cost reimbursements.

Redistribution Policies that have the effect of changing the pattern of consumption by different income classes, thereby allowing one group (the poor, the middle-class, the rich) to consume a larger share of GDP.

Regressive A regressive policy is one that redistributes costs and benefits disproportionately in favor of those at the top. A regressive tax is one that takes a proportionately larger share of income from those at the bottom (such as gasoline, SSI, or cigarette taxes). (See **Progressive**.)

Regulatory Balloon The observation that any regulation pushing costs down on one side is apt to exert pressure pushing costs up in some other direction.

Regulatory Capture The subtle takeover of a regulatory agency by the industry it was meant to regulate, so that it tends to represent the interests of the industry rather than the public.

Reimbursement The process of paying for the costs incurred, especially through a third party.

Reinsurance Acceptance by a second insurer (the reinsurer) of all or part of the risk undertaken by the first insurer; usually used to cover very large losses and protect against bankruptcy. For example, a reinsurer might agree that if total losses exceed the $5 million in expected claims by more than $1 million, they will, for a price, pick up 90 percent of the extra losses.

Relative Value Scales A list of point scores for each service to be used in setting reimbursement.

Rents Profits in excess of those necessary to call obtain the requisite supply of inputs in the market. Compensation above competitive amounts obtained by professionals who are able to control supply.

Retention Ratio Agreement A contract specifying an allowed ratio of premiums to medical expenses, with some fraction of any excess underwriting gains to be returned to the firm or used to reduce premiums in the following year.

Retrospective Review Monitoring records after discharge and disallowing (refusing to pay for) any services that do not meet specified standards of medical necessity and timeliness.

Revolving Door Term used to describe staff that leave a regulatory agency to work within the industry that is supposed to be regulated, and vice versa. Such changes in employment can compromise the agency's objectivity.

Risk The chance or probability that an event will occur.

Risk Adjustment The process of setting the capitation rate for an insurance policy based on the health status and expected medical costs of an individual or group purchasing the plan.

Risk Aversion The extent to which an individual is willing to pay to reduce variation in losses or income due to random events.

Risk Pooling Forming a group so that individual risks can be shared among many people.

Risk Selection Enrollment of healthier-than-average persons into an insured group.

Sanitary Revolution The 19th-century campaign to clean up the environment and change personal behavior to conform to Victorian notions: "cleanliness is next to godliness."

Scarcity Scarcity exists when the quantity of a good or service available is insufficient to satisfy demand at a zero price. An economic good is thus any good or service that is scarce relative to our wants for it.

Selection Bias A disproportionate share of above- or below-average persons in the group.

Self-Insurance A health plan funded and controlled by the firm itself, so that no risk is transferred to an insurance company, although benefits may be administered by an outside party. Self-insurance often enables a firm to avoid regulations governing purchased health insurance.

Service Benefits If the insurance company contracts directly with the doctor or hospital to provide the service rather than setting up some form of financial reimbursement, this is a service benefit. Blue Cross provides service benefits through its contracts with hospitals. An advantage of a service benefit to the insurance company is that they usually get a discount off the price that the patient would have to pay directly for the services rendered. An advantage to the consumer is that they obtain complete medical care as a service, without having to file insurance forms or pay and wait for reimbursement from the insurance company.

Shared-Income Hypothesis Income becomes more and more important as a determinant of health care spending as the unit of observation increases in size from the individual to the nation.

Social Insurance Pooling funded through taxes for protection against risks provided by the government for all (or almost all) of the citizens in a society. Social Security in the United States and the National Health Service in England are examples of social insurance plans.

Spend-Down The process of spending or giving away assets by elderly persons so as to qualify for Medicaid reimbursement of long-term care expenses.

Stock The amount at a point in time (i.e., total assets, population).

Stop-Loss A limit on the maximum amount a person would ever have to pay is known as a stop-loss. If a family has a $1,000 stop-loss, then the insurance company will pay everything after the family's out-of-pocket expenses reach $1,000.

Subcapitation Carving out a specialized service (physical therapy, mental health) and paying the specialized provider on a per-member per-month basis.

Subsistence Having barely enough food and other resources to sustain life.

Sustainable Growth Rate A formula limiting the annual increase in total Medicare physician fees to the growth rate of GDP. For health policy, "sustainable" means that the growth rate is long-run affordable by the government, somewhere in the range of GDP + 0% to GDP + 1%.

Tertiary Care Specialized medical care delivered in technologically sophisticated hospitals.

Third-Party Administrator An organization that processes claims for a self-insured firm but bears no financial risk for losses.

Third-Party Transaction An exchange that is indirect and often pools the funds of many individuals with money collected and disbursed by a third party such as an insurance company, voluntary nonprofit organization, or government agency.

Time-Series Analysis Statistics using multiple observations of an individual or group over time; statistical analysis of the dynamics of change.

Trade-off The idea that every individual will voluntarily sacrifice some of one good or service in exchange for a sufficient increase in the amount of some other.

Transaction Costs All costs, monetary and nonmonetary, whether counted or not, of carrying on trade.

Triple-Option A complete array of plans consisting of an HMO, a PPO, and an indemnity plan, offered by an insurer as a package. The package as a whole is experience rated, so that any one option may be significantly over- or underpriced to create cross-subsidies between plans.

Two-Party Transaction An exchange between a buyer and seller, usually trading money for goods or services.

Underwriting Gains (Losses) The amount by which premiums received exceed (or fall short of) benefits paid out.

Universal Health Insurance A national plan providing health insurance or services to all citizens or to all residents.

Usual, Customary, and Reasonable (UCR) A method for setting the maximum allowed fee for each service based on usual charges by other physicians in the area, the customary charge by this particular doctor over the preceding year, and "reasonable" adjustments for severity or special conditions.

Utilization The number of services used, often expressed per 1,000 persons per month or year.

Utilization Review (UR) Monitoring of medical records to determine if services are appropriate and should be paid for.

Variability The extent of random changes over time or between persons.

Voluntary Organization A nonprofit organization, such as a hospital or social service agency, governed by a board of concerned citizens rather than owners or elected officials.

Welfare Loss The decline in social welfare (total value of consumption/production) due to monopoly supply restrictions, price controls, rationing, taxes, or other interventions that cause misallocation of resources. Also known as *deadweight losses*.

Welfare Triangle The reduction in consumer's surplus caused by a reduction in quantity sold due to monopoly supply restrictions, price controls, or other distortion.

Willingness to Pay (WTP) How much a person is willing to give up in order to obtain some item or specified improvement in quality of life.

Withhold A pool of money for providers that is held back and distributed by the HMO only if total expenses for the year end up being at or below acceptable levels.

Workers' Compensation A mandatory insurance program covering the costs of medical treatment and disability due to work-related accidents and illness.

Wrap-Around An insurance policy designed to create a more comprehensive set of coverages sold with an underlying base policy.

INDEX